Health Promotion

Praise for the book

Health Promotion: Planning and Strategies makes an important contribution to the growing literature in the health promotion arena, with its comprehensive coverage of contemporary philosophical, research and practice issues. The book is suited both for advanced independent study in the field and as a text for a comprehensive, advanced course. A growing number of health promotion education programmes employ problem based learning methods, and this book will be a favourite source for students engaged in exploring health promotion on their own. It is suited, also, as a bookshelf reference work for even the most experienced professional. The book's unique strengths are its level of detail and thorough referencing, especially in its treatments of healthy public policy and health education, both subjects that receive relatively little emphasis in most other texts. The healthy public policy chapter provides the best treatment of this topic of which this reviewer is aware. The book makes abundant use of cases and examples from the United Kingdom to illustrate key points, but includes also material drawn from other places, enhancing its relevance to the international audience.

Professor Maurice B Mittelmark
President of the International Union of Health Promotion and Education

Health Promotion

Planning and Strategies

KEITH TONES
and
JACKIE GREEN

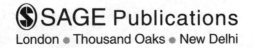
SAGE Publications
London • Thousand Oaks • New Delhi

ISBN 0-7619-7448-2 (hbk)
ISBN 0-7619-7449-0 (pbk)
© Keith Tones and Jackie Green 2004
First published 2004
Reprinted 2004, 2005

SAGE Publications Ltd
1 Oliver's Yard
55 City Road
London EC1Y 1SP

SAGE Publications Inc
2455 Teller Road
Thousand Oaks
California 91320

SAGE Publications India Pvt Ltd
B–42 Panchsheel Enclave
PO Box 4109
New Delhi 110 017

British Library Cataloguing in Publication data
A catalogue record for this book is available from the British Library

Library of Congress Control Number: 2003108063

Typeset by C&M Digitals Pvt. Ltd., Chennai, India
Printed and bound in Great Britain by
Athenæum Press Limited, Gateshead, Tyne & Wear

Contents

List of Boxes, Figures, Illustrations and Tables

LIST OF BOXES

LIST OF FIGURES

LIST OF ILLUSTRATIONS

LIST OF TABLES

Acknowledgements

Every effort has been made to trace all the copyright holders, but if any have been inadvertently overlooked the publishers will be pleased to make the necessary arrangement at the first opportunity.

The BBC, Sir Antony Jay and Mr Jonathan Lynn for *Lies, Damned Lies and Statistics?* in Chapter 1.

Palgrave for Figure 2.4: Accounts of health.

Margaret Whitehead for Figure 2.6: The main determinants of health.

Oxford University Press for Figure 2.7: Some interrelationships in the complex system of lifestyle, environment and health status.

Margaret Whitehead for Table 2.15: Determinant of Differentials.

Lippincott, Williams and Wilkins for Figure 4.2: Dignan and Carr's planning model.

Professor Anthony S. Blinkhorn for *I Spat* (illustration in Chapter 4).

McGraw Hill for Figure 4.3: Precede/proceed.

IUHPE for Figure 4.6: Public health decision making model (PABCAR).

Sage Inc. for Figure 4.7: Bracht et al.'s community organisation model.

Oxford University Press for Figure 4.8: A planning framework for incorporating community empowerment into top-down health promotion programmes.

Palgrave for Figure 5.3: Doyal and Gough's theory of human need in outline.

WHO for Figure 5.8: Information Profile.

Routledge for Figure 5.9: Beatie's Model of Health Promotion.

Routledge for Figure 6.1: Health promotion – alternative approaches.

Oxford University Press for Figure 6.2: Health education and health promotion.

BUGA UP for Figure 8.1.

Professor Carl Parsons for Figure 9.1: The eco-holisitic model of the health promoting school.

CCDU for Figure 9.7: Appropriate learning strategies.

Introduction: A Distinctive Voice
for Health Promotion

Those who are enamoured of practice without science are like a pilot who goes into a ship without a rudder or compass and never has any certainty where he is going.

Leonardo da Vinci

It is well recognized that concepts of *health* and *health promotion*, are both essentially contested: their philosophical basis and the principles governing definition and practice are all open to multiple interpretations. We will explore several of these different conceptions – and misconceptions – in this book. However, we think it important at the outset to assert that it is not our purpose to provide a detached and distant summary of the manifold variations in philosophy and theory. Although, hopefully, our approach will be eminently logical, we will not adopt a neutral stance. We provide our own version of what we believe should be the distinctive voice of health promotion.

DEFINING HEALTH AND ITS DETERMINANTS

The problematical nature of health

Our opening chapter seeks to lay the foundations for building a theory and ideology of health promotion. It starts with a brief consideration of what Dubos (1979) famously described as the 'mirage of health' – a phantasmagoric state well worth pursuing but which tends to evaporate when attempts are made to achieve it or even to capture its essence. Numerous texts and philosophical tracts have, over many decades – even centuries – been devoted to analysing health and actively propagating particular concepts of it. Despite the difficulties associated with what Lowel S. Levin has described as 'shovelling smoke', it is important for all health promoters to make the effort to at least formulate a working definition in order to provide a comfortable basis for their professional practice. However, limitations on space limit the extent of our discussion.

Accordingly, we merely offer a simple working model that might help with the important task of operationalizing the notion of health as a precursor to more extensive analysis of the meaning of health promotion. In this context, we acknowledge the existence of a dichotomy between a 'positive' approach to conceptualizing health and a 'disease-focused' definition. Importantly, though, we do not view these two 'Manichean' formulations as mutually exclusive. Indeed we assert that such notions as self-actualization, coherence and, above all, empowerment are central to both perspectives. In fact, we will argue that empowerment is the main *raison d'être* of health promotion. Following the classic formulation of World Health Organization (WHO), we also accept that health involves physical, mental and social aspects. We also consider it important to distinguish between an individual dimension of social health and the health of society in general. Indeed one of the urgent imperatives of health promotion is to take account of 'sick societies' and associated remedial measures such as the development of social capital.

Defining health and its determinants

Given the continuing debate and discussion about the nature and scope of what might be called the 'wider public health workforce' (which includes both lay and professional people), decisions about where conceptual boundaries should be drawn become increasingly important if health promotion is not to be regarded as an idiosyncratic study of everything! In other words, a reasonably well constructed 'ring fence' is needed to establish the limits to our health promotion aspirations.

Furthermore, just as a clear conceptualization of the nature of health and the role of health promoters are important precursors to effective practice, it is essential to have a sound understanding of the factors that contribute to health – and to ill health. Action should be based on evidence of need; effective action is proportionate to the degree of understanding of causal factors. We, therefore, follow our critical analysis of the philosophical and technical nature of health promotion with a review of key determinants of health and illness. This includes epidemiological analysis and consideration of lay perspectives. We are especially interested in the often heated confrontation that occurs between those who emphasize the importance of lifestyle influences on health and illness, and those who assert the primacy of broader and more fundamental structural factors. We argue that, as social and environmental factors and individual behaviour are intricately interrelated, it is unhelpful to focus on one approach rather than the other. Problems tend to arise from taking a myopic view – that is, blindness to either broader structural influences or individual capabilities, dispositions and behaviour leads to ineffective health promotion. However, in practice, there still tends to be an overemphasis on individual factors, which means that environmental, social and economic factors are frequently ignored. Accordingly, we seek to restore the balance and emphasize the importance of health promotion focusing on root causes and avoiding a victim-blaming tendency.

A further issue concerns the means of 'measuring' health and its determinants. The capacity to address this in a robust way underpins both the assessment of need and evaluation of the effectiveness of interventions. However, there are tensions between different approaches – deriving from conflicting ideological and epistemological positions. We consider these different positions and the relative emphasis on professionally led or participative methods of assessment and how they relate to the core values of health promotion.

THE IDEOLOGY OF HEALTH PROMOTION

Just as personal and socio-cultural values underpin people's predilections for one or other model of health – frequently causing them to focus on and emphasize associated explanations of the causes of health and ill health – those values will result in different approaches to health promotion being privileged or discounted. In short, health and health promotion are socially constructed. Explanations of health promotion and preferences for particular strategies and methods are, ultimately, ideologically determined. The notion of ideology is therefore particularly important to an explanation of why certain approaches are preferred (sometimes with almost religious zeal) while others are rejected (often with equal zeal). We examine in some detail the meaning of ideology and how it may provoke the several clashes and skirmishes that not infrequently exist between rival groups of theoreticians, philosophers and practitioners. We note especially the centrality of power to understanding different ideological positions. We also note both cultural and political power operating at different levels, both in their overt forms and their more insidious presence as manifested in false consciousness.

Our analysis of ideology leads us back to a further consideration of the opposing positions of Asclepius and Hygeia in the form of the different value positions of a medical model and other conceptualizations of the purpose of health promotion. We highlight the apparent conflict between the long-established preventive model of health education and health promotion and various 'social'/positive/radical models. Although there is often a genuine difference in interests and values, it is not unreasonable that those in the medical and associated professions should be interested in illness, disease and its prevention. Moreover, it is certainly eminently desirable that disease should be treated, cured and prevented. Whatever one's prime interest in the nature of health, most people do not feel well (or 'healthy') if they are suffering. It is hypocritical for people to lambast medicine unless they rigorously refuse medical help and treatment. There are, however, frequently significant ideological differences between a 'medical' approach to health promotion (that is, prevention) and what we characterize as an empowerment approach. These differences are founded on deep-seated views of the world generally and the nature of humanity and human agency. Importantly, they have to do with beliefs about the locus of power.

As mentioned above, our stance here is not neutral. Our formulation of health promotion's distinctive voice is encapsulated by the notion of empowerment. Accordingly, we argue that the model that should (ethically and ideologically) characterize health promotion is an empowerment model. We discuss the nature and underlying philosophy of this model at some length. Hopefully we move beyond mere posturing and rhetoric. Indeed, throughout the book, we seek to show how empowerment – at the levels of social groups, communities and individuals – may be operationalized and translated into particular strategies and specific methods. Of course, empowerment does not just happen – there is a reciprocal relationship between individuals and their environment. Not only must individuals be 'strengthened' in some way, but their socio-economic, physical and cultural environments must be conducive to their making empowered choices.

THE CASE FOR CRITICAL HEALTH PROMOTION

Perhaps the most significant feature of the empowerment model that we espouse in this book is the recognition that health promotion should operate as a kind of militant wing of public health. Essentially it is a political endeavour and concerned with addressing issues of fundamental importance – particularly the pursuit of social justice and achievement of equity. This approach, therefore, almost inevitably subscribes to critical theory in arguing for ideological and political commitment. The result is an *a priori* challenge to the focus on individualism that has, with justification, been vilified as victim-blaming. As clinical medicine inevitably focuses on individuals and their component parts, it is not surprising that the preventive model mentioned above has been associated with a victim-blaming tendency. Merely working with individuals does not constitute individualism (despite rather illogical views to the contrary); victim-blaming occurs when the broader environmental factors that impact on the individual are ignored. It is therefore just and proper that medicine in general and prevention in particular should be concerned with individual conditions and influencing individuals' health and illness-related actions. It is, however, essential that the primacy of broader social, cultural, economic and environmental influences should be accepted. It follows, therefore, that those working in medical services should be prepared to contribute to both individual empowerment and taking political action to challenge adverse environmental circumstances. If this happens, there need be no difference between preventive and empowerment models, merely a difference in emphasis. Indeed, it is one of our firm contentions that subscribing to an empowerment model provides the most effective means of achieving the goals of preventive medicine.

EFFECTIVE PROGRAMME PLANNING

This book is predicated on the view that effective health promotion depends on systematic programme planning. Although perhaps at first glance this assertion might not seem entirely compatible with our commitment to empowerment, we do not make the assumption that planning is necessarily 'top-down', but, rather, argue that many programmes derive from

community or client concerns and all programmes should maximize the opportunities for the involvement of all 'stakeholders'. It is, of course, a fact that many, if not most, past examples of systems approaches to planning interventions do originate with health professionals and many owe their origins to concerns about controlling and preventing disease (a prime example being a number of heart disease prevention programmes). However, it is ideology that ultimately drives the shape and character of interventions, and an empowerment ideology requires participation.

Furthermore, we do not reserve the term 'programme' for only large-scale interventions involving multiple settings and using the whole panoply of available strategies and methods. We also use the term for any planned health promotion encounter. It might thus refer to bedside patient education, group work in a community context or a school-based enterprise. However, we would argue that all such situations will not only benefit from planning but also need systematic planning that involves certain key components if outcomes are to be achieved.

We do not necessarily advocate the use of any particular planning model (although some have been designed for particular purposes and ought, logically, to have greater relevance). Accordingly we describe a number of planning models, together with a 'systems checklist' identifying important elements and processes. We also discuss the kinds of information that will usually be needed to develop good programmes, making particular reference to health needs assessment, the construction of community profiles and the importance of participatory processes. In the context of discussing the ways in which programme planners (including community participants) might generate solutions to problems and meet the health needs that have been identified, we explore and examine key features of different settings, such as hospitals and schools. We note the peculiar characteristics and requirements of settings and emphasize the importance of intersectoral working and the establishment of coalitions.

THE KEY ROLE OF THEORY

We assert our faith in the development and application of theory, following the maxim that, 'there is nothing so practical as a good theory'. A distinction is made between *normative* theory and *analytical* theory and models derived from these. The former variety of theory applies to the logical, comprehensive and critical consideration of what, for example, would be involved in translating an empowerment model of health promotion into practice. It would embody its concern for what would be ethically and ideologically sound and its application to programme development and implementation. Analytical theory, on the other hand, provides explanations of causes and provides guidelines for the development of effective tactics to achieve given ideological goals. A sound body of theory has traditionally been seen as distinguishing the 'professional' from the 'artisan'. While it might well be the case that, in George Bernard Shaw's words, 'the professions are enemies of the laity' (*The Doctor's Dilemma*, 1911), the greater theoretical depth of professional education increases the applicability of their knowledge and their capacity to make sound decisions in novel situations. There is no reason for professionals alone enjoying the benefits of theoretical understandings! It is certainly the case that these theoretical understandings can help programme planners generate sound solutions to problems in conditions of uncertainty. Last but not least, in an age when we can be swamped with information as a result of the mediation of a search engine, we need theory as a companion and guide.

UNDERSTANDING THE FACTORS GOVERNING HEALTH CHOICES

We have argued that effective health promotion requires an understanding of health and the determinants of health. It also requires insight into the determinants of health and illness behaviour. As it happens, there are very rich and relevant bodies of theory describing and explaining the factors that contribute to health- and illness-related decision making at both community and individual levels. Accordingly we aim to provide a comprehensive review of key principles and associated research relating to:

- how social systems change
- the psychological, social and environmental factors that typically determine the adoption and maintenance of health actions.

In particular we use the health action model (HAM) to provide a coherent framework that will incorporate other significant models and accommodate specific research findings. We also demonstrate how the key constructs of empowerment – at both environmental and individual levels – relate to such components as beliefs, motivation, normative pressures, personality traits and factors that may facilitate or militate against behavioural intentions and minimize the likelihood of 'relapse'.

THE RESURRECTION AND REVITALIZATION OF HEALTH EDUCATION

One of the most significant theoretical assumptions that gives our conceptualization of health promotion its distinctive voice is a simple but valuable way of encapsulating the notion of health promotion. We argue that it is useful to conceptualize health promotion as a synergistic interaction between education and policy or, more particularly, between health education and healthy public policy. The importance of public policy in achieving health outcomes has been thoroughly canvassed and documented and has formed part of the lexicon of health promotion since before the Ottawa Charter (WHO, 1986). Most health educators would also agree that a supportive environment will maximize the impact of their educational activities and this is undoubtedly true. What is rarely stated is that, without education, *significant* health-promoting policies (such as greater equality in the distribution of wealth within a nation) will not take place.

Healthy public policy

We begin our discussion and justification of this argument with a critical discussion of healthy public policy. We seek to describe the essential features of a rather vague notion that has been likened to an elephant in that it is hard to define but easy to recognize! We remind readers of the WHO position and discuss what is involved in developing policy – both the rhetoric and reality. We consider the function of advocacy and the factors involved in adoption and implementation of policy. We also give some thought to the important matter of health impact assessment – analysis of the ways in which policies of all kinds can have an effect on public health, for good and, often, for ill!

Varieties of health education

The relationship between education and health has a long history. It has its normative theories and its analytic theories. For instance, philosophers have emphasized that, to qualify as an *educational* intervention, the endeavour must be voluntaristic. People must be helped to understand rather than prodded into particular behaviour. Indeed disagreement with the teacher based on understanding would be considered a laudable outcome. 'True' education – doubtless for obvious reasons – has always been a rare commodity. Various philosophically incorrect activities have been much more common and attempts to coerce and persuade characterize most early health education efforts. The predominance of these efforts has resulted in the marginalization of health education – largely due to its politically incorrect association with a victim-blaming tendency to concentrate on changing individual behaviour. However, we argue that it is more meaningful to adopt a technical definition of education (that is, any planned activity or set of activities that bring about learning) that can then be applied to a range of health-promoting programmes. It would thus include not only such health-promoting activities as patient education, but also a variety of interventions of a radical and empowering nature. We, therefore, spend some time examining these variations on an educational theme. These include a relatively brief reference to cognitive learning – frequently ignored, but which, to a greater or lesser extent, is common to all initiatives. We consider the substantial research into the use of persuasion and attitude change and its particular relevance to our commitment to empowerment. We pay special attention to the use of radical, emancipatory approaches that were typified by the work of Paolo Freire. We also refer to the whole package as critical health education.

One or other of the above-mentioned strategies would not only be involved in, but would be essential to, the success of health promotion – including the implementation of healthy public policy. As we point out, Freirean methods seek to raise critical consciousness with a view to generating sufficient public indignation and pressure to bring about policy change. Advocacy and lobbying have also been closely associated with the exertion of pressure on powerful agencies in an attempt to generate healthy policy. Effective advocacy and lobbying typically draw on the educational armamentarium associated with persuasion and attitude change. This in itself creates an interesting persuasion paradox. If participation and the empowerment imperative should govern health promoters' work with their clients and the general public, does a different set of rules apply to their attempts to influence politicians and the powerful gatekeepers of policy? An intriguing ideological dilemma!

METHODS AND STRATEGIES

Assuming that health needs have been satisfactorily identified and information about the beneficiaries of the planned health promotion programme has been accumulated – firmly located within the context of sound theory – the health promoters'

thoughts must turn to the strategies and methods needed to achieve the programme objectives. They should ideally, of course, be consistent with the ideological requirements of an empowerment model of health promotion. Following our systematic planning approach, we therefore critically reflect on the kinds of strategies that might be used, together with their potential for achieving the programme goals and their limitations.

We have selected two apparently different and sometimes conflicting strategies by way of illustration. We compare and contrast the use of mass media with community development. In reviewing mass communication, we also reiterate the importance of theory by showing how both normative and analytical models may be applied to explaining media effects.

Mass media

Over the years, there has been a tendency in public health to consider mass media as a panacea, offering the attractive prospect of yielding dramatic and substantial changes in the health-related practices of a substantial number of people over a short period of time. At the same time, researchers and theorists have asserted exactly the opposite and stressed the limitations of mass media. We will examine these counter claims together with certain key theories that seek to explain the factors that determine the nature, extent and conditions under which mass media may achieve results. We argue that, apart from politicians' cynical desire to be seen to be doing something to address difficult problems, the inflated expectations of mass media derive from making false comparisons between selling soap powder and 'selling' health. Accordingly we provide a critical review of social marketing theory and seek to limit the aspirations of health promoters while urging them to follow the technical requirements of marketing to base their campaigns on such essential activities as audience segmentation and pretesting.

We also consider it important to examine the ideological dimensions of media and its use of myth in advertising and political manipulation. Our conclusions in general are that health promotion should not concentrate on a marketing approach to changing audience behaviour. If we accept the tenets of uses and gratification theory, people are resistant to direct manipulation, but tend to 'use' mass media to meet their perceived needs and gratify their prejudices. On the other hand, health promoters should seek to work with mass media producers via the process of consultative collaboration in order to develop healthy media policy.

However, most important of all, health promotion should concentrate its efforts on media advocacy – that is, using the consciousness-raising and agenda-setting potential of mass media to influence political systems and address the major environmental determinants of health and illness.

We complete this section by listing the key principles governing successful mass media use.

Working with communities

Community development is a long-standing, and perhaps the best known, strategy to empower people living in communities or neighbourhoods. We provide a critique of this strategy, compare it with alternative non-formal approaches and consider some specific mechanisms. We argue that many of these approaches might merely result in 'gilding the ghetto' and propose the need for an alternative strategy that might best achieve the aims of critical health promotion. This would incorporate Freirean techniques, the use of media advocacy and the development of coalitions with interested parties.

The settings approach

We feel that it is important to also give some quite detailed consideration to what has become known as the 'settings approach' to health promotion. A setting is not just a location or agency in which health education might be 'delivered'. Rather, it involves a holistic consideration of the setting, its context and ethos. We review the approach and illustrate this by focusing on the 'Health Promoting Schools' initiative.

Methods for facilitating learning

The various strategies mentioned above may make a greater or lesser contribution to meeting the programme needs identified in the process of systematic planning. Inevitably, however, more specific activities and interventions will be used – typically within the context of given settings and/or as part of broader strategies, such as community development. The selection of methods to achieve learning will inevitably be guided by the type of learning, but should also include consideration of the characteristics of the learner, 'teacher' and contextual factors. We exemplify these methods by discussing the contribution of various approaches, including peer education and the creative arts.

EVALUATION

This book, as we have noted, is based on the assumption that systematic planning is essential for achieving effective health promotion outcomes. We have offered alternative models for programme planning, but all models must inevitably consider ways in which to assess whether or not the programme has worked. Accordingly we devote the final chapter to a discussion of evaluation. We argue that the purpose of evaluation is to measure the extent to which certain valued goals have been achieved. We also note that, contrary to popular perceptions, evaluation is not merely a series of technical activities. It is imbued with ideological concerns and issues. For instance, the differential power of stakeholders can determine not only whether or not a programme gets under way in the first place, but also what its form might be and even which research methodology ought to be used. In short, paradigm wars may be waged before, during and after the development of programmes and their evaluation.

We seek to provide some insight into the main research paradigms and, in particular, the challenge to the dominant logical-positivist stance by radical approaches associated with interpretivism. We discuss aspects of critical theory, realistic evaluation and utilization-focused evaluation. We aim to consider the relevance of opposing schools of thought and their often vitriolic arguments about the proper way to evaluate health promotion.

We also consider variations in the meaning of effectiveness and, in particular, the notions of efficiency and efficacy (as well as a few brief observations about cost-effectiveness). However, our main concern is to emphasize that there is a quite fundamental difference between health-promotion programmes and their evaluation requirements and other interventions, especially those associated with medicine. This distinction is based on the facts that health-promotion programmes may operate for relatively long periods of time and are frequently highly complicated. Thus, we examine the nature of this complexity and the kinds of indicators that might be needed to demonstrate success – or failure. Somewhat controversially, we insist that traditional epidemiological indicators are never appropriate.

We also argue that the 'gold standard' randomized controlled trial (RCT) should rarely, if ever, be used to evaluate health promotion. The major arguments for this assertion centre on the ideological premise that health promotion should be concerned with empowerment and must involve the participation of the public, clients and patients. They are also based on the requirement of critical health promotion that research should lead to action. This often entails action research – a fluid, constantly changing process of intervention, evaluation and formative change. Furthermore, it could be argued that all but the very simplest programmes need illumination, that research results should provide a real understanding of what actually happened during the intervention if future programmes are to improve. Given the complexity of most health-promotion programmes, illumination is of paramount importance.

We are at some pains to point out that abandoning the RCT does not mean abandoning the quest for validity. Indeed, given the power imbalance between the two research traditions, it becomes more rather than less important to secure sound evidence of success. We argue, therefore, for a new gold standard. We propose that this be provided by a judicial principle that uses evidence eclectically, but tends to place greater emphasis on qualitative methodology supported by triangulation. One of the main components of triangulation is the use of relevant theory.

We have argued for the pre-eminence of theory in the whole planning process. It is of special importance in relation to evaluation. The choice of appropriate theory supports the choice of research design adopted and the selection of methodology. Appropriate theory contributes to the interpretation of evidence and generalization to practice. Evaluation itself should contribute not only to improvements in practice, but also to the building of health-promotion theory that, as we noted earlier, facilitates effective decision making at many levels.

Our final thoughts on evaluation are concerned with an issue of considerable current interest – evidence-based health promotion. We consider the nature of evidence and its relationship to theory. We also consider access to evidence and the translation of evidence into practice.

With our discussion of evaluation we have come full circle. Our early discussion of the nature and meaning of health and its determinants – and the ideological factors associated with these – determine our programme aims and objectives. They also influence our choice of strategies and methods. They also influence our philosophy and practice of evaluation. Again, evaluation contributes to the evidence needed to develop effective programmes in different contexts for different individuals and groups. Our commitment to an empowering, critical health promotion defines what is or is not acceptable in both the design and evaluation of programmes. Our view is that empowerment is the most appropriate approach to achieving a number of desirable health outcomes and, furthermore, the process of evaluation should contribute to this empowerment process.

1

Health and Health Promotion

Man and his species are in perpetual struggle – with microbes, with incompatible mothers-in-law, with drunken car-drivers, and with cosmic rays from Outer Space... The 'positiveness' of health does not lie in the state, but in the struggle – the effort to reach a goal which in its perfection is unattainable.

Gordon, 1958, in Dubos, 1965: 349

HEALTH AS A CONTESTED CONCEPT

A major concern of this book is that of providing insight into the factors contributing to the effective and efficient design of health-promotion programmes. This goal cannot readily be achieved without at least acknowledging that health is what Gallie (1955) famously described as an essentially contested concept. Its many, often conflicting, meanings are socially constructed. Indeed, as we noted earlier, Lowell S. Levin remarked that the task of defining health is akin to shovelling smoke. It is difficult, to say the very least, to provide precise definitions, largely because health is one of those portmanteau words that mean many things to most people. All we can securely say is that health is, and apparently always has been, a significant value in people's lives. Even though it has rightly been described as a mirage – worth pursuing but unattainable – if we do not acknowledge the contentious nature of health and have a sound understanding of the determinants of our preferred conceptualization of health, it is unlikely that we will be able to develop incisive strategies for promoting it.

Defining health: contrasting and conflicting conceptualizations

A number of different, approaches to defining health may be readily identified. One such approach, for example, contrasts lay interpretations with those of 'professionals', typically medical professionals. Another approach emphasizes the positive dimensions of health and contrasts this with disease-focused definitions. This positive dimension may be variously described in terms of 'well-being' or 'quality of life'; it may include an assertion of the importance of interpreting health in a holistic way and might also include reference to the importance of individuals and groups establishing harmonious relationships with their environment.

THE WHO DEFINITION OF HEALTH: ORIGINS

On 21 March, 1946 a Sub-Committee... submitted a 'Draft of Preamble' to the Convention of the World Health Organization. The first paragraphs of Annex 10 read as follows: 'The States parties to this World Convention recognize these fundamental truths, which are deemed to be basic to the acceptable inter-relationship of all peoples in a world at peace. The right to health is one of the fundamental rights to which every human being, without distinction of race, sex, language or religion, is entitled.

Health is not only the absence of infirmity or disease but also a state of physical fitness and mental and social wellbeing.'

Turner, 2001: 23

Some all-embracing 'philosophical' formulations define health as synonymous with the 'good life' (see, for instance, Buchanan, 2000).

Perhaps the best-known definition of all comes from the World Health Organization that famously not only emphasized the positive in its reference to wellbeing, but increasingly adopted a political posture centring on equity and empowerment and asserting that health is a human right.

The confrontation of Hygeia and Asclepius

One of the most persistent distinctions between interpretations of health has been embodied in Greek mythology in the persons of Hygeia and Asclepius. Hygeia was a goddess who symbolized the virtues of wise living and wellbeing; Asclepius was a physician who lived in the twelfth century BC and came to represent the medical view of health. As Dubos (1979: 131, noted: 134)

The myths of Hygeia and Asclepius symbolize the never-ending oscillation between two different points of view... For the worshippers of Hygeia, health is the natural order of things, a positive attribute to which men are entitled if they govern their lives wisely. According to them, the most important function of

medicine is to discover and teach the natural laws which will ensure to man a healthy mind in a healthy body. More sceptical or wiser in the ways of the world, the followers of Asclepius believe that the chief role of the physician is to treat disease, to restore health by correcting any imperfection caused by the accidents of birth or of life.

While Asclepius is in Luther's words only 'God's body patcher', the serene loveliness of Hygeia in the Greek marble symbolizes man's lost hope that he can some day achieve a state of harmony within himself and with the surrounding world.'

As we will indicate later in this chapter, these 'two different points of view' still figure prominently in contemporary debates about the purpose of health promotion.

Health, adaptation and actualization

Arcadia is a fiction; utopias unattainable. Humanity rarely, if ever, achieves stasis. People are constantly engaged in an often problematic process of adaptation to their environments – to their physical, material, economic and social circumstances. The dynamic interaction between individuals and their

A MEDICAL PERSPECTIVE ON HEALTH

... disease can only reasonably be defined as the absence of health... [the author therefore].... feels compelled to accept the consequent proposition that health is indeed the absence of disease. ... an individual is healthy when his level of function does not impede or determinably threaten to impede the performance of an acceptable social role.

Smith, 1977

environments is recognized within WHO statements on the primary purpose of health promotion, defined as enabling people to gain control over their lives and their health. The central tenet of Dubos' influential perspective on health is that positive health is a mirage – it is evanescent and unattainable but worth pursuing. If health means anything, it resides in the pursuit, in engaging with these constantly changing and typically unpredictable environmental forces.

Aspects of Maslow's (1970) notion of self-actualization resonates with Dubos' perspective on the nature of health. He (1970: 46) defines it as follows:

> Self-actualization... refers to man's desire for self-fulfillment, namely, to the tendency for him to become actualized in what he is potentially. This tendency might be phrased as the desire to become more and more what one idiosyncratically is, to become everything that one is capable of becoming... In other words, 'What a man *can* be, he *must* be.'

Apart from providing a useful operational definition of psychological health and his emphasis on the importance of self-esteem, Maslow's work has considerable relevance for the empowerment imperative of health promotion.

Coherence, commitment and control: health as empowerment

In an article published posthumously, Antonovsky (1996) declared his concern regarding health promotion's obsession with risk factors. He urged health promoters to adopt a 'salutogenic model' as a basis for practice and for the development of a clear and distinct identity.

Negentropy and the sense of coherence

'Salutogenesis' is a key concept that focuses on the 'salutary' – that is, health-enhancing – rather than 'pathogenic' – that is, disease-causing aspects of health. It also incorporates Antonovsky's main theory about the factors that determine the extent to which people become healthy and experience wellbeing. Central to this theory is the challenge posed by the complexities and uncertainties of the world – complexities that are encapsulated in the notion of entropy. In addition to its definition in physical science, 'entropy' refers to the level of disorder within systems. At a psychological level, it refers to *perceptions* that disorder exists. People's worlds may thus be more or less chaotic in reality or they may only *think* that they are disordered and, thus, meaningless. Both situations are

considered to be undesirable and two remedies are possible:

- changing the situation so that it is less chaotic
- changing people's perceptions and beliefs about the situation so that it becomes more meaningful.

It is worth noting, however, that to modify perceptions without providing the means with which to change the chaos is a risky strategy!

The salutogenic approach is, therefore, designed to be substantially and essentially 'negentropic'. A major task of health promotion is thus to reduce entropy and perceptions of entropy and, in so doing, generate a sense of coherence, which is a central attribute of a healthy person.

Antonovsky (1979: 123) defines coherence as follows:

> ... a global orientation that expresses the extent to which one has a pervasive, enduring though dynamic feeling of confidence that one's internal and external environments are predictable and that there is a high probability that things will work out as well as can reasonably be expected.

Health and empowerment

The concept of empowerment will receive further consideration on a number of occasions in this book. For the present, we will simply observe that two of the three key requisites of a sense of coherence are concerned with beliefs about control and these figure prominently in conceptualizations of empowerment. Two further points about empowerment will be made at this juncture. First, we might choose to describe empowerment (or, indeed, some of the other constructions of health discussed above) as synonymous with (positive) health. In other words, to be healthy is to be empowered!

Alternatively, we might wish to define empowerment instrumentally – that is, as a means to achieving (positive) health. This, of course, is an issue that cannot be resolved empirically and will doubtless remain a matter for personal preference.

There is a third way. Empowerment could be viewed as both a terminal and an instrumental value. The standpoint adopted here is that, whatever the definition of positive health, empowerment will necessarily be a key component. Furthermore, in respect of the Asclepian disease prevention and management dimension, we will assert that it is certainly not only a key component, but the most important component.

The second major observation at this stage relates to the potentially dramatic conflict between empowerment and a sense of meaningfulness – both

---

MEANINGFULNESS IN ARCADIA – OR POTENTIAL UNFULFILLED?

A time there was, ere England's grief began,
When every rood of ground maintained its man;
For him light labour spread her wholesome store,
Just gave what life required, but gave no more;
His best companions, innocence and health;
And his best riches, ignorance of wealth.

Goldsmith, 'The Deserted Village', 1770

Full many a flower is born to blush unseen,
and waste its sweetness on the desert air.
Some village-Hampden, that with dauntless breast
The little tyrant of his fields withstood;
Some mute inglorious Milton here may rest,
Some Cromwell guiltless of his country's blood.

Gray, 'Elegy Written in a Country Churchyard', 1751

---

of which feature in Antonovsky's negentropic sense of coherence. In short, while the feeling that 'all is for the best in the best of all possible worlds' will doubtless make people feel better, it may well be delusory. Consider Downie and Macnaughton's (1998: 13) reference to 'the quiet life of honest toil' being frequently promoted in literature as 'the life of true health and wellbeing', and their inclusion of a stanza from Goldsmith's 'The Deserted Village' by way of illustration. Apart from the Arcadian touch, Goldsmith's illustration is not so much one of idyllic health, but, rather, false consciousness. The landed gentry would doubtless have approved! In the context of empowerment, Thomas Gray provides a rather more apposite image.

HEALTH: A WORKING MODEL

As may be seen from Figure 1.1, for all practical purposes, health is defined as having both positive and negative aspects. The term wellbeing is used as shorthand for the positive dimension. We are quite clear that preventing and managing disease and disability is a laudable goal in its own right and a central concern of those who are professionally involved in the business of healthcare and health promotion. On the other hand, it is equally clear that the more positive dimensions must figure prominently in the formulation of a satisfactory definition of health. In the first place, those involved in medicine cannot ignore its importance. Second, it is the major focus of

interest for a wide variety of non-medical professionals working in fields such as social work, education and the arts. Perhaps most important of all, however, is the fact that those measures that result in the achievement of positive goals are frequently more effective in achieving preventive outcomes than the more limited tactics employed by espousing a narrow version of the medical model.

Being all that you can be

The three components that make up WHO's holistic conception of health are featured in the model. Following Maslowian self-actualization principles, it is tempting to argue that maximal health status involves 'being all that you can be'. Healthy individuals would thus be those who had fulfilled their mental, physical and social potential. It is clear that the attainment of complete mental, physical and social health is logically and practically impossible. Furthermore, it would be feasible to achieve high levels of potential in relation to one component of health at the expense of others. For example, the degree of commitment required to achieve maximal physical growth and development might not only militate against social health and, possibly, be inconsistent with cultural norms, it might also be viewed as evidence of obsessional neurosis! Equally, a lifestyle characterized by sloth and self-abuse might lead to considerable happiness and a very successful social life, but result in an early death.

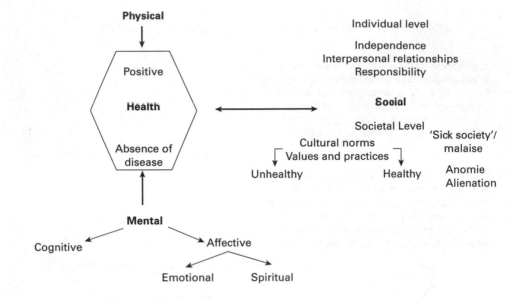

Figure 1.1   A working model of health

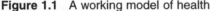

Accordingly, health must involve some kind of balance between mental, physical and social components. How, though, is such a balance to be determined? Two interesting possibilities come to mind:

- individuals themselves make the decision
- society makes the decision for them.

As the second option is inconsistent with the principles of empowerment (which are intrinsically healthy), only the first option is a serious contender. We will, however, emphasize later in this book the importance of healthy individuals being guided by commitment to a considerate way of life. Thus, individuals should be in a sufficiently empowered position to enable them to choose the course of action of their choice, provided only that the rights of other people are not damaged.

Mental, social and spiritual health

The definition of physical health is relatively straightforward. On the one hand, it is associated with minimizing disease and disability; on the other hand, it may involve having a sufficient level of fitness necessary for achieving other (more important) life goals or/and the experience of high-level wellness or, more realistically, the feelings of wellbeing (allegedly) associated with a high degree of physical fitness. Wellbeing may thus be associated with fitness, but is by no means an identical dimension of health. A person might, for example, exhibit high levels of fitness, but limited feelings of wellbeing or, alternatively, high levels of wellbeing but minimal fitness!

Defining mental health is a rather more complicated and problematic matter and cannot therefore be extensively discussed here. We will have to content ourselves with making just two observations. First, it is useful to consider mental health as having both cognitive and affective dimensions. The affective dimension includes emotions and feelings and most discourse on mental health centres on this aspect. The cognitive dimension rarely features in definitions of mental health, but might be incorporated in a holistic model. 'Being all you can be' in cognitive terms refers to the extent to which individuals fulfil their intellectual potential. The reasons for failure to fulfil intellectual potential have been a source of considerable study and evidence of inequity has been a source of outrage. It thus is intimately associated with broad-based health-promotion initiatives designed to address general social inequalities. Second, many people have asserted that any serious consideration of positive health must include the spiritual dimension. This particular interpretation of health is itself open to several interpretations, but features in Figure 1.1 in the context of mental health and wellbeing. It has both a cognitive element, consisting of the doctrinal aspects of, for instance, a religious system, and the emotional commitment associated, in this case, with the value system central to the notion of faith – that is, '… an illogical belief in the occurrence of the improbable' (an observation attributed to the American journalist H.L. Mencken)!

Social health: individual and society

The social dimension of health is, like mental health, quite complicated and so cannot be explored in depth in this chapter. As can be seen from Figure 1.1, there are two categories. The first of these refers to the social health of the individual; the second is concerned with the health of society itself. Three main aspects of individual social health have been identified.

- **Independence** A socially mature individual acts with greater independence and autonomy than a relatively immature individual.
- **Interpersonal relationships** A socially healthy individual is characterized by the capacity to relate to a number of significant others and cooperate with them.
- **Responsibility** A person who is socially mature accepts responsibility for others.

The health of society

The distinction between the social health of individuals and the health of society is recognized in everyday parlance with references to 'sick societies' and 'social malaise'. We will make further reference to this dimension of social health later in this chapter and at a number of points in this book when we consider health promotion's concerns with the prevalence of powerlessness, meaninglessness, normlessness, isolation and self-estrangement in 'sick societies' and its commitment to addressing human rights.

PROMOTING HEALTH: COMPETING IDEOLOGIES

No science is immune to the infection of politics and the corruption of power.

Dr Jacob Bronowski, *The Ascent of Man*
(BBC2, 1973)

Defining health promotion

A key issue in defining health promotion is whether it is viewed as an umbrella term, covering the activities of a range of disciplines committed to improving the health of the population, or as a discipline in its own right. Bunton and Macdonald (1992: 6) suggest that 'recent changes in the knowledge base and the practice of health promotion are characteristic of paradigmatic and disciplinary development'. They take a discipline to involve an ordered field of study embracing associated theories, perspectives and methods. A discipline would be expected to have its own ideology that would also inform standards of professional practice. Prior to our analysis of the ideology of health promotion and the values integral to different models, we will briefly clarify the distinction between health education and health promotion.

Although the generic use of the term 'health promotion' to describe any activity that improves health status can be traced back earlier, Terris (1996) noted that in 1945 Henry Sigerist described the four tasks of medicine as the promotion of health, prevention of illness, restoration and rehabilitation of the sick (cited by French, 2000). However, it was not until the late 1970s that this term began to be applied in a more specific way to a concept, movement, discipline and, indeed, profession. While a systematic account of the history of health promotion is beyond the scope of this text, we should note that the roots of contemporary health promotion are in health education.

The earliest examples of health education in the context of public health would now be described as health propaganda. This typically took the form of pamphleteering, which was intended to generate political change in support of a variety of environmental health measures designed to combat squalor and provide clean water supplies. Early health education was thus seen as an adjunct to public health efforts. Indeed, Naidoo and Wills (1994: 63) note that, by the 1920s, health education had become associated with 'diarrhoea, dirt, spitting and venereal disease!' With this increasing focus on personal rather than public health, health educators continued their adjuvant role, but now acted as handmaidens to the medical profession. Their activity during this period essentially involved giving information and persuading people using mass communication strategies.

The dominant themes in the early health education journals of the 1950s and 1960s centred on methods of delivering information in ways that would attract attention and interest people in the substantive content of health messages. The primary concern

BLAMING THE VICTIM – IGNORING THE EFFECTS OF POVERTY

Being poor is stressful. Being poor is worrisome; one is anxious about the next meal, the next dollar, the next day. Being poor is nerve-wracking, upsetting. When you're poor it's easy to despair and it's easy to lose your temper. And all of this is because you're poor. Not because your mother let you go around with your diapers full of bowel movement until you were four; or shackled you to the potty chair before you could walk. Not because she broke your bottle on your first birthday or breast-fed you until you could cut your own steak. But because you don't have any money.

Ryan, 1976: 157

was very much with the technicalities of delivering information. The assumption was that if people were given the 'right' knowledge, they would act appropriately. As we will see in Chapter 3, this grossly underestimated the complexity of the task.

Two broad paths can be traced in the subsequent development of health education. One – the preventive approach – sought ever more sophisticated ways of achieving behaviour change by means of the application of psychological theory. The other, which was more in tune with progressive educational philosophy, was concerned with enabling people to make informed choices – the so-called educational approach.

In the period following the Lalonde report (1974), a renewed interest in the importance of the social and environmental influences on health status – both directly and indirectly by shaping behaviour – brought health education under fierce critical scrutiny (see, for example, Navarro, 1976, Ryan, 1976). Of particular concern were the emphasis on individual responsibility and the failure to recognize constraints on individual behaviour – most notably their economic and material circumstances. Health education was accused of 'victim-blaming' – a term attributed to Ryan. The essence of victim-blaming lies in attempts to persuade individuals to take responsibility for their own health while ignoring the fact that they are victims of certain social and environmental circumstances. Accordingly, Ryan argued that the fundamental factors governing health were power and money.

The emergence of health promotion was as a response to the need to address the environmental as well as the behavioural determinants of health. In effect it marked a shift from being concerned with healthy choices to making 'the healthy choice the easy choice'.

We will review different models of health promotion at a later point in this chapter and also WHO's interpretation of health promotion. However

we should at this point note briefly that health promotion includes efforts to tackle the social and environmental determinants of health by means of healthy public policy. The scope of health promotion can therefore be summed up in a simple formula:

health promotion = health education ×
healthy public policy

The contribution of the World Health Organization (WHO) to the definition of health promotion

The evolution of health promotion has been accompanied by considerable debate about its nature and purpose – debate that has exposed its core underlying values. WHO has been a major voice in shaping the development of health promotion and it is pertinent at this point to summarize the main issues that have emerged from the key documents. Not only have these documents been a source of reference for health-promotion practice, they have also been assimilated into professional training courses – that is, they have become part of the doctrine of health promotion.

As mentioned above, WHO has taken a holistic view of health from its inception. The well-known definition of health as 'a state of complete physical, mental and social wellbeing and not merely the absence of disease or infirmity' was featured in the WHO's Constitution (WHO, 1946). The 'Health for All' movement was launched at the Thirtieth World Health Assembly in 1977. The following year saw the *Declaration of Alma Ata* (WHO, 1978), which identified primary healthcare (PHC) as the principal means of attaining 'Health for All' targets. Primary healthcare – as distinct from primary medical care – was envisaged as embracing all the services that impact on health, including, for example, education, housing and agriculture.

A number of key issues in the *Declaration* have informed subsequent thinking. In addition to emphasizing the importance of a holistic view of health, the following assertions figure in many WHO publications and declarations:

- health as a fundamental right
- the unacceptability of inequality in health within and between nations
- health as a major social goal
- the reciprocal relationship between health and social development
- the need to involve a number of different sectors in working towards health
- the rights and duties of individuals to participate individually and collectively in their own healthcare
- education as the means of developing communities' capacity to participate.

In January 1984, WHO set up a new programme on 'health promotion'. A discussion document on health promotion (WHO, 1984) saw it as a 'unifying concept' bringing together 'those who recognize the need for change in the ways and conditions of living, in order to promote health'. It defined health promotion as 'the process of enabling people to increase control over, and to improve, their health'.

Basic resources for health were identified. Income, shelter and food were acknowledged to be a primary requisite for health. Importance was also attached to the provision of information and life skills, the creation of supportive environments providing opportunities for making healthy choices and the creation of health-enhancing conditions in the economic, physical, social and cultural environments.

The document outlined the key principles of health promotion as:

- the involvement of the whole population in the context of their everyday life and enabling people to take control of, and have responsibility for, their health
- tackling the determinants of health – that is, an upstream approach, which demands the cooperative efforts of a number of different sectors at all levels, from national to local
- utilizing a range of different, but complementary, methods and approaches – from legislation and fiscal measures, organizational change and community development to education and communication
- effective public participation, which may require the development of individual and community capacity
- the role of health professionals in education and advocacy for health (WHO, 1984).

Action was therefore seen to require an integrated effort to encourage individual and community responsibility for health along with the development of a health-enhancing environment. The document reflected a commitment to voluntarism and formally acknowledged the risk of dictating how individuals should behave. This is referred to as 'healthism' – a notion that we will return to later. Other potential problems included an overemphasis on individual behaviour rather than the social and economic determinants of behaviour and the possibility of increasing social inequality if the varying capacity of different social groups to exercise control over their health was not tackled. A further concern was that health promotion might be appropriated by particular professional groups to the exclusion of others and lay people.

A series of major international conferences followed. The Ottawa Charter, developed at the First International Conference on Health Promotion (WHO, 1986), built on many of the key principles set out in the WHO discussion document and has been a constant source of reference since. It identified three broad strategies for working to promote health:

- **advocacy** to ensure the creation of conditions favourable to health
- **enabling** by creating a supportive environment, but also by giving people the information and skills that they need to make healthy choices
- **mediation** between different groups to ensure the pursuit of health.

The Ottawa Charter listed five main action areas that have been central to the conceptual framework of health promotion:

- build healthy public policy
- create supportive environments
- strengthen community action
- develop personal skills
- reorient health services.

There is potentially some tension between individual and societal responsibility for health, between individual and collective responsibility and between voluntarism and control. The Ottawa Charter handled this by seeing individuals as having responsibility for their own health, but also a collective concern for the health of others. However, there is an overriding societal responsibility to create the conditions that enable people to take control of their health. Recognition that health is created where people 'learn, work, play and love' heralded the 'settings approach' to health promotion.

The Second International Conference on Health Promotion in Adelaide (WHO, 1988) focused on healthy public policy as a means of creating supportive environments that would be health-enhancing in themselves and would also – in the words of the much-used phrase – contribute to making the healthy choice the easy choice. In particular, it acknowledged the importance of addressing the needs of underprivileged and disadvantaged groups and emphasized the responsibility of developed countries to ensure that their own policies impacted positively on developing countries. It saw healthy public policy as 'characterized by an explicit concern for health and equity in all areas of policy and an accountability for health impact'. The Adelaide Conference identified the need for strong advocates and also saw community action as a major driving force.

The Sundsvall Conference (WHO, 1991) addressed the issue of supportive environments for health. In addition to the physical environment, it recognized the importance of the social environment and the influence of social norms and culture on behaviour. It also noted the challenge to traditional values arising from changing lifestyles and the increasing social isolation and lack of a sense of coherence. The need for action at all levels and across sectors was recognized and, in particular, the capacity for community action. The key elements of a 'democratic health promotion approach' were seen to be empowerment and community participation. The importance of education as a means of bringing about political, economic and social changes was recognized as well as its being a basic human right.

The Jakarta Declaration on Leading Health Promotion into the 21st Century (WHO, 1997) was developed at the Fourth International Conference on Health Promotion. It viewed health both as a right and as instrumental to social and economic development. It envisaged the 'ultimate goal' of health promotion as increasing health expectancy by means of action directed at the determinants of health in order to:

- create the greatest health gain
- contribute to reduction in inequities
- further human rights
- build social capital.

The Jakarta Declaration built on the commitments of the previous documents and provided clear endorsement of the value of comprehensive approaches and involving families and communities. It called for strong partnerships to promote health including – for the first time – the involvement of the private sector.

Overall, the priorities for the twenty-first century were to:

- promote social responsibility for health
- increase investments for health development
- consolidate and expand partnerships for health
- increase community capacity and empower the individual
- secure an infrastructure for health promotion.

The first resolution on health promotion, which was passed at the Fifty-First World Health Assembly in May 1998 (WHO, 1998c), incorporated the thinking of the Jakarta Declaration.

As it moved into the twenty-first century, WHO (1998) identified the following key values underpinning the 'Health for All' movement:

- providing the highest attainable standard of health as a fundamental human right
- strengthening the application of ethics to health policy, research and service provision
- equity-orientated policies and strategies that emphasize solidarity
- incorporating a gender perspective into health polices and strategies. (1998: v).

The Fifth Global Conference on Health Promotion held in Mexico in 2000 focused on 'bridging the equity gap'. It issued a Ministerial Statement signed by some eighty-seven countries, including the United Kingdom (WHO, 2000b), that acknowledged that 'the promotion of health and social development is a central duty and responsibility of governments that all sectors of society share' and concluded that 'health promotion must be a fundamental component of public policies and programmes in all countries in the pursuit of equity and health for all.'

A strong theme to emerge from the Mexico conference was the need to 'work with and through existing political systems and structures to ensure healthy public policy, adequate investment in health, and facilitation of an infrastructure for health promotion' (WHO, 2000b: 21). This was felt to require:

- democratic processes
- social and political activism
- a system of equity-orientated health impact assessment
- reorientation of health services
- improved interaction between politicians, policy makers, researchers and practitioners
- strengthening existing capacity for implementing health-promotion strategies and supporting synergy between different levels (local, national and international).

While the primary concern of these documents is with identifying appropriate action, they are underpinned by clear values. Indeed, it could be said that unless activity is consistent with these values, it should not be regarded as 'health promotion'. These values include equity and empowerment – the twin pillars of health promotion – along with health as a right, voluntarism, autonomy, participation, partnerships and social justice. Consideration of rights and responsibilities, power and control generates some interesting paradoxes in relation to health education and policy interventions, which we discuss more fully below.

Ideology, social construction and competing discourses

Theories and models

Before further discussion of the 'medical model' or 'empowerment model' of health promotion, it is useful to note Morrow and Brown's (1994) distinction between two varieties of theories and models derived from theories. They suggest two categories – normative and empirical. In the words of these authors, normative models represent: 'modes of theorizing that legitimate different ethical, ideological, or policy positions with respect to what *ought* to be' (our emphasis). Accordingly, assertions that the main purpose of health promotion should be the pursuit of social justice and its major concern should be remedying inequalities are normative assertions. Theories and models that represent ideologies are, therefore, also normative. On the other hand, models that seek to explain how people make health decisions (such as the health action model (HAM) discussed in Chapter 3) are essentially empirical.

Defining ideology

The original meaning of 'ideology' was merely the scientific study of human ideas. It has been transformed over time into a complicated concept that includes cognitive, affective and action dimensions. Although ideologies are value-laden – and it is not unusual for the term to be used synonymously with values systems – the contemporary construction of the word ideology is much more complicated than this.

Eagleton (1991) listed 'more or less at random' some sixteen definitions in current use – and these were not necessarily mutually compatible. They ranged from 'the indispensable medium in which individuals live out their relations to a social structure' to 'false ideas which help to legitimate a dominant political power'.

De Kadt, discussing the ideological dimensions involved in implementing WHO's 'Health for All' agenda, states that ideologies are an amalgam of fact and unsubstantiated assertion. He observes that, 'comprehensive ideologies (as opposed to partial ideologies) are commitment-demanding views about societies, their past history and present operation, which contain a strong evaluative element and hence provide goals for the future' (De Kadt, 1982: 742).

In order to clarify the central meaning of 'ideology', Eagleton contrasts the emotionally charged nature of ideology, which has a 'partial and biased view of the world', with an 'empirical' or 'pragmatic' approach to discussing issues. There is, of course, a tendency for those espousing political causes to describe their 'pragmatic' construction of reality as rational and based on common sense whereas opponents' views are characterized by ideological zealotry involving, as Eagleton (1991: 3) notes, their:

… judging a particular issue through some rigid framework of preconceived ideas which distorts their understanding. I view things as they really are; you squint at them through a tunnel vision imposed by some extraneous system of doctrine. There is usually a suggestion that this involves an oversimplifying view of the world – that to speak or judge 'ideologically' is to do so schematically, stereotypically, and perhaps with the faintest hint of fanaticism.

Eagleton (1991: 4) provides a sardonic illustration of these alternative constructions of similar political events:

What this comes down to is that the Soviet Union is in the grip of ideology while the United States sees things as they really are … to seek some humble, pragmatic political goal, such as bringing down the democratically elected government of Chile, is a question of adapting oneself realistically to the facts; to send one's tanks into Czechoslovakia is an instance of ideological fanaticism.

Ideology and values

Belief systems and doctrine are major parts of the territory of ideology. However, values and value systems feature with equal prominence. Rokeach defines values as, 'an enduring belief that a specific mode of conduct or end-state of existence is personally or socially preferable to an opposite or converse mode of conduct or end-state existence' (Rokeach, 1973: 10). Following Guttman's (2000) review, the major ethical values assumed to underpin health promotion (or, more specifically, 'public health communication interventions') are:

- beneficence, or, 'doing good'
- non-maleficence, or, 'doing no harm'
- respect for personal autonomy

- justice or fairness
- utility and the public good
- (possibly) community involvement and participation.

As we will see, the extent to which these values are actually central to the ideology of health promotion will depend on the preferred model. At this point, it is interesting to note Pellegrino's (1993: 1160) observation that the principle of autonomy fits particularly well with American culture: '[The] ... individualist temper of American life ... emphasizes privacy and self-determination'. Thus, the empowerment model of health promotion would, at first sight, appear to be eminently acceptable to a US population. However, while self-empowerment may chime with the individualistic values of America, aspects of *community* empowerment and the implementation of policy designed to remedy inequity would certainly not be compatible with such a culture. Moreover, what Guttman calls 'market autonomy', although apparently related to individual autonomy and personal choice, privileges the wealthy at the expense of the poor (Milio, 1981, and Deetz, 1992).

The centrality of power

Given our emphasis on empowerment in this book, it is axiomatic that individual and community power are pivotal to the ideology of health promotion and central to the design of health promotion programmes. Questions of power feature prominently in discussions of ideology. Giddens (1989: 727) is quite explicit about this:

> Ideologies are found in all societies in which there are systematic and engrained inequalities between groups. The concept of ideology connects closely with that of *power*, since ideological systems serve to legitimize the differential power which groups hold.

In Fairclough's (1995: 18) laconic phrase, ideology is in fact, 'meaning in the service or power'.

Eagleton (1991: 5–6) provides a comprehensive account of the mechanisms whereby a dominant group exerts its power and creates 'false consciousness':

> A dominant power may legitimate itself by *promoting* beliefs and values congenial to it; *naturalizing* and *universalizing* such beliefs so as to render them self-evident and apparently inevitable; *denigrating* ideas which might challenge it; *excluding* rival forms of thought, perhaps by some unspoken but systematic logic; and *obscuring* social reality in ways convenient to itself. [our emphasis]

The relevance of ideology is not only measured in terms of the ways in which the power of dominant social groups is legitimized. More significant for health promotion are the ways in which subordinate groups are 'de-powered' by dominant groups. Indeed, the radical ideology underpinning the model of health promotion proposed in this book is substantially concerned with empowering subordinate and oppressed social groups. Pursuing the matter of false consciousness, Eagleton (1991: xiii) reminds us of the subtle and potentially insidious ways in which people may be de-powered:

> The most efficient oppressor is the one who persuades his underlings to love, desire and identify with his power; and any practice of political emancipation thus involves that most difficult of all forms of liberation, freeing ourselves from ourselves.

He does, however, caution against exaggerating the power of this 'hegemonic' process and optimistically notes that nobody is ever wholly mystified. Despite a capacity for self-delusion, human beings are at least moderately rational and, unless the process of domination provides sufficient gratification over time, the dominated will rebel. If this were not true, health promotion's emancipatory strategies for critical consciousness raising would be doomed to failure.

Ideology, discourse and narrative

Discourse analysis and health messages
'Discourse' is, 'a pattern of talking and writing about or visually representing an event, object, issue, individual or group' (Lupton and Chapman, 1994: 38). The notion of discourse has its roots in linguistics. It is more than mere language, rather the thought underlying language. Accordingly, 'discourse analysis' is not merely the recording and classification of content or topics. Instead, it involves penetrating beneath the surface of language or images and seeking out subtexts and meanings relating to wider beliefs and value systems – often their social and political contexts. It is often useful to separately identify subordinate narratives under the general rubric of discourse and Figure 1.2 shows the relationship between ideology, discourse and narrative.

Lupton and Chapman's (1994) analysis of health and medical news provides a good example of three varieties of competing narrative derived from the discourse of smoking and featured in newspaper coverage of 'National No Smoking Day' in Britain. These represented smokers and smoking as follows:

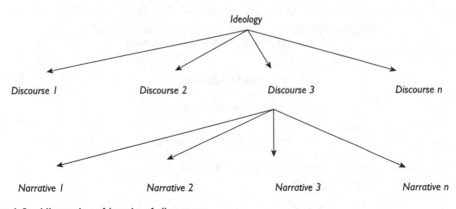

Figure 1.2 Hierarchy of levels of discourse

- **Outcasts and (recalcitrant) deviants** An article in *The Times* described the now familiar pattern of bands of smokers huddled together outside various offices and other buildings from which they had been banned. One recalcitrant smoker commented, 'I've smoked for almost 40 years and no one but me is going to decide when I quit.'
- **Castigation of role models** A photograph of the late Princess Margaret looking pale and drawn (but without a cigarette) together with the headline 'HOW MANY DID YOU HAVE TODAY?' accompanied by text that noted her return from a Caribbean holiday with the comment, 'Butt who'd have known from her fagged out look last night?'
- **The nanny state** The then minister Virginia Bottomley was lambasted by Conservative backbench members of Parliament after she launched 'No Smoking Day'. Their discourse along the lines of freedom for the individual was encapsulated by a photograph of the minister with the heading 'GOLDEN VIRGINIA' and reference being made to her 'best headmistressy tones'.

This kind of discourse analysis has special relevance for health promotion in relation to the development of policies designed to restrict 'unhealthy' media advertising – and to the construction of health promotion messages used, for instance, in media advocacy (more on this in Chapter 8).

Ideology and discourse – an example from family planning A study by Sternberg (2002) of Nicaraguan men's involvement in sexual and reproductive health provides a convincing demonstration of the ways in which sexuality is socially constructed. The research was based on detailed analysis of transcripts of focus group interviews. One of the main issues researched was that of male involvement in family planning. He highlights five major ideological dimensions, which are listed in the box below. It should be noted that Sternberg elects to use the term 'discourse' rather than 'ideology' in his analysis.

A few further points of clarification should be made in connection with Sternberg's analysis. First, medical discourse does not represent an 'official' medical consensus on contraceptive methods, but, rather, lay perspectives on what some of the men themselves view as 'medical matters'! Again, the term 'pro-feminist discourse' refers to an acceptance by some of the men of women's rights – an acknowledgement that is consistent with the 'official' position encapsulated in the notion of 'Western progressive' discourse.

It is perhaps worth noting that power is central to the discourses portrayed. Indeed, some writers have portrayed the Catholic religion, patriarchy and medicine as examples of dominant ideologies. De Kadt (1982) also refers to feminism as a radical ideology that challenges the dominant power positions of all three! Our preference here, however, is to use discourse as a subordinate component of ideology. Thus, Catholicism can legitimately be defined in ideological terms, whereas the doctrinal notion that contraception is sinful is best categorized as discourse – informed by Catholic ideology more generally.

Medical discourse and the preventive model

The history of health promotion has been marked by a struggle to distance itself from the medical

FIVE MAJOR IDEOLOGICAL INFLUENCES ON MEN'S INVOLVEMENT IN FAMILY PLANNING

Catholic discourse

Discursive positions

- Contraception is sinful.
- Vasectomy prevents a man from doing his duty by procreating.
- Marriage is for having children.
- It is sinful not to have all the children you can afford.
- The purpose of life is procreation.

Traditional patriarchal discourse (machismo)

Discursive positions

- Women who use certain family planning methods will be unfaithful.
- If a woman becomes pregnant it is her fault for not taking precautions.
- A man has a right to decide when and if a woman should become pregnant because he pays the bills.
- Vasectomy feminizes a man.
- A man should leave a woman who does not want to become pregnant.

Medical discourse

Discursive positions

- Artificial methods such as the Pill are harmful.
- Vasectomy weakens a man.
- Condoms reduce sexual sensation.
- The Pill and the IUD are not safe, reliable methods.
- Contraception has benefits for women's health.

Pro-feminist discourse

Discursive positions

- Women have the right to choose whether or not they want to become pregnant.
- Men often force women to have children against their will.

Western progressive (liberal feminist) discourse

Discursive positions

- A responsible man is one who has only the number of children he can afford.
- A couple should decide together the number of children they want.
- Vasectomy and condoms allow men to play a role in family planning.

Sternberg, 2002: 256

model that has dominated twentieth-century discourse on health and illness. Some would contend that this break is more evident in the rhetoric than in the practice of health promotion (Kelly and Charlton, 1995). Although the medical model has been referred to at a number of points so far, it is worthwhile considering – in the context of our discussion about ideology, power and control – the nature of the model and the origins of concern about its applicability to health promotion. The key features of the medical model have been variously seen as including:

- a mechanistic view of the body
- mind–body dualism
- disease as the product of disordered functioning of the body or a part of it
- a focus on pathogenesis – that is, the causes of disease
- the pursuit of the causal sequences of disease and an emphasis on micro-causality
- specific diseases having specific causes.

The medical model is therefore very much in tune with modernist rational thought and characterized by a reductionist view of the causes of ill health, together with a mechanistic focus on micro-causality.

The medical model is inextricably linked with medical practice and, more generally, biomedicine. It shares common ideological origins and has acquired added authority as a result of its association with the power and authority of the medical profession. The dominance of medicine has itself been the subject of an extensive sociological critique – for example, its role in supporting a capitalist value system (Navarro, 1976, and Doyal and Pennell, 1979); monopolization of healthcare (De Kadt, 1982); the comodification of health and appropriation of authority over the areas that influence health (Illich, 1976); and maintaining gendered power structures in society (Doyal and Pennell, 1979, and Ehrenreich and English, 1979).

The medical model belongs to a group that Rawson (1992: 210) has termed 'iconic model' – that is, 'simplified descriptions of some aspect of known reality, portraying a literal or isomorphic image of nature'. It is possible, in principle, to identify a number of different models within medical practice and, equally, the medical model can be recognized within a range of different types of professional practice. It is also worth noting, in passing, that the ascendancy of high-tech medicine in the twentieth century and marginalization of preventive medicine has not gone unchallenged within medicine itself. The work of McKeown is well known in this regard (see, for example, McKeown, 1979). The emergence of 'The New Public Health' has been an attempt to retreat from an emphasis on individual responsibility for health and health actions and refocus on the factors that collectively influence health status. However, critics such as Petersen and Lupton (1996) contend that 'The New Public Health' has not entirely freed itself from the ethic of individual responsibility. Nor has it mounted an effective challenge to the increasing disparity in wealth and power within many societies.

Application of the medical model to health promotion leads to an emphasis on prevention – particularly primary prevention. This association with prevention effectively 'rebadges' the medical model as the preventive model.

The dominant concept is that of risk, whether viewed as a 'property of individuals or as an external threat' (Petersen and Lupton, 1996: 174). Furthermore, the conceptualization of risk is often narrow, ignoring the wider social and environmental determinants of health. The emphasis is on individual responsibility, which – as noted above in our comments on 'victim-blaming' – places the onus on

LEVELS OF PREVENTION

- **Primary prevention** aims to prevent new cases of a disease from developing by reducing exposure to causal and risk factors.
- **Secondary prevention** aims to reduce the consequences of disease and increase the chances of cure by early diagnosis and treatment, often as a result of screening procedures.
- **Tertiary prevention** aims to halt the progress, or reduce the complications, of established disease by effective treatment and rehabilitation.

A fourth level of prevention has been recognized (Beaglehole et al., 1993): **primordial prevention**. It aims to prevent the emergence of social, economic and cultural patterns known to be associated with disease in cultures that already have healthy traditional ways of life.

Table 1.1 *Levels of prevention*

Level of prevention	Aim of health education
Primordial	Persuade people not to abandon healthy lifestyles and ways of living.
Primary	Persuade individuals to adopt healthy lifestyles and reduce exposure to risk. Persuade individuals to use preventive services, such as immunization.
Secondary	Persuade individuals to seek screening. Raise awareness of the early signs and symptoms of diseases. Persuade people to seek early treatment. Persuade people to comply with treatment.
Tertiary	Persuade people to comply with treatment. Persuade people to comply with rehabilitation advice. Encourage resumption of an appropriate lifestyle.

individuals to reduce their exposure to risk by avoiding risky behaviour and contact with risks in the environment. O'Brien (1995: 196) notes that the focus on risk leads to health being:

> constructed as a series of encounters with risk factors in diet and behaviour, at work and at play, in public and private networks, factors that can be monitored and correlated, channelled and controlled, prioritized and targeted.

Attempts to influence behaviour primarily take the form of health education interventions. The role of health education in relation to the different levels of prevention is summarized in Table 1.1.

The preventive model has a number of consequences. As we noted above, it results in an essentially 'victim-blaming' approach in its disregard for the social, environmental and political factors that shape and, indeed, constrain behavioural choices. Illich's (1976) critique of the extension of medical control beyond legitimate concern with disease to include ordinary aspects of human experience – so-called 'social iatrogenesis', or medicalization of life – is well known. Including within the medical remit exposure to risk and, along with it, a whole range of behavioural and lifestyle factors extends the notion of medicalization even further and brings substantial areas of life under expert, rather than autonomous, control. Kelleher, Gabe and Williams

(1994: xii) note that, along with the decline in organized religion, this has led to:

> doctors being cast more and more in the role of secular priests whose expertise encompassed not only the treatment of bodily ills but also advice on how to live the good life, and judgements on right and wrong behaviour.

Moreover, the acknowledgement of expert authority over areas of life normally managed by individuals, families and communities erodes confidence in their capacity to take responsibility for their own health. By undermining self-reliance, communities and cultures are disempowered. Illich (1976: 42) refers to this as 'cultural iatrogenesis', which he sees as:

> destroy[ing] the potential of people to deal with their human weaknesses, vulnerability, and uniqueness in a personal and autonomous way.

Horrobin's (1978: 25) riposte to Illich accepts the existence of some undue dependence on the medical profession in matters of sickness, but notes the remarkable resistance of the healthy to accept medical advice and overexaggeration of the power of medicine to influence people. He quotes John Owen's sixteenth-century verse:

> God and the doctor we like and adore
> But only when in danger, not before;
> The danger o'er, both are alike requited,
> God is forgotten, and the doctor slighted.

Furthermore, he contends that Illich's (1976: 29) portrayal of society as 'an ignorant and unwilling victim of medical imperialism' is a misrepresentation. Similarly, O'Neill's (2002) thought-provoking Reith Lectures drawing attention to the lack of trust in contemporary society suggests that the acceptance of treatment or advice cannot be taken as indicative of trust when no effective alternatives are available to people.

Notwithstanding these arguments, medicine is still accorded considerable expert power. Deference to such authority provides further legitimation. It reinforces the dominance of the medical model and, ipso facto, the preventive model, even when the view espoused is at odds with the experiences of individuals.

What, then, is the source of this medical authority? De Kadt (1982: 746) suggests that:

> Expertise and the 'life and death' responsibilities of the physician are used to provide ideological justification for physician dominance in the doctor–patient (healing) context.

Parsons' (1958) concept of the 'sick role' throws further light on the doctor–patient interaction. When people are ill, they are unable to fulfil their normal social roles and everyday activities. Diagnosis will medically legitimate their adoption of the sick role which exempts them from their normal social obligations. However, there is a concomitant obligation to attempt to get better, by seeking and complying with medical advice. The sick role therefore requires submission to medical authority and compliance with a therapeutic regimen.

Formalization of the 'at risk' role within the preventive model makes equivalent demands in terms of an obligation to modify behaviour and exposure to risk (Baric, 1969). Individuals are held responsible for their exposure to risk and failure to act accordingly may be attributed to ignorance at best or deliberate fecklessness at worse. Unlike the sick role, the at risk role does not confer any rights. The outcome of this is twofold. On the one hand it labels as deviant those who cannot or choose not to comply with admonitions on how to live their life, and holds them responsible for the consequences. The categorization of more and more areas of life as healthy or unhealthy effectively creates its own dogma about ways of living, coupled with the associated moral sanction of disapproval if unhealthy options are chosen. As Petersen and Lupton (1996: 178) note:

> The idealization of the 'normal', 'healthy' subject as one endowed with certain 'natural' capacities and inclinations fails to recognize the multiplicity of possible subject positions, and can serve to coerce, marginalize, stigmatize and discriminate against those who do not or cannot conform with the ideal. This ideal denies difference – whether this is based on social class, gender, sexuality, 'race' ethnicity, physical ability, or age – and the kinds of personal commitments and demands that are required of those who are called upon to conform to it.

On the other hand, it creates a remorseless pressure to improve health (Bunton and Burrows, 1995: 208):

> The contemporary citizen is increasingly attributed with responsibilities to ceaselessly maintain and improve her or his own health by using a whole range of measures. To do this she or he is increasingly expected to take note of and act upon the recommendations of a whole range of 'experts' and 'advisers' located in a range of *diffuse* institutional and cultural sites.

An overemphasis on keeping healthy has been referred to as 'healthism' – a term attributed to Crawford (1980: 368), who defines it as:

> the preoccupation with personal health as a primary – often the primary – focus for the definition and achievement of wellbeing; a goal which is to be attained primarily through the modification of lifestyles, with or without therapeutic help.

Despite healthism's emphasis on positive health, its focus on individual responsibility can be seen to have some parallels with victim-blaming. The no fault principle enshrined in the notion of the sick role does not apply and is replaced by a 'your fault dogma'. Those, therefore, who fail, or refuse, to seek health-promoting ways of life become 'near pariahs' (Crawford, 1980: 379). Furthermore, preoccupation with health elevates it in status to a super value – health becomes an end in itself rather than a means of achieving other values and positive health behaviour acts as a hallmark of good living.

Reference to our earlier discussion of health promotion will indicate that the preventive model and healthism are both inconsistent with the two central tenets of health promotion – equity and empowerment. The emphasis on individualism and lack of attention to the social and environmental factors that impinge on health – both directly and indirectly as a result of their influence on behaviour – could, in fact, increase rather than reduce the health gap in society. Health gains will inevitably be greatest in those who are most able to make changes by virtue of their relatively advantaged position.

However, even though we have argued that a preventive model is inconsistent with the values position of health promotion, we should finish on a word of caution and not throw the baby out with the bathwater. Rejection of the preventive model does not necessarily imply rejection of the need for biomedical knowledge or appropriate preventive action. Horrobin (1978) argues that it is inadequate knowledge and insufficiently rigorous criteria that have been responsible for the unnecessary use of screening procedures rather than the inexorable spread of medical knowledge cited by Illich (1976). Furthermore, evidence about cause is necessary to much health promotion practice – indeed, any attempts to influence behaviour in the absence of evidence that this will be beneficial would be unethical. The problem lies not so much with a biomedical interpretation per se but with too exclusive a reliance on it and dismissal of other perspectives – that is, with the imbalance of power and the dominance of medical expert authority. Reference to the discussion of empowerment in Chapter 3 also draws attention to the importance of knowledge and the ability to access and interpret accurate knowledge as key components of empowerment. Such knowledge and understanding can give people greater control over their own lives. It also enables them to enter into a circle of shared understanding with professionals and contributes to breaking down power structures and facilitating dialogue.

Education and the discourse of voluntarism

Health education is a key component of health promotion. Self-evidently, education itself has a long history in terms of its philosophy and ideology and the technical aspects that determine effective practice. In other words, and returning to Morrow and Brown's (1994) conceptualization, both normative theory and empirical theory underpin it. There is also the considerably contentious question as to what education *ought* to be for! We propose the following 'empirical' definition, which centres on the process of learning:

> health education is any planned activity designed to produce health- or illness-related learning.

'Learning' has frequently been defined as a relatively permanent change in capability or disposition – that is, the change produced is not transitory and, after the educational intervention, people are capable of achieving what they were not capable of achieving before the intervention and/or feel differently about ideas, people or events. Accordingly, effective health education may result in the development of cognitive capabilities such as the acquisition of factual information, understanding and insights. It may also provide skills in problem solving and decision making and the formation or development of beliefs. It might also result in the clarification of existing values and the creation of new values – and, quite frequently, in attitude change. Health education also aims to foster the acquisition of health-related psycho-motor or social interaction skills. It may even bring about changes in behaviour or lifestyle or create the conditions for the adoption of healthy public policy.

One of the most important and enduring sources of ideological argument centres on the question of rationality and voluntarism. For example, Hirst (1969) asserted unequivocally that the central purpose of *all* education should be rationality. The educational philosopher Baelz (1979: 32) contrasts education with manipulation and with indoctrination:

> The educator encourages his [sic] pupil to develop the capacity to think for himself, while the indoctrinator

wishes to make it impossible for his pupil ever to question the doctrine that he has been taught.

The concept of doctrine is equated with the notion of dogma and typically refers to some creed or body of religious, political or philosophical thought that is offered for acceptance as truth. Etymologically speaking, the reference to teaching or instruction is highly appropriate, but the intention would be that those who had been thus instructed would actually *believe* the doctrine presented – a fact also included in the dictionary definition's reference to a 'credo'. The notion of doctrine is thus not far removed from the notion of 'dogma' (from *dokein* – to seem good). The purpose of indoctrination is therefore to present a body of ideas in an appealing way such that the ideas are accepted. The distinction between indoctrination and education is therefore fundamental.

Health education, voluntarism and choices for health

For many health educators, voluntarism is an ideological sine qua non. Note, for instance, Green and Kreuter's (1999: 27) influential definition:

> Health education is any combination of learning experiences designed to facilitate *voluntary* actions conducive to health… *Voluntary* means *without coercion* and with the full understanding and acceptance of the purposes of the action. [Our emphasis]

Faden and Faden (1978) made the point even more forcibly in their discussion of the ethics of health education. They cited the Society of Public Health Educators' (SOPHE) *Code of Ethics* (1976), noting its affirmation of the importance of voluntary consumer participation:

> Health educators value privacy, dignity, and the worth of the individual, and use skills consistent with these values. Health educators observe the principle of informed consent with respect to individuals and groups served. Health educators support change by choice, not by coercion.

According to the educational model of health education, coercive strategies and techniques are, therefore, unacceptable. Coercion occurs when an individual's or group's freedom of action is constrained. Faden and Faden (1978) cite Warwick and Kelman (1973), who defined coercion as a process forcing individuals to act or refrain from acting under the threat of severe deprivation – and clearly involving the application of power to reward or punish. It frequently results from externally imposed sanctions or other barriers.

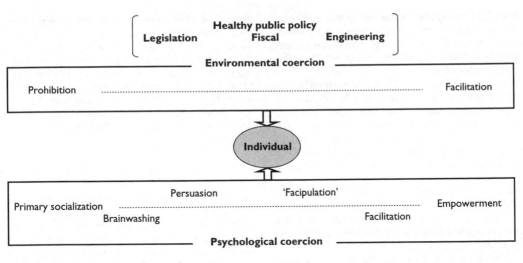

Figure 1.3   A spectrum of coercion

It is important, then, to recognize the existence of two varieties of coercion. The first of these is externally imposed. For instance, it involves the implementation of policy measures imposing a potentially wide range of various restrictive regulations, in the form of legislation, fiscal measures and environmental engineering. Examples of such 'healthy public policies' would include removal of cigarette vending machines, smoke-free areas; redesigning roadways and traffic-calming measures, the inclusion of vitamins in popular food products, regulation of the food industry to reduce the fat content of products, increases in the price of alcohol and so on. An interesting example of Japanese health legislation was the banning of the Pill in order to promote the use of condoms as a device to control the spread of HIV (Jitsukawa and Djerassi, 1994). The attraction of these various coercive strategies is doubtless self-evident, but McKinlay (1975: 13, in Guttman, 2000: 85) summarized it succinctly as follows:

> One stroke of effective health legislation is equal to many separate health intervention endeavours and the cumulative efforts of innumerable health workers over long periods of time.

The second form of coercion is perhaps less obvious and may be designated as psychological rather than environmental manipulation. It involves the use of certain techniques to create a particular kind of learning that lacks the element of genuine informed choice that characterizes the principle of voluntarism. Figure 1.3 locates examples of these techniques on a continuum ranging from high degrees of coercion to maximal potential for facilitating 'free' choice. Accordingly, 'brainwashing' is seen as highly coercive while 'facilitation' is, by definition, seeking to assist learners to achieve their own goals. 'Persuasion' is generally viewed as an intervention concerned with achieving the goals of the persuader rather than helping the persuadees to make up their own minds.

In the case of psychological coercion or 'persuasion', personal choice is modified in some way without the knowledge of the person in question. Faden and Faden (1978) in proposing this latter description had in mind Warwick and Kelman's (1973) definition of persuasion as a 'form of interpersonal influence, in which one person tries to change the attitudes or behaviour of another by means of argument, reasoning, or, in certain cases, structured listening'. In fact, it is somewhat misleading to define coercion of this kind solely in terms of the persuadee's lack of knowledge of what is going on. 'Insight' might be a better term as it is clear that, in many instances, individuals are well aware that someone is trying to influence them. Indeed, the most blatant form of psychological coercion, brainwashing, leaves the unfortunate recipient under no illusion that some fairly dramatic coercive techniques are being applied!

It may at first glance seem surprising, that brainwashing has been partnered with primary socialization. This represents both an expression of doubt about the power of brainwashing to fundamentally affect firmly grounded values and, at the same time, seeks to acknowledge the potentially greater power of the processes of 'shaping', conditioning and modelling that are part and parcel of the child-rearing experience.

At a more mundane level, people exposed to persuasive advertising also know that the advertiser is seeking to influence them. They may, however, lack insight into the influence process – for instance, why the advertiser is manipulating certain images or using certain presenters. This lack of insight into the psychodynamics of the attempt to influence militates against the principle of voluntarism, albeit in a rather more subtle way than the deliberate presentation of misleading information or the partial presentation of evidence supporting the attitude or behaviour change the persuader is seeking to induce.

Warwick and Kelman use the term 'structured listening' to refer to a type of interpersonal encounter that, at first glance, does not seem to involve coercion. It is particularly interesting as it serves as a reminder of the way in which a technique, that would be, considered eminently educational – non-directive counselling – may, with a few apparently minor modifications, be employed as a persuasive tool. Effective counselling depends on the deployment of such social skills as active listening, empathy, appropriate self-disclosure and the constant supply of unconditional positive regard. Janis (1975) has noted how the replacement of the ethically unexceptionable unconditional positive regard with what he terms 'quasi unconditional positive regard' can be a compelling device for influencing attitude and behaviour change – in a non-voluntaristic way. This technique involves implying that the highly rewarding positive strokes supplied by the health educator will be rationed and made contingent on the client adopting certain healthy practices. This apparently benevolent method will presumably be all the more powerful as it is difficult to detect the overt attempt to influence.

Rather like structured listening, the coined term 'facipulation' has been used for a persuasive method cosmetically concealed under a cloak of educational respectability (Constantino-David, 1982). Essentially it refers to the subtle process whereby 'leaders' actually manage to manipulate their clients under the guise of 'facilitation' with the intention, conscious or otherwise, of promoting the leaders' own political and ideological agenda.

Facilitation would usually be viewed as fundamentally voluntaristic and therefore ethical. After all, its concern is, by definition, to help people achieve the objectives that they have set for themselves. However, voluntaristic choice is not necessarily consonant with the ethics of health promotion. For instance, the term 'facilitation' might reasonably describe any enabling process, irrespective of its goals. Training individuals to achieve their felt needs to become better terrorists might be appropriate to certain revolutionary ideologies, but is certainly inconsistent with the aims of health promotion! As we will note later, freedom to choose applies only to those objectives that do not militate against the key values of health promotion.

Limits to freedom of choice

One of the avowed aims of an empowerment model of health promotion is to remove obstacles to rational decision making and freedom of choice. In some instances, overcoming such barriers is relatively simple – for example, the barrier created by ignorance. Others are more substantial – consider, for example, the case of addiction or other compulsive behaviours that sap freedom of choice. As McKeown (1979: 125) pointed out:

> it is said that the individual must be free to choose [whether he wishes to smoke]. But he is not free; with a drug of addiction the option is open only at the beginning.

Environmental barriers to voluntaristic action have received considerable recognition in recent years and, in part, have contributed to the formulation of the contemporary ideology of health promotion. Indeed, probably the greatest progress in health promotion in recent years has been its acknowledgement of the fact that material, social and cultural environments can both damage health and limit people's capacity to take action to promote their own health and the health of their communities. It is quite apparent that various natural disasters, such as famine and war, may both damage health directly and indirectly by removing the possibility of making empowered health-related decisions. Indeed, Keys (2000) has offered a very plausible account of how a natural disaster in AD535–536 (probably a major volcanic eruption or an asteroid colliding with the Earth) triggered dramatic and enduring climatic change. This allegedly not only had a direct impact on health but also contributed to various plagues and, ultimately, had a major effect on sociopolitical systems that resulted in the collapse of empires and 'resynchronized world history'.

Although less dramatic, poverty and inequality (buttressed by appropriate ideology) damage individuals' and communities' capacity for action and are now recognized as being major determinants of public health. On a smaller scale, lack of access to affordable healthy food will largely nullify the effects of health education initiatives. Less obviously, the complementary effects of culture and child-rearing may effectively block choice and genuine decision making. For instance, in the process of socialization, cultural values may result in certain foods being classified as 'taboo', thus creating a moral imperative forbidding consumption, regardless of the nutritional advantages of the food in question.

In the face of these many and varied psychological and environmental obstacles to the achievement of health, it is not surprising that often draconian measures have been proposed, usually under the rubric of implementing 'healthy public policy'. As is apparent from Figure 1.3 above, most of these policy measures are essentially coercive and typically involve fiscal, economic and legislative measures together with environmental changes – all of which militate against freedom of choice. Although it is argued that healthy public policy makes the healthy choice the easy choice, it may effectively make the healthy choice the only choice! How can such attacks on freedom be reconciled with the discourse of voluntarism, which characterizes an 'educational model'?

The fact is, of course, that unbridled freedom is only the prerogative of the despot and, possibly to a lesser extent, of certain privileged groups. There are inevitably and appropriately limitations on freedom of choice. It could well be argued that 'true' education should encourage people to think in a systematic way about what is of most importance to them in their lives so that they might consistently act in accordance with the values they have clarified. It is also important that educated individuals should be helped to make decisions rather than uncritically absorb dogma. There are, however, obvious limitations to freedom of choice. As noted elsewhere (Tones, 1987) all values are not equally acceptable in a given society: a decision to rape and pillage would not normally be considered acceptable, even if the individual had decided to wholeheartedly espouse antisocial behaviour as part of a programme of self-improvement.

Health promotion would certainly not subscribe to unfettered freedom of choice. It is avowedly committed to certain major values and has its own ideology to which most nations subscribe (or to which they at least pay lip-service) and has been incorporated in the various doctrines and discourse propagated by WHO, as we have seen. This position is, or should be, non-negotiable. While cultural sensitivity is part of a concern for people in general, where cultural peculiarities are inconsistent with the overriding values of health promotion, they must be challenged. In the context of the principles of voluntarism, we must therefore observe two

major qualifying principles. People should have a right to self-fulfilment, provided that this does not impede others' right to fulfilment and/or otherwise damage the wellbeing of the community at large. A good deal of consideration has, in fact, been given to the question of imposing limitations on liberty. The resulting ideological principles are most usefully expressed in terms of utilitarianism and paternalism. These principles provide support for the occasional overriding of personal liberty, either for the greater good or because some people seem incapable of exercising choice.

Utilitarianism, paternalism and the justification of coercion

There are two broad approaches to defining the ethics of interventions. One of these supports the principle that the integrity of a moral principle should be of prime consideration whatever the consequences. For example, it is always wrong to deliberately provide inaccurate information, even if this might seem to be in the interests of the recipient of that information. The alternative view is that it is the results of actions that are most important (Guttman, 2000). This latter moral principle is generally described as utilitarianism.

There is an obvious and generally acceptable rationale underpinning actions based on the principle of utilitarianism. In short, people's freedom of action should be respected, so long as it does not interfere with the general good (for example, Mappes and Zembary, 1991). Indeed, it provides a simple baseline value for health education that legitimately espouses the imperative of self-actualization: maximize whatever mix of mental, physical and social potential for growth you care to choose. However, personal gratification should not limit others' equal right to self-actualization.

It follows logically, therefore, that it is quite legitimate to use many of the varieties of coercion identified in Figure 1.3 above where individuals' actions can be shown to damage the public generally. The restrictions on smoking in public places, for example, is therefore entirely justifiable in that it is not merely a public nuisance, but puts non-smokers at risk as a result of passive smoking. Less clear-cut perhaps is the argument that seeks to restrain self-destructive behaviour on the grounds that the prudent in society should not have to pay for the excesses of the imprudent. More generally, economic arguments have indicated how self-inflicted illness damages the economy in terms of reduced productivity due to working days lost and increases the burden on already hard-pressed health services. Legislation can therefore be justified. For instance,

---

LIES, DAMNED LIES AND STATISTICS ?

Prime Minister: Cholera killed 30,000 people in 1837 and we had the Public Health Act. Smog killed 2500 in 1952 and we had the Clean Air Act. Certain drugs kill half a dozen people and they are withdrawn from sale. Cigarettes kill 100,000 people a year and what do we get?

Sir Humphrey: Four billion pounds a year, 35,000 jobs in the tobacco industry, a flourishing cigarette export business helping our balance of trade, 250,000 jobs related to tobacco – newsagents, packing, transport ...

Prime Minister: They're just guesses!

Sir Humphrey: No, they're facts!

Prime Minister: So your statistics are facts and my facts are statistics? ... Humphrey we're talking about 100,000 deaths a year.

Sir Humphrey: Yes but cigarette taxes pay for one third of the cost of the National Health Service. We're saving many more lives than we otherwise could – because of those smokers who voluntarily lay down their lives for their friends ... they are national benefactors!

Yes, Prime Minister, 1990

---

in the UK, legislation enforcing seatbelt use and the wearing of protective headgear by motorcyclists has been in place for some time and is demonstrably effective. The situation regarding smoking is more equivocal – doubtless because a substantial number of smokers feel less in control of that particular behaviour. Certainly many arguments have been adduced to demonstrate that smokers cover the cost of their morbidity and early mortality as a result of the finances levied by taxation and should actually be treated as social benefactors, just as the fictitious civil servant Sir Humphrey Appleby pointed out to the Prime Minister seeking to introduce legislation to ban all advertising of cigarettes (see box).

The cost–benefit analysis of smoking is a matter for health economics and so will not be debated here. However, a serious point is frequently made that those indulging in high-risk activities should be allowed to do so, providing that this does not damage the wellbeing of others and that possible social and medical costs are covered by insurance. The financial argument would not, of course, apply to those who impose a financial burden on the state because of illness for which they cannot be blamed. Wikler (1978: 234), however, compares diabetics (who cannot be blamed for their illness) with smokers and suggests that the distinction is by no means clear-cut. Smokers could only be blamed for their condition if their actions were truly deliberate and voluntary.

If the smoker's behaviour is less than voluntary, if it is the result of irresistible commercial or societal conditioning or of psychological need, then the smoker is, morally speaking, in the same position as the diabetic. His need becomes deserving, and the resulting burden is not especially unfair.

The principle of utilitarianism, then, does not prove as unambiguous as it first appears. The question of limitations to free choice again proves problematic and leads us to consider the second principle, which may justify coercive methods. If people are not really responsible for their actions, then society must make decisions on their behalf, for their own good. These decisions will inevitably involve the restriction of liberties and involve some degree of coercion. This principle of paternalism (Nikku, (1997), though, proves even more difficult to justify than the appeal to utilitarianism. Beauchamp (1978: 244) cites John Stuart Mill's (1961) treatise on liberty and his assertion that utilitarianism is the only justification for coercion:

The only purpose for which power can be rightfully exercised over any member of a civilized community, against his will, is to prevent harm to others. His own good, either physical or moral is not a sufficient warrant. He cannot rightfully be compelled to do or forbear because it will be better for him to do so, because it will make him happier, because in the opinion of others, to do so would be wise, or even right. These are good reasons for remonstrating with him, or reasoning with him or persuading him or entreating him, but not for compelling him.

However, as Daniels (1985: 157, in Guttman, 2000: 52) indicates:

Even a view that holds the individual to be the best architect of his ends and judge of his interests rests on important assumptions about the information available to the agent, the competency of the agent to make these decisions rationally, and the voluntariness of the decisions he makes. It is because these assumptions are not always met that we require a theory of justifiable paternalism.

Pollard and Brennan (1978), in discussing the basis for governmental intervention in cases of self-regarding behaviour – that is, behaviour affecting only the individual but not others – cite Dworkin's (1972: 71) justification of paternalistic behaviour on the grounds that some adults may not be capable of rational thought because, 'at some point in the future the individual will see the wisdom of the paternalistic intervention, even though at present he or she is not aware of its value.'

The intervention thus, in some way, protects the 'real' will of the individual. At first glance such a proposition looks distinctly dubious. However, it is undoubtedly true that most societies routinely take responsibility for certain categories of individual. For instance the very young, the insane and those having a substantial degree of mental impairment would routinely be protected in many societies. Again, the notion of protecting someone's real will is not as Machiavellian as it might appear. For instance, it would seem fairly clear that a substantial majority of smokers would prefer not to smoke and it is appropriate to recall McKeown's (1979: 125) observation that, 'the critical decision to smoke is taken not by consenting adults but by children below the age of consent.' Paternalistic intervention to limit people's freedom to choose to smoke might make some sense ethically. Furthermore, even if suicide were, legal, a depressed person might be legitimately prevented from taking his or her life on the reasonable supposition that, when no longer depressed, (s)he would not wish to do so.

Wikler (1978: 232) poses the question, 'Is there, then, a case for paternalist coercion for health?' and answers it as follows:

It depends on whether the behaviour slated for change is involuntary or not, whether there exists a practical, non-intrusive way to find out if it is voluntary or not, whether actual policies and programmes can be made subtle enough to distinguish in practice between voluntary and involuntary behaviour; and whether pressure can be applied to specific behaviours without the need to take on whole cultures. It also depends on whether those making and executing policy in this area can distinguish between involuntary actions and actions which are merely different from their own; whether they can restrain themselves from enforcing their views in subjects on which they are not expert; whether the coercive methods they use inflict greater intrusions and privations than the behaviours they attempt to eradicate; and whether allowing health professionals to exercise paternalistic power within these strict limits will lead inexorably to abuses and unjustified restrictions on liberty. These questions are empirical, not philosophical, and those who would want to justify coercive lifestyle reform programmes on paternalist grounds would do well to engage in the research needed for answers. Alternatively, one might despair of fashioning a paternalist defence of coercion in health behaviour change and switch to one of the other potential lines of argument.

Beauchamp (1978) critically appraises the argument advanced by his namesake Dan Beauchamp that the state should adopt a paternalistic stance, then rejects it! The notion, however, merits some further consideration. It relates to the general concept of 'distributive justice'. Distributive justice is about the ways in which both social goods and burdens are distributed – for example healthcare and the taxation needed to pay for it. Dan Beauchamp advocates social justice, asserting that all people have an *entitlement* to health protection and minimum standards of income (incidentally, a position equivalent to WHO's association of health with human rights). He (1976: 488) compares the idea of social justice with the prevailing (North American) preference for market justice, which he views as, 'the primary roadblock to dramatic reductions in preventable injury and death ... the marketplace is a pervasive ideology protecting the most powerful or the most numerous from the burdens of collective action ... [it] is fatally deficient in protecting the health of the public.'

The question of choice versus coercion in the interest of public health is very real. On the one hand, the principle of voluntarism urges freedom of choice unless good reason can be provided for coercive measures on the basis of utilitarianism, paternalism or 'social justice'. On the other hand, it seems particularly difficult to reach consensus about when, where and to what extent these principles can be used to justify coercive interventions in the interest of public health. Those of a left-wing orientation might object to any infringement of liberty of disadvantaged people, but wholeheartedly support paternalistic (or should it be 'maternalistic'?) measures by the nanny state on the grounds of social justice and equity. Equally, the more tough-minded advocates of market forces would object vocally to interventions that restricted their own freedom of action, but might well subscribe to utilitarian restriction of the liberty of people of a different political persuasion!

We may be able move some way towards resolving this dilemma by promoting self-empowerment. However, we should take account of Beauchamp's (1978: 450) noteworthy observation that, 'Public health should – at least ideally – be suspicious of behavioural paradigms for viewing public health problems since they tend to "blame the victim" and unfairly protect majorities and powerful interests from the burdens of prevention.' Accordingly, our later analysis and discussion of empowerment will emphasize the importance of *community* participation and *community* empowerment.

Health promotion and the discourse of empowerment

The assertion that health promotion's main concern should be that of empowerment is becoming increasingly acceptable, although this acceptance often takes the form of lip-service rather than practice and policy! Certainly, as noted above, most of the key pronunciamentos published by WHO since the inception of 'Health for All by the Year 2000' have placed emphasis on individuals gaining control over their lives and their health and on the importance of active participating communities.

It is axiomatic from our earlier discussion that empowerment is based on the principles of voluntarism. Assuming that due attention is paid to the various caveats mentioned in that discussion, there remain two major ideological questions to be addressed.

- Should *all* people have a right to power, to be in control?
- Can all people be trusted to exercise power?

Assuming that health promoters subscribe to the WHO-endorsed empowerment ideology, only one key question remains: how can people who lack power become more powerful and actually gain a reasonable degree of control over their lives? How can they compete with, and resist coercion by, those who already have power?

Further reflections on power

Empowerment, by definition, has to do with people acquiring a degree of power and control. Self-empowerment thus describes the extent to which individuals have power and control over their interactions with their physical and social environment. By analogy, an empowered community is an identifiable group of people who also possesses power and control. It is a matter of some importance to understand the different circumstances under which people acquire power, wield it and yield to it.

REFLECTIONS ON FATE, CHANCE AND FREE WILL

... many have held and hold the opinion that events are controlled by fortune and by God in such a way that the prudence of men cannot modify them, indeed, that men have no influence whatsoever. Because of this, they would conclude that there is no point in sweating over things, but that one should submit to the rulings of chance.

Nonetheless, so as not to rule out our free will, I believe that it is probably true that fortune is the arbiter of half the things we do, leaving the other half or so to be controlled by ourselves. I compare fortune to one of those violent rivers which, when they are enraged, flood the plains, tear down trees and buildings, wash soil from one place to deposit it in another. Everyone flees before them, everybody yields to their impetus, there is no possibility of resistance. Yet although such is their nature, it does not follow that when they are flowing quietly one cannot take precautions, constructing dykes and embankments so that when the river is in flood it runs into a canal or else its impetus is less wild and dangerous.

Niccolo Machiavelli (1469–1527),
The Prince, 1961: 130.

A TYPOLOGY OF INFLUENCE

Force   The individual or group is obliged to comply by removing all choice.

Coercion   Compliance is achieved by the threat of deprivation where conflict exists regarding values or courses of action.

Manipulation   This is a 'subconcept' of force. Compliance results in the absence of recognition by those who comply of the source of nature of the demand made.

Influence   This term is used when an individual or organization succeeds in causing others to change their intended actions, but without overt or tacit threat of deprivation.

Authority   This form of power operates when people comply because they accept that commands are reasonable in terms of their own values or because an appropriate and acceptable procedure has been adopted.

                                                                          Bachrach and Baratz, 1970: 28

Definitions of power and related concepts

The notion of power may manifest itself at macro, meso and micro levels. All three levels have some degree of relevance for health promotion. Studies of power at the micro level are concerned with influences on, and exerted by, individuals or small groups; meso-level power might refer to the power exerted by organizations or communities; the influence of national policy would be a macro-level influence – and, of course, the kinds of ideological controls discussed above. Its essence has been subjected to detailed analysis and debate.

Naturally, there are a number of different ideas associated with power. For instance, concepts such as 'control', 'authority' and 'influence' may be used almost interchangeably with power. Corwin (1978), for instance, defines 'authority' as legitimized institutionalized power (and uses the term 'coercion' to refer to the illegitimate use of power). He posits a continuum of control ranging from a situation in which there is a capacity for applying a high level of sanction through to an opposite in which control is limited to minimal sanction capability delivered in relatively informal circumstances. Corwin employs the term 'influence' to describe this latter circumstance. He also identifies a further kind of authority, which he calls 'consensual authority', which is when power and control depend on the outcome of negotiation based on the differential possession of resources.

Bachrach and Baratz (1970) also acknowledge that variations in the nomenclature and meaning of these various terms and offer a useful typology of influence (see box).

The classic Weberian analysis identifies three forms of power:

- **social power** based on such factors as prestige, family status, lifestyle and patterns of consumption
- **economic power** based on a group's relationship to the mode of production, its position in the labour market and general life chances
- **political power** based on affiliation to parties, bureaucracy and legal structure.

Corwin (1978: 65) also provides a useful introduction to the notion of 'social power'.

Social power is the probability that a person or group can realize its will against opposition. Since power pervades most social relationships, it can be observed when armies fight, corporations bribe politicians, employers direct their employees, a political candidate sways voters, teachers evaluate their students, prison guards shoot rebellious prisoners, parents set examples for their children, and unions negotiate with management.

Lukes (1974) reminds us that dominant groups shape people's needs and wants – by means of mass media, 'indoctrination' at the school or, more powerfully, socialization, for example. Lukes' analysis is clearly consistent with our earlier discussion of the often subtle means whereby dominant ideologies are perpetuated, including the creation of false consciousness. These observations are not only relevant to our discussion of ideologies in general, but, as we noted earlier in this chapter, more particularly, to questions of utilitarianism and paternalism. They also have an important bearing on our later examination of the assessment of health needs.

Moreover, these two notions underpin thinking about empowerment, bearing in mind Kindervatter's (1979: 62) definition of empowerment as, 'People gaining an understanding of and control over social, economic and/or political forces in order to improve their standing in society.' A clear understanding of the different constructions of power also has special significance in, for example, determining the success or failure of lobbying and advocacy for the implementation of healthy public policy at macro and meso levels.

At this juncture, though, we will move to an individualistic view of power. For, while it is important at the level of discussing politics and 'healthy public policy' to adopt a sociological stance, we must also consider the direct, interpersonal exercising of power individuals are subject to. After all, continuing pressure is placed on individuals – either face-to-face or via mass media – to adopt healthy or unhealthy practices. We will consider these processes in greater detail later in this book, but it is convenient to extend our review of power a little here and consider this individual perspective.

Five varieties of power: an individual perspective One of the classic, and still valid, analyses of power at the micro level was provide by French and Raven (1959), who distinguished five varieties of power. This scheme (which has similarities to Weber's analysis of charismatic, traditional and rational–legal power) is frequently used to illuminate interactions when analysing small group dynamics and discussing leadership functions. Their analysis comprises the following five varieties of power.

- **Legitimate power** authority is derived from legitimate status formally bestowed by a given social system.
- **Expert power** authority derives from the actual and perceived expertise of the individual in question. It may or may not be associated with legitimate authority or be an informal adjunct of referent power (see below).
- **Reward power** authority derives from the individual's capacity for providing rewards.
- **Coercive power** authority derives from the individual's capacity to sanction.
- **Referent power** authority derives from the referent's individual characteristics, which, for some reason, are valued by the person who is influenced.

Stardom and charisma Alberoni (1962, in McQuail, 1972) also discusses the characteristics of individuals who, despite lacking legitimate authority, nonetheless can exert quite a powerful influence over other people. He describes this 'powerless "élite"' as 'stars'. Their, 'institutional power is very limited or non-existent, but [their] doings and way of life arouse a considerable and sometimes even a maximum degree of interest.' He likens their personal characteristics to Weber's (1968: 241) notion of charisma:

> By charisma we mean a quality regarded as extraordinary and attributed to a person ... The latter is believed to be endowed with powers and properties which are supernatural and superhuman, or at least exceptional even where accessible to others; or again as sent by God, or as if adorned with exemplary value and thus worthy to be a leader.

It is sometimes said, with a degree of acrimony, that many celebrities in contemporary society are 'famous for being famous'! It is certainly the case that these charismatic characters may well exert a quite dramatic degree of influence on people. They may influence taste and preferences and act as models. This phenomenon will be revisited in Chapter 7 when we consider the influence of source credibility and attractiveness in persuading individuals to adopt healthy or unhealthy courses of action.

The concept of referent power also merits some further comment. The individual's influence is bestowed on him or her by 'followers' on account of that person's perceived expertise or reward value. The concept has some points in common with the notion of charismatic leadership. It also relates to opinion leadership and the principle of 'homophily', both of which feature in the communication of innovations theory, which will be considered in Chapter 3.

French and Raven's conceptual scheme provides a bridge between the broader sociological perspective on power and the meso- and micro-level perspectives of social psychology and attitude change theory. It is, for example, consistent with the 'Yale-Hovland' approach that guided research into the relative effects of source, message, audience and channel on the recipients of persuasive communications (Hovland, Janis and Kelley, 1953). In short, the source of a communication may play a significant part in determining the beliefs, attitudes and even behaviour of its recipients. Of more direct relevance to the study of empowerment are those investigations that have examined the effect of message source on an individual's compliance and conformity. Perhaps the best-known – and most alarming – of such studies is the work of Milgram,

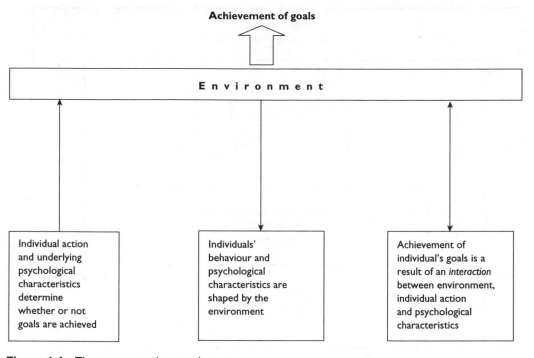

Figure 1.4   Three perspectives on human agency

who demonstrated that, under the influence of an authority figure, 65 per cent of a group of 'ordinary' people were prepared to administer a 450-volt electric shock to an experimental subject. Many of them did this even while experiencing obvious concern and conflict (Milgram, 1963). As Higbee and Jensen (1978: 27) point out:

> people find it extremely difficult to refuse any request by an experimenter. In experimental settings people have tried to balance a marble on a steel ball and eat a large number of dry soda crackers, dump out cans of garbage and sort it into piles of similar material, add adjacent numbers on sheets containing random digits, tearing up each sheet after completing it, and continuing for five and a half hours until the *experimenter* gives up, and pick up a poisonous snake, put their hands into nitric acid, and throw acid into an assistant's face (the people *thought* they were doing these things).

We might legitimately conclude that empowered individuals would be more able and willing to resist pressure and not submit to unreasonable demands,

particularly those, that run counter to their existing values.

While analyses such as French and Raven's are undoubtedly useful in designing health promotion programmes, it is essential to ask how someone comes to wield legitimate authority, how they are in a position to reward, how they acquire the power to coerce, how they acquire expert authority or come to be treated as referents by their communities. The first three and, to some extent, the fourth of these questions relate directly to our earlier discussion of ideology. In short, the possession of wealth provides power. As we also noted earlier, power does not only rely on the crude application of force and coercion, but can also be exerted by the ideological control of culture and the hegemony of political and state institutions.

Self-empowerment, community empowerment and reciprocal determinism

Earlier in this chapter, we emphasized the dramatic effects an oppressive environment can have on

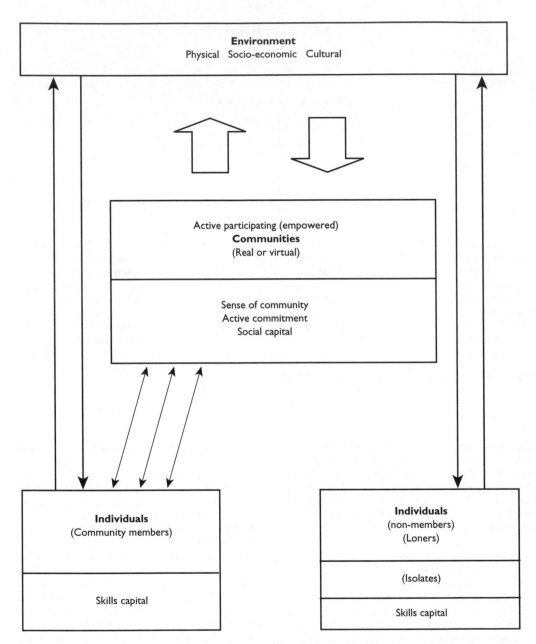

Figure 1.5   Reciprocal determinism and empowerment of communities and Individuals

individuals' health and their capacity to make choices. It is therefore self-evident that empowerment – people's opportunities to make genuinely free choices – is not possible unless physical, socio-economic and cultural circumstances are favourable. Thus, it is imperative that empowerment policy and the ensuing strategies must engage with the thorny question of environmental change.

On the other hand, it is clear that individuals are, in many situations, capable in principle of making choices even when the environment is not especially conducive to individual action. Three different perspectives on human agency can be identified (see Figure 1.4 on page 33).

In the first situation, the focus of attention is centred on individuals and those characteristics that explain their behaviour. The theorist may be interested only in psychological phenomena or even be effectively blind to the existence of the environment. Some forms of counselling may be characterized by this approach.

In the second instance, individuals are viewed as being largely controlled by their circumstances – directly or indirectly.

The third formulation of human agency asserts that humans (and animals) interact with their environments. They are, on the one hand, affected by environmental forces but, on the other, typically capable of having at least some impact on the various physical, socio-economic and cultural factors that influence them. The ideology and practice of empowerment ultimately derives from this last standpoint and has been a central feature of social learning theory. Its major exponent and advocate is Bandura (1986) who described the interactive process as 'reciprocal determinism' and contrasted it with the Skinnerian emphasis by referring to this latter theorist's assertion that, 'A person does not act upon the world, the world acts upon him' (Skinner, 1971: 211). Bandura argues that a process of 'triadic reciprocality' operates when humans engage with life. In short, there is an often complicated system of interaction between psychological factors (such as beliefs and attitudes), behaviour and the environment. A more comprehensive account of this system is given, and discussed, in Chapter 3.

We should also note that this archetypal psychological analysis of human agency is by no means inconsistent with the broader perspectives of sociology. For instance, Giddens (1991: 204) observes that, 'actors are at the same time creators of social systems yet created by them.'

Individual and community dimensions of empowerment

The logic of reciprocal determinism for an empowerment model of health promotion is inescapable. If empowerment is about facilitating voluntaristic decision making and achieving free choices (or those that are consistent with moral imperatives), then it must operate at both the level of the environment and at the level of the individual. Furthermore, it is important to recognize that the environment itself has many levels – from macro to meso, from the level of national policy to the level of regional organizations and institutions down to the level of the neighbourhood or village. In short, individuals exist within a web of social systems. At the same time, they may be intimately involved at the neighbourhood level with a social system of particular significance for health promotion – the community. Figure 1.5 gives an indication of this complexity within the context of commenting on both individual and community empowerment.

As may be seen from Figure 1.5, the community may mediate individual agency in relation to the general physical, socio-economic and cultural environment. The community is an especially important social system within the lexicon of empowerment and health promotion. Following the doctrine of the Ottawa Charter and related developments of WHO, an active, empowered community is perhaps seen as the most important of the desirable empowerment outcomes of health promotion activities. In short, it enables the people to take an active part in influencing policy. Three key features of an empowered community are also shown, namely: a sense of community – that is, a therapeutic feeling of identification with fellow community members – an active commitment to achieve community goals and what is increasingly termed 'social capital' (see Chapter 2 for more about this).

Individual or self-empowerment, on the other hand, comprises a cluster of attributes related to a personal capacity for voluntaristic action (Tones and Tilford, 2001: 40).

> Self-empowerment is a state in which an individual possesses a relatively high degree of actual power – that is, a *genuine* potential for making choices. Self-empowerment is associated with a number of beliefs about causality and the nature of control that are health promoting. It is also associated with a relatively high level of realistically based self-esteem together with a repertoire of *life skills* that contribute to the exercise of power over the individual's life and health.

Clearly, a community is composed of its membership – and it is arguable whether or not a community is more than the sum of the individuals making up this membership. In all events, a community is generally considered to be beneficial for its individual members, and the characteristics and capabilities of these individuals will contribute to the power of the community as a whole.

Figure 1.5 makes a distinction between 'real' and 'virtual' communities. The former represents a

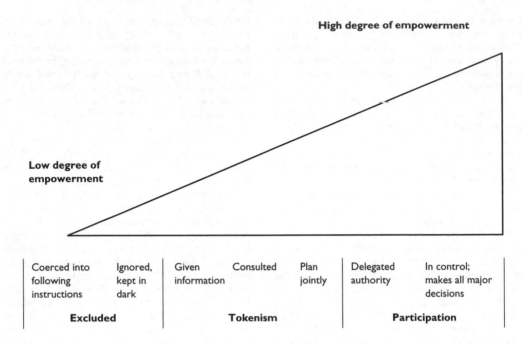

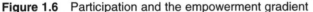

Coerced into following instructions	Ignored, kept in dark	Given information	Consulted	Plan jointly	Delegated authority	In control; makes all major decisions
Excluded		**Tokenism**			**Participation**	

Figure 1.6   Participation and the empowerment gradient

traditional idea of community as a group of people within a relatively small geographical area having a sense of identity and a network of relationships. A virtual community may lack the narrow geographical dimension of a real one, but otherwise have a shared identity. For instance, we can realistically talk about the gay community. What may be lacking, however, are interpersonal relationships. On the other hand, a virtual community may actually have more power at its disposal than a real community and, moreover, with the advent of technology such as the Internet, may benefit from different kinds of interaction.

Although often ignored in discussions of communities, Figure 1.5 reminds us that some individuals may not be part of any community – real or virtual. We have labelled as 'non members' individuals who exist in relative isolation because no community exists. By contrast, and borrowing terminology from the domain of sociometry, we have used the term 'loner' to distinguish people who do not wish to belong to a community from those whose felt need is to belong, but who are not accepted or rejected – so-called isolates.

Figure 1.5 (see page 34) also notes that individuals are affected by, and in turn affect, their environments at different levels without the mediation of community groups.

We might also note that environments do not exert their effects in a unidimensional way. It is more realistic to consider any given environment as exerting both facilitative and inhibitory influences of different strengths on communities and individuals. The sum total of both positive and negative pressures might be described in terms of these macro or meso influences 'making the healthy choice the easy choice' or, alternatively, being fundamentally oppressive. The specific, technical, detailed aspects of both community and individual empowerment will be explored at some length in Chapter 3.

One of the factors most closely associated with empowerment – with respect to both ideological and technical aspects – is that of participation. WHO has frequently commented on the importance of an active, participating community and the desirability of individual involvement in decision making is virtually taken for granted as a healthy development.

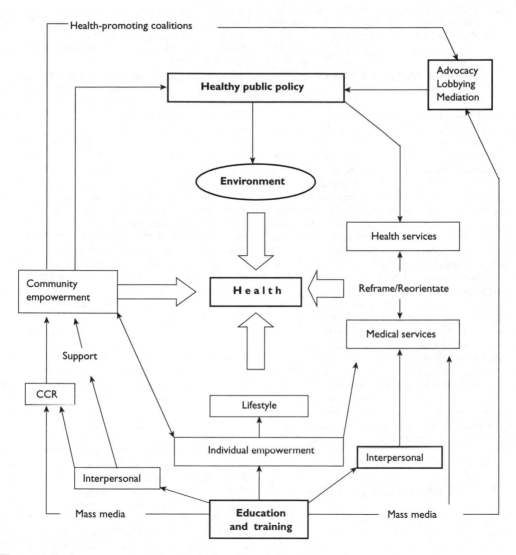

Figure 1.7   An empowerment model of health promotion

We will also note in Chapter 5 the centrality of participation to the needs assessment process. How does participation actually contribute to empowerment? It is almost a matter of common sense! A community that takes action – that is, participates in action to influence policy at local or national level – feels that it has actually achieved something, even if the outcome is not dramatic. Similarly, individuals who are actively involved are likely to experience at least some degree of control. Obviously there are many different degrees of involvement and Figure 1.6 indicates an assumed relationship between degrees of participation/involvement and empowerment. It draws on the classic analyses of Arnstein (1971) and Brager and Specht (1973).

It should be noted that Figure 1.6 applies equally not only to communities but also settings such as health promoting hospitals and health promoting schools and, at the micro level, interactions between individuals, such as doctor and patient.

An empowerment model of health promotion

We have considered the medical discourse associated with public health and a preventive model of health promotion or, rather, health education. We have also explored ideas related to the discourse of voluntarism, which might be said to give rise to an educational model of health promotion. Both of these models are limited in that they are inconsistent with the ideological thrust of health promotion. They are also technically limited in their capacity to explain what would be involved in achieving the empowerment goals of health promotion. Figure 1.7 seeks to identify the main components of an empowerment model of health promotion and their interrelationships.

The central dynamic of the empowerment model is the interplay of education and healthy public policy. The development and implementation of policy is the essential precursor to the creation of health-promoting environmental influences. The relationship is multiplicative, as we noted earlier in the 'formula' health promotion = health education × healthy public policy. The empowering function of education not only strengthens individual capabilities for health-related action, but also makes a major contribution to the establishment of healthy public policy.

Action to achieve healthy public policy

We discussed the five action areas of the Ottawa Charter earlier in this chapter, including the imperative to reorientate health services. Accordingly, Figure 1.7 not only shows policy initiatives addressing physical, socio-economic and cultural circumstances, but also indicates how policy initiatives are necessary to improve service provision in the most appropriate way to meet the health needs of particular populations. It also urges policymakers to make services user-friendly (partly to maximize the likelihood of these services being used appropriately). More importantly, however, the focus should be less on reorientation and more on reframing. In other words, the main *raison d'être* of most health-promoting services (as opposed to sickness services) should not be health in any formal sense.

For example, their prime concern might be transport, housing, economic development. However, all of these have a major impact on health (and on disease).

Two major action strategies are included in the model. One is the traditional means of seeking to influence policy, such as lobbying. Advocacy is defined here as lobbying of those who exercise power by those who have power but who are doing so on behalf of the relatively powerless. The term 'mediation', which was incorporated within the Ottawa Charter list of major actions, refers to the process of mediating between competing interests. By way of illustration, we might consider the different concerns of the owners and producers of mass media programmes and health professionals. The main goal of the former is to entertain the public and advertise products in order to make profits. The interests of the health promoters, on the other hand, are to control advertising and the representation of health issues (for example, in soap operas) in ways, that are considered to be damaging to the public health.

The second – ultimately the most powerful – means of producing policy change is to create a sufficient level of public pressure so that decisionmakers and politicians at national or local level feel obliged to change. Within a democracy this might, in the last analysis, result in change by means of the ballot box. In other, more dangerous, circumstances, change might occur via revolution.

The catalyst for change is health education, but emphatically not the variety of health education that has been tarred with the brush of victim-blaming! Rather, following the precepts of critical theory, it might usefully be called 'critical health education' and its purpose is radical and political. Again, the nature of education and its technology will be reviewed in Chapters 7 and 8 and particular attention will be devoted to its radical and critical manifestations.

Health education and individual empowerment

Figure 1.7 includes an analysis of the essential contribution made by education to individual action. A training function has also been included in the model to demonstrate the continuing importance of providing skills – not only to communities, but also to the professionals who work in the various services to which reference was made above. This training would include awareness-raising of the health-promoting role of the organizations, as well as making available the competences needed to communicate with clients and the general public, providing appropriate education and analysing the impact of policy on health – and making appropriate adjustments in the interest of effectiveness and efficiency.

We earlier reviewed the traditional health education function. We noted that its purpose was to persuade individuals to adopt behaviours that would result in the prevention of disease, both with regard to lifestyle and making proper use of medical services. The role of critical health education is not primarily that of persuasion (which is both ethically dubious and of limited effectiveness, but one of empowerment and support. Empowered individuals are more likely to make an efficient contribution to community action, which, in turn, contributes to their empowerment, as we mentioned earlier. They are also more likely to engage with the various services contributing to health in an assertive and productive fashion. They are almost certainly more likely to adopt a lifestyle conducive to achieving the objectives of preventive medicine than if they were not empowered! Indeed, one of our more forceful assertions here is that the successful adoption of an empowerment model of health promotion is not only more likely to achieve positive health outcomes in an ethical fashion, but also be more efficient in attaining the important outcomes associated with the prevention and management of disease and disability.

The empowerment model: critiques and reservations

The empowerment model of health promotion is advocated here both on grounds of ideological soundness and practical effectiveness. It is not without its critics, however. For instance, some might reasonably argue that empowerment is a fashionable term distinguished by its lack of clarity in conceptualization and use (the same criticism could, of course, be levelled at health promotion itself and even the notion of public health). A second objection derives from the assertion that empowerment lacks a theoretical base. This assertion is fundamentally incorrect, as we are in the process of demonstrating!

What is undoubtedly more problematic is translating the rhetoric into action. For instance, Mayo and Craig (1995: 2) cite the Bruntland Commission's conviction that the prerequisite for sustainable development is securing the effective participation of citizens, the World Bank's inclusion of empowerment as a main objective of community participation and the Human Development report definition of participation in terms of people having constant 'access to decision-making and power'. They also remind us that functionalist sociologists such as Parsons (1967) considered that power in society was a 'variable sum' and thus 'the powerless could be empowered, and could then share in the fruits of development, alongside those who had already achieved power.' Mayo and Craig argue that an alternative, and perhaps more convincing, viewpoint is that power is a 'zero sum'. Accordingly, the powerful will be reluctant to yield their power in the interest of empowering the powerless and will utilize the various ideological devices discussed earlier to keep the powerless in their place!

Croft and Beresford (1992: 20) observe that participation is at the heart of social policy and political debate, but 'generates enthusiasm and hostility in equal proportion' and is frequently handled in both a 'superficial' and 'depoliticized' way. It needs very careful scrutiny. Grace (1991) considered that empowerment in general has 'major problematic contradictions and inconsistencies' and, critically reviewing the discourse of empowerment, argued that it was not dissimilar to the discourse of marketing! De Kadt adopted a similarly sceptical note when he contrasted WHO's rhetoric about participation with the reality at grass roots level. He referred to Werner's (1980) review of forty rural health programmes in Latin America, which concluded that genuine community participation was a rare event. On the other hand, there were many examples of, 'handouts, paternalism and superimposed, initiative-destroying norms' (De Kadt, 1982: 94).

The superficial concern demonstrated by oligarchy is, of course, well recognized in the failure of 'trickle-down' theories of wealth creation. It is also apparent in the neo-liberal, New Right attack on welfare and the nanny state with its emphasis on the efficiency of the private market and the illusory freedom of the individual from the state that such measures allegedly create. A lack of true empowerment can also characterize the self-help movement, despite its several benefits. Although self-help initiatives may well be empowering in their contribution to demedicalization, they may also minimize the need to look for radical solutions to health problems by reducing state expenditure.

It should hopefully be clear from the observations made in this chapter that power and politics are central to health promotion. It would be a mistake to underestimate the difficulties of challenging power structures. Nonetheless, we believe that sophisticated analysis grounded in sound theory can result in the development of empowering strategies that can achieve results. In Chapter 3, the notion of empowerment will be operationalized and its theoretical and technical basis subjected to critical scrutiny.

2

Health and its Determinants – Issues of Assessment

'It is a capital mistake to theorize before you have all the evidence. It biases the judgement.'

'I should have more faith,' he said; 'I ought to know by this time that when a fact appears opposed to a long train of deductions it invariably proves to be capable of bearing some other interpretation.'

Sir Arthur Conan Doyle, *A Study in Scarlet*, 1888

INTRODUCTION

Green and Kreuter (1991) trace their initial motivation to develop a planning model for health education to their observation that, in practice, they could frequently discern no apparent reason for choosing the health issue to be addressed, nor the target population to be reached. Furthermore, the intervention strategy selected was also often simply a preferred method of working rather than the most strategic option to achieve defined outcomes. They assert that, 'The systematic and critical analysis of priorities and presumed cause–effect relationships can start the planner on the right foot in health promotion today' (1991: 25). What is required, therefore, is:

1 an analysis of health issues/problems
2 prioritization
3 analysis of the determinants.

Health promotion, as noted in Chapter 1, is characterized by its multisectoral nature and the involvement of a variety of different professional groups. Furthermore, a central tenet of health promotion is the importance of involving communities. The differing ideological positions and values of the various professional and lay groups will inevitably influence the way in which the determinants of health and causal factors are defined, the evidence that is accepted to support their existence and the ways in which priorities are identified and framed. The purpose of this chapter is to consider approaches to assessing the health status of communities and the broad range of factors that influence this as a basis for establishing needs and setting priorities for action.

The chapter falls into two broad sections. The first focuses on the assessment of health, beginning with a consideration of the role of epidemiology, before presenting a case for drawing on multiple professional and lay perspectives. The second section identifies the major determinants of health status.

EPIDEMIOLOGICAL PERSPECTIVES

Epidemiology has been viewed as a 'primary feeder discipline' for health promotion by virtue of its contribution to setting the agenda and its role in driving the system (Tannahill, 1992: 97). As we shall see, there is considerable criticism of over-reliance on epidemiological perspectives, which are often equated with a biomedical interpretation of health. However, for now, we will confine the discussion to consideration of its scope and potential contribution.

Epidemiology has typically been defined as 'the study of the distribution and determinants of disease in human populations' (Barker and Rose, 1984: v). While this draws attention to the focus of epidemiology being on populations rather than individuals, it will be immediately apparent that this interpretation conforms to a negative model of health. More recent definitions signal some move towards including a positive dimension – for example, 'the study of the distribution and determinants of health-related states or events in specified populations, and the application of this study to control of health problems' (Last, 1988, in Beaglehole et al., 1993: 3). This particular example also emphasizes the action-orientated role of epidemiology.

Unwin et al. (1997) identify three categories of information needed as a basis for planning interventions to improve the health of populations and communities:

- basic demographic information
- the health status of communities
- determinants of health in the community.

Kroeger (1997) further lists nine key epidemiological questions that can inform the planning process. These can be organized under four key headings, as shown in the box below.

Descriptive epidemiology

As we demonstrated in Chapter 1, health is both a contested concept and a subjective state and has been said to be as impossible to define as love, truth and beauty. It is not without difficulty, then, that epidemiology seeks to measure health objectively. Basch (1990) asserts that some composite indicator of health status is desirable but, ultimately, unattainable and a best estimate is therefore obtained by looking at levels of ill health. Descriptive epidemiology is essentially concerned with charting the disease burden of communities, together with the patterns of distribution of diseases – classically in relation to time, place and persons. There is frequently a heavy reliance on the use of routinely collected official health data, such as mortality and morbidity statistics, together with basic population data.

NINE EPIDEMIOLOGICAL QUESTIONS

Identification

 1 What are the main health problems?

Magnitude and distribution

 2 How common are they?
 3 When do they generally occur?
 4 Where do they occur?
 5 Who is affected?

Analysis

 6 Why does the problem occur?

Action and evaluation

 7 What measures could be (were) taken to deal with the problem?
 8 What results were anticipated (achieved)?
 9 What else could be done?

Derived from Kroeger, 1997

Mortality rates

The collection of data on vital events has its origins in the civil registration of births, marriages and deaths. Registration in England and Wales began in 1837, subsequent to the Births and Deaths Registration Act of 1836. Prior to this, the only records were in parish registers.

Because of the legal requirement to register deaths, mortality data are regarded as providing a complete representation. Deaths are recorded by underlying cause – confirmed either by a medical practitioner or an inquest. The death certificate requires identification of the immediate cause of death together with any underlying cause, defined as 'the disease or injury which initiated the train of events leading to death' (Unwin et al., 1997: 12). Other significant conditions contributing to death can also be recorded. The production of mortality statistics is based on coding of the underlying cause of death according to the International Classification of Disease (ICD). Distinguishing between the immediate cause of death and underlying cause can be a source of error. Death rates are expressed in a number of different ways, as summarized in the box.

Clearly each of the various mortality rates will create a different overall picture. The actual rates provide insight into the burden of mortality, but, given that the level of mortality is influenced by the age structure of the population, they are of little use when comparing populations with different age structures. The standardized rates, although artificial constructs, compensate for variations in age structure and can be used for comparative purposes. It is important, therefore, that appropriate rates are selected according to the intended purpose.

Morbidity rates

An important distinction in morbidity rates – and indeed health-related behaviour – is between incidence and prevalence. *Incidence* represents the number of new cases within a particular time period. *Prevalence*, in contrast, includes all the cases – either at a point in time (point prevalence) or over a defined period in time (period prevalence). Prevalence is often depicted as a pool together with the factors that contribute to filling and emptying the pool, as shown in Figure 2.1.

Morbidity data, unlike mortality data, are not complete in the sense that only those who come into contact with the health services will be routinely recorded. They are regarded as representing the tip of the clinical iceberg (Last, 1963) and below the surface are those who are self-medicating, using

---

Mortality rates

Actual rates

Crude mortality rate	number of deaths per thousand people.
Age-specific mortality rate	number of deaths per thousand people in a specific age group.
Infant mortality rate	number of deaths in the first year of life per thousand live births.
Under five mortality rate	number of deaths in the first five years of life per thousand live births.
Sex-specific rates	number of deaths per thousand women/men.
Cause-specific rates	numbers of deaths from a specific cause per thousand people.

Constructed rates

Age standardized mortality rates	the death rate that would exist in a population if it had the same age structure as a standard population (for example, national population, European standard population, Segi World Population, WHO World Standard Population (Ahmad et al., 2001)). A direct method of standardization.
Standardized mortality ratio (SMR)	the ratio of the *actual* number of deaths in a population to the number of deaths that would be *expected* if that population had the same levels of mortality as a reference population. The ratio is multiplied by 100. A SMR greater than 100 indicates a level of mortality higher than the reference population. An indirect method of standardization.

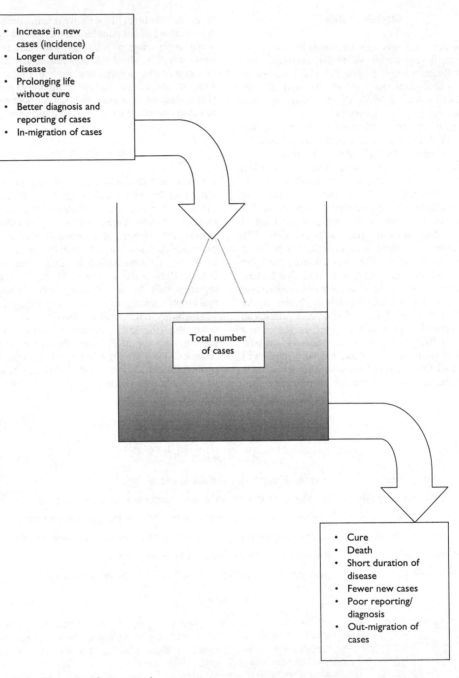

- Increase in new cases (incidence)
- Longer duration of disease
- Prolonging life without cure
- Better diagnosis and reporting of cases
- In-migration of cases

Total number of cases

- Cure
- Death
- Short duration of disease
- Fewer new cases
- Poor reporting/ diagnosis
- Out-migration of cases

Figure 2.1   The prevalence pool

alternative therapy, with subclinical symptoms or just putting up with their symptoms. The volume under the surface is likely to be greater the less serious – and, ipso facto, the more common – the condition. It will also be influenced by the availability of services and cultural factors associated with their usage. The main sources of routinely collected morbidity data are summarized in the box.

ROUTINE MORBIDITY DATA IN THE UK

- Hospital activity data.
- General practice data.
- Cancer registrations.
- Notification of infectious disease.
- Sexually transmitted diseases.
- HIV/AIDS.
- Congenital anomalies.

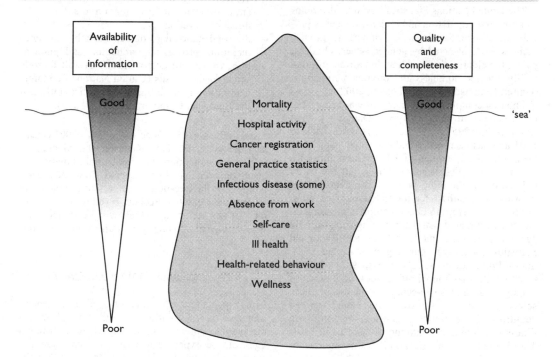

Availability of information		Quality and completeness

Good   Mortality   Good   'sea'

Hospital activity

Cancer registration

General practice statistics

Infectious disease (some)

Absence from work

Self-care

Ill health

Health-related behaviour

Wellness

Poor   Poor

Figure 2.2   The data iceberg

Given that the majority of day-to-day illnesses never bring people into contact with the health service, they will go un- or under-reported. Figure 2.2 applies the notion of the clinical iceberg to the availability of data and their completeness in what might be referred to as a 'data iceberg'.

Relatively little routine information is available on minor illnesses, states of wellbeing or health-related behaviour. Obtaining data on these is therefore usually dependent on surveys. In Great Britain, the General Household Survey, for example, asks each year about:

- long-standing illness, disability or infirmity and the extent to which this limits activities

- acute sickness or restricted activity during the preceding two weeks
- use of health services
- general health during the preceding year.

It also includes, on a more occasional basis, questions about health-related behaviour, such as contraceptive use and smoking.

Population data

Beaglehole et al. (1993) note that the central tool of epidemiology is the comparison of rates.

Rate = number of events in a population (numerator) ÷ size of the population (denominator)

In order to calculate rates, it is essential to know the size of the population and, for comparative purposes, the characteristics of that population. Such information is typically obtained by a census, which has been defined as 'a complete count or enumeration of a population conducted under the auspices of some governmental authority' (Ginn Daugherty and Kammeyer, 1995: 293).

The United Nations Statistics Division also notes that national population and housing censuses provide valuable information on vulnerable groups, such as those affected by gender issues, children, youth, the elderly, those with an impairment or disability and the homeless and migrant populations (United Nations Statistics Division, 2002).

The first complete modern census was carried out in Sweden in 1749 (Ginn Daugherty and Kammeyer, 1995). The UK census dates back to 1801 and has been conducted every ten years since then, with the exception of 1941. The nature of a census is such that it attempts to count the entire population. It therefore provides the denominator information required for the calculation of rates. Despite the attempt to obtain complete coverage, it has been estimated that there was, in fact, only 98 per cent coverage in the 1991 UK census (National Statistics, undated a) – omitting the so-called 'missing million'. The census also provides the opportunity to collect additional information on a range of demographic and socio-economic factors – those selected tend to vary over time and between countries. For example, a question on long-term illness was introduced into the UK census in 1991. The United Nations Economic Commission for Europe and the Statistical Office of the European Communities suggest that the topics included in

a census should result from a balanced consideration of:

- the needs of the country, national as well as local, to be served by the census data
- the achievement of the maximum degree of international comparability, both within regions and on a worldwide basis
- acceptability of questions to respondents and their ability to provide the required information without an undue burden being placed on them
- the technical competence of the enumerators (if any) to obtain information on the topics by direct observation
- the total national resources available for enumeration, processing, tabulation and publication, which will determine the overall feasible scope of the census (United Nations Economic Commission for Europe and Statistical Office of the European Communities, undated: 7).

A list of the areas included in the UK's 2001 census is provided in the box. Kerrison and Macfarlane (2000) draw attention to two potential limitations of health data obtained by the census. First, the precise wording of the questions is important in relation to the response elicited. Second, it relies on the accuracy of self-reporting, which will be subject to a whole range of potentially contaminating or distorting factors.

Life expectancy, DALYs and QALYs

Life expectancy is frequently used as a general indicator of a population's health status. It means the average number of years individuals of different ages can be expected to live if current mortality rates apply (Beaglehole et al., 1993). Within the UK, for example, the indicator of health used in

---

AREAS INCLUDED IN THE UK CENSUS 2001

- Household accommodation and car ownership.
- Demographic characteristics (age, sex, marital status).
- Health/long-term illness/provision of care.
- Qualifications.
- Household relationships.
- Cultural characteristics (such as ethnic group).
- Migration.
- Employment.
- Workplace and journey to work.

National Statistics, undated b

the government's 'quality of life barometer' is life expectancy – currently seventy-five years for men and eighty for women, although for women the last eleven years are likely to be in poor health compared with only eight years for men (Department for Environment Food and Rural Affairs, 2001).

Mortality can be considered premature if individuals do not survive to an expected age and the shortfall is equivalent to lost years of life. The total number of life years lost due to different causes of mortality can be calculated. The use of this as a measure of disease burden and for comparative purposes clearly attaches more weight to deaths occurring in younger age groups.

The well-known health promotion maxim of adding life to years not just years to life draws attention to the issue of *quality* of life. The quality adjusted life year (QALY) is a way of assigning a numerical value to a health state. It is based on the premise that, if a year of good-quality life expectancy is given the value of one, then a year of poor-quality or unhealthy life must be worth less than one. It therefore combines the length and quality of life into a single index (Bowling, 1997a).

It should be emphasized that the notion of quality is essentially applied to negative health states. There are several different ways of assessing quality of life (for a more detailed discussion see Bowling, 1997a, Bowling, 1997b, and Edgar et al., 1998). The EuroQol Group has developed the EQ-5D as a standardized instrument for measuring health outcome (EuroQol, undated). It uses five dimensions of health (mobility, self-care, usual activities, pain/discomfort, anxiety/depression) and each dimension comprises three levels (some, moderate or extreme problems). Given the subjective nature of quality of life and the various philosophical interpretations of health and wellbeing referred to in Chapter 1, it will come as no surprise that there is considerable debate about attempts to measure these factors objectively.

The primary aim of developing QALYs was to provide utility rating to compare the health benefits of different interventions. The Wanless report (2002), for example, notes that the NHS currently spends £500 million per year on statins (drugs that reduce cholesterol) for the primary and secondary prevention of coronary heart disease. While acknowledging that statins can be effective in lowering cholesterol levels and reducing risk, the report comments that lifestyle factors create the risk in the first place. The cost-effectiveness of smoking cessation is estimated to be between £212 and £873 per QALY compared with £4000 to £8000 per QALY for statins.

This use of QALYs has been much criticized. The criticisms are both technical, on account of their method of construction, and ethical (for a full analysis, see Edgar et al., 1998). The use of QALYs as a means of prioritization of healthcare has been viewed as unjust because it is essentially ageist – systematically favouring interventions that improve the health status of the young by virtue of their longer life expectancy. It also arbitrates on the basis of the capacity to benefit rather than on the basis of actual need – a point we will return to in Chapter 5. However, arguments in defence of QALYs identify the need for a single index of health with which to compare the outcomes of different interventions in order to deploy limited resources to achieve maximum benefits for the community (Williams and Kind, 1992).

Disability-adjusted life year (DALY), in contrast, is concerned with the loss of life due to premature death and disability. A premature death in this context is defined as one that occurs before the age that the person could be expected to reach if they were a member of a standard reference population with a life expectancy equal to the world's longest-surviving population – that is, Japan (WHO, 1999).

This concept was introduced in the *World Development Report 1993* (World Bank, 1993) as a means of measuring the global burden of disease and the effectiveness of health interventions. A DALY is 'calculated as the present value of the future years of disability-free life that are lost as the result of the premature deaths or cases of disability occurring in a particular year' (World Bank, 1993).

The value of the time lived includes a factor to account for the dependency of the young and the elderly on adults. Based on a consensus judgement, the value increases from zero at birth to a peak at age twenty-five and then decreases with age. A comparison of estimated costs per DALY saved by tackling different issues is provided in Table 2.1.

The allocation of resources based on DALYs is surrounded by similar arguments to those about QALYs. In addition, the greater value attached to adult life as opposed to that of children or the elderly, attracts particular criticism (Abbasi, 1999). However, DALYs do perform a useful function in documenting disease burden, which formerly had been overly reliant on mortality statistics. The use of DALYs, for example, has revealed the magnitude of the contribution of neuropsychiatric conditions, which account for 11 per cent of the global disease burden – an issue that had been overlooked by analyses of mortality statistics as such conditions are not major causes of mortality (WHO, 1999).

Table 2.1   *Cost-effective interventions for women aged 15–44, 1990*

Main causes of disease burden	Cost per DALY saved (in US dollars)
Unwanted pregnancy	15–150
Maternal causes	60–110
STDs	10–15
HIV	3–5

Source: World Bank, 1993, in Campbell et al., 1999

Positive health

Much of the foregoing has focused on mortality and morbidity. The application of this information to the assessment of health is predicated on the assumption that the absence of disease is indicative of health. Yet, we noted in Chapter 1 that health is more than just the absence of disease. Catford's (1983) early attempt to identify positive health indicators provides examples of individual behaviour and health knowledge, socio-economic conditions and aspects of the physical environment.

Although it moves the focus of attention upstream, away from disease towards its determinants, this analysis is still located within a disease causation continuum. The factors identified can only be deemed healthy by virtue of their contribution to prevention of disease and do not of themselves influence positive wellbeing. Surveys such as the Health Survey for England (MIMAS, 2001) collect data on these upstream determinants and subjective assessments of health. The survey was established in 1991 to monitor trends and progress towards national health targets. The core and non-core topics included in the survey are listed in the box.

Kemm (1993) notes the relative ease of defining negative rather than positive health states and the greater success of epidemiology in handling the former rather than the latter. Bowling (1997a: 5) suggests that positive health:

implies 'completeness' and 'full functioning' or 'efficiency' of mind and body and social adjustment. Beyond this there is no one accepted definition. Positive health could be described as the ability to cope with stressful situations, the maintenance of a strong social

---

TOPICS INCLUDED IN THE HEALTH SURVEY FOR ENGLAND

'Core' topics:

- general health
- smoking and drinking behaviour
- blood pressure
- height and weight
- anthropometric measures
- prescribed medication
- use of health services.

'Non-core' topics:

- cardiovascular disease (1991–94, 1998, 1999)
- asthma and other respiratory diseases (1995–97, 1999)
- lung function (1995–97)
- atopic conditions (1995–96)
- eating habits (1993–94, 1997, 1999)
- physical activity (1991–94, 1997, 1999)
- accidents (1995–97)
- General Health Questionnaire (1991–95, 1997)
- generic health state measures – EuroQol and SF-36 (1996)
- disability (1995)
- contraceptive use (1992–95, 1997)
- psychosocial health (1999)
- social support, religion and cultural identity (1999)
- Children's Strengths and Difficulties Questionnaire (1997, 1999).

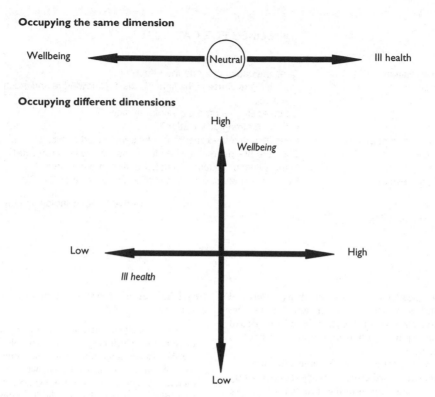

Figure 2.3 Dimensions of wellbeing and ill health (derived from Kemm, 1993, and Downie et al., 1996)

support system, integration in the community, high morale and life satisfaction, psychological wellbeing, and even levels of physical fitness as well as physical health.

Both authors are in agreement that the components of wellbeing require both precise definition and the formulation of criteria. A key issue is whether positive and negative states are opposite ends of the same dimension with some neutral midpoint or, as argued by Downie et al. (1996), they occupy different dimensions. These alternative conceptualizations are shown in Figure 2.3. Kemm (1993) asserts that there is little evidence to support positive health being viewed as a distinct dimension, although there may be theoretical reasons for doing so. Furthermore, positive and negative health may occupy the same dimension for some aspects, such as objective physical health, but different dimensions for subjective health.

A number of different scales exist for assessing aspects of quality of life and wellbeing. Some derive from professional perspectives, some – such as the Nottingham Health Profile – have incorporated lay

views in their development. There is considerable variation in the conceptual underpinnings of the various instruments and their validity and reliability (for a detailed analysis see Bowling, 1997a).

Analytic epidemiology

While the patterns of distribution of disease revealed by descriptive epidemiology may generate tentative hypotheses about causation, analytic epidemiology focuses specifically on exploring cause-and-effect relationships. One of the best-known early examples is the work of John Snow, who, by meticulously mapping cholera outbreaks in London during 1848–49 and 1853–54, was able to demonstrate that cholera was spread by contaminated water (Chave, 1958). Although derided by the miasmatists, who favoured the view that such diseases were caused by the miasma emanating from filth and putrefying material, and well in advance of Koch's discovery of the micro-organism that causes cholera in 1884, Snow's work provided evidence to support the general introduction

GUIDELINES FOR CAUSALITY

Temporal relation	Does the cause precede the effect?
Plausibility	Does it make sense in the light of existing knowledge and mechanisms of action?
Consistency	Do other studies produce similar findings?
Strength	Is there a strong association?
Dose–response relationship	Does increase in exposure produce increased effect?
Reversibility	Does the risk decrease when the possible cause is removed?
Study design	Is the evidence robust and derived from strong studies?
Judging the evidence	How many lines of evidence lead to the conclusion?

Derived from Beaglehole et al., 1993

of public health measures, such as improved water and sanitation – over and above the renowned removal of the handle of the Broad Street water pump to halt an outbreak of cholera in the vicinity.

The evidence for causality is subject to epistemological debate. Furthermore, many contemporary health problems are not the product of simple cause-and-effect relationships. Analysis is often concerned with multiple causes and, in some instances, multiple effects. Frequently, the focus is, therefore, on complex multifactorial webs.

Moon and Gould (2000) identify three main conditions that must be present if observed associations are to be judged as causally linked. First, do the levels of exposure and disease vary in the same way – that is, co-variation? Second, does cause precede the effect – that is, temporal precedence? Third, have other possible explanations and confounding factors been eliminated?

A number of different types of epidemiological studies are used to explore causality. These range from observational studies, such as ecological and cross-sectional studies, which are regarded as relatively weak in their capacity to demonstrate causality, to the more robust case control and cohort studies. Intervention or experimental studies are more able to control for confounding variables and may take the form of randomized controlled, field or community trials. Beaglehole et al. (1993) provide a useful set of guidelines for assessing causality and these are listed in the box above.

We will give further consideration to the complexity of causal relationships in health promotion programmes when we discuss evaluation in Chapter 10. However, returning to the subject of disease causation,

Beaglehole et al. (1993: 71) define the cause of a disease as:

an event, condition, characteristic or a combination of these factors which plays an important role in producing the disease. Logically a cause must precede a disease. A cause is termed *sufficient* when it inevitably produces or initiates a disease and is termed *necessary* if a disease cannot develop in its absence. [Our emphasis.]

It therefore follows that, in many instances, well-recognized causal factors are neither necessary nor sufficient. Take smoking, for example. Some people who have never smoked will develop lung cancer, so smoking cannot be seen as necessary, and some people who smoke do not develop lung cancer, hence smoking is not sufficient. There is, however, indisputable evidence that smoking is an important causal factor that increases the probability of developing lung cancer and, conversely, that this will be reduced by smoking cessation. Thus, it becomes important to think in terms of probability and risk.

The term 'risk factor' is applied to those factors that are associated with the development of a disease, but not sufficient in themselves to cause it – often with the underlying intent of identifying factors that can be modified to prevent disease occurring. 'Relative risk' is the ratio of the rate of the disease in those exposed to a particular factor to the rate in those not exposed (see the box opposite). It indicates the number of times *more likely* it is that an individual exposed to the factor will develop the disease. It is useful in establishing the strength of the association and also in graphically encapsulating the levels of additional risk incurred by individuals.

ASSESSMENT OF RISK

Relative risk (x)   = rate of the disease in those exposed to the risk factor ÷ rate of the disease in those not exposed

Attributable risk (rate)   = rate of the disease in those exposed to the risk factor – rate of the disease in those not exposed

Population attributable risk   = attributable risk × proportion of the population exposed to the risk factor

Table 2.2   *Relative and attributable risk of smoking*

Cause of mortality	Annual mortality rate per 100,000 men current smokers				Relative risk of smokers 25+	Attributable risk for smokers 25 + per 100,000
	Non-smoker	1–14	15–24	25+		
Lung cancer	14	105	208	355	355/14 = 25.4	355 – 14 = 341
Bladder cancer	13	29	29	37	37/13 = 2.8	37 – 13 = 24
Ischaemic heart disease	572	802	892	1025	1025/572 = 1.8	1025 – 572 = 453
Cerebral thrombosis	93	93	150	143	143/93 = 1.5	143 – 93 = 50

Source: Data derived from Doll et al., 1994

In contrast, the notion of 'attributable risk' acknowledges the fact that many diseases develop independently of exposure to risk factors. In order to assess the amount of disease that is actually attributable to exposure, the rate in those not exposed to the risk factor (that is, those who would have developed the disease regardless of exposure) is subtracted from the rate in those exposed (see box for formula).

A related concept is the 'population attributable risk', which is derived by multiplying the attributable risk by the proportion of the population exposed to the risk factor. This indicates the amount of disease that would be avoided if exposure to the risk factor was completely eliminated. Reference to Table 2.2 (derived from Doll et al., 1994) shows that although the relative risk among heavy smokers for lung cancer is much higher than for heart disease, indicative of a stronger causal relationship, more actual deaths from heart disease can be attributed to smoking.

Establishing the potential and feasibility of prevention rests on the capacity to identify modifiable risk factors. Conventionally, different levels of prevention are distinguished:

• **primary prevention** is concerned with preventing the development of disease by reducing exposure to risk factors – environmental and behavioural

• **secondary prevention** in contrast, focuses on early diagnosis – for example, by screening – to improve the prospects of treatment

• **tertiary prevention** includes measures to reduce the consequences of illness and is often seen as integral to a rehabilitation programme.

A further issue is whether it is preferable to target preventive interventions at the population in general or high-risk groups (Rose, 1992). Arguments in favour of the high-risk approach include its greater cost-effectiveness and the fact that people who are known to be at high risk may be more motivated to change. However, it presupposes that it is both possible to identify those at risk and that the disease will not occur in those who do not fall within this category. Nor would such an approach contribute to changing general norms, so it might be more difficult for individuals to make changes. Furthermore, health and health behaviour is influenced by a broad range of social and environmental factors that can only be tackled at the population level. Even when focusing on specific behaviour, the whole population approach has the capacity to achieve a significant reduction in disease. Although major change may be achieved at the population level, it requires many individuals to make changes and relatively few of them will gain any personal benefit – referred to by Rose (1992) as the 'prevention paradox'. Charlton notes that a population-wide approach potentially labels the whole population as being at risk. It also creates the new category of the 'worried-well'. As Illich (1976: 97) cautioned, 'The concept of morbidity has been enlarged to cover prognosticated risks ... People are turned into patients without being sick. The medicalization of prevention thus becomes another major symptom of social iatrogenesis.'

THE NEED FOR ALTERNATIVE PERSPECTIVES

Two key questions are often asked when assessing the utility of health information.

* Is it necessary?
* Is it sufficient?

Both are pertinent to the selection of information to identify priority health issues and assess health needs. Furthermore, the answers to both will be influenced by issues of ideology, epistemology and, not least, practicality.

Epidemiological approaches to assessing health status and identifying the determinants of health are consistent with a modernist emphasis on rationality and faith in the scientific method. De Kadt (1982) suggests that perspectives on health are informed by the dominant conceptions of medicine. Of particular relevance are its mechanistic nature, together with a focus on micro-causality. As a consequence, attention is directed towards individuals who become sick and, by inference, their unhealthy lifestyles rather than the social, economic and environmental factors that are responsible for these lifestyles. Krieger (2001) states that the early epidemiology and public health of the mid to late nineteenth century clearly recognized that population health is shaped by both social and biological processes. However, increased interest in personal preventive measures in the late nineteenth and early twentieth centuries signalled a shift in emphasis for mainstream modern epidemiology. Criticism of this shift has come from within epidemiology itself as well as from other fields, such as sociology and anthropology. Moon and Gould (2000: 143) draw on an editorial in the *Lancet* (Anonymous, 1994) to suggest that:

> the discipline's focus is now so far 'downstream' that it has lost sight of what is going on up river. The result is an exclusion of the *contexts* in which disease happens unless they are immediately measurable and the *voices* of those people whose social conditions threaten their health...

They are critical of the way in which modern epidemiology is consistent with, and upholds, dominant value systems. Furthermore, they challenge the methodological assumptions associated with its positivist methodological position – particularly its reductionist principles and the lack of attention to context. While accepting that there is some value in identifying causal factors, they assert that they reveal little about the structural factors that influence people's lives.

The emergence of 'social epidemiology' in the 1950s was distinguished by its explicit focus on the *social* determinants of health – a position reflected in the 'new public health' movement. 'Critical epidemiology', furthermore, 'places an emphasis on the social and power relations that shape disease definition and disease causation' (Moon and Gould, 2000: 7).

Issues of micro-causality are undoubtedly relevant to understanding the factors that impact on health status, such as is the case with exposure to the tubercle bacillus and the development of tuberculosis. However, they are not sufficient. They need to be understood within the context of the social and environmental factors – such as overcrowding, social class, poverty and urbanization – that are also associated with the development of the disease. Furthermore, Kelly and Charlton (1995) caution against reification of the social system and a simple deterministic view of the relationship between social factors and ill health, which merely replicates the type of thinking integral to a biomedical approach – albeit further upstream. They note the tension in health promotion discourse between free will and determinism – that is, between *agency* and *structure* – and call for an understanding of the reciprocal relationship between the two.

The application of science and rationality to the analysis of the determinants of ill health, or even positive health states, assumes that there is an objective reality. A postmodern understanding, in contrast, views reality as both contextual and contingent. Rather than one objective reality, there are multiple perspectives and interpretations of reality. Graham's work on smoking provides a useful example. Smoking is strongly linked to social disadvantage. An 'outsider's' view of mothers in low-income households smoking is that this is irrational by virtue of the cost and health risks incurred. However, an 'inside view' is that, for the mothers themselves, smoking can be part of their coping strategy. Graham's (1987) study revealed that, from the mothers' perspective, smoking was associated with breaks from their caring role, which enabled them to recharge, and was also a means of coping when things got too much. Looking at the issue from the perspective of the mothers transforms apparently irrational behaviour into a rational response to their situation.

Furthermore, contrary to the customary view that science and the scientific method is concerned with the objective pursuit of truth, in fact, science itself is socially constructed, both in its focus and its methods. The breadth of scientific enquiry is restricted by the limits of current paradigms (Kuhn, 1970). The construction of problems – the ways in which they are framed and the determinants explored – are all socially shaped (Petersen and Lupton, 1996). How far upstream will, or should, the quest for determinants go? What risk factors are regarded as legitimate areas of enquiry? What evidence will be accepted?

Official statistics form the basis of much epidemiological and, indeed, sociological enquiry. It is appropriate at this point to consider the nature of official data.

Official health data – reality or myth?

The characteristics of official health statistics are that they generally include large data sets that have been collected regularly by official agencies over long periods of time. It is a truism that data do not exist in their own right, but are constructed. There are clearly issues concerning the technicalities of data collection, its representativeness and completeness. As we have already noted, official health data will only include those who have come into contact with services, registered vital events or been included in official surveys. Consulting a doctor or taking time off work will inevitably be influenced by a range of social and cultural factors. The collection of some official data – such as mortality and census data – attempts to include all cases, whereas surveys will only involve a sample.

The way in which data are classified and categorized is also socially constructed. For example, in relation to certification of death, 'old age', which featured prominently as a cause of death in the late nineteenth century, becomes an inadequate descriptor in our more biomedically enlightened times – more specific causal explanations are required. There is a well-known tendency towards underreporting of emotionally charged issues, such as suicide and AIDS. Furthermore, at what point in the temporal sequence of causality do we identify a single cause? For a child dying in one of the least-developed parts of the world is it measles, malnutrition or poverty? For a man dying prematurely in a rundown inner-city area, is it lung cancer or smoking or unemployment? Interestingly, the tenth revision of the *International Classification of Disease* introduced a set of codes for factors that influence health status and contact with health services. When even ostensibly objective issues such as mortality and morbidity can be seen to be socially constructed, assessing 'quality of life' becomes even more problematic. Classifying people by gender, ethnic group and socio-economic status provides further evidence of social construction.

Official data, then, are not facts in their own right, but are constructed. The ways in which they are constructed will be influenced by both technical and ideological issues. The Radical Statistics Health Group lists a series of questions to consider when assessing the quality of official health data (see the box).

May (1993) identifies three schools of thought in relation to official statistics:

- **realist** considers official statistics to be objective indicators of phenomena
- **institutionalist** sees official statistics as artificial constructs revealing more about an institution's priorities in collecting data than the phenomena they purport to represent
- **radical** extends the institutionalist view to include discretionary practices embedded

---

CONFRONTING THE STATISTICS

- How were the data collected?
- How were the data coded and classified?
- How were the data tabulated and analysed?
- How were the statistics selected and interpreted?
- What has been left out or ignored?
- It can't be true – my experience was different? (Is it atypical?)

Radical Statistics Health Group, 1987: 188–189

within and replicating the power structure and dynamics of society.

By way of example, let us take the use of waiting lists for hip replacement surgery as an indicator of prevalence and need. A realist interpretation would presuppose that individuals would have equal access to general practitioners, who would refer them to hospital for treatment and the length of the waiting lists would simply be the product of the number of individuals requiring treatment and the period required for throughput.

An institutionalist view would question the way in which the hospital constructed the waiting list for treatment. For example, have treatment waiting lists been kept short by having a long waiting period prior to consultation?

A radical view would locate this last question within the context of any national imperative to reduce waiting lists and political pressure to demonstrate more efficient services. Changes in these contextual factors would inevitably influence the comparability of data over time.

Conspiracy theorists would subscribe to the view that statistics are deliberately manipulated to suit an agenda rather than being the unconsciously biased products of systems and practices. Huff's delightfully subversive *How to Lie with Statistics* (1979) identifies a number of tactics. These include:

- using a sample with an in-built bias, such as self-selected respondents
- choosing the 'right' average – if a distribution is skewed, the median will be less affected than the mean, so, for example, a few high-earners would raise the mean earnings but not the median
- using very small samples
- manipulating graphs:
  - unnumbered axes
  - plotting means to obscure highs and lows
  - changing the vertical scale or cutting off the bottom of graphs to exaggerate trends
  - using pictorial representation
- tacitly implying associations when none has been proved
- assumptions about causality.

The danger in seeing official data merely as social constructs is that it can lead us to reject them as having no inherent value. We then have a limited capacity to assess health status and identify problem issues. The evidence that exposed, and continues to document, the effects of social inequality, for example, drew substantially on official health data. Without this insight, it would have been difficult to mount an argument in favour of tackling social inequality. What is needed is the *critical* use of health data that takes full account of the ways in which they have been constructed. This is aptly summed up by Roberts (1990: 13):

> An over-reverent approach to figures supports the empiricist fallacy that figures are merely given objective facts, a proper understanding of which compels one conclusion and one only. An oversceptical approach sustains the equally erroneous belief that statistics are mere mystification, a way of obscuring truth and legitimizing error, that they are born in deception and formed of quantified ideology.

The lay perspective

The lay perspective introduces a completely different dimension. Lay knowledge is rooted in the direct and vicarious experience of individuals and communities and their cultural understandings. It is interpreted within the context of people's real lives and day-to-day experiences. The earlier reference to the 'clinical iceberg' would indicate that most of our individual and collective experiences of ill health and health occur below the surface. There, it is effectively hidden from the reaches of routine data-collection systems and, hence, does not feature in most accounts of health.

Faith in the value of lay knowledge about health and ill health has been central to the development of the self-help movement – a movement that challenged medical, and, indeed, expert hegemony. Furthermore, community activists have used their own insights, derived by means of what has been termed popular or lay epidemiology, to mount campaigns to tackle what they perceive to be the cause of local health problems. Williams and Popay (1994) provide a number of high-profile examples, such as tackling the problems of toxic waste and environmental pollution, but, equally, lay epidemiology can support the case for local measures, such as improved housing and traffic-calming measures.

Frankel et al. (1991) see lay epidemiology as being concerned with the interpretation of health risks by lay people as a result of observation and discussion within their own personal networks and the public arena, as well as information derived through the media. Moon and Gould (2000: 7) note that, although critics have challenged this approach as being 'anecdotal, uninformed and even dangerous', it provides direct insight into the ways in which health and ill health are commonly experienced, understood and managed. Roberts' (1998) work on injury prevention provides a useful example of this. Participatory research involving children and families revealed how they manage to successfully negotiate what are intrinsically dangerous environments and the expense that this incurs in relation to children's loss of freedom and parental anxiety. It also enabled the antecedents of accidents and near accidents to be identified rather than the sequelae that feature in routinely collected data based on hospital admissions. Clearly, the former has much greater relevance for planning health promotion.

Lay interpretations of health are complex and multidimensional. Far from being trivial, they demonstrate coherent and sophisticated understandings. A number of major studies have explored these understandings (for example, Herzlich, 1973, Blaxter and Patterson, 1982, Williams, 1983, and Cornwell, 1984) and the following key dimensions can be identified:

- the absence of disease, illness, pain
- a reserve for coping with stress and illness
- functional ability to allow tasks to be performed
- an ideal state, including positive wellbeing.

Basch (1990) adds to this list:

- conformity to expected norms.

Lay recognition of the absence of disease, illness and pain as integral to health is noteworthy as the professional discourse on wellbeing does not always explicitly address this issue.

There is some interplay between professional and lay accounts of health, though. For example, the germ theory is fully integrated into most Western lay interpretations of disease. It is interesting to note, however, that lay accounts might include such reductionist explanations, but they also go further, addressing issues associated with meaning, such as 'Why me?' and 'Why now?' (Williams and Popay, 1994). A full understanding of health and ill health will necessarily seek to incorporate these hitherto often private accounts.

The premise underpinning our earlier discussion of risk was that, from an epidemiological perspective, it can be measured objectively. In the same way that health and illness are not simple biological states, but are socially constructed, lay interpretations and perceptions of risk are also complex. As we will explore more fully in Chapter 3, they derive from the interplay of a plethora of psycho-social and cultural factors.

Frankel et al. (1991) note that lay perceptions of risk are often in tune with mainstream epidemiological analyses. For example, with regard to coronary heart disease, there is lay understanding of an association with both hereditary factors and adverse social circumstances – issues that rarely feature in health education campaigns. Frankel et al. raise the interesting question as to why there was a rapid and dramatic reduction in egg consumption in the UK in the late 1980s in response to concerns about salmonella infection when years of warning about the harmful effects of the cholesterol content of eggs brought about little change. They propose that there are different lay conceptualizations of risk. At one end of the spectrum, the risk is both immediate and easily imagined and therefore to be avoided – encapsulated as 'bad/poisonous behaviour'. At the other end of the spectrum, risks are perceived to be less immediate and less specific. Some behaviour associated with this type of risk, such as smoking, are acknowledged to be harmful, but may also have desirable aspects – hence, they are termed 'bad/desirable behaviour'. They suggest that the advertising industry attempts to keep behaviour away from the bad/poisonous end of the spectrum by emphasizing the desirable elements. Individuals may also use humour to the same effect – for example, 'naughty but nice' and 'what's your poison?'

The biomedical model has often been criticized because of its expert-led, top-down orientation. However, even interpretive approaches – which purport to provide greater insight into the experiences of lay people – may still remain an essentially expert analysis of that experience. A true commitment to including the lay perspective involves going beyond seeing people merely as research subjects. It requires an egalitarian approach to seeking their active involvement at all stages of the research process – not least in formulating the priority issues to address.

Pathogenesis or salutogenesis

Regardless of whether or not they conform to a reductionist, biomedical or more interpretive position, the majority of studies of the determinants of health and ill health are located within a pathogenic paradigm. As Kelly and Charlton (1995: 82) note:

> The social model of health is, in this regard, no different to the medical model. In the medical model the pathogens are microbes, viruses or malfunctioning cellular reproduction. In the social model they are poor housing, unemployment and powerlessness. The discourse may be different but the epistemology is the same. The social model is not, in our view, an alternative to the discredited medical model. It is a partner in crime and a very close modernist relative.

Antonovsky (1984) asserts that the fundamental assumption of this paradigm is that individuals are in a state of balance or homeostasis and that when this state is challenged by microbial, physical or chemical factors or psycho-social stressors, regulatory mechanisms come into play to restore homeostasis. He identifies a number of consequences of this thinking:

- the tendency to think dichotomously about people, classifying them as healthy or diseased
- a focus on disease states or risk factors
- the search for cause or multifactorial causes
- the assumption that stressors are bad
- mounting wars against specific diseases
- ignoring the factors associated with wellness.

In proposing a salutogenic paradigm, Antonovsky advocates a radical change in perspective concerning what is involved in staying healthy. This shifts the focus away from specific diseases and towards those general factors involved in health, and in moving along what he terms the 'health-ease/dis-ease continuum' Antonovsky (1984: 117). He does not, however, totally abandon the pathogenic paradigm, but offers salutogenesis as an *additional* perspective.

> I am not proposing that the pathogenic paradigm be abandoned, theoretically or institutionally. It has immense achievement and power for good to its credit. I have attempted to point to its limitations, to the blinders involved in any paradigm.

Salutogenesis focuses on the factors associated with successful coping, which are envisaged as buffers mitigating the effects of stressors. While there are numerous individual coping variables, Antonovsky (1987: 19) proposes the 'sense of coherence' (SOC) as an overarching explanatory variable.

> The sense of coherence is a global orientation that expresses the extent to which one has a pervasive, enduring, though dynamic feeling of confidence that:
>
> 1 the stimuli deriving from one's internal and external environments in the course of living are structured, predictable and explicable
> 2 the resources are available to one to meet the demands posed by these stimuli and
> 3 these demands are challenges, worthy of investment and engagement.

These three components of the SOC are called comprehensibility, manageability and meaningfulness.

In considering how a strong SOC helps people to cope with stressors, Antonovsky (1984) attempts to identify generalized and specific resistance resources. The features that such resistance resources have in common are:

- **consistency** the greater the consistency of life experiences, the more they will be comprehensible and predictable

- **underload–overload balance** demand is appropriate to capability
- **participation in decision making** the emphasis here is on active participation rather than control.

Early formulations of the SOC suggested that it was the product of early life experiences and that, by adulthood, it was more or less a fixed part of a person's makeup. Such a view offers little to those seeking to improve health. However, Antonovsky subsequently accepted that movement along the SOC can occur even in adulthood, albeit within fairly narrow limits. While he still subscribes to the view that macrosocial change is the only way to achieve substantial change in SOC for most people, he accepts that changes in everyday life can make some difference (Antonovsky, 1984).

Whose voice counts?

The validity of different accounts of health is the subject of debate, caught up in epistemological questions concerning ways of knowing and what constitutes truth.

Beattie (1993) provides a useful analysis of 'different ways of knowing' based on modes of thought and the focus of attention. Modes of thought are seen as ranging from 'hard' mechanistic approaches consistent with the natural sciences to 'soft' humanistic approaches associated with sociological enquiry. Similarly, lay perspectives are often regarded as prerational and trivial in contrast to the rational, and therefore supposedly serious, view of the so-called experts. The focus of attention ranges from individuals to collectives. Figure 2.4 provides an overview of the relationship between these and identifies four models.

Beattie equates each model with different sociopolitical philosophies and attempts to identify cultural bias within the various accounts of health as summarized in Table 2.3.

One of the characteristic features of health promotion is its concern with holism – a view of health that includes positive wellbeing in addition to the absence of disease, a broad conceptualization of the determinants of health and an emphasis on participation. Its information needs, therefore, are necessarily broad and include a range of different professional interpretations deriving from different disciplinary bases and including the lay perspective.

Much of the literature on lay perspectives draws on a discourse of conflict, couched in such terms as 'mounting a challenge' to biomedical interpretations and 'struggle over meaning'. Sociological accounts are also frequently expressed in this vein. Debate about the relative merits of the contributions

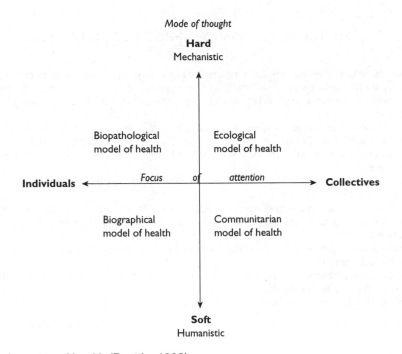

Figure 2.4 Accounts of health (Beattie, 1993)

Table 2.3 *Accounts of health – socio-political philosophies and cultural bias*

Account of health	Socio-political philosophy	Cultural bias
Biopathological	Conservative	Subordination
Biographical	Libertarian	Individualism
Ecological	Reformist	Control
Communitarian	Radical pluralist	Cooperation

Source: Beattie, 1993

of different research disciplines and perspectives is helpful in so far as it exposes the strengths and limitations of the various approaches and their respective utility – particularly when this results in positive attempts to redress shortcomings by seeking complementary approaches. It becomes damaging when it is merely a contest between different epistemological positions and methodologies in laying claims to the truth and different accounts of health are afforded different status.

A narrow and partial analysis of health problems cannot provide a secure basis for identifying priority issues and their determinants. Green and Kreuter (1991: 50) suggest that priorities are 'generally based on an analysis of data indicating the pervasiveness of the problems and their human and economic cost'. Mainstream epidemiological

diagnoses, as we have noted, are concerned with objectively assessing the magnitude and distribution of diseases and health states together with the factors that contribute to them. Green and Kreuter argue strongly that a wider view is needed and problems should be defined from the outset in broad social terms. They offer two main reasons for this. Involving communities helps to ensure that their priority social and quality of life concerns are addressed and so avoids missing the mark in relation to social targets. It also contributes to encouraging community participation. They see the relationship between social and epidemiological diagnoses as complementary, operating in what they term either a 'reductionist' or an 'expansionist' way. Starting with an analysis of social problems, a reductionist approach would analyse the health and non-health factors that contribute to, or cause, the problem. The expansionist approach, in contrast, starts with an epidemiologically defined issue and works towards identifying the way this 'fits' into the larger social context. Green and Kreuter suggest that this avoids any tendency towards oversimplification.

While recognizing its contribution, Tannahill (1992) also cautions against an overemphasis on epidemiology as a driver in health promotion programme planning. He suggests that it neglects

THE LEEDS DECLARATION – PRINCIPLES FOR ACTION

- There is an urgent need to refocus upstream, to move away from focusing predominantly on individual risks towards the social structures and processes within which ill health originates.
- Research is needed to explore factors that keep some people healthy despite living in the most adverse circumstances.
- Lay people are experts and experts are lay people – lay knowledge about health needs, health service priorities and health outcomes should be central to public health research.
- The experimental model is an inadequate gold standard for guiding research into public health problems.
- Not all health data can be represented in numbers – qualitative data have an important role to play in public health research.
- There is nothing inherently 'soft' about qualitative methods or 'hard' about quantitative methods – both require rigorous application in appropriate contexts and hard thinking about difficult problems.
- An openness to the value of different methods means an openness to the contributions of a variety of disciplines.
- Public health problems will only be solved through a commitment to the application of research findings to policy and practice.
- Research funding should address the new directions that follow from these principles.

Nuffield Institute for Health, 1993

methodological issues by focusing on 'what to' rather than 'how to', creates an incomplete view of health, takes a narrow view of outcomes and leads to unsound programme planning. Of particular concern is the translation of single-issue problems into single-issue programmes, which ignores, on the one hand, the broader determinants and, on the other, that there may be factors common to a number of different conditions. For example, tobacco would be a common issue in relation to coronary heart disease, cancers and addiction, and all three are influenced by socioeconomic status. Programmes that address single issues in isolation – so-called 'vertical programmes' – therefore risk duplication of messages and inefficiency.

Our position is that we need multiple complementary perspectives to identify priority health issues and their determinants, as encapsulated in The Leeds Declaration (see the box).

DETERMINANTS OF HEALTH

Major improvements in health in the latter part of the nineteenth century have been attributed to improvements in the environment and general living and working conditions. The development of the germ theory and the improved possibility for immunization towards the end of the nineteenth

century shifted the emphasis towards personal preventive services. The introduction of insulin and sulphonamide drugs in the 1930s heralded the dawn of the therapeutic era (Ashton and Seymour, 1988). The numerous subsequent technological developments in the biomedical field and faith in their capacity to improve health led to the rise of high-tech medicine An increasingly technological view of health resulted in a shift in emphasis away from public health and community-based services and towards hospitals – so-called 'disease palaces'. Green (1996), for example, notes that, in North America, over 90 per cent of expenditure on health is on medical care and less than 10 per cent on promoting healthy behaviour, lifestyles and environments, even though these account for between 50 and 71 per cent of all preventable premature mortality before the age of 75.

The Lalonde Report (1974) is frequently cited as the seminal document in challenging the narrow, technically focused emphasis on disease and advocating a broader, social model. It (1974: 31) recognized the need for a simple conceptual framework to bring order to the many and various factors influencing health:

to organize the thousands of pieces into an orderly pattern that was both intellectually acceptable and sufficiently simple to permit a quick location, in the pattern, of almost any idea, problem or activity related to health; a sort of map of the health territory.

ELEMENTS OF THE 'HEALTH FIELD CONCEPT'

- **Human biology** includes all those aspects of health, both physical and mental, which are developed within the human body as a consequence of the basic biology of man [sic] and the organic makeup of the individual.
- **The environment** includes all those matters related to health which are external to the human body and over which the individual has little or no control.
- **Lifestyle** consists of the aggregation of decisions by individuals which affect their health and over which they more or less have control.
- **Healthcare organization** consists of the quantity, quality, arrangement, nature and relationships of people and resources in the provision of healthcare.

Lalonde, 1974: 31–32

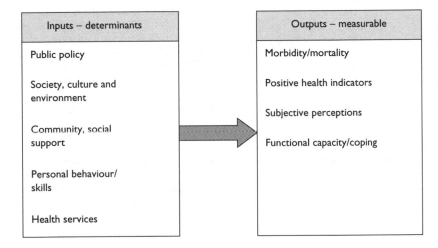

Figure 2.5 The expanded health field concept (derived from Raeburn and Rootman, 1989)

This was achieved using the 'health field concept', which identified four main elements – human biology, environment, lifestyle and healthcare organization (see the box).

The health field concept therefore marked a radical break from the increasing emphasis on high-tech medicine, elevating as it did the other three categories to equal standing. The concept itself is both simple and comprehensive. It was designed to provide insight into the factors associated with sickness and death and identify courses of action to improve health. The health field concept was also expected to encourage an analysis of any health problem in relation to all four categories. It could

therefore be used to identify areas for research and guide policy and planning.

Some fifteen years after the publication of the health field concept, Raeburn and Rootman (1989) noted that the development of health promotion within this framework had focused particularly on lifestyle with insufficient attention being given to the influence of the environment. They also suggested that it was implicitly concerned with reduction of morbidity and mortality.

To address these limitations, they proposed an expanded model that includes both inputs and explicit outputs (see Figure 2.5). The output side moves beyond morbidity and mortality to include functional capacity, positive health indicators and subjective perceptions. The input side is derived from the five action areas of the Ottawa Charter. With the exception of human biology, the other elements of the original health field concept are present. The reasons offered for its omission are that it is both a 'given' and an issue that falls under the aegis of health services rather than within the wider domain of policy, planning and research to promote overall health and wellbeing.

Lifestyle and environment

The relative importance of lifestyle and environment as determinants of health has been the subject of much debate – a debate that has contributed to defining health promotion as a discipline.

Lifestyle

The recognition of chronic diseases as the major cause of death in the more highly developed parts of the world in the mid twentieth century – against a backdrop of escalating healthcare costs – brought renewed interest in the role of prevention. In the UK, documents such as *Prevention and Health: Everybody's Business* (Department of Health and Social Security, 1976) identified lifestyle as a key factor in improving health status. Green et al. (1997) acknowledge the importance of lifestyle, too, when they contend that, in developed nations, a large proportion of deaths are associated with a relatively small number of behavioural risk factors. In the United States, for example, the ten leading

causes of death have been causally related to one of three main behavioural risk factors, namely smoking, dietary practices and alcohol use.

Despite widespread recognition of the importance of lifestyle factors, there is little agreement about the meaning of the term. The WHO Health Education Unit (1993) identifies the following different interpretations:

- patterns of consumption and general living relevant to health
- freely chosen habits and behaviour
- general way of living – the product of living conditions and individual patterns of behaviour determined by socio-cultural factors and personal characteristics (O'Brien, 1995).

The ways in which the construct has become blurred over the years is succinctly encapsulated by Sobel (1981: 1, in O'Brien, 1995: 197): 'If the 1970s are an indication of things to come, the word lifestyle will soon include everything and mean nothing, all at the same time.'

O'Brien's analysis of the appropriation of 'lifestyle' identifies three major influences:

- new systems of product marketing that segment the population into groups on the basis of lifestyle characteristics and consumption patterns (see the box for examples)
- counterculture movements and alternative lifestyles as markers of ideological commitments
- critiques of modernization and a reemphasis on self-determination.

EXAMPLES OF LIFESTYLE CATEGORIES

Northern and Yorkshire RHA 'super profiles':

- affluent achievers
- country life
- thriving greys
- settled suburbans
- nest-builders
- producers
- senior citizens
- urban venturers
- hard-pressed families
- have-nots
- unclassified.

Lister et al., 1994

Green and Kreuter (1991: 12) draw on anthropological, sociological and psychological interpretations to define lifestyle as:

> patterns of behaviour that have an enduring consistency and are based in some combination of cultural heritage, social relationships, geographic and socio-economic circumstances, and personality.

They are critical of the widespread and erroneous use of the word 'lifestyle' for any kind of behaviour and note that it has even been applied to temporary behaviour or single acts. Antonovsky (1996) also notes that an examination of the literature on lifestyle and health reveals little more than a list of behavioural risk factors.

Green and Kreuter (1991: 13) also suggest that the term 'lifestyle' should only be used to describe 'a complex of related practices and behavioural patterns, in a person or group, that are maintained with some consistency over time.'

They argue that greater precision in the distinction between behaviour and lifestyle supports a more holistic and comprehensive approach to promoting health. If behaviour is understood within the context of the complex web that makes up a lifestyle, it immediately becomes evident that attempts to change that behaviour will need to have regard for the social, environmental and cultural circumstances that sustain that lifestyle. Furthermore, it demands sensitivity to possible knock-on effects for other aspects of the lifestyle. They also suggest that the use of the terms 'behaviour', 'action' or 'practice' to describe targets signals greater realism than the more aspirational term 'lifestyle', which is notoriously difficult to influence independently of the wider environmental context. This raises the issue of the relationship between lifestyle and environment, which we will explore more fully along with a consideration of environmental factors.

Much of the literature on lifestyle is located within a pathogenic paradigm and focuses on the association between risk behaviours and disease (Antonovsky, 1996). In contrast, the focus within a salutogenic paradigm would be on the identification of those aspects of lifestyle that actively promote health – so-called 'salutary factors' – rather than the absence of risk factors. The recent interest in 'social capital' makes some move towards incorporating this salutogenic perspective.

Environment

The health field concept's interpretation of 'environment' placed considerable emphasis on the *physical* aspects of the environment with only passing reference being made to the *social* environment. Its central defining criteria for environmental factors are that they are external to the body and outside our immediate control. More recently there has been much greater emphasis on social, cultural and economic aspects, particularly in the context of inequality.

Environmental factors can influence health either directly or indirectly. Simple examples of direct effects include exposure to toxic materials, shortage of food, lack of safe drinking water and overcrowding. Others factors will operate in a more indirect way. For example, lack of facilities for exercise in the environment will be associated with lower levels of physical activity and poorer heart health, while poor access to health services will be associated with low levels of uptake and so on.

Environmental factors may also interact with each other – in some instances creating vicious circle effects. Poverty is associated with poor housing, diet, education and healthcare, for example, leading to fewer life chances overall. Even ostensibly random occurrences, such as natural disasters, disproportionately affect poorer communities. It is estimated that, of the 80,000 deaths that occur each year because of natural disasters, 95 per cent occur in poorer countries (WHO, 2001). Equally, global warming – itself the product of atmospheric pollution – is predicted to affect water supplies and food production, resulting in population displacement as well as causing changes in some disease patterns. Again, the major effects are anticipated to be felt to the greatest extent by the world's most vulnerable populations.

Our earlier discussion of the term 'lifestyle' indicated that it is heavily influenced by the environment. The Lalonde Report discusses the validity of using free choice as the basis for distinguishing between lifestyle and environmental factors in the health field concept. The premise is that individuals can make choices about their lifestyle, but can do little about the environment. The Lalonde Report (1974: 36), while accepting that the environment does affect lifestyle, concludes that:

> the deterministic view must be put aside in favour of faith in the power of free will, hobbled as this power may be at times by environment and addiction.

However, there has been increasing doubt about whether or not behaviour can legitimately be seen to be under autonomous control. Green and Kreuter (1991: 12) see it as 'socially conditioned, culturally embedded and economically constrained'.

O'Brien (1995: 192) draws on earlier sociological interpretations of lifestyle to identify two main

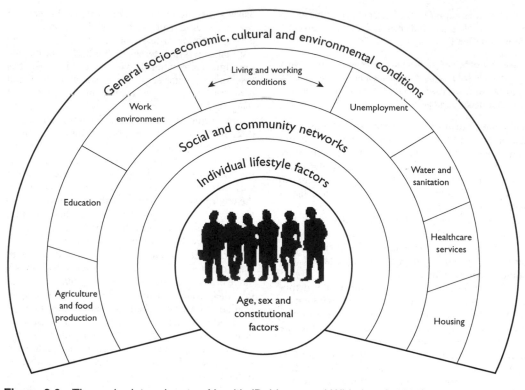

Figure 2.6   The main determinants of health (Dahlgren and Whitehead, 1991)

elements in its construction – political, economic and cultural resources and the psycho-social characteristics of the individual or groups – that is, a combination of environmental and personal factors, with the former having the major influence: '"Lifestyle" implied "choice" within a constrained context and the contexts were held to be more important than the choices.'

There is clearly tension between recognizing humans as autonomous free agents and taking a deterministic view of environmental factors. This tension between agency and structure is also evident in decisions about the relative merits of environmental or lifestyle approaches to health promotion. Clearly, the two are inextricably linked. The PRECEDE planning model (Green and Kreuter, 1991) recognizes the interrelationship between behaviours and environment. It identifies factors in the environment and conditions of living that facilitate actions by individuals or organizations – 'enabling factors'.

Diagrammatic representation of the health field concept – which has typically shown the four elements of lifestyle, environment, human biology and healthcare organization as discrete entities – has perhaps reinforced the tendency to see them as independent variables. Nesting the main determinants within each other, as depicted by Dahlgren and Whitehead (1991), is more indicative of their broad interrelationships and the respective positioning of macro and micro determinants, as shown in Figure 2.6.

Green et al. (1997) provide a more detailed analysis of the complex interrelationships, as shown in Figure 2.7.

An alternative approach acknowledges the relative importance of the various major determinants of health at different stages of the lifespan – for example, the powerful early influence of primary socialization. This conceptualization is central to the notion of the 'health career', which charts individuals' progress through the lifespan and the ways

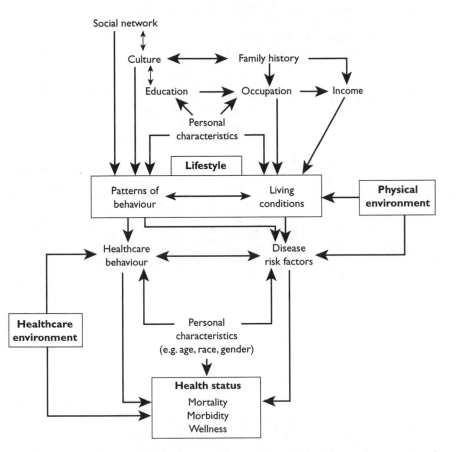

Figure 2.7 Some interrelationships in the complex system of lifestyle, environment and health status (Green et al., 1997)

in which different factors come into play over time (Tones and Tilford, 2001). The focus is on individuals and their cumulative experience rather than a more general overview of determinants. Figure 2.8 represents the health career as a coaxial cable, with the central core being made up of an individual's values, attitudes and beliefs. The health career analysis can assist in ascertaining the key influences on individuals at different stages in their life and also identifying opportunities for intervention.

Social capital

There is an increasing body of evidence suggesting that social support is protective against ill health, while social isolation and exclusion are associated with higher levels of ill health – indeed, some 100 articles per year were cited in the Current Contents

journal abstracting service from 1989–91 (Gottlieb and McLeroy, 1992). The box provides examples of some of the major prospective studies to have demonstrated the association. Similarly, Mittelmark (1999a) cites Schwartzer and Leppin's (1992) meta analysis of eighty studies, which demonstrated the negative association between social integration/social support and morbidity/mortality.

Stansfield (1999) makes the important distinction between social networks and the functional aspects of support. A measure of social networks would include the number and frequency of contacts – taking account of the closeness of the contacts – and the density of the network. The quality of the support would include positive emotional and practical support and also any negative, undermining aspects of close relationships. Over and

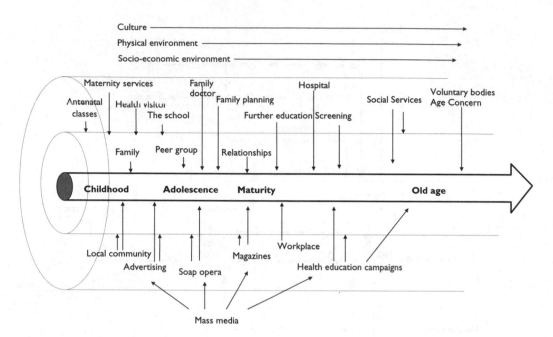

Figure 2.8   The health career (Tones and Tilford, 2001)

MAJOR STUDIES DEMONSTRATING THE EFFECT OF SOCIAL SUPPORT ON MORTALITY

- Alameda County Study, Berkman and Syme, 1979.
- Tecumseh Study, House et al., 1982.
- Durham County Study, Blazer, 1982.
- North Karelia Study, Kaplan et al., 1988.
- Kuopio Study, Kaplan et al., 1994.
- In Sweden, Welin et al., 1985 and Orth-Gomér and Johnson, 1987.
- In relation to mortality from cardiovascular disease, accident and suicide, Kawachi et al., 1996.

Derived from Stansfield, 1999

---

above offering direct support and encouraging health-enhancing behaviour, social connectedness, in itself, has been shown to have a positive effect on health status, possibly by acting as a buffer for stressors.

Mittelmark (1999a: 447) suggests that the anticipated benefits of strengthening social ties are 'better-functioning individuals, families, neighbourhoods and work groups, and improved physical and mental health'. He also summarizes the various

pathways that have been proposed to explain how social ties affect health. These include:

- sources of information to help avoid high-risk or stressful situations
- positive role models
- increased feelings of self-esteem, self-identity and control over the environment
- social regulation, social control and normative influences

- sources of tangible support
- sources of emotional support
- perceptions that support is available
- buffering actions of others during times of stress.

While the emphasis in the literature is on the health-enhancing consequences of social ties, Mittelmark also draws attention to the emerging evidence (spearheaded by fields such as gerontology) that they may also be a source of social strain. Such strain would derive from actions by persons in an individual's social network, such as excessive demands, criticism, invasion of privacy and meddling, that, 'intended [or] unintended, cause a person to experience adverse psychological or physiological reactions' (Mittelmark, 1999a: 448).

Furthermore, he contends that social support and social strain are not opposite ends of the same continuum – and so not mutually exclusive – but separate constructs. It follows, then, that there can be four permutations – high support/high strain, high support/low strain and so on.

The notion of 'social capital' has been applied to the social resources within a community and is currently enjoying a good deal of popularity. The concept was first explored by Bourdieu (1980) and further developed by other authors such as Coleman (1988, 1990) and Fukuyama (1999). However, the term is particularly associated with Putnam and his early work on local government in Italy (Putnam, 1993). For Putnam (1995: 67), social capital:

> refers to features of social organization such as networks, norms and social trust that facilitate coordination and cooperation for mutual benefit... life is easier in communities blessed with a substantial stock of social capital... networks of civic engagement foster sturdy norms of generalized reciprocity and encourage the emergence of social trust. [They] facilitate coordination and communication... and allow dilemmas of collective action to be resolved. Finally, dense networks of interaction probably broaden the participants' sense of self, developing the 'I' into the 'we' ...

This interpretation encompasses more than just the existence of community networks and the resources available. It also includes the social norms of trust and reciprocity, a sense of belonging and willingness to engage in civic activity.

Fukuyama (1999) – writing from the perspective of an economist – provides an interesting interpretation of social capital. He notes that the usual definitions of social capital actually refer to *manifestations* of social capital rather than to its basic constructs. Thus, his (1999: 1–2) definition is as follows:

> social capital is an instantiated informal norm that promotes cooperation between two or more individuals.

The norms that constitute social capital can range from a norm of reciprocity between two friends, all the way up to complex and elaborately articulated doctrines like Christianity or Confucianism. They must be instantiated in an actual human relationship: the norm of reciprocity exists *in potentia* in my dealings with all people, but is actualized only in my dealings with *my* friends. By this definition, trust, networks, civil society, and the like which have been associated with social capital are all epiphenomenal, arising as a result of social capital but not constituting social capital itself.

According to Fukuyama (1999: 2), the norms that constitute social capital are 'related to traditional virtues like honesty, the keeping of commitments, reliable performance of duties, reciprocity, and the like.' Notwithstanding the potential for cooperation, which can extend beyond the immediate group, social capital can have negative effects (just as, 'physical capital can take the form of assault rifles or tasteless entertainment, human capital can be used to devise new ways of torturing people.') Moreover, a group's internal cohesion may be achieved by treating outsiders with suspicion, hostility or even hatred. According to the author, organizations such as the Ku Klux Klan and the Mafia, because they have shared norms and cooperate, actually have social capital, but they produce 'abundant negative externalities for the larger society'. 'Good' social capital results in 'positive externalities' – that is, it will be beneficial to external individuals and groups. Furthermore, if a group's social capital produces positive externalities, the 'radius of trust' will extend beyond the group itself. Fukuyama sees modern society as a series of overlapping radii of trust – from friends, family and cliques up to large organizations and religious groups. Small radii of trust and within-group solidarity reduce the capacity for cooperation with outsiders and may be typical of more traditional social groupings. Campbell et al. (1999: 97) refer to the warning by Pahl (1995) that:

> romanticized views of past community life in England serve to conceal the fact that these idealized cohesive communities were often organized around socially exclusive and repressive hierarchies characterized by, among other things, greater repression of women.

The large variety of overlapping social groups in modern societies may make it easier to transmit information, have greater resources and be readier to innovate than was the case in the past. Fukuyama asserts that social capital is an important feature of modern economies and underpins modern liberal democracy.

There has been considerable recent interest in the notion of social capital as a means of improving health prospects and particularly as a response to the adverse effects of social exclusion, which we will discuss below. Social capital is viewed as a prerequisite for an active participating community. Gottlieb and McLeroy (1992) make related points in their examination of the meaning of social health, which for them includes social integration or involvement (quantity and quality of relationships), social support (functional content of relationships, such as emotional support) and social networks (the structure of relationships with other people within a social system). However, to date, there has been comparatively little research on the effects of community-level networks and relationships on health (Campbell et al., 1999). Neither is there a consensus on the components of social capital. Commonly used measures are the levels of civic participation and social trust (Cooper et al., 1999). For example, Kawachi (1997) reports high levels of trust being associated with both lower mortality rates and higher levels of reported good health in the United States. Furthermore, bowling league membership (used by Putnam (1995) as indicative of levels of social participation) also correlated with lower mortality rates.

Campbell et al. (1999) describe an exploratory qualitative study in the UK to assess the applicability of Putnam's conceptualization of social capital to the UK context as well as the variations in social capital between different communities with comparable socio-economic status but different health experiences. They conclude that:

- the social capital constructs of trust and civic engagement may be particularly relevant to health status
- sources of social capital may cross the geographically defined boundaries of communities
- some network types (diverse and geographically dispersed) might be more health-enhancing than others
- Putnam's typology of social networks needs to be expanded to include informal networks
- the provision of community facilities does not constitute social capital – the processes by which such facilities are established and run require consideration
- Putnam's notion of community cohesion should be reconsidered in the light of the high levels of mobility and plural nature of contemporary communities
- there are major differences within communities in the ways in which social capital is created, sustained and accessed.

Hyppä and Mäki (2001) used the concept of social capital to account for differences in active life and mortality between groups in an area of Finland. The Swedish-speaking minority has a longer active life than the Finnish-speaking majority, yet the two groups have similar profiles of socio-demographic variables, socio-economic circumstances and availability of healthcare and similar exposure to conventional risk factors. The better health prospects of the Swedish-speaking community were attributed to higher levels of social cohesion due to its small size, strong institutional network, cultural activity and geographic stability.

Coulthard et al. (2002: 1) suggest that the main indicators of social capital are:

- social relationships and social support
- formal and informal social networks
- group memberships
- community and civic engagement
- norms and values
- reciprocal activities, such as childcare arrangements
- levels of trust in others.

Fukuyama (1999) distinguishes two broad approaches to measuring social capital:

- a census of the groups and group membership in a given society
- a survey of levels of trust and civic engagement.

Putnam, for example, draws on group membership (derived from the number of groups, bowling leagues, sports clubs, political groups and the membership of groups) as an indicator of the level of civic engagement and social capital in society. He is sceptical about the contribution of 'mailing list' organizations to social connectedness on the grounds that the members do not actually meet and their ties are to a common ideology or symbols rather than to each other (Putman, 1996). Fukuyama identifies a number of additional relevant variables:

- the internal cohesion of groups
- the radius of trust and the extent to which this encompasses the whole group plus or minus outsiders
- group affiliation and the extent to which this engenders distrust of outsiders.

Survey data on levels of trust and civic engagement can also be used to gauge levels of social capital. Questions on civic engagement already feature in national surveys in the United States. A module of questions to assess social capital has recently been developed for use in the General Household Survey in Britain (Coulthard et al., 2001). Each of the main topic areas is explored by means of a series of questions that focus on the following five aspects of social capital:

NEIGHBOURHOOD AND COMMUNITY INVOLVEMENT

View of the local area:

- 87 per cent enjoyed living in the local area
- 60 per cent felt very safe walking during the daytime
- 33 per cent felt fairly safe walking during the daytime
- 26 per cent felt a bit unsafe or very unsafe walking after dark
- 20 per cent never went out alone after dark
- 15 per cent had been victims of crime in the last year.

Civic engagement:

- 59 per cent felt well informed about local affairs
- 56 per cent felt that communities could influence decisions in the area
- 26 per cent felt that they personally could influence decisions in the area
- 21 per cent were involved in a local organization
- 27 per cent had been involved in action to solve a local problem
- 18 per cent felt civically engaged – well informed, believed that they could influence decisions and agreed or strongly agreed that local people can affect decisions relating to their neighbourhood
- 16 per cent were not civically engaged – they had not been involved in an organization in the area, had not been involved in any action to solve a local problem, did not feel well informed, did not feel that they could influence decisions affecting the neighbourhood, either alone or working with others.

Neighbourliness:

- 27 per cent spoke to neighbours daily
- 19 per cent spoke to neighbours once a week
- 46 per cent knew most or many people in their neighbourhood
- 48 per cent knew a few people in their neighbourhood
- 6 per cent knew nobody
- 58 per cent felt that they could trust most or many people in their neighbourhood.

Social networks:

- 27 per cent spoke to relatives daily
- 82 per cent spoke to relatives at least once a week
- 30 per cent had at least five close friends living close by
- 27 per cent had no close friends living in their local area
- 44 per cent had no relatives they felt close to living close by
- 66 per cent had a satisfactory friendship network – saw or spoke to friends at least once a week and had at least one close friend who lived nearby
- 52 per cent had a satisfactory relatives network
- 20 per cent had neither.

Social support:

- 97 per cent could get help if they were ill in bed
- 93 per cent could get a lift if they needed to be somewhere
- 86 per cent could borrow £100 if in financial difficulty
- 58 per cent had at least five people they could turn to in a serious personal crisis
- 18 per cent had at least three people they could turn to in a serious personal crisis
- 2 per cent had nobody.

Source: derived from Coulthard et al., 2002

- view of the local area
- civic engagement
- reciprocity and local trust
- social networks
- social support (Coulthard et al., 2001: 7).

Commissioned as part of the Health Development Agency programme of research on social capital, the General Household Survey 2000/2001 incorporated this module of questions, becoming one of the first national surveys in Britain to address this issue. The box provides a selection of the key findings of this survey of social capital (Coulthard et al., 2002). Of the variables included, a high 'neighbourliness' score showed the strongest association with the other measures of social capital.

INEQUALITY AND SOCIAL EXCLUSION

Exposure to a plethora of different determinants throughout the course of life will inevitably result in some variations in health experience. A central concern of health promotion – one that is driven by a vision of health as a basic human right, together with a commitment to the fundamental value of social justice – has been to reduce inequality in health, both within and between nations. There is a vast body of literature on inequality that addresses the key issues of social class, gender, ethnicity, age, disability and unemployment – many of which are interrelated and mediated through poverty and

social exclusion. However, we will confine ourselves here to key definitional issues.

While some variation in health experience is unavoidable, much of it can be attributed to unequal opportunities – that is, social inequality. The use of the term 'equity' introduces greater precision here. Whitehead (1990: 5) makes the important distinction between *inequality*, which can simply apply to any variation, and *inequity*, which is applied to variations deemed to be both avoidable and unjust:

> The term 'inequity' has a moral and ethical dimension. It refers to differences which are unnecessary and avoidable but, in addition, are also considered unfair and unjust. So, in order to describe a certain situation as inequitable, the cause has to be examined and judged to be unfair in the context of what is going on in the rest of society.

The box below provides a simple checklist for assessing which differences in health are inequitable. However, in many industrialized countries, the term 'inequalities in health' is often taken to be synonymous with inequity (Leon et al., 2001).

There is considerable evidence that social class is a key determinant of health status. Within the UK, such evidence has accumulated throughout the twentieth century – from the early work of Rowntree at its dawn to the Acheson report (1998) at its close. The box provides some key facts.

WHICH HEALTH DIFFERENCES ARE INEQUITABLE?

Determinant of differentials	Potentially avoidable?	Commonly viewed as unacceptable?
Natural biological variation	No	No
Health-damaging behaviour if freely chosen	Yes	No
Transient health advantage of groups who take up health-promoting behaviour first (if other groups can easily catch up)	Yes	No
Health-damaging behaviour where choice of lifestyle is restricted by socio-economic factors	Yes	Yes
Exposure to excessive health hazards in physical and social environment	Yes	Yes
Restricted access to essential healthcare	Yes	Yes
Health-related downward social mobility (sick people move down social scale)	Low income – yes	Low income – yes

Source: Whitehead, 1992: 4

SELECTED KEY FACTS ON HEALTH INEQUALITIES IN THE UK

- Life expectancy at birth for a baby boy in social class V is sixty-eight years compared with nearly seventy-eight years for social class I – nine years less.
- An unskilled man is three times more likely to die from coronary heart disease before reaching the age of sixty-five than a professional man.
- Children in social class V are five times as likely to die as a result of injury than their peers in social class I – 83 per 100,000 for social class V and 16 per 100,000 for social class I.
- Of men in unskilled manual households, 44 per cent smoke compared to 15 per cent of men in professional households. Among women, 32 per cent smoke in unskilled households and semi-skilled households compared with 14 per cent in professional households.
- Children in receipt of free school meals (indicative of disadvantaged backgrounds) have lower educational achievement than others.

Derived from Department of Health, 2001

Social class has typically been measured as occupational class. The main government classification system – the social class based on occupation (Registrar General's Social Class) – was based on grouping occupations according to the levels of skill involved. Using this system, the population could be divided into six classes, as shown in the box below. This broad pattern of categorization was introduced in 1921 and, apart from subdividing class III into manual and non-manual in 1971, has remained substantially unchanged.

A new social classification system has recently been introduced to reflect the changing patterns of work – the National Statistics Socio-economic Classification (NS SEC) – see the box. Although still based on occupation, it focuses on employment conditions and, particularly, the amount of control people have over their own and other people's work rather than on skill. It also includes a category for the long-term unemployed and those who have never had paid work. The publication of statistics based on the new system began in 2001.

SOCIO-ECONOMIC CLASSIFICATIONS

Social class based on occupation

I   Professional occupations
II   Managerial and technical occupations
III Skilled occupations:

   (N)   non-manual
   (M)   manual

IV   Partly skilled occupations
V   Unskilled occupations

National Statistics Socio-economic Classification (NS SEC)

1   Higher managerial and professional occupations
     1.1   Employers and managers in larger organizations
     1.2   Higher professionals
2   Lower managerial and professional organizations
3   Intermediate occupations
4   Small employers and own account workers
5   Lower supervisory, craft and related occupations
6   Semi-routine occupations
7   Routine occupations
8   Never worked and long-term unemployed

National Statistics, 2001

Much of the evidence on health inequality is based on occupational class. However, there has been some debate about its relevance for groups such as women, the unemployed, the elderly and children, and concern that occupational class may not fully reflect their circumstances. For example, married women have often been classified by their husband's occupation. This conceals their own employment status and may fail to fully recognize the effects of paid employment and working conditions on women's health. It also overlooks their contribution to the family's standard of living (Whitehead, 1987).

Sacker et al. (2000) note that, using the NS SEC, occupational class emerged as the most important influence on mortality for men, but was less sensitive to variation in mortality for women, even when allocated by their own occupation. A better indicator for women was found to be the household level of social and material advantage and lifestyle measured using the Cambridge scale (see, for example, Prandy, 1990), which is based on choices of friendships.

A further issue concerns what occupational class actually measures. Family members are usually classed according to the occupation of the head of the household and, although they may not be directly exposed to occupation-linked factors, will also share the variation in health associated with social class – childhood injuries, for example, show a marked social gradient (Roberts and Power, 1996). Occupational class, therefore, clearly encompasses a whole constellation of factors over and above different occupational conditions. These would include levels of income, housing, area of residence, education, and lifestyle. Nichols (1979) also notes that occupational class incorporates a cultural element and reflects status within the community The landmark Black Report analysed possible explanations for variation in health status with social class and concluded that, although genetic and cultural factors might make some contribution, the major underlying factor was material inequality and deprivation (Department of Health and Social Security, 1980).

An analysis of male mortality trends in England and Wales between 1971 and 1991 (Drever et al., 1996) shows an overall decline in mortality for social classes I–IV, but not for V, in which there was a slight increase. For all the major causes of mortality there was a gradient across the social classes, and this was steeper in 1991 than in 1971.

Income has frequently been identified as a key determinant of social variation in mortality. Poverty influences physical health as it limits access to good-quality nutrition and housing, but also has an effect on mental health (Shaw et al., 1999). Yet, against a backdrop of overall improvement in general prosperity and health status, differentials seem to be widening – a pattern not untypical of industrialized nations. A key factor would seem to be income inequality (Davey Smith, 1996). Indeed, Wilkinson (1994) states that life expectancy has increased most in industrialized nations where income differences have narrowed and mortality is more closely related to income inequality *within* countries than absolute differences in income *between* countries (Wilkinson, 1997).

This raises the issue of absolute and relative poverty. *Absolute* poverty exists when insufficient resources are available to provide the basic essentials of life, such as food and shelter. The World Bank, for example, has used the notional 1 dollar per day as an absolute minimum survival budget. However, this level has little meaning in the context of advanced industrialized societies. Some countries, such as the United States, have defined an official poverty line based on the cost of a basic food basket. The Canadian Council on Social Development (2001) provides an analysis of different ways of defining poverty and notes the debate over which items should be regarded as necessities. A key issue concerns whether a poverty line should be set in relation to a basic survival budget or a level of income that would enable people to participate in society.

Relative poverty, in contrast, involves comparing individuals or groups with some notional norm (Calman, 1997) and focuses on comparative conditions of living.

> Adam Smith himself closely embraced a relative definition of poverty, arguing that to be poor was to have to go without what was needed to be a 'creditable' member of society.
>
> Canadian Council on Social Development, 2001

An article by Frank (2000) in the *New York Times Magazine* drew attention to the importance of relative poverty/affluence in people's lives:

> Consider a choice between the two scenarios:
>
> World A: You earn $110,000 per year and others earn $200,000.
>
> World B: You earn $100,000 per year and others earn $85,000.
>
> The figures for income represent real purchasing power. Although in absolute terms individuals would be better off in Scenario A, a majority of Americans choose Scenario B.

There are several different ways of establishing relative poverty levels. For example, the proportion of income needed to cover the basic necessities of life, the proportional relationship to the median income and measures based on 'market baskets', which would include items in line with community norms.

A national survey of poverty and social exclusion in Britain published by the Joseph Rowntree Foundation (Gordon et al., 2000) used a variety of measures of poverty. These included not being able to afford what are generally perceived to be 'necessities'. The box gives a list of items that over half of the adult population regard as necessities. It is clear that the interpretation of what constitutes a necessity goes beyond the basic survival needs of subsistence diet, shelter, clothing and fuel to include participating in social customs, fulfilling obligations and taking part in activities.

ITEMS PERCEIVED AS NECESSITIES

Item	% considering item 'necessary'
Beds and bedding for everyone	95
Heating to warm living areas of the home	94
Damp-free home	93
Visiting friends or family in hospital	92
Two meals a day	91
Medicines prescribed by doctor	90
Refrigerator	89
Fresh fruit and vegetables daily	86
Warm, waterproof coat	85
Replace or repair broken electrical goods	85
Visits to friends or family	84
Celebrations on special occasions such as Christmas	83
Money to keep home in decent state of decoration	82
Visits to school, such as sports day	81
Attending weddings, funerals	80
Meat, fish or vegetarian equivalent every other day	79
Insurance of contents of dwelling	79
Hobby or leisure activity	78
Washing machine	76
Collect children from school	75
Telephone	71
Appropriate clothes for job interviews	69
Deep freezer/fridge freezer	68
Carpets in living rooms and bedrooms	67
Regular savings (of £10 per month) for rainy days or retirement	66
Two pairs of all-weather shoes	64
Friends or family round for a meal	64
A small amount of money to spend on self weekly, not on family	59
Television	56
Roast joint/vegetarian equivalent once a week	56
Presents for friends/family once a year	56
A holiday away from home once a year, not with relatives	55
Replace worn-out furniture	54
Dictionary	53
An outfit for social occasions	51

Derived from Joseph Rowntree Foundation, 2000

There has been no tradition of routinely collecting official data on poverty in the UK – partly due to the difficulties of defining levels of poverty. The receipt of social security benefits has been used as a proxy indicator. However, there have been moves to redress this (for a detailed discussion, see Kerrison and Macfarlane, 2000). The Department of Social Security Analytical Services Division (1999), has developed a series of low income indicators. These are based on percentage levels of both mean and median incomes before and after allowing for housing costs. The New Policy Institute also reports regularly on a series of fifty indicators of poverty and social exclusion (Rahman et al., 2000). The South East Public Health Observatory has developed an online tool that provides support in relation to methodologies for assessing inequality and deprivation (Carr-Hill and Dixon-Chalmers, 2002).

Whereas absolute poverty is a central issue in the developing world, poverty in urban, industrialized countries has been defined (Supplementary Benefits Commission, 1979, cited in Dahlgren and Whitehead, 1991) as:

a standard of living so low that it excludes and isolates people from the rest of the community. To keep out of poverty they must have an income which enables them to participate in the life of the community.

This definition draws attention to the issue of social exclusion, which is receiving considerable attention. The concept of social exclusion encompasses material deprivation and relative poverty, but also includes the process of marginalization of some individuals and groups from social and community life (Shaw et al., 1999). This process is not solely restricted to economic factors, but would also include other forms of cultural and social discrimination. Major groups of socially excluded people are the unemployed, ethnic minorities, refugees, the elderly, lone parents and their children and those, especially children, with disability.

A report by the Terence Higgins Trust (2001) notes that the groups primarily affected by HIV in the UK are those marginalized or socially excluded by society. They attribute this to low self-esteem among those excluded, which is associated with risk-taking and social exclusion, making sexual health a low priority. Furthermore, people with HIV may experience further exclusion on account of their HIV status and this may influence the way in which they access appropriate care.

Clearly, social exclusion exerts a powerful psycho-social influence and there are obvious links with the notion of social capital. Kawachi (1997) demonstrates lower levels of social trust in states with a higher 'Robin Hood Index' – a measure of income inequality based on the proportion of aggregate income that would have to be redistributed to level up earnings. Similar findings are obtained for participation in voluntary associations. However, Lynch et al.'s (2000) analysis of income inequality and mortality cautions against an exclusive emphasis on psycho-social effects and the lack of social cohesion, which, they allege, is akin to victim-blaming at the community level. They propose that the main causes of health inequality are material – including access to both private and social resources, such as education, healthcare, social welfare and work.

Raphael's (2001: 30) analysis of social inequality and heart disease in Canada provides a concise summary of the interaction between these various elements.

Social exclusion is a process by which people are denied the opportunity to participate in civil society; denied an acceptable supply of goods or services; are unable to contribute to society, and are unable to acquire the normal commodities expected of citizens. All of these elements occur in tandem with material deprivation, excessive psycho-social stress, and adoption of health-threatening behaviours shown to be related to the onset of, and death from, cardiovascular disease.

The concept of deprivation can apply both to individuals and areas and includes material and social elements (Krieger, 2001). There is some evidence that, independently of an individual's level of deprivation, living in a deprived area has an adverse effect on health (Shaw et al., 1999).

There are some composite indicators of deprivation that can be used to assess the overall levels of deprivation within different areas. The Jarman and Townsend indices have been used widely in the UK and draw on census data (see the box). The Jarman index has been much criticized – both on account of its method of construction and also because it is biased towards classifying areas in London as being deprived rather than those in the North (Talbot, 1991). This has been attributed to the skewed distribution of single-parent families and highly mobile populations, for example, which tend to be more concentrated in the inner London area. Attempts to measure levels of deprivation on a large geographic scale often obscure smaller pockets of deprivation. There is considerable interest, therefore, in small area analysis. The Department of the Environment, Transport and Regions (DETR) has developed its Index of Multiple Deprivation (DETR, 2000). It identifies six different domains:

- income deprivation
- employment

THE JARMAN AND TOWNSEND INDICES OF DEPRIVATION

Jarman underprivileged area score (UPA)

Derived from GPs' views about factors that influence their workload.

- Percentage of children under five.
- Percentage of unemployment.
- Percentage of ethnic minorities.
- Percentage of single-parent households.
- Percentage of elderly living alone.
- Overcrowding factor.
- Percentage of lower social classes.
- Percentage of highly mobile people.
- Percentage of unmarried couple families.
- Poor housing factor.

The above ten items were originally included in the Jarman UPA score, but the last two are omitted from the Jarman UPA8 score.

Townsend combined deprivation indicator

- Percentage of economically active residents aged 16–59/64 who are unemployed.
- Percentage of private households that do not possess a car.
- Percentage of private households that are not owner occupied.
- Percentage of private households with more than one person per room.

Derived from Whitehead, 1987.

- health deprivation and disability
- education, skills and training deprivation
- housing deprivation
- geographical access to services.

Each domain is assessed using a series of indicators and the weighted domains are combined to produce an overall index of multiple deprivation for each electoral ward.

Carr-Hill and Dixon Chalmers (2002) emphasize that these various indices are artificial constructs and only partial or proxy measures of phenomena such as deprivation. They caution against reification, which can occur when operational constructs used as approximate measures become substituted for the actual meaning of the concepts they purport to measure. While their argument focuses on the measurement of deprivation, it would apply equally to other indicators of health status.

SUMMARY AND CONCLUSIONS

It is axiomatic that planning interventions to promote health requires understanding of the current health status of populations and the factors that influence it. This chapter began by looking at the role of epidemiology in contributing to this understanding. In particular, we noted its capacity to assess the health of populations, communities and subgroups within them, explore cause-and-effect relationships and identify modifiable risk factors. However, while acknowledging the relevance of this contribution and major achievements – for example, in providing convincing evidence of the effects of social inequality on health – we have discussed a number of the limitations of epidemiology. The focus tends to be on morbidity and mortality rather than positive health states and wellbeing. This is, in part, attributable to the relatively greater ease with which we can define ill health and obtain relevant data for it, although it is also held to reflect a biomedical ideological position and a positivist epistemology.

For some, the reductionism and attention to micro-causality inherent in biomedical approaches leads to an emphasis on downstream behavioural risk factors rather than a more upstream focus on the structural factors that affect people's lives. While there has been some attempt to redress these issues with a move towards developing positive indicators of health and the emergence of the fields of social and critical epidemiology, there is a strong argument that a more complete understanding of a complex multidimensional concept such as health necessarily needs to draw on multiple perspectives.

Rather than engage in sterile debate on the relative superiority of biomedical and interpretivist approaches, we would contend that they offer complementary insights. Tension arises from the unequal power positions of those subscribing to different methodologies and the dominance of biomedicine. This has been challenged from both professional and lay quarters. In that health is essentially a subjective experience, the lay perspective is particularly relevant.

We have also noted the tendency to focus on the factors that disrupt health rather than consider what is involved in staying healthy. The seminal work of Antonovsky has led the way in calling for a move towards such a salutogenic paradigm.

The emergence of health promotion as a discipline placed emphasis on environmental influences on health – both directly and in terms of shaping behaviour and lifestyle. Notwithstanding the debate about the primacy of agency or structure, it is clear that there is a reciprocal relationship between the two elements. The complexity of the interrelationship has become more evident as our conceptualization of the environment has broadened. While the contribution of social and socio-economic aspects of the environment have been recognized for some time, the recent resurgence in interest in social capital focuses attention on social connectedness and opportunities for civic engagement.

Equity is a fundamental goal of health promotion and one that accords with health being seen as a basic human right. Material deprivation and absolute poverty have been implicated as key sources of inequity in health. In industrialized countries, the notion of relative poverty is currently receiving considerable attention, along with the related issue of social exclusion.

The measurement of health and quality of life and their determinants is undoubtedly challenging. It calls for complementary multidisciplinary perspectives and the inclusion of lay views. It also requires the extension of routine data collection systems to include quality of life issues and indicators of the major determinants of health over and above the conventional focus on morbidity and mortality. We will consider the process of systematic programme planning in Chapter 4 and the issue of needs assessment in Chapter 5.

To conclude this chapter we should note that the capacity to assess the health of communities and identify key determinants underpins rational planning processes. Clearly, the way such assessment is approached should reflect the ideology and values of health promotion.

3

Determinants of Health Actions

To every human problem there is a neat and easy solution – and it's wrong.

H.L. Mencken (www.lhup.edu/~dsimanek/mencken.htm)

CHANGE AT THE MACRO LEVEL – THE ADOPTION OF INNOVATIONS

Social systems and social change

Macro-level analysis focuses on relatively large aggregations of individuals. Whereas it is relatively easy to define one individual, it is difficult to provide a precise and meaningful distinction between aggregates containing various numbers of individuals. There is, for example, no very clear distinction between an organization and a community in terms of numbers. Moreover, a region in one large industrialized country may be considerably larger than a small nation state. The difficulty is compounded by the fact that the definition of 'community' may actually be contested. Accordingly, the term 'social system' will be used here to refer to any social group, large or small. The meso level will be viewed as part of an inclusive macro system and, of course, individuals will exist within each of these two levels.

A detailed discussion of models of social change is beyond the scope of this chapter. Accordingly, further discussion will be limited to commenting on what is probably the most commonly used theoretical analysis – and one that has been consistently applied to the adoption of health innovations.

Communication of innovations theory

Communication of innovations theory is concerned with the factors relating to the adoption of innovations within social systems (Rogers and Shoemaker, 1971, and Rogers, 1995). 'Innovations' are practices that are new or are *perceived* to be new by members of the social system. A number of key principles have been derived from this theory and the wide variety of research studies on which it is based (for instance, Rogers and Shoemaker in the original 1971 text commented that their model was grounded in 1084 publications from a number of disciplines). A major generalization resulting from

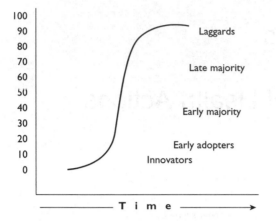

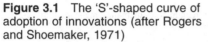

Figure 3.1 The 'S'-shaped curve of adoption of innovations (after Rogers and Shoemaker, 1971)

these various studies is that the cumulative rate of adoption of innovations describes a sigmoidal curve (see Figure 3.1).

The following points should be noted:

- the adoption process starts slowly, gathers speed until the majority of people in a population are adopters and then tails off
- the steepness of the adoption curve will depend on the relative attractiveness of the adoption in question – that is, innovations that have zero attraction, except to a handful of people who seem inclined to try any novelty, will approximate to a horizontal line!
- persuading the final few per cent of a population to adopt the innovation becomes increasingly difficult (even when the innovation is seized on eagerly by the populace at large) – doubtless it is true that a few people are against most things all of the time!

Assuming that the innovation is ultimately adopted, the theory proposes that individuals first of all become aware of the existence of an innovation and (probably) understand its implications. They then adopt a positive attitude to the innovation – probably as a result of persuasion and interpersonal influence. They make a decision to adopt and, provided that nothing untoward happens, put the innovation into practice. As a result of their subsequent experience, they either continue happily in the new way or abandon it and return to their former activities. The final implementation stage of the adoption process is increasingly considered to be of major importance as evidence accumulates of the failure of apparently successful

community-wide projects to be sustained and become part of routine practice.

The relative steepness of the curve in Figure 3.1 describes an innovation that has been very popular. It is, of course, important for effective programme planning that we understand what contributes to popularity. Five key features have been identified:

- nature of the social system
- channel
- perceived characteristics of the innovation
- leadership
- community participation.

Nature of the social system

Social systems differ in a number of ways. Although different social systems may be more or less ready to adopt particular innovations, it is assumed that some communities are inclined to react more readily than others. For instance, certain communities are labelled 'traditional' (and therefore conservative) and more reluctant to change than 'modern', cosmopolitan social systems. Certainly the nature and extent of geographical isolation, together with the existence or lack of communication systems, might be expected to reduce the speed of change.

Channel

It might be assumed that communities having extensive and sophisticated mass media would be inclined to change more rapidly than those without (witness, for instance, the inroads made by global marketing and the appearance of Coca-Cola and McDonalds in the most unlikely places!). Certainly, mass media are effective in awareness-raising, but, on the other hand, interpersonal influence is more important in changing attitudes and providing skills.

Characteristics of the innovation

It is well recognized, and indeed common sense, that people's perceptions of the nature and implications of the innovation they are being asked to adopt will be a highly significant factor in determining whether or not they are willing to take the risk. The following features tend to be associated with adoption rather than rejection:

- simplicity
- possibility of trying the innovation prior to permanent commitment

- 'observability' – that is, the possibility of observing the effects of the innovation within a short period of time
- compatibility with existing practices
- relative advantages of new practices – anticipated benefits with minimal costs.

Leadership and the principle of homophily

The competence of the change agents used to influence the community will contribute to the likelihood of adoption. Ideally, they would collaborate with opinion leaders, who act as referents and models for the community. The powerful principle of 'homophily' offers an explanation of the status and influence of opinion leaders, as well as advice for change agents who, by definition, cannot aspire to opinion leadership as such. Rogers and Shoemaker (1971: 14) define it as follows:

> Homophily is the degree to which pairs of individuals who interact are similar in certain attributes, such as beliefs, values, education, social status and the like. A further refinement of this proposition includes the concept of empathy ... the ability of an individual to project himself into the role of another.

The leadership characteristics mentioned above will be seen to parallel our earlier comments on power and, in particular, French and Raven's (1959) analysis. They also relate to the notion of credibility of the source, to which further reference will be made in later discussions about attitude change theory. It is also worth commenting here that it is simplistic to think only in terms of change agents and opinion leaders. A number of individuals in a community would exercise differing degrees of influence and thus be described in leadership terms. For instance, Tagdhisi (1992) discussed the influences of six different kinds of leaders in an Iranian village:

- religious leaders
- traditional leaders
- *behvarz* (primary healthcare workers)
- schoolteachers
- literacy movement trainers
- *baseej* (militia).

Community participation

One particular factor likely to influence the adoption of an innovation is of especial importance – not least because of its centrality to the ideological commitments of health promotion. In short, it concerns the extent to which the community is involved in defining its own needs (a point to which we will return in the context of our review of needs assessment) and in identifying ways of meeting those needs. Figure 3.2 (page 78) sets out the relationship between this degree of participation and the anticipated rate of adoption of a given innovation.

Further explication of the application of communication of innovations theory and, indeed, other models of social system change is beyond the scope of this chapter (see, for instance, Bartholomew et al., 2001, Goodman et al., 1997, Oldenburg et al., 1997, and Parcel et al., 1990). Our concern now is to shift focus from the macro to the micro level, to examine influences on individual health actions.

CHANGE AT THE MICRO LEVEL – INFLUENCES ON INDIVIDUAL HEALTH ACTIONS

A thorough understanding of broader social and environmental influences on health and illness-related behaviours is, of course, invaluable. However, in the last analysis it is individual people who make decisions and the sum total of their decision making that ultimately determines social action. For instance, why exactly might people be motivated to adopt an innovation once they have become aware of its existence? What does it mean when we say that adoption is influenced by people's perceptions of the innovation's characteristics? Are we really talking about perceptions or would 'beliefs' be a more accurate description? What are the psycho-social dynamics involved in an individual ultimately making a decision to adopt and then either maintain the new practice or reject it?

It is the purpose of this next part of the chapter to provide a detailed examination of the various psychological, social and environmental determinants of health or illness-related choices and behaviour.

The health action model

A veritable plethora of models and theories is available to those wishing to understand individual decision making. While they have many features in common – even though the terminology may differ – they typically have particular emphases and their own peculiar orientations. Many were developed for general use, but have been found to have special relevance for health behaviour, while others were constructed with health education, health promotion and public health in mind. They include the following important models:

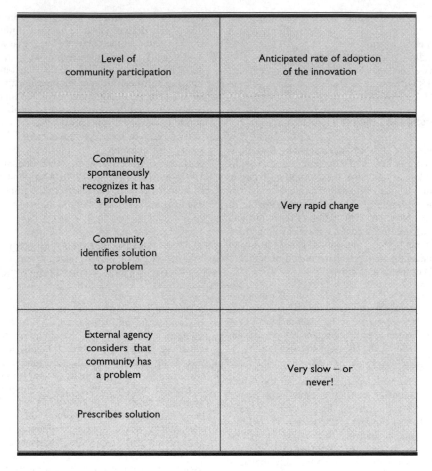

Level of community participation	Anticipated rate of adoption of the innovation
Community spontaneously recognizes it has a problem Community identifies solution to problem	Very rapid change
External agency considers that community has a problem Prescribes solution	Very slow – or never!

Figure 3.2   Participation by rate of adoption

- health belief model
- theory of reasoned action
- theory of planned behaviour
- transtheoretical model
- social learning theory
- protection motivation theory.

For further details, see Winett et al., 1989, Conner and Norman, 1996, Sarafino, 1990, and Bennett and Murphy, 1997. A number of texts on patient education also utilize a psychological approach (for example, Rankin and Stallings, 2001).

It is not possible here to review the models listed above. Accordingly, one particular model will be used to identify the constructs that are central to understanding health and illness-related behaviour and particularly relevant to planning health promotion programmes. The model in question is the 'health

action model' (HAM) which was initially devised by Tones in the early 1970s to provide a theoretical base for the emerging specialist professional practice of health education (Tones, 1979, 1981). It was subsequently modified to take account of the shift in emphasis that took place with the emergence of health promotion (with its emphasis on healthy public policy and related macro influences). As will be apparent, it draws eclectically, pragmatically (and unashamedly!) on a number of key models and theories. It is reproduced as Figure 3.3.

The health action model (HAM) identifies key psychological, social and environmental influences on individuals adopting and sustaining health- or illness-related actions. It comprises two major sections – the systems that contribute to 'behavioural intention' and the factors that determine the likelihood of that behavioural intention being translated

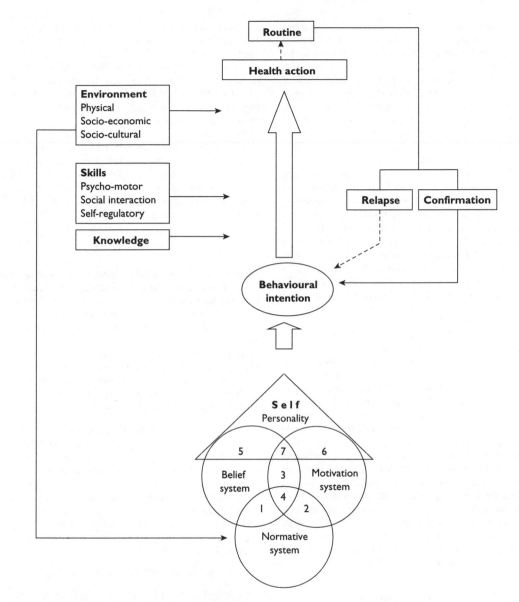

Figure 3.3 The health action model (HAM)

into practice. The first of these sections has traditionally been associated with health *education*, while the second is of major importance to health *promotion*. However, as we will see, the imperatives of health promotion – especially empowerment – are centrally represented in the first of these two sections.

In short, four interacting systems – concerned with beliefs, motivation, normative influences and the self – all determine the likelihood of a given

individual developing an *intention* to adopt a particular course of health- or illness-related action. Whether this happens or not will depend on a number of enabling or facilitating factors, including the knowledge and skills necessary to adopt the health action. Of special importance – as should now be apparent – is the availability of a supportive environment that 'makes the healthy choice the easy choice'. An alternative way of expressing the importance of these enabling factors is to assert that health promotion is charged with removing those psychological, behavioural and environmental barriers that militate against people making healthy choices.

The health actions in question may include actions related to positive health outcomes and/or actions designed to prevent disease. In both cases, the actions do not only relate to individual health, but also may contribute to the health of the public – for instance by empowering individuals to undertake political actions that contribute to healthy public policy. HAM acknowledges the difference between single time, discrete health actions and routines. A discrete health action might be involved when, for example, only one visit is necessary to a clinic to have a child immunized or a potential political activist writes a letter of complaint to a member of Parliament. Usually, though, benefits only accrue when health actions become part of a routine – for instance, when individuals routinely build exercise into their lifestyle or the political activist continues to stir up public indignation at breaches of human rights.

When a single-time choice has been made or, more commonly, when a routine has been undertaken, two outcomes are possible. The first is that the health action in question is not problematical and results in confirmation of the behavioural intention. Alternatively, the innovation may be rejected and the individual relapses. The notion of relapse is traditionally associated with addictive or quasi-addictive behaviour, such as giving up smoking or other drugs. However, it could equally be applied to those actions that involve discomfort or inconvenience. The transtheoretical model is especially concerned with questions of maintenance and relapse. Usefully, it notes how those who initially relapse will frequently try again (and even again and again!) before finally being confirmed in a healthy way of life (Prochaska and DiClimente, 1984, and Prochaska et al., 1997).

The belief system

The K-A-P formula

One of the simplest attempts to explain the adoption of particular behaviour is encapsulated in the K-A-P 'formula'. It is based on the reasonable assertion that knowledge alone does not lead to behaviour – it is usually necessary, but rarely sufficient. Accordingly, the provision of knowledge (K) has to be supplemented by persuasive techniques designed to bring about a change in attitude(s) (A) before the target person or population will adopt appropriate practices (P).

The model is, of course, amazingly naïve, but so-called KAP surveys are still in evidence. They might, for example, ask about the sexual practices of a community, check whether sexually active people know which practices are desirable and which might result in HIV/AIDS and whether or not they have positive or negative attitudes to unsafe or safer sexual practices.

As will be apparent from Figure 3.3 earlier in this chapter a much more sophisticated constellation of constructs is necessary if behaviour is to be understood and influenced. One of the most important of these is the concept of belief, which in HAM is presented as part of a belief system – that is, a complex of interacting elements.

Beliefs defined

To understand how beliefs operate, it is essential to make some conceptual distinctions, particularly between knowledge and attitude. As with knowledge, beliefs are cognitive constructs, whereas attitudes are affective – that is, they refer to a person's evaluation of some object, person or activity. Attitudes, therefore, refer to feelings and, for example, might indicate the degree of importance attached to skimmed milk, a domineering doctor or healthy exercise. Fishbein (1976) provides an unequivocal definition of belief as follows:

> A belief is a probability judgement that links some object or concept to some attribute. The terms 'object' and 'attribute' are used in a generic sense and both terms may refer to any discriminable aspect of an individual's world. For example, I may believe that Pill A (an object) is a depressant (an attribute). The content of the belief is defined by the object and attribute in question, and the strength of the belief is defined by the persons's subjective probability that the object–attribute relationship exists (or is true).

On the other hand Fishbein (1976: 103) notes:

> An attitude is a bipolar evaluative judgement of the object. It is essentially a subjective judgement that I like or dislike the object, that it is good or bad, that I'm favourable or unfavourable towards it. [The term 'object'] … is used in a generic sense. Thus I may have attitudes towards people, institutions, events, behaviours, outcomes, etc.

Beliefs are, thus, subjective probabilities and will frequently operate in parallel with objective probabilities. By way of example, epidemiological data might suggest that cancer is a major cause of mortality – a statistical observation mirrored by individuals' beliefs about seriousness. On the other hand, subjective and objective interpretations might operate independently. For example, there may be no objective/scientific evidence that the fumes from a local industrial site contribute to lung disease in an adjacent neighbourhood. Moreover, statistical analysis might also reveal that the prevalence of lung disease in the neighbourhood is neither more nor less than in the population at large. The members of the community, on the other hand, are:

- convinced that they have a real problem of 'chesty coughs' (their non-specific lay version of lung disease)
- consider it is self-evident that these 'chesty coughs' are due to the fumes from the incinerators in the factory.

The health belief model

The health belief model (HBM) is probably the most frequently used model of all those purporting to explain health-related decision making. Originated by Hochbaum (1958) and developed by Rosenstock (1966, 1974), the model was devised to explain variations in the utilization of preventive medical services and was based on pioneering work by Lewin (1951).

In its earlier manifestation, it is essentially a model of the expectancy–value/value–expectancy variety. In other words, it argues that decision making depends on individuals believing that a particular course of action will result in the likelihood of a valued outcome being achieved. It is neither possible nor desirable here to provide a full review of this model – more complete analyses can be found in Becker (1984) and Scheeran and Abraham (1996) – but it is useful to record the four major beliefs emphasized by it:

- belief in personal susceptibility to a negative event
- belief that the event is serious
- belief that the recommended preventive measure will be effective in reducing the threat of the negative event
- belief that the recommended measure will not entail too heavy a cost.

Two additional elements of the HBM deserve note:

- cues to action
- health motivation.

The originators of the model considered that these four beliefs alone might need some additional trigger to jolt into action those who were already predisposed to certain courses of action by their beliefs. A general factor – health motivation – was

included in a later version of the model. It was considered that the explanatory value of the HBM might be improved if a measure of people's general health motivation were to be included. The formulation is eminently logical as common sense suggests that individuals would not take action to avoid an unpleasant event if they did not believe it was likely to happen to them or, if it did, it would be insignificant. Again, it might well be assumed that people would not follow health education advice if they did not believe it would work and if the disadvantages outweighed the benefits. As Scheeran and Abraham (1996: 51) rightly observe in their thorough analysis of the model:

> The HBM has provided a useful theoretical framework for investigators of the cognitive determinants of a wide range of behaviours for more than thirty years. Its commonsense constructs are easy for non-psychologists to assimilate and apply and it can be readily and inexpensively operationalized. It has focused researchers' and healthcare professionals' attention on modifiable psychological prerequisites of behaviour and provided a basis for practical interventions across a range of behaviours.

How effective are the HBM beliefs in explaining health-related behaviour? A completely comprehensive model that incorporates every social, psychological and environmental influence on health choices would account for 100 per cent of the difference in people's health actions (the variance). The evidence suggests that HBM explains *some* of the variance, but not a lot!

Belief hierarchies and the notion of salience

One of the particularly useful formulations in Fishbein and Ajzen's (1975) seminal work is the demonstration that beliefs may be either 'salient' or 'latent'. The phenomenon of salience is relevant for health education strategies. Translating latent beliefs into salient beliefs, say in the course of group discussion or face-to-face interaction, might alter the belief–attitude dynamic, reduce uncertainty and result in commitment to adopting a healthy course of action.

Figure 3.4 provides an example of a typical hierarchy of beliefs associated with stopping smoking. These beliefs may be salient or latent.

There are several self-evident lessons for health promotion. For instance, it is inefficient, even pointless, addressing higher-order beliefs without first ensuring that necessary precursor concepts and subordinate beliefs have already been acquired. It is also apparent that a kind of mental balance sheet is

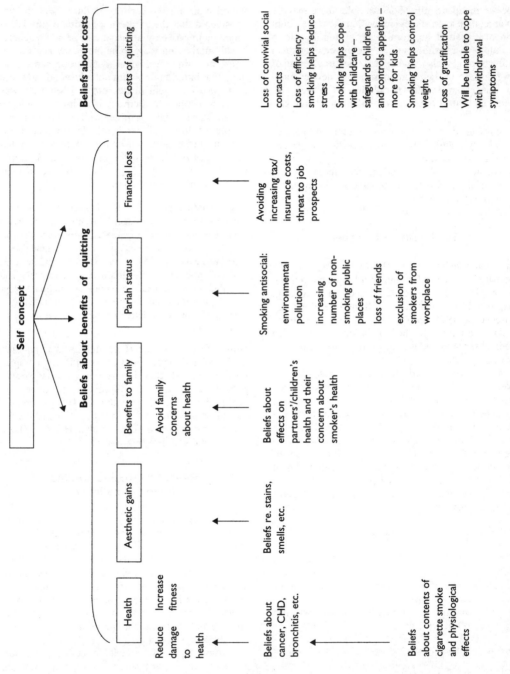

Figure 3.4 Example of a belief system concerning stopping smoking

operating and that the outcome will depend on the ultimate balance and relative strengths of the beliefs about the positive and negative outcomes of giving up smoking. This will reflect the relative strengths of the various motivational forces that determine action.

The motivation system

Whereas the belief system is cognitive, the motivation system is affective – it is concerned with feelings. 'Motivation' refers to goal-directed behaviour and its psychological underpinning. It defines the push and pull forces that impel individuals towards the achievement of pleasure and away from undesirable outcomes.

Different kinds of motivation can be identified and operate at different levels. Four kinds are included in the motivation system: values, attitudes, drives and emotional states.

The values dimension

There is a reasonably clear consensus in psychology about the definition of values and their origin. The doyen of research in this area is Rokeach (1973: 3) who makes five assertions about the nature of human values:

- the total number of values is relatively small
- everyone possesses the same values to different degrees
- values are organized into value systems
- values are created and influenced by culture, society and its institutions and personality
- values play a part in virtually all phenomena investigated by the social sciences – psychology, sociology, anthropology, psychiatry, political science, education, economics and history.

In relation to other psychological and social constructs – all of which are of importance in explaining health- and illness-related decisions – values have a transcendental quality, in so far as they energize attitudes and underpin behaviour. In Rokeach's (1973: 13) words, 'values are guides and determinants of social attitudes and ideologies on the one hand and of social behaviour on the other.'

As with beliefs, values typically occupy hierarchies having superordinate and subordinate levels. Rokeach, for example, usefully distinguishes 'terminal values' from 'instrumental values'. Moreover, he (1973: 14) links these with self-esteem – that major, higher-order value that has special prominence in empowerment theory and health promotion generally.

Terminal values are motivating because they represent the supergoals beyond immediate, biologically urgent goals. Unlike the more immediate goals, these supergoals do not seem ... to satiate – we seem to be forever doomed to strive for these ultimate goals without quite ever reaching them... there is another reason why values can be said to be motivating. They are in the final analysis the conceptual tools and weapons that we all employ in order to maintain and enhance self-esteem. They are in the service of what McDougall (1926) has called the master sentiment – sentiment of self-regard.

There are also two kinds of instrumental values: moral values and competence values. Interestingly, one of the examples of an intrapersonal competence value that figures prominently in Rokeach's discussion has to do with self-actualization, which, as we noted earlier, can be viewed as a healthy state in its own right or as the peak of a hierarchical motivational structure.

The attitude dimension

The concept of attitude is central to social psychology. Reference was made earlier to Fishbein's definition of attitude, but a number of alternative and influential formulae can also be found. Perhaps the most common of these makes reference to disposition or readiness for action. Occasionally, the term is used to describe a psychological construct having not only affective but also cognitive and 'conative' elements. The cognitive dimension involves 'beliefs', the affective dimension is concerned with feelings and the conative aspect with the action implications of a given attitude. In HAM we follow Fishbein and Ajzen in limiting the conative element to 'behavioural intention'. As we will see, this is viewed as the product of the belief, motivation and normative systems and, depending on the availability of 'empowering' knowledge, skills and environment, may or may not be translated into actual behavioural outcomes or health actions.

Again, attitudes operate within a hierarchical system based on values and may be more or less salient or latent. Figure 3.5 provides a review of the values associated with stopping smoking and thus complements the belief hierarchy presented in Figure 3.4 above.

Inspection of Figures 3.4 and 3.5, however, reveals that the combined force of values and beliefs ought to generate an overwhelmingly negative attitude to smoking and a resounding positive attitude to stopping. The fact that this does not always happen is due to the third key element in the motivation system – that cluster of often primitive feelings that are here variously described as drives and emotional states.

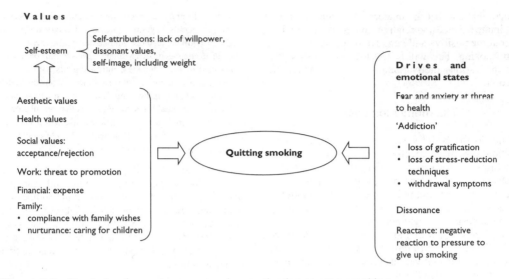

Figure 3.5   Example of a system concerning motivation to stop smoking

Drives, acquired drives and emotional states

In addition to values and attitudes, a third motivational category is identified in HAM. This includes the concepts of drive and emotional state. A detailed review of the complicated and sophisticated field of motivation is not appropriate here. However, at the risk of being simplistic, we could try to sum up the term 'drive' as a kind of primary motivation that is considered to be innate or instinctive. It energizes readily recognized behaviour that frequently has survival value. The most instinctive of these are hunger, thirst, sex and the avoidance of pain.

It is assumed that drives typically exert a greater influence over behaviour than motivation derived from values and attitudes. Indeed, Maslow's (1954) pyramid viewed physiological needs for 'air, food, water, sleep, etc.' as providing a foundation for his motivational hierarchy. Although self-actualization and the achievement of various values were also located at the top of the hierarchy, the physiological needs must be satisfied before higher-order needs can be fully achieved.

Whereas there is clearly evidence that the achievement of values goals might, for some people, override the need for food or sex, it would be unwise to rely on this! As WHO has observed, the need for peace, safety and security must be satisfied before people consider adopting behaviour that will improve their health.

The term 'acquired drive' is used to refer to what are normally termed addictions. Again, we must avoid oversimplification, but the power of dependence on various substances generally has more in common with the traditionally defined innate drives than it does with values.

Again, the term 'emotional state' cannot be accorded a precise definition. For instance, while fear is undoubtedly an emotional state, it could equally qualify as a drive, both in respect of its innate qualities and its effects on the individual experiencing it. On the other hand, anxiety would not normally be considered a drive, though it has been defined as a 'fractionated fear response' – that is, a watered-down version of pure fear. In all events, it can exert a powerful effect on decision making and behaviour and so should be considered as qualitatively different from a value.

Consider, for example, the case of breastfeeding. Factor analytic research typically reveals two major value-related factors that influence the decision to breastfeed or use bottles. They are the value associated with health and the value associated with social convenience. 'Embarrassment' is a major factor associated with the rejection of breastfeeding (see, for instance, Martin, 1978). The definition of 'embarrassment' is by no means clear and this emotional state may vary in its strength from somewhat demure modesty at the prospect of breastfeeding in front of friends to an almost neurotic anxiety that seems to have its roots in a failure to come to terms with sexuality.

It is doubtless apparent that an external representation of danger – perhaps in the form of a poster produced by the shock horror school of health education – might succeed in its intention to generate anxiety or even fear. Similarly, the stimulus may come from an individual's own thought processes and imagination. In all events, the assessment of the nature of the threat associated, for instance, with beliefs about vulnerability, may generate some degree of autonomic arousal and feelings ranging from mild concern to panic and terror. These feelings may well be revealed – if not verbally then, in all probability, non-verbally.

One final example of an emotional state that frequently contributes to intention to act is that of 'cognitive dissonance' (Festinger, 1957). It is best described as a state of unease that results from simultaneously holding two or more cognitions (beliefs) that are psychologically inconsistent. The theory posits that individuals experiencing the uncomfortable emotional state of dissonance will be motivated to act to remove it. The dissonance phenomenon has been extensively researched and some further comments will be made in our discussion of attitude change in Chapter 7. However, the position adopted here is that dissonance is but one of many different emotional states that may contribute to behavioural intentions. Its impact can be demonstrated in laboratory situations, but, in real-life situations, it will typically compete with a highly complicated system of drives and values in its effect on behavioural intention. One such competitor is encapsulated in the notion of social pressure, to which we now turn.

The normative system

The normative system describes the network of social pressures that might be brought to bear on an individual's intention to adopt or reject health actions. As may be seen from Figure 3.6, it is conceived as a hierarchical set of influences ranging from the proximal impact of close family and friends to the increasingly distal effects of community and the further reaches of the social system. It is assumed that the effect of significant individuals, close family and friends will typically be more powerful than community pressure, which, in turn, will have more influence than national norms conveyed by mass media.

Interpersonal influences

The potential power of interpersonal pressure exerted face to face needs little further explication here. Those individuals who exert a direct effect are commonly described as 'significant others'. In addition to close friends or partners, individual professionals

might well play an important part in influencing attitudes and behaviour (our earlier discussion of the nature of leadership has already suggested the characteristics that might result in the 'other' being considered 'significant'). The relative importance of family and significant friends will, of course, depend on the nature of existing relationships. However, at the levels of both research and anecdote, the impact of a passionately antismoking partner is well documented!

Peer pressure

One of the conventional axioms of health promotion is that the peer group exerts a disproportionate and draconian effect on its members. As this influence is also typically assumed to be unhealthy, it is deemed necessary to provide young people with an armamentarium of skills that will enable them to resist this social pressure. Even limited experience of working with youth (or indeed old age!) leads to the conclusion that people frequently do not actually want to resist the persuasive influence of their peers. In effect, a much more sophisticated view of the nature of peer group pressure is essential if appropriate education and health promotion is to be designed (see, for instance, Michell's (1997) demonstration that there is no such thing as *the* peer group, there are peer *groups* (plural), having different characteristics and status).

Social norms, the community and the lay referral system

As noted above, the assumption reflected in Figure 3.6 is that the influence of community norms will be less powerful than that of family, friends and peer groups, but will have more impact than more distal norms conveyed by mass media. Of course, family, friends and peer groups may also be an integral part of the community. As we comment elsewhere, a genuine community, by definition, has common norms and a network of contacts and relationships, which, traditionally, include extended families. Where such a community exists, the extent of its social influence will be substantially greater than in a social system characterized by anomie (normlessness).

Due to the effects of socialization, it is likely that community norms will be reinforced by families and adopted by individuals. In fact, following earlier observations about the subtle and powerful effect of dominant ideologies and following the assumptions inherent in the notion of false consciousness, normative pressures may reinforce the status quo and, thus, the social power structure. The

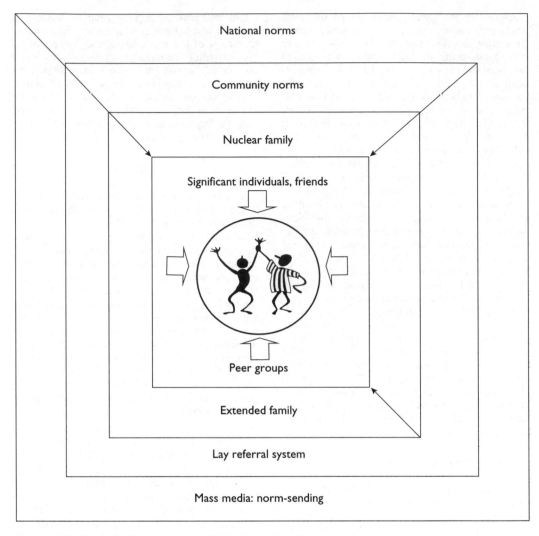

Figure 3.6   Social influences on individual health actions

implications of this analysis have some relevance for one particular situation where social pressure plays a key part – the lay referral system. This has its origins in sociological analyses of the factors associated with compliance with medical advice and the appropriate use of health services.

The lay referral system and pressure to comply

The notion of a lay referral system (LRS) has been influential in providing insights into the effects of community norms on the adoption of 'appropriate'

health- and illness-related behaviour. Freidson (1961: 146–7) writes:

> the process of seeking help involves a network of potential consultants from the intimate and informal confines of the nuclear family through successively more select, distant and authoritative lay-men [sic] until the 'professional' is reached. This network of consultants which is part of the structure of the local lay community, and which imposes form on the seeking of help, might be called the 'lay referral structure'. Taken together with the cultural understandings involved in the process we may speak of it as the 'lay referral system'.

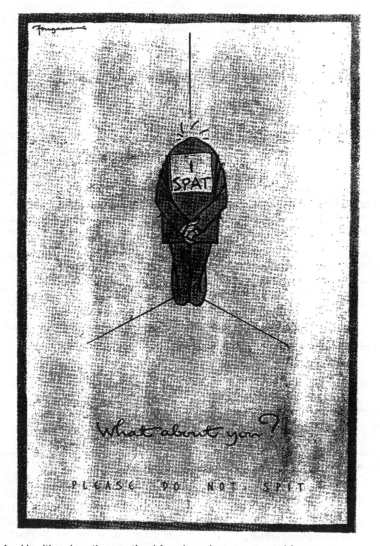

Illustration 3.1   Health education method for changing unacceptable norms

The LRS emphasizes two key factors that will determine the extent to which individual members of a community will make use of health services, namely, structure and culture. The interaction of these two factors is considered to differentially influence utilization of health services (see Table 3.1 opposite).

Label and libel – the nature of stigma

It is appropriate at this point to refer to a particularly important effect of social pressure on individual health – the question of stigma.

One of the major barriers preventing individuals seeking available help for curable and preventable conditions is the cultural conceptualization of particular diseases and the emotional reactions to these. To the extent that diseases are associated with culpable or antisocial actions or are considered to be due to the intervention of supernatural forces, anticipated public opprobrium – which may even take the form of violence – may militate against help-seeking behaviour. Such diseases as leprosy, TB and AIDS will immediately spring to mind in this regard. Following the formula for the power of social pressure discussed above, the existence of a

Table 3.1   *The lay referral system and service utilization*

Lay referral structure	Lay culture	
	Congruent with professional	Incongruent with professional
Loose truncated	A: medium high utilization	B: medium low utilization
Cohesive extended	C: highest utilization	D: lowest utilization

close-knit community will increase the perceived threat of disclosing the particular condition.

A comment by a respondent to a survey on TB in Nepal (Pool, 1992: 108) provides a flavour of the anticipated effects of stigma:

> if it is discovered in my district ... they would make me separate from the community as if I had leprosy. Where I live there isn't anywhere nearby to get good treatment and so leprosy people whatever they've touched isn't eaten, in fact anything they've touched or used is not touched or used by other people.' (... a student from the remote district of Mugu where there are few medical services).

Mass media pressures

More detailed analysis of the nature and effectiveness of mass media will be provided in Chapter 8. For the present, we will merely assert that the impact of the mediated norms of the larger culture transmitted in this way are likely to be considerably less effective than the other social influences discussed above.

Beliefs, motivations and normative pressures – interaction effects

Reference to Figure 3.3 (see page 79) above indicates that several points of overlap exist between these separate systems and the nature of the interaction is signalled by the various 'segments' numbered from 1 to 7.

Normative beliefs and motivation to comply

The normative system discussed above actually exerts its effect on behavioural intention via the mediation of both the belief and motivation systems. HAM follows the practice adopted by Fishbein and Ajzen (1975) as it is both theoretically satisfying and practically useful to separately identify

beliefs about normative pressures and motivation to conform to those pressures. According to Fishbein, individuals have a set of (salient and latent) beliefs about the likely reactions of key individuals to their intentions to act. However, this anticipated approval or disapproval by significant others will only affect their intention to act if they are also concerned about this approval or disapproval. If the others are not actually significant, they will have no influence. Segment 1 indicates beliefs about the reactions of others and segment 2 indicates motivation to comply.

In HAM, Fishbein and Ajzen's formulation has been extended to the remaining potential influences included in the motivation system. Accordingly, beliefs about the likely reactions of peer groups, awareness and beliefs about the nature of social norms and national norms transmitted by mass media will also contribute to intention to act, provided that the individual in question is also motivated to conform to these various social pressures.

According to the 'pressure gradient', the motivational effect of mass media norm sending is unlikely to be as powerful as interpersonal pressures, and any effect is likely to result from the individual's evaluation of the information content of the message.

Community norms – statistical and coercive characteristics

As with each of the systems identified in Figure 3.3 above, it would be possible for a researcher or onlooker to provide a relatively objective view of the reality of the factors contributing to an individual's intention to act and identify beliefs about that reality and the motivational levels associated with the beliefs. Similarly, it is possible to provide an objective view of what is 'statistically' normal in any given social system together with people's beliefs about normality and, of course, their motivation to conform to those perceived norms (Baric, 1969, 1974, 1975, and Baric et al., 1976).

Interaction of belief and motivation systems

The above discussion of the normative system describes a *particular* case of the mutual effects of beliefs and motivation. The belief and motivation systems in general routinely interact as a two-way influence process. As we emphasized earlier, beliefs represent subjective probabilities. These internalized probabilities may then trigger emotional states or generate attitudes to particular courses of action as a result of becoming 'affectively charged' by personal values. The strength of the ensuing intention to act will depend on the combined strength of beliefs and motivations that interact in a multiplicative fashion.

The most common health education interventions probably operate in a manner designed to influence people's beliefs in order to generate a level of motivation that will result in some approved action or actions. However, it is important to recall that, although beliefs influence motivation, motivation also influences beliefs. In short, people frequently engage in autistic thinking – that is, they typically believe what it is comfortable to believe. When faced with uncomfortable facts and experiences, they may well selectively attend to information that confirms their prejudices or is otherwise threatening. They may reinterpret and distort messages or indulge in defensive avoidance and denial. Earlier discussion of the phenomenon of dissonance also showed specifically how people may resort to autistic thinking in order to reduce the discomfort experienced when beliefs about self and behaviour are in conflict. Marcel Proust's observation (cited by Sutherland, 1987) provides an excellent example of the impermeability of human defences to unpalatable facts:

> The facts of life do not reach the place where our beliefs are to be found; nor do they bring them into existence; they cannot destroy them; they can inflict on them the continual violence of contradiction but they cannot weaken them; a family assaulted by successive avalanches of misery and sickness will not lose its faith either in the clemency of its God or in the skill of its physician.

We should also note that individuals may not only hold beliefs that *generate* motivation, but may actually have beliefs *about* motivation. This phenomenon is represented by segment 3 in Figure 3.3 above. For instance, in Marsh and Matheson's (1983) survey of adult smoking attitudes and behaviour, one of the most important factors determining whether or not smokers intended to quit smoking in the future was the belief they held about the unpleasant withdrawal symptoms they expected to experience and their anticipated loss of gratification. Thus, beliefs about effects significantly reduced their intention to act.

Segment 4 in Figure 3.3 also refers to individuals' beliefs about affect. In this case, it indicates their beliefs about the level of their motivation to comply with (or resist) normative pressures – for example, the degree of discomfort they expect to experience if they do not comply with a partner's wishes or choose to confront the smoking norms of their workmates.

Segments 5 and 6 indicate the relationships of belief and motivation systems respectively with the self. Segment 5 refers to what is normally described as the 'self concept' – that is, the sum total of individuals' beliefs about themselves as persons interacting with other persons and living in a given environment. Segment 6 describes what elsewhere we term 'self sentiment', which is the sum total of feelings individuals might have about themselves as people. This key motivational component is more commonly described as self-esteem. As we will see, it plays a central part in the principles and practice of health promotion.

The final segment – segment 7 – acknowledges the fact that individuals will typically be able to articulate their beliefs about the feelings they have about themselves – for example, acknowledging that their self-esteem is unrealistically low.

The triangle in Figure 3.3 describes the totality of the individual self and his or her personality as it might be revealed by observers, researchers or, more technically, in the results of various personality tests and profiles. This final influence on individual intentions to act will now be subjected to scrutiny.

EMPOWERMENT: A CRITICAL REVIEW OF THE DYNAMICS

In Chapter 1, we discussed ideological issues underpinning the definition and practice of health promotion. We examined the discourse of empowerment and argued that an empowerment model of health promotion should govern theory and practice. We now consider what might be involved in operationalizing empowerment so that we understand how philosophy might be translated into practice. Therefore, we will focus on what could be called the anatomy and dynamics of empowerment. We will do so within the framework of HAM, which, in short, locates self-empowerment within the interlocking systems of beliefs, motivations and normative influence. The conceptualization of empowerment, which concentrates on the facilitating or inhibiting effects of the physical, social and economic environment, shifts the focus on to the systems that determine whether or not 'empowered' intentions are translated into practice.

Defining the self concept

As we observed above, segment 5 in Figure 3.3 refers to the self concept. A number of these beliefs have especial significance for health status. For instance, body image (segment 6), can influence the self both positively and negatively. Moreover, low self-esteem may result in mental and physical illnesses, such as those associated with eating disorders. On the other hand, mental illness may create low self-esteem. Other beliefs contribute indirectly to health and our emphasis here will be on beliefs about susceptibility to negative outcomes and, more particularly, on beliefs about control, which are central to the process and state of empowerment. Nonetheless, given the importance of the notion of the self and the considerable amount of research, past and present, it is appropriate to give further consideration to this construct.

Defining the self

It is important to make the distinction between the self as perceived by an individual himself or herself and the self as he or she might appear in a pen portrait drawn by an external observer or be delineated in more objective fashion by a psychometric test. As mentioned above, segment 5 in Figure 3.3, refers to the former and represents the personal formulation of self and the extent to which individuals accept the accuracy and truth of that particular formulation.

From the perspective of health promotion theory and practice, there are two key issues. The first of these is the extent to which the self concept is a global construct rather than comprising an aggregate of different component parts (such as sexual attractiveness or intelligence). The second issue concerns the relationship between the self concept and self-esteem – including the possible tension between the formulation of an ideal self and an actual, perceived self.

The increased interest in the self concept in recent years – and the varieties of the subordinate concepts – are revealed by the number of instruments designed to measure these. For instance, Keith and Bracken's (1996) historical and evaluative review of instrumentation identifies some twenty scales and instruments in current use. In all events, the contemporary view is that the self concept has a structure that is derived from the substantial body of information that people have accumulated about themselves. This structure is multidimensional and hierarchical. It becomes increasingly differentiated over time as a result of age and experience. Shavelson and Marsh (1986), Song and Hattie (1984) and Hattie (1992) have produced influential taxonomies that illustrate both the differentiation and the hierarchical structure. Figure 3.7 summarizes this structure and, in relation to the 'academic' category, emphasizes, not only

the importance of school-related achievement, but also general intellectual competence and skills. It also indicates the importance of the interpersonal context (note, for instance, our earlier observations about peer group influence) and, of course, the prime importance of body image and the associated attributes of confidence and self-esteem. It is doubtless self-evident that taxonomies of this kind are essentially culturally constructed and, because of the origins of most of the research, tend to reflect North American values and ideals.

The self concept, susceptibility and risk taking

As mentioned earlier, beliefs about susceptibility to disease and its sequelae are a key feature of the HBM. In it, beliefs about susceptibility when associated with beliefs about the seriousness of disease generate a level of perceived threat (in HAM terms, an emotional state associated with the fear drive). This, in turn, allegedly leads to preventive action, provided beliefs about the benefits of that action are considered to outweigh the costs. Perception of susceptibility thus signals a specific belief about the self. The belief in question relates to risk. However, as with other beliefs, it reflects – and, quite frequently, may distort – objective reality. Accordingly, the unthinking use of this belief about vulnerability to predict cautious, preventive decision making may very well lead to dramatically inappropriate conclusions. First of all, a substantial amount of productive research effort has been devoted to the description of *objective* risk – that is, to the use of statistical techniques to accurately record the probabilities of particular activities and circumstances resulting in accidents or other negative consequences. Second, it is clear from equally sound research that individuals' perceptions of risks and beliefs about vulnerability are only imperfectly related to objective risk. For instance, there is a clearly demonstrated tendency to overestimate the likelihood of the unlikely and underestimate the real frequency of relatively common threats (Slovic et al., 1982, Lichtenstein et al., 1978, Weinstein, 1982, 1984, and Kasperson et al., 1988). One broad set of factors contributing to these misperceptions of threat has to do with faulty information processing and a lack of decision-making skills (Janis and Mann, 1977). For instance, the so-called 'availability heuristic' results in risk appraisal being biased by frequently reported, but not necessarily frequently occurring, events.

Again, affective factors often influence the interpretation of risk. The intuitive observation that young people consider themselves immortal is

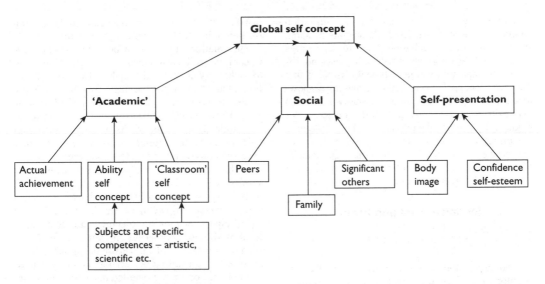

Figure 3.7 A taxonomy of the self

supported by academic research demonstrating that there is a tendency for people to underestimate the extent of their personal vulnerability to harm – what Weinstein (1982) termed 'unrealistic optimism' – a phenomenon often closely related to wish fulfilment!

By contrast, when frequent reporting of dangerous situations and disasters is accompanied by, for example, extensive media coverage in full and gory Technicolor, the availability heuristic can introduce the dread factor into beliefs about personal vulnerability. A further discussion of the inflation of perceptions of risk and associated feelings of threat is to be found in 'Social amplification of risk' theory (Kasperson et al., 1988).

An additional problem with a naïve interpretation of susceptibility is the fact that some individuals actively pursue risk. They would, by definition, not pursue it unless they believed that they were susceptible to some negative outcome. There are various explanations of the motivation for deliberate risk-seeking. One suggestion is that some individuals enjoy the physiological effects. To put it somewhat crudely, it would seem that they become addicted to these. Note, for instance, Delk's (1980: 134) reference to high-risk behaviour as, 'a form of tension-reduction behaviour with addictive qualities related to the build-up of intoxicating stress hormones'. This might well explain the attractions of ever more enervating theme park and fairground rides as on such rides there is adrenaline arousal accompanied by a belief that there is no real danger.

However, it would not account for other circumstances where risks are taken only when there is genuine danger. Lyng (1990) offers an interesting explanation of this phenomenon – one that is of particular interest in the context of our discussion of empowerment and control. He employs the term 'edgework', which is seen as a way of handling, 'the problem of negotiating the boundary between chaos and order.'

Lyng's analysis could be said to have a certain authority as it is based on participant observation as a jump pilot! He (1990: 856) asserts that all edgework involves:

> a clearly observable threat to one's physical or mental wellbeing or one's sense of an ordered existence. The archetypal edgework experience is one in which the individual's failure to meet the challenge at hand will result in death or, at the very least, debilitating injury.

He also argues that many features of drugtaking and even binge drinking do not involve self-destructive behaviour as such but, rather, an attempt to demonstrate mastery and control – both concepts that are central to the notion of empowerment, as we will demonstrate later.

The psychological analysis of susceptibility and risk taking described above poses a serious challenge for the HBM. It may also create a dilemma for those who espouse a narrow preventive model of public health. The paradoxical pursuit of control in hazardous circumstances can result in serious casualties, even when a damage-limitation approach is used and individuals are taught about safety procedures, including how to use drugs 'safely' and deal with an overdose. It poses no difficulty for an empowerment model, provided that there is evidence that risktakers are making empowered decisions. Clearly, if the casualty rate is so high as to impose too heavy a burden on society or risktakers put other people at risk, then, following the principle of utilitarianism, coercive measures may prove necessary. However, in the vast majority of circumstances, empowerment is healthy – both in positive and preventive terms.

Empowerment and health

Self-esteem and health

As we noted above, self-esteem is the affective counterpart of the self concept in the HAM. Indeed, a number of instruments to which reference was made in the discussion of the self concept above focus on self-esteem, such as Coopersmith's self-esteem inventories, the culture-free self-esteem inventories and Rosenberg's self-esteem scale.

It is virtually axiomatic that self-esteem has a significant effect on health – both directly and indirectly. For instance, self-esteem is typically considered a key feature of mental health and therefore worth pursuing in its own right. It may also contribute indirectly to health by contributing to intentions to undertake healthy or unhealthy actions. For instance, at a commonsense level, individuals who respect and value themselves will, other things being equal, seek to look after themselves by adopting courses of action that prevent disease. Less obviously perhaps, and pursuing earlier observations about cognitive dissonance, there is strong evidence that people enjoying high self-esteem are less willing to tolerate dissonance and more likely to take rational action to reduce that dissonance, by, for example, rejecting unhealthy behaviour (Aronson and Mettee, 1968). Again, those having low self-esteem are more likely to conform to interpersonal pressures than those enjoying high self-esteem (Aronson, 1976). Clearly, it would generally be considered unfortunate when such social pressure results in 'unhealthy behaviour'. In terms of empowerment, though, any unthinking yielding to social pressure would be considered unhealthy!

It is also worth noting that various aspects of the self concept contribute differentially to self-esteem. It is generally considered that a discrepancy between the ideal self and actual self is likely to generate low self-esteem (unless, of course, the individual has a sufficient belief in his or her capability to remedy that discrepancy – in which case, successfully bridging the gap will actually enhance self-esteem).

The relationship between body image and self-esteem is well recognized. Although, Hoge and McScheffrey (1991) and Marsh and Holmes (1990) found that children's self-esteem was more strongly related to social acceptance than physical appearance, Harter (1985; 1993) found the reverse to be true. Indeed, she reported that students' scores on global self-worth correlated above 0.60 with their perceived physical appearance, compared with 0.45 with their perceived social acceptance. This is not surprising given the widespread dissatisfaction with body image – particularly among young women – and its relationship with eating disorders and the use of cigarette smoking to achieve and maintain a level of slimness bordering on anorexia. However, such discrepancies are not surprising as self-esteem must reflect prevailing personal and cultural values and norms. For a more detailed discussion of social acceptance and the 'social self concept', see Berndt and Burgy (1996).

Self-esteem, then, can be influenced in various ways, one of the most important of which is a belief about being in control.

The case of learned helplessness and hopelessness

The phenomenon of learned helplessness was demonstrated by Seligman (1975: 9). 'Helplessness is the psychological state that frequently results when events are uncontrollable.' Even if something pleasurable happens to an individual, the sense of uncontrollability and the consequent helplessness will result if this 'reward' is not contingent on an individual's own actions (Seligman, 1975: 74).

> organisms, when exposed to uncontrollable events, learn that responding is futile. Such learning undermines the incentive to respond, and so it produces profound interference with the motivation of instrumental behaviour. It also proactively interferes with learning that responding works when events become uncontrollable, and so produces cognitive distortions. The fear of an organism faced with trauma is reduced if it learns that responding controls trauma; fear persists if the organism remains uncertain about whether trauma is controllable; if the organism learns that trauma is uncontrollable, fear gives way to depressions.

Lack of control therefore has three main effects:

- **cognitive** it disrupts the ability to learn
- **conative** it saps motivation to take action
- **affective** it produces emotional disturbance.

Seligman speculated on the physiological mechanisms affected by learned helplessness. At the time, this speculation seemed somewhat fanciful, but more recently interest has grown in the notion of 'biological transition'. For instance, Brunner (in Brunner et al., 1996) argued for a quite direct link between the lack of control experienced by the lower grades of civil servants in the second Whitehall Study (Marmot, in Brunner et al., 1996: 290) and specific physiological effects, postulating the existence of a pathway linking:

> the chronic stress response of the hypothalamic pituitary adrenal system with resulting elevated levels of corticosteroids to central obesity, insulin resistance, poor lipid profile and increased tendency for the blood to clot.

Again, Karasek and Theorell's (1990) 'job demand–control model' argues that a combination of heavy demands and limited decision latitude to moderate these demands results in 'job strain', which, in turn, creates various negative health consequences, including the dramatic and peculiarly Japanese *Karoshi* – stress death from overwork!

In all events, the general notion of helplessness is convincing. However, its original formulation was criticized, largely on the grounds that, clearly, individuals do not always subside into helplessness when they experience uncontrollability, even after frequent exposure to circumstances in which there is little consistency in the relationship between behaviour and the outcomes of that behaviour. Accordingly, a modification of the theory was suggested by Seligman and other researchers (Abramson et al., 1978, and Miller and Norman, 1979). The modification involved an emphasis on an individual's 'attribution of causality' – that is, their beliefs about what causes particular outcomes.

Empowerment and social malaise

The above comments relate in general to individual health. However, as will be apparent from the reference above to false consciousness, the pathological effects of disempowerment can be applied to notions of social health and, conversely, to social malaise. We will therefore return to this theme in the context of later discussions of *community* empowerment.

Indirect effects of empowerment on health – beliefs about control

As we have noted before, empowerment can be viewed as a health state in its own right – for both individuals and communities. A lack of empowerment can be seen as unhealthy and/or have direct negative physiological effects. More commonly, empowerment is considered to have an indirect effect on health by influencing individual and community action. In this context, it is viewed as involving both *actual* possession of power and *beliefs* about having power. Different kinds and levels of beliefs have been identified (see, for instance, Sarafino, 1990, and Lewis, 1987). The hierarchy below exemplifies these different levels.

- **Informational control** refers to the possession of information necessary for taking action.
- **Cognitive control** follows both Sarafino and Lewis' conceptualizations. According to Lewis, it relates to the acquisition of information that allows the intellectual management of an event and, thus, possibly reduces its threatening properties. In Sarafino's (1990: 113) words, it is:

> the ability to use thought processes or strategies to modify the impact of a stressor. These strategies can include thinking about the event differently or focusing on a pleasant or neutral thought or sensation. While giving birth, for instance, the mother might think about the event differently by going over in her mind the positive meanings the baby will give to her life.

- **Decisional control** refers to having opportunities to make decisions.
- **Behavioural control** indicates the possession of skills necessary for translating decisions into action. It can also be applied to the possession of skills to enhance 'cognitive control'.
- **Existential control** a term employed by Lewis in the context of patient education. It refers to a belief about the meaningfulness of circumstances rather than control proper.
- **Contingency control** of particular interest as it approximates to the concepts of 'locus of control' and 'self-efficacy'. It refers to individuals' beliefs that the outcomes of decision making and action are actually under their own control – that is, are contingent on their decision making.
- **Locus of control** perhaps the best-known and most influential conceptualization of control. It was developed by Rotter (1966) in the context of social learning theory. He named it 'perceived locus of control' (PLC) to emphasize the fact that it referred to a *subjective* probability rather than the *actual* degree of control possessed by individuals.

The purpose of empowerment strategies is, of course, to foster internality. Perhaps the most important aspect of this notion is the fact that beliefs or expectancies are generalized: they refer to a general tendency to believe that one is in charge of one's life (internal PLC) or, by contrast, generally powerless (external PLC). We should also note that there are two varieties of externality. First, a belief that one is controlled by chance, luck or fate and, second, that one's life is controlled by 'powerful others'.

Health locus of control

Of particular interest to health promotion is a variant on the notion of PLC in the form of 'health locus of control' (HLC). This originated with the work of Kirscht (1972), who developed measures of PLC specifically orientated towards health, and Wallston et al. (1976), who subsequently developed a more sophisticated version in the form of the 'multi-dimensional health locus of control scale (MHLC). Parcel and Meyer (1978) also produced a special version of MHLC for children.

The concept of perceived locus of control has been subjected to considerable scrutiny and, in 1982, Wallston and Wallston reported that, at the time of writing, there had been over 1000 published papers, in addition to 'a myriad of unpublished theses, dissertations and studies investigating the construct.' Researchers have examined the relationship between PLC and HLC and a range of health-related topics (such as health knowledge, smoking, birth control, weight loss, information-seeking and compliance, seatbelt use and so on). Some results were encouraging, though Wallston and Wallston considered that their (1982) review of *health* locus of control was disappointing.

A thorough review by Norman and Bennett (1996) also concluded that the predictive power of HLC is weak. Wallston himself concurs with this opinion, but, with a touch of irritation, voices his opinion that critics 'do not properly understand or appreciate the theoretical underpinnings of the construct' (1991: 251). Wallston makes the very important point that it is essential to consider HLC together with individuals' health values and other important constructs in any prediction equation, such as specific measures for 'self-efficacy', for example. In short, 'An individual's health behaviour is multidetermined; there is no sense kidding oneself that HLC is the most important determinant.'

Self efficacy – specific beliefs about control

The concept of self-efficacy is one of the most useful, and applicable, notions in social psychology. It is attributed primarily to Bandura (1977, 1982,

1986, 1992). Its relevance can be appreciated from Bandura's (1982: 122–3) own definition:

> Perceived self-efficacy is concerned with judgements of how well one can execute courses of action required to deal with prospective situations ... Self-percepts of efficacy are not simply inert estimates of future action. Self-appraisals of operative capabilities function as one set of proximal determinants of how people behave, their thought patterns, and the emotional reactions they experience in taxing situations. In their daily lives people continuously make decisions about what course of action to pursue and how long to continue those they have undertaken. Because acting on misjudgements of personal efficacy can produce adverse consequences, accurate appraisal of one's own capabilities has considerable functional value. Self-efficacy judgements, whether accurate or faulty, influence choice of activities and environmental settings. People avoid activities that they believe exceed their coping capabilities, but they undertake and perform assuredly those that they judge themselves capable of managing.

Self-efficacy is one of the most valuable and practical features of social cognitive theory (SCT) – an extension and elaboration of social learning theory. Its importance is reflected in the fact that it has been added to Fishbein and Ajzen's theory of reasoned action as a kind of bolt-on extra. The revised model was rebranded as the *Theory of Planned Behaviour* (Ajzen, 1991, and Conner and Sparks, 1996). It also forms a key part of the so-called 'ASE' (attitude social norm efficacy) model devised by researchers in the Netherlands (Kok et al., 1992), which emphasizes self-efficacy.

As noted earlier, SLT/SCT offers a simple but effective model of successful human agency. It includes the formula: action is the product of response efficacy and self-efficacy where response efficacy is the belief that a particular course or courses of action will result in the achievement of some desired outcome. It follows that self-efficacy refers to the individual's conviction that he or she is actually capable of undertaking the actions necessary to achieve the outcome. Self-efficacy, like PLC, is therefore what was described earlier as a contingency belief, though self-efficacy differs from PLC in its specificity. Perhaps due to this specificity, it is clear that single measures of self-efficacy can correlate substantially with behavioural outcomes. For instance, de Vries (1989) demonstrated a correlation of 0.71 with smoking outcomes. Self-efficacy is also useful in predicting outcomes in the field of rehabilitation. For example, Ewart (1992: 287) stated that interventions to improve self-efficacy enabled patients 'to cope more effectively with the many challenges posed by heart attack'. Holman and Lorig

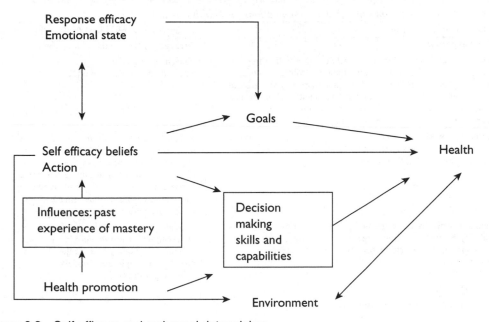

Figure 3.8 Self efficacy and reciprocal determinism

(1992: 305) asserted that, 'perceived self-efficacy to cope with the consequences of chronic disease is an essential contributor to developing self-management capabilities.'

The notion of 'reciprocal determinism' is also central to the formulation. In other words, there is a reciprocal relationship between the environment and the individual – each influences the other and outcomes depend on the results of that interaction. The interaction is expressed diagrammatically in Figure 3.8.

The assumption is made that individuals not only have beliefs about the nature of the health action and about the likelihood of their performing it, they also have beliefs about the extent to which they possess the skills and capabilities they need to achieve the health action goals. Self-efficacy beliefs can be influenced by, and also create, particular emotional states, such as shame or anxiety at the prospect of failure or failing to take any action because of lack of confidence.

As we mentioned above, response efficacy is also an affective factor related to an acceptance that the health action is a worthwhile goal. Active goal setting will occur to the extent that individuals believe they are capable of achieving them. Furthermore, they will have beliefs about the

relationship between the environment and the health action. They must accept that there is a reasonable probability of their being able to overcome any environmental barriers before they commit themselves to action. Typically, it will be necessary to have certain capabilities and skills related to the attainment of the desired outcome, including decision-making skills. If individuals do not believe that they possess these competences, their commitment to change will be reduced.

Self-efficacy beliefs will depend substantially on past experience of mastery – of success or failure. The role of health promotion is threefold. First, it aims to influence efficacy beliefs directly. Second, it aims to exercise an indirect influence by providing the competences and skills needed to carry out a health action and/or cope with environmental barriers. Third, it aims to remove those environmental barriers that militate against the formation of efficacy beliefs.

Influences and implications for health promotion

Bandura argues that there are four general factors influencing self-efficacy beliefs. They are (in

Table 3.2 *Influences on self-efficacy – implications for health promotion*

Influences on self-efficacy	Examples of implications for health promotion
Direct experience	Arrange experience through role play
Physiological state 'People rely partly on information from their physiological state in judging their capabilities. ... Fear reactions generate further fear through anticipatory self arousal. By conjuring up fear-provoking thoughts about their ineptitude, people can rouse themselves to elevated levels of distress that produce the very dysfunctions they fear'	Anticipatory guidance Stress management techniques
Verbal persuasion 'is widely used to try to talk people into believing they possess capabilities that will enable them to achieve what they seek'	Various, well-recognized attitude change techniques, such as using credible sources, appropriate message style, right level of emotional arousal, minimizing reactance. *Beware*: changes may be short-lived and this strategy is not empowering and of dubious ethicality!
Vicarious efficacy information 'information conveyed by modelled events ... people judge their capabilities partly by comparing their performances with those of others'	A recommended strategy involving observational learning. People's efficacy beliefs can be changed after they observe credible/'homophilous' models achieving success
Direct experience	

Source: Quotations are from Bandura, 1986: 399ff

descending order of power) direct experience, vicarious experience, verbal persuasion and physiological state. These are listed in Table 3.2 in conjunction with implications for health promotion.

Personality and behavioural intention

Personality is included in the portrayal of 'self' in the HAM. It is considered to be one of the factors contributing to behavioural intention. Personality differs from other psychological constructs in that it refers to the relatively fixed and enduring attributes of the individual. These attributes may be described in terms of 'traits', which may be further classified into 'types' and 'profiles'. Despite some earlier dalliance with attempts to link personality with health-related behaviour, traditional analyses of personality have not been considered to be particularly useful in health promotion, although an article in the *Financial Times* (20 March 2002) recorded an example of the use of psychoanalytical personality theory in the promotion of cigarettes!

> In exchange for a large fee, the psychoanalyst A.A. Brill explained to Bernays' (an adviser to the advertising industry – and, incidentally, a nephew of Sigmund Freud) 'that the cigarette was a symbol of the penis and male sexual power. Inspired by this insight, Bernays briefed the press about an imminent women's rights protest, and then persuaded a group of wealthy debutantes to take part in New York City's Easter day parade and, at his signal, light up some Lucky Strikes. The photographs in the following day's papers were

captioned 'torches of Freedom', and sales of cigarettes to women soon began to rise.

We will make some further reference to the use of 'depth psychology' in advertising in our discussion of mass media in Chapter 8. We will therefore limit ourselves here to noting four instances where aspects of personality do seem to affect intentions and action to a greater or lesser extent.

Coherence, hardiness and resilience

The existence of a 'Hardy Personality' has been identified (for example, Kobasa, 1979) and it is of interest to our present discussion as its three major characteristics have special relevance to our discussion of empowerment and, in its reference to 'challenge', to radical health promotion. Hardiness has three main features:

- a sense of **personal control** to all intents and purposes, this is identical to locus of control
- **commitment** a sense of purpose and involvement with community and life in general
- **challenge** change is viewed as opportunity.

In addition to its similarity to Antonovsky's 'sense of coherence' (SOC, to which reference was made in Chapter 1), it is also virtually synonymous with the notion of 'resilience', which was used by Garmezy (1983) to describe children who grow to be competent and well-adjusted adults despite adverse circumstances. Studies of resilient children have recorded, with some surprise, a tendency for them to recover rapidly from adversity, be well adjusted, have good social skills and, above all, a sense of personal control and relatively high self-esteem. All this despite experiencing horrific circumstances, including being raised by dysfunctional families, being abused and even growing up in concentration camps (see, for instance, Werner, 1987). It is difficult to account for such phenomena when they are so inconsistent with the received wisdom of theories of learned helplessness. To the extent that such characteristics do reflect personality, it would seem necessary to have recourse to explanation in terms of inherited, 'temperamental' traits.

Type A and B personalities

Another contender for the title of personality type is related to the Type A and Type B behaviour patterns that are considered important by some researchers because of their associations with a predisposition, or not, to coronary heart disease (Friedman and Rosenman, 1974).

A full description of these personality types is not necessary here. However, we should perhaps note that their importance rests on a robust association with heart disease. A Type A personality has been defined as, 'an excess of free-floating hostility, competitiveness, and time urgency' (Bennett and Murphy, 1997: 20) and its significance has been demonstrated by such studies as that of the Western Collaborative Group Study. This research demonstrated that those assessed as Type As carried twice the risk for heart disease as Type Bs, after controlling for other risk factors such as smoking (Rosenman et al., 1975).

The sensation-seeking personality

Another psychological construct having pretensions to a personality trait or type – and relevance for health promotion – is the concept of 'sensation seeking'.

It is assumed that individuals vary in the extent to which they actively seek sensations and Zuckerman (1990) developed a sensation-seeking scale (SSS). Bearing in mind earlier observations about risk taking and phenomena such as edgework, the reality of this personality characteristic is of some importance to health promoters (and creates still more tension for the HBM's notion of susceptibility). Table 3.3 provides a flavour of the operationalization of sensation seeking.

Thuen (1994) assessed the relationship between a modified sensation-seeking scale and injury related behaviour and concluded that there was indeed a strong relationship, 'well above ... the typical correlations between personality trait and behaviours.'

Table 3.3 *Sample items from the sensation-seeking scale (SSS)*

Categories of sensation-seeking	Examples
Thrill and adventure seeking	*'I would like to try parachute jumping'*
Experience seeking	*'I like to try new foods I have never tried before'*
Disinhibition	*'I often like to get high (drinking liquor or smoking marijuana)'*
Boredom susceptibility	*'I like people who are sharp and witty, even if they do sometimes insult others'*

Source: Thuen, 1994

Radicalism v. conservatism and related social characteristics

One final example of personality traits relevant to health promotion relates to social values. It is not that relevant to the adoption of preventive health actions, but, rather, to the ideological values that underpin policy development and implementation.

Cattell (1966) identified two of his sixteen personality factors that might predispose individuals towards particular models of health promotion. One of these (Factor Q.1) he called radicalism v. conservatism. Measures to assess this trait included such items as, 'Our greatest need today is that all people should learn birth control', and, 'People who are certain to pass on serious hereditary defects should be compulsorily sterilized.' Cattell also identified a related trait that described a 'tough-minded v. tender-minded' tendency (rather esoterically termed *Premsia* v. *Harria*!)

Eysenck (1960) incorporated these traits into a two-dimensional model that he argued would help explain political orientation. For instance, a tough-minded radical would favour communism, while tough-minded conservatism would characterize a fascist tendency. Readers might care to experiment with applying this typology to professional colleagues of their acquaintance!

TRANSLATING INTENTION INTO PRACTICE: REMOVING BARRIERS AND EMPOWERING COMMUNITIES

The discussion so far has centred on self-empowerment and examined various psychological characteristics associated with those personal capabilities and characteristics that help an individual gain control over his or her life and health. However, bearing in mind the paramount importance of reciprocal determinism, it is not possible to seek to facilitate individuals' empowerment without paying due attention to the nature of the environment. Indeed, to do so is merely to engage in a more sophisticated form of victim-blaming. Accordingly, we will now consider what is involved in translating behavioural intentions into action.

Assuming that the complex of multiple influences between self, belief, motivation and normative systems have resulted in an intention to act, it is imperative to consider what more is needed to maximize the chances of individuals achieving the goals they have set for themselves. However, let us not forget – and taking account of the principles of self-efficacy – that an individual's beliefs about the nature and strength of environmental barriers and deficits may cause the intention to act to be aborted. Returning to HAM (shown in Figure 3.3 on page 79), it will be seen that three kinds of facilitating factors may be necessary before intention is translated into practice (or, conversely, three kinds of barriers may need to be removed). These will now be reviewed.

Facilitating health actions – knowledge and skills

Different functions of knowledge

In terms of HAM, it is important to clarify the two different contributions made to health choices by knowledge. The first concerns the acquisition of information that may influence the formation of beliefs – this may, ultimately, contribute to an intention to act. The second of these merely involves providing the information that people who are already committed to taking action need to help them translate their intention to act into practice.

With regard to the first of these two contributions made by knowledge, it is important to remember that knowledge alone, although necessary, will very rarely be *sufficient* to lead to behaviour. As we noted earlier, knowledge rarely leads to practice without, at the very least, a shift in attitude. We might also observe that, frequently, a positive attitude to making a particular health choice may lead to a search for knowledge to clarify and support the tentative intention to act. In such a case, it would not be a K-A-P progression, but, rather, an A-K-I-P progression (from attitude to knowledge to intention to practice!) It is often said that knowledge is power, but this is true only up to a point. Knowledge may play but a small part in empowering progress from intention to action. For example, while it is true that knowing about the existence of family planning clinics offering contraceptive advice might be essential to the routine adoption of condom use, social skills would also be necessary to interact confidently and assertively with professional staff – and, more importantly, to negotiate condom use with a partner.

The importance of skills

There is no precise definition of skills in general – apart from an implication that they are goal-directed and would be applied to some practical purpose. However, a number of specific skills can be precisely identified, together with the conditions needed to acquire proficiency. The box contains a summary of the key skills of concern to health promotion.

SKILLS FOR EMPOWERMENT

Cognitive skills

- **Literacy** As Freire famously demonstrated, de-powered people view the ability to read and write as virtually magical. The possession of these skills is intrinsically empowering, apart from their specific use in writing letters of complaint to members of Parliament and so on. Despite the current inappropriate and sloppy use of the term, 'health literacy' is clearly an important application of the general skill (being able to read and comprehend written health-related communications, for example).
- **Decision-making skills** i.e. competences associated with cognitive problem-solving, such as using a *minimax* strategy to calculate the costs and benefits of particular courses of action.

(Continued)

(Continued)

Psycho-motor skills

- Skills involving the integration of perception and movement, such as the kinds of hand-eye coordination involved in the correct use of a condom, using a hypodermic syringe in the control of diabetes, administering first aid procedures, such as those necessary in connection with a harm minimization strategy for substance misuse.

Social interaction skills

- **Life skills** The term 'life skills' is used to describe the use of skilled responses to a range of social situations (the term 'health skills' may also be used to refer to specific health-related scenarios). Although, 'life skills' also incorporates applied knowledge and understanding, its emphasis is on the acquisition and practice of various skills, but particularly social interaction skills, such as how to deal with housing officials or how to work in groups and organize for radical social action.
- **Assertiveness** Because of its history and nature, assertiveness and assertiveness training occupies a special place in radical health promotion. It comprises a valuable package of the knowledge and skills needed to achieve desired goals while, at the same time, recognizing other people's needs and rights. It is, therefore, not only technically relevant to empowerment, it is also congruent with its philosophy. Indeed, the word 'assertiveness' derives from the Latin *asserere*, meaning 'to declare one's slave free by the laying on of hands'. Highly appropriate!

Empowerment – the role of the environment

The significance of environmental factors in determining health status has been emphasized on a number of occasions in this book and will, therefore, be mentioned only briefly here. Clearly, failure to address physical, social, economic and cultural circumstances is to unwittingly blame the victim whose health suffers from those circumstances and whose scope for action is dramatically impeded by them. Although the empowerment techniques that are involved in fortifying individuals – by influencing their beliefs (predominantly about self) and furnishing them with skills – are an essential part of the empowering process, people will not find themselves in control of their lives and health so long as barriers remain and the environment in which people live and work does not actively conspire 'to make the healthy choice the easy choice'.

The physical environment ranges from the drastic effects of natural and man-made disasters and the debilitating effect of squalor and preventable disease to access to clean water supplies and user-friendly health services, from smoke-free public places to wide availability of condoms – in a machine or (as was the case in certain African workplaces) in the pay packet. As we described earlier at some length, the socio-economic environment includes the prevalence of poverty and its byproducts and, particularly, the insidious effects of inequalities and inequity. The socio-cultural environment includes those various normative practices that are intrinsically unhealthy and inconsistent with global imperatives validated by international organizations such as the United Nations and WHO.

The empowerment model of health promotion to which we subscribe in this book (described in Chapter 1), is premised on a need for action for self-empowerment, but, importantly for empowerment, directed at social and environmental change. One of the main strategies is the Ottawa Charter principle of the creation of 'active participating communities'. We now consider factors associated with the empowerment of communities and their relationships with the larger social system. First, we will consider the meaning of sick and healthy societies.

Healthy societies and communities

In our discussion of the determinants of health in Chapter 2, reference was made to the popular notion of social capital. As we noted, social capital is typically viewed as a feature of a healthy society, just as financial capital can be considered to contribute to *economic* 'health'. It will doubtless be apparent that, although some difference in emphasis may be discerned, the key features of social capital are virtually synonymous with what has been described previously in terms such as sense of community, trust and participation. We will not, therefore, repeat our earlier observations about social capital, but give some thought to the meaning of these parallel ideas and concerns.

At one level, it can be argued that a healthy society or community is an empowered one. Accordingly, it is important to look more closely at what are considered to be the key features of such a community. As it happens, some people might consider that a community is, by definition, healthy – or at least if the standard definition is used, which characterizes a 'genuine' community as a relatively small aggregate of people (probably in a relatively small geographical locality or neighbourhood) that has both a tightly knit network of relationships and a common sense of identity. The reference to a sense of identity is more commonly described as a 'sense of community' and this is frequently seen as highly desirable. However, while a sense of community might well be a feature of an empowered one, the converse is not necessarily true. Indeed, individuals may recognize that they are part of a social group and, for instance, take some comfort from their awareness of sharing a common predicament. This is not empowering, particularly if we accept the premises of social control by means of false consciousness!

Another paradox related to the apparently healthy effects of a sense of community is illustrated by consideration of religious communities. The phenomenon was revealed by Maton and Rappaport's (1984) investigation into empowerment among members of a 'Christian, non-denominational religious setting'. The members of the community in question clearly demonstrated their access to 'social capital' and were undoubtedly active. They enjoyed the benefits of a sense of coherence in terms of emotional meaningfulness, but, in their dependence on God, it is arguable whether or not they were really empowered, in the sense of being in control of their lives. As Banfield (1958: 109) puts it, 'Where everything depends upon luck or the caprice of a saint ... on divine intervention, there is no point in community action. The community, like the individual, may hope or pray, but it is not likely to take its destiny into its own hands.'

In a more secular context, Kindervatter (1979: 62) emphasizes the key elements of an empowered community as being, 'People gaining an understanding of and control over social, economic and/or political forces in order to improve their standing in society.' Rappaport (1987: 130) declared that empowerment was not just an individual attribute but also:

an organizational, political, sociological, economic, and spiritual [construct]. Our interests in racial and economic justice, in legal rights as well as in human needs, in healthcare and educational justice, in competence as well as in a sense of community, are all captured by the idea of empowerment. The reason we care about fostering a society whose social policies appreciate cultural diversity ... is that we recognize that it is only in such a society that empowerment can be widespread. We are as much concerned with empowered organizations, neighbourhoods, and communities as we are with empowered individuals.

Participation and empowerment

Reference was made earlier to the Ottawa Charter's emphasis on the virtues of empowered, participating communities. The question might legitimately be asked whether empowered communities generate participation or participation creates empowerment – and, ultimately, action. Kieffer (1984: 31) considered that the empowered state consisted of 'an abiding set of commitments and capabilities which can be referred to as participatory competence.' The effects of this were believed to be:

- the development of a positive self concept
- a more critical understanding of the surrounding social and political environment
- the cultivation of individual and collective resources for social and political action.

Additional discussion of empowering communities features in our discussion of community development in Chapter 8.

Empowerment and the avoidance of relapse

It can be seen from HAM that the single time choice of a specific health action is not the end of the story. Although there are instances where they are all that is required – for instance, attendance at a clinic for a one-off vaccination – the more common requirement is that the health action should be sustained and become adopted as a 'routine'. Once this has happened, the results of that choice may be confirmed. 'Outcome efficacy' may be confirmed and individuals may continue to enjoy the benefits of the health action to which they have committed themselves. Not unusually, though, an individual may discover that the anticipated benefits fail to materialise result or actual loss of gratification or discomfort may be experienced. In short, relapse may occur.

Relapse is traditionally associated with various kinds of addiction (a term that, we admit, is open to several interpretations) and it is worth, at this juncture, giving some thought to the applicability of a popular explanatory model – the 'transtheoretical model' (see above). We will also consider its relationship to the conceptual schema used in HAM.

A useful summary of the model is provided by Prochaska et al. (1997) and its origins are revealing. Prochaska and colleagues carried out detailed analyses of some 300 different theories of psychotherapeutic interventions and identified 10 processes of change. The model scanned these theories and processes (hence, 'trans'), then combined and reformulated them.

While the model can be applied to any behaviour, it has been most frequently applied to those health actions involving the sacrifice of gratification and the experience of discomfort, which create the consequent likelihood of relapse. So, smoking, alcohol and substance misuse, eating problems and obesity feature prominently in research using the model.

A key feature of TTM is its assumption that individuals move through a series of stages but may relapse at almost any time. However, there is a high level of probability that many will move again from a stage of (temporary) 'precontemplation' and proceed through the various stages once more until, hopefully, they will be successful. The reason for the phrase 'revolving door model' being used as a synonym for TTM is thus doubtless apparent.

Another point of considerable importance is that interventions designed to achieve behaviour change must be tailored to the individual and, therefore, take account of the particular stage that they have reached in their behaviour change career. Rollnick et al. (1992) provide a good example of such tailoring in their use of the technique 'brief motivational interviewing'.

Prochaska et al. (1997) provide an extensive list of approaches and techniques that have been used to maximize success and minimize the chance of relapse – including not only individual methods, such as 'consciousness-raising' and 'counterconditioning', but also what they term 'social liberation' – broader, 'primary preventive' social measures to influence social norms that foster unhealthy behaviour.

How does the TTM relate to HAM? Clearly, it relates well to the confirmation/relapse pathway that follows the period of 'trying out' the health action in question. The process of developing a routine – especially where the health action is problematic – may take some time. Following Prochaska's comment about the move from 'maintenance' to 'termination', it may take between six months and five years! On the other hand, as the precontemplation stage describes the state existing prior to the formation of an intention to adopt a healthy course of action, HAM's analysis of the complex of beliefs, motivations, norms and factors associated with self and personality demonstrates that, at this point, the TTM analysis is somewhat superficial!

Returning to our focus on empowerment, one of the empowering approaches to minimize relapse involves attribution theory and, more specifically, reattributing individuals' perceptions of the nature of the barriers to maintain their avoidance of negative behaviour, such as overeating or other 'addictions'.

As we mentioned earlier, one of the factors influencing adult males' intentions to give up smoking was the belief that they would be unable to cope with the loss of gratification and the side-effects of their dependence on tobacco (Marsh and Matheson, 1983). However, Davies (1992) has suggested (admittedly, a decidedly idiosyncratic point of view!) that it is unhelpful to view behaviour such as substance misuse or overeating in terms of overwhelmingly powerful drive-like states. The title of his book – *The Myth of Addiction* – is revealing. What seems to be necessary is a reattribution of beliefs! Of course, those who believe they are suffering withdrawal symptoms and consider that they crave their chosen substance, would doubt the truth of Davies' view! As we mentioned earlier, our view is that the motivation system comprises qualitatively different motivators, requiring qualitatively different methods to achieve given outcomes.

'DON'T BLAME HIM, HE'S JUST A POOR SEX ADDICT'

When Valerie Harkess was faced with her toughest question (why *did* you go back and sleep with Alan Clark...) she opted for the twentieth-century equivalent of seeking sanctuary in a holy place. 'I suppose I was addicted to him,' she said. In other words – I need help, not condemnation. I have taken the vows of victimhood. You cannot touch me here....

(Continued)

(Continued)

The general implication is that if you're in the grip of an addiction you are not culpable. What you do might be reprehensible, but the blame for it resides not in you but in your disease.... So though Michael Douglas might once have been described as a fornicator and libertine, he now issues a press release stating that he has checked into a clinic to have treatment for sex addiction. Poor thing, we are supposed to think, how brave he is to fight it. Where can we send our donations to help us to stamp out this terrible illness?...

Oddly enough there doesn't seem to be a similar get-out for money – no counsel has *yet* dared to step forward and argue that his client is hopelessly addicted to used notes and is conscientiously attending meetings of Cashaholics Anonymous. This is probably because the compulsive acquisition of money is socially sanctioned anyway, so that moral distinctions are reserved for ways of getting hold of it. But in almost every other sphere of moral action the rule holds good. If you're hooked, you're off the hook.

Sutcliffe, 1994

Empowerment and self control

We have already reiterated the point that a number of different, empowering life skills are frequently necessary to facilitate individuals' intentions to adopt health practices. HAM incorporates one particular class of life or health skills that are similar to some of the intervention measures identified by Prochaska. These are skills derived from a long tradition of work in behaviour modification and are here termed self-regulatory skills.

Empowerment is ultimately concerned with self-determination and, at the risk of saying this one too many times, environmental factors may limit the possibility of self-determination. On the other hand, individuals can exercise a good deal of personal control. In short, freedom of will can be a reality. Central to the achievement of personal control are 'self-referent cognitions' – that is, beliefs about oneself – that also include 'meta cognitions' – the uniquely human capacity to think about thought and reflect on reflections.

The paramount importance of Bandura's application of the concept of self-efficacy in understanding how people can successfully interact with their environment doubtless needs no reiteration either. Not surprisingly, Bandura (1989: 1182) comments on the importance of self-efficacy beliefs in relation to self-regulation.

Self-generated influences operate deterministically on behaviour the same way as external sources of influence do. Given the same environmental conditions, persons who have developed skills for accomplishing many options and are adept at regulating their own motivation and behaviour are more successful in their pursuits than those who have limited means of personal agency. It is because self-influence operates deterministically on action that some measure of self-directedness and

freedom is possible ... Self-regulatory functions are personally constructed from varied experiences not simply environmentally implanted ... Through their capacity to manipulate symbols and to engage in reflective thought, people can generate novel ideas and innovative actions that transcend their past experiences. They bring influence to bear on their motivation and action in efforts to realize valued futures.

With respect to our current discussion, the 'valued futures' mentioned by Bandura above include freedom from addictions. Traditionally, behaviour modification has been employed to deal with these powerful drives. It has its roots in behaviourist attempts (typically in competition with counselling interventions derived from psychoanalysis) to deal with various kinds of mental illness, such as phobias and compulsive behaviour. Following, for example, Skinnerian 'operant conditioning theory', psychologists were concerned to shape unwanted and unhealthy behaviour into that which was acceptable to therapists, their clients (and society as a whole). Many of the methods used – such as counter conditioning by means of electric shock – would seem to be diametrically opposed to the ethics and practice of empowerment. However, more recent developments have switched the emphasis away from 'therapist control' to 'client control'. This was doubtless partly due to the problems of finding enough psychologists to meet clients needs, but also reflected an acceptance of the importance of self-regulation. In fact, in its review of the morality of health education interventions, the Society of Public Health Education (SOPHE, 1976) agreed that *client contract* behaviour modification (our emphasis) was ethically acceptable along with communication and community development. In short, the DIY version of behaviour modification aimed to put clients in charge of their own 'therapy' and this approach has become integrated into various health-promotion methods concerned with fostering behaviour change.

Kanfer and Karoly (1972) were among the first to address the apparent paradox of employing behaviour modification techniques to achieve voluntaristic outcomes. They pointed out, for instance, how certain tactics that achieved desired behaviour change goals, at least in the short term, did not involve genuine self-control – that is, empowered decision making. They (1972: 408) noted, too, that genuine self-control occurs only when:

> an individual alters or maintains his behavioral chain in the absence of immediate external supports ... Once an obese person has put a lock on the refrigerator or the alcoholic mixed an emetic in his drink [external factors] are sufficient to account for the resulting behaviour.

Returning to observations made in Chapter 1 on voluntarism, it is interesting to note the parallel between these coercive measures at the micro level and the coercive potential of healthy public policy. This may go considerably further than making 'the healthy choice the easy choice' by seeking to make it the only choice!

Before considering the key skills needed to achieve self-regulation of behaviour, it is worth recalling that the kinds of behaviour currently under consideration are those where:

- a change in relatively recently adopted health actions occur as a result of significant reduction in gratification or the experience of significant aversive consequences
- where the emergence of a competing motivation of superior strength results in an undesirable behaviour.

An example of the first situation is provided by experience of negative effects after giving up smoking or when vigorous exercise proves painful. The second situation is illustrated by times when the sex drive overrides the motivating force of moral value and/or concern at the prospect of infection in the context of an unanticipated romantic encounter.

Self-regulatory skills – a model

Figure 3.9 (on page 104) seeks to describe key features of self-regulation in the particular context of combating relapse.

An essential feature of many, if not most, situations where people are seeking to change their behaviour is the provision of 'anticipatory guidance'. This term can be used to describe the whole

package – including the provision of skills. It is used here to refer to providing 'cognitive control' – that is, a degree of empowerment by giving individuals a grasp of what will be involved in the aftermath of choice. More important is the use of methods to generate appropriate self-efficacy beliefs – for example, by using models, those who have successfully moved through the 'maintenance' stage and reached 'termination' (for instance, ex-smokers who have not smoked for more than one year), in group discussions with clients.

A recommended and standard procedure for achieving self-control is the formulation of a contract between trainer and client. As with any contract, there is a process of negotiation and mutual agreement about the responsibilities and commitments of trainer and client, including what the client is prepared to do. The contract might actually be written or merely involve a verbal discussion. The procedure might involve contingency contracting. Examples of this include a cash deposit that will only be refunded once the target behaviour has been attained.

It is usually agreed that three key processes are involved in the acquisition of a repertoire of self-regulatory skills:

- self-monitoring
- self-evaluation
- self-reinforcement.

It is generally accepted that, in order, ultimately, to handle motivational problems, clients should first of all be involved in conscious monitoring of behaviour and associated feelings. Monitoring involves paying attention to, and correctly interpreting, external environmental cues and internal, physiological events. For example, clients might ascribe the surge of excitement and gastronomic arousal to the display in the pâtisserie window prior to their succumbing to temptation!

'Proprioception' – the interpretation of internal states – is not only part of acquiring motor skills, it is also important in acquiring self-control skills. The individual learns to become aware of autonomic responses and associated thought processes. In self-monitoring, therefore, feedback is received from external stimuli, one's own behaviour and internal cognitive, affective and autonomic processes.

Self-evaluation consists of comparing self-monitored data with some standard of performance and judging the adequacy of the overall performance. This judgement then serves as a discriminating stimulus for either positive or negative reinforcement. In other words, the performance in the pâtisserie may serve as a cause of self-congratulation or harbinger of guilt!

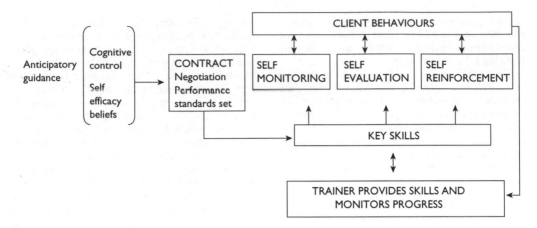

Figure 3.9   Self regulation of health actions

Perhaps the most problematic of the three processes is that of 'self-reinforcement'. The key task is somehow to override the reinforcing qualities of the unwanted behaviour with some replacement reinforcer. The powerful gratifications delivered by the cream cake must somehow be reduced and/or replaced with a more powerful reinforcer. Unfortunately, it is often difficult to find a really enticing alternative. For instance, some of the suggestions offered in leaflets designed to help smokers quit their habit are distinctly uninspiring, such as,

to take your mind off your need for a cigarette, doodle with a paperclip, suck a mint or take a brisk walk!

Thoresen and Mahoney (1974) devote many pages to self-reinforcement and note four major categories, as shown in the box.

Readers may experience some doubts about the widespread applicability or acceptability of the tactics described in the box and less demanding reinforcement schedules would be more commonly used, such as public praise from peers or even self-satisfaction at meeting goals.

FOUR CATEGORIES OF SELF-REINFORCEMENT

- **Positive self-reward** The self administration or consumption of a freely available reinforcer only after performance of a specific, positive response, such as treating oneself to a special event after having lost weight
- **Negative self-reward** The avoidance of, or escape from, a freely avoidable aversive stimulus only after performance of a specific, positive response, such as removing an uncomplimentary pig poster from one's dining room whenever a diet is adhered to for a full day
- **Positive self-punishment** The removal of a freely available reinforcer after the performance of a specific, negative response, such as tearing up a dollar bill for every 100 calories in excess of one's daily limit
- **Negative self-punishment** The presentation of a freely avoidable aversive stimulus after the performance of a specific, negative response, such as presenting oneself with a noxious odour after each occurrence of snacking

Thoresen and Mahoney, 1974: 22

THE TRULY FREE INDIVIDUAL

the truly 'free' individual is one who is in intimate contact with himself [sic] and his environment (both internal and external). He knows 'where he's at' in terms of the factors influencing both his actions and his surroundings. Moreover, he has acquired technical skills that enable him to take an active role in his own growth and adjustment. He is no mechanical automaton passively responding to environmental forces. He is a personal scientist, a skilled engineer capable of investigating and altering the determinants of his actions.

Thoresen and Mahoney, 1974: 144

Self-reinforcement will frequently be supplemented by attempts to break the stimulus–response link between situation and gratification. Dieters might be advised not to shop when hungry and smokers might be advised to break habitual links. Roberts (1969), for instance, claimed success in reducing smoking by having his clients restrict their smoking to a special 'non-smoking chair', which is, preferably, located in a rather uninspiring setting such as a chilly outhouse away from family and friends. This stratagem not only breaks the stimulus–response link, but adds a dash of negative reinforcement!

One of the important issues in developing self-regulatory skills is the extent to which a skilled counsellor/trainer should be involved. For instance, as Kok et al. (1992) point out, it is important that attributions *after* failure should not lead to disillusionment. They cite Hospers et al. (1990), who demonstrate that people whose attributions of their failure are 'internal, stable and uncontrollable' are likely to feel that they lack the willpower to lose weight. The task of the trainer would be to change the attribution to 'unstable, internal and controllable' in order to reduce that expectation of failure and the associated guilt or anger that might be felt. Successful counselling would thus create higher persistence, hopefully leading to ultimate success. Attempts have been made to provide mediated help and guidance for individuals via booklets and computers, for example, that are based on targeting individuals and tailoring messages to their apparent needs, often in the context of a 'stages of change' analysis. Success in this endeavour would certainly be cost-effective, but the potential of such approaches must still be treated with a degree of scepticism.

PROGRAMME PLANNING AND THE DETERMINANTS OF ACTION

In this chapter, in our discussion of communication of innovations theory, we have examined in some detail major factors governing the adoption of new practices at the level of social systems. However, the bulk of the chapter has paid particular attention to the determinants of individual health actions – especially from an empowerment perspective. It will doubtless be self-evident that any systematic and thoughtful attempts at devising effective interventions and programmes must categorically take account of these various influences on individuals and social systems. Indeed, understanding the determinants of health actions is essential if we are to develop effective and efficient interventions to influence those underlying factors that govern our health- and illness-related choices.

This principle does not apply only to individual behaviour change. Indeed, in accordance with our commitment to empowerment, we need to understand which characteristics of individuals and social systems can be influenced in order to enable them to gain control over their environmental and social circumstances.

Empowerment and the principle of reciprocal determinism are central to this endeavour. We are all influenced by our environments at macro and meso levels and many of us are in a position to reciprocate and exercise power over our physical, social and economic circumstances. Regrettably, too many people have little influence in these areas and react passively to those circumstances. Understanding the determinants of powerlessness is therefore of special importance and using that understanding to develop empowering health promotion programmes must constitute our major *raison d'être*.

In the chapters that follow, we will be discussing models that might be used in planning efficient health promotion programmes. In Chapter 5, we seek to demonstrate that it is not only necessary to understand the determinants of health action but also important to use such 'evidence', together with other strategic information, for our programme planning.

4

A Systematic Approach to Health Promotion Planning

Lose this day loitering – t'will be the same story
Tomorrow – and the next more dilatory;
Each indecision brings its own delays,
And days are lost lamenting o'er lost days.

Are you in earnest? seize this very minute –
Boldness has genius, power and magic in it.
Only engage, and then the mind grows heated –
Begin it, and then the work will be completed!

Johann Wolfgang von Goethe (1749–1832)
from *Faust* translated by John Anster

CONTENT OF CHAPTER 4

INTRODUCTION

The basic premise of this chapter is that well-planned interventions are more likely to be effective than any others. A number of recent developments have placed greater emphasis on the importance of a systematic approach to health promotion planning. These include the need for greater economic accountability, a target-driven climate and the general move towards evidence-based practice. Furthermore, within the UK, the adoption of market principles for commissioning services that accompanied the health service reforms of the early 1990s led to a contract culture that required greater attention to the formal planning and costing of health promotion activity and quality assurance than was the case previously.

Speller et al. (1998) identify strategic planning, programme management and monitoring as three of the key functions of health promotion that should be considered in quality assessment. There is also an ethical imperative to make explicit the rationale for interventions and the assumptions, values and principles on which they are based.

It will be clear from the earlier chapters that health promotion can involve a wide range of different interventions, used either on their own or in combination, to achieve health gain. Green and Kreuter (1991) summarize the purpose of health promotion as intervening to reduce or prevent an increase in the proportion of the population engaged in negative health behaviour or exposed to negative health conditions and, conversely, to increase the proportion that exhibits positive health behaviour or is exposed to positive health conditions. Sustainability is achieved by maximizing the conditions that enable individuals or groups to assume control over their health. Such support can range from putting policies in place to changing organizational practices and creating a supportive social climate.

Bartholomew et al. (2001) note that health promotion programmes may be directed at a number of different levels – individual, interpersonal, organizations, community, society and supra-nation. Given the breadth of health promotion and the numerous options concerning possible interventions, the selection of an appropriate course of action can be perplexing and is often influenced either by ideological considerations or custom and practice. However, a number of models exist that provide a guide through the complexity.

This chapter identifies the stages in the process of rational planning and provides examples of planning models. It also considers the issue of quality and health promotion. There is increasing recognition that tackling the complex factors that influence health status is not just the responsibility of the health sector, but requires the coordinated response of a number of different sectors. The participation of communities is also integral to effective health promotion. This chapter concludes by considering intersectoral collaboration and partnership working.

HORIZONTAL AND VERTICAL PROGRAMMES

Before providing an overview of selected planning models, we should note that practitioners are not always in a position to begin with a blank canvas. They may be appointed to a designated programme or required by managerial directives to address particular issues. Such programmes are often defined in terms of disease and are referred to as 'vertical programmes'. The first English national health strategy, *The Health of the Nation* (Department of Health, 1992), set targets for five key areas – coronary heart disease and stroke, cancers, mental illness, HIV/AIDS and sexual health and accidents. The strategy was criticized on account of its vertical disease orientation. French and Milner (1993: 98), for example, contended:

it is confined to a set of largely biomedical disease reduction targets and does not address structural

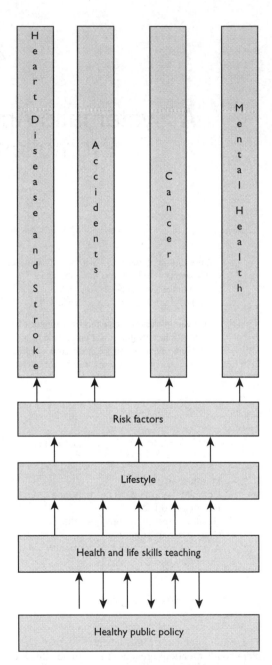

Figure 4.1 Horizontal and vertical programmes

influences on poor health or positive wellness, nor the resource commitment necessary to tackle the massed ranks of poverty, poor environment and crumbling social infrastructure...

Furthermore, it was felt that the emphasis on national targets, although providing a focus for activity, did not encourage the identification of local needs and flexibility in setting local targets (Department of Health, 1998).

The subsequent strategy, *Saving Lives: Our Healthier Nation* (Department of Health, 1999), focused on four areas – cancer, coronary heart disease and stroke, accidents and mental health. However, it gave much greater attention to the underlying *horizontal* influences on health status, particularly inequality in health. It also recognized the need for local targets and local partnerships to promote health.

Our earlier discussion of the determinants of health in Chapter 2 and the factors associated with changing behaviour in Chapter 3 would indicate that there are common issues across these vertical programmes. Lifestyle factors, such as smoking, would be common to both cancers and cardiovascular disease. Similarly, at a more fundamental level, personal attributes, such as locus of control, self-esteem and life skills, will exert an influence on lifestyle. Furthermore, environmental factors will have an impact on lifestyle, as well as direct effects on health status. There is strong evidence linking poverty with all four programme areas. It is clear that not only are programmes more likely to be effective if they tackle these cross-cutting or *horizontal* issues, but also that reorientation towards a horizontal approach should lead to greater efficiency. Figure 4.1 illustrates how horizontal programmes can be applied to vertically defined problems. It also draws attention to the reciprocal relationship between environment and life skills. The exercise of democratic rights requires appropriate life skills and can be instrumental in achieving healthy (or healthier) public policy. Conversely public policy will limit individuals' freedom of choice and behaviour and may also determine what opportunities exist to develop life skills.

PLANNING MODELS

I have a cunning plan.

Richard Curtis and Ben Elton, *Blackadder*

The overall purpose of systematic planning is to identify goals and the most effective means of achieving them. This involves making strategic decisions about the most appropriate courses of action together with operational decisions about the deployment of resources and ensuring that all the necessary elements are in place. Dignan and Carr (1992: 4) note that:

> Effective planning requires anticipation of what will be needed along the way towards achieving the goal. This statement implies that the goal is defined, as are the necessary steps involved in reaching the goal. Perhaps most importantly, it requires an understanding of the steps and how they interrelate.

We noted in Chapter 1 the wide range of activities that can be included under the health promotion umbrella. It follows that comprehensive health promotion programmes will need to include an appropriate combination of methods and involve a number of different sectors. Programmes are more likely to be successful if planning is approached in an inclusive way, involving all the major stakeholders. Not only does this create a bigger pool of experience to draw on, but it also establishes collective ownership of the programme. Furthermore, exclusivity runs counter to health promotion's commitment to participation. It is important at the outset, therefore, to identify the stakeholder community.

'Stakeholders' are all those individuals, groups or organizations with an interest in the initiative. They include those affected by the impact of an initiative and those who are in a position to influence its success. The different groups of stakeholders are outlined in the box.

The relative power and influence of the different stakeholders should be assessed together with their perceptions of, and willingness to support, the initiative. Such a stakeholder analysis can be instrumental in identifying potential alliances and partners and mobilizing the support required to get initiatives up and running.

The terminology associated with planning tends to be used somewhat loosely and interchangeably within health promotion literature. In the interests of clarity, we have defined the way we have used

STAKEHOLDERS

- **Primary stakeholders** are the potential beneficiaries – those who are directly affected, either positively or negatively, by the initiative.
- **Secondary stakeholders** are those involved in implementing the initiative.
- **Key stakeholders** are those whose support is essential to the continuation of the initiative – for example, fundholders.

PLANNING TERMINOLOGY

Programme
delineates the area that is being addressed. This is an umbrella term that includes all the activities involved in developing and running, for example, a coronary heart disease programme or a community development programme.

Strategy
the preferred course of action for achieving immediate or longer-term goals. It is selected tactically on the basis of evidence, theory or experience. The term can be used at all levels – for example, an 'overall programme strategy' or an 'implementation strategy'.

Plan
an outline of all the various components and how they relate to each other.

Aim
a broad statement of what is intended to be achieved. Aims can be developed at different levels – for example, overall programme aims, educational aims, policy aims.

Objective
precise and detailed statements of the intended outcomes that will contribute to the overall aim.

Intervention
the activities or collection of activities that will contribute directly to the desired change.

Method
specific approaches or techniques used.

the terms here in the box. It is not altogether surprising that the etymological origins of some of these terms derive from military campaigning, given the compelling need within this context to be decisive, establish clear goals and ensure that action is coordinated at all levels in pursuit of these goals. For example, 'strategy' is defined as the 'management of an army or armies in a campaign; art of so moving or disposing troops or ships as to impose upon the enemy the place and time and conditions for fighting preferred by oneself' (Fowler, 1929).

Hubley (1993: 207) identifies four questions, the answers to which should inform the planning process.

Where are we now?
Where do we want to go?

How will we get there?
How will we know when we get there?

These four questions are integral to the planning model proposed by Dignan and Carr (1992) shown in Figure 4.2.

The process begins with a needs assessment. This involves a community analysis to identify the programme's focus and the characteristics of the community, followed by a more specific, targeted assessment to identify the determinants of any problems and the key issues that will need to be addressed to achieve change. The goals and objectives for the programme should then be identified, along with resource implications and any potential obstacles. The actual methods to be used in the intervention can then be selected. The logistics of implementation

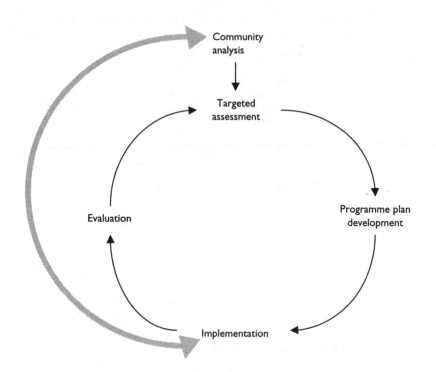

Figure 4.2   Dignan and Carr's planning model (Dignan and Carr, 1992)

should be considered and monitoring and evaluation systems put in place.

The apparent simplicity of this model belies the complexity of the decisions required at each stage. There is fuller discussion of these issues at relevant points in this book – indeed, its structure reflects the various stages of the planning process. We have already discussed the determinants of health and health-related decisions in Chapters 2 and 3. Chapter 5 will consider needs assessment in more detail. Chapters 6, 7, 8 and 9 will address different methods and Chapter 10 evaluation. Our purpose in this chapter, however, is to focus on the planning process itself and the adoption of a systematic approach.

There are several different planning models. While conforming to the same broad outline as Figure 4.2, they vary in the level of detail and their relevance for particular purposes. We outline some examples below.

Precede-proceed

One of the best-known planning models is the precede–proceed model (Green and Kreuter, 1991), as shown in Figure 4.3.

A particular strength of this model is the attention given to identifying the multiple factors that affect health status as a basis for focusing on the subset of factors that need to be addressed by the proposed intervention. Indeed, the model is premised on the view that there are multiple determinants of health and that efforts to improve it require multidimensional and multisectoral action.

The starting point of the model is an assessment of the quality of life and any social problems experienced by the population. It then identifies any specific health problems that contribute to quality of life and establishes which of these should be prioritized. These are then analysed to establish both environmental and behavioural risk factors. The attention given to the environment acknowledges its importance in supporting health-related behaviour as well as its direct influence on health. Further analysis identifies the plethora of factors that influence health behaviour. These are grouped as follows:

- **predisposing factors** personal factors that influence motivation to change, such as knowledge, beliefs, attitudes, values

Precede

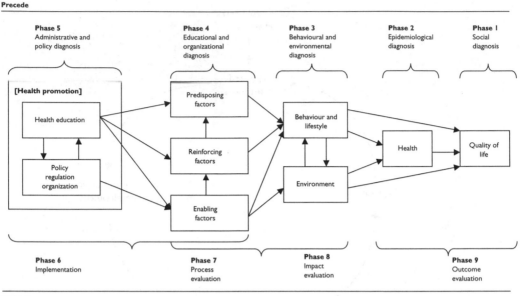

Figure 4.3   Precede–proceed (Green and Kreuter, 1991)

- **enabling factors** factors that support change in behaviour or environment, such as resources and skills, and also any barriers
- **reinforcing factors** the feedback received from adopting the behaviour.

In essence, these various phases lead to a diagnosis of all contributory factors. Two key considerations influence the selection of factors to focus on in developing an intervention. The extent to which they contribute to the problem is clearly of fundamental importance. However, the resources available and the organization's capacity to deliver health promotion programmes will also be influential.

An appropriate combination of methods can then be selected and the intervention implemented. Evaluation will include process, impact and outcome measures. Although presented as a linear sequence, the evaluation findings should feed back into the earlier stages, creating a more cyclical process.

The various phases of the model draw on a range of different disciplines. Phases 1, 2 and 3, for example, will draw on epidemiological methods and information; phases 3 and 4 social and behavioural theory; designing interventions will require

educational, political and administrative theory; and implementation will draw on political and administrative science and community organization theory.

Logical frameworks

Logical frameworks have their origin in military planning, but were adapted for use by USAID in 1969 and have subsequently been used by other aid programmes in response to demands for more effective planning (Nancholas, 1998). Figure 4.4 provides an overview of the logical framework, or LogFrame, matrix.

The vertical hierarchy corresponds to the stages in developing the LogFrame. It starts with the goal, which is usually expressed in very broad terms, such as reducing teenage pregnancy. The next level is the purpose, which is a statement of the desired achievement of the project. The purpose should make a direct contribution to the goal. Each LogFrame should contain only one goal and one purpose, which are often expressed in behavioural terms. Pursuing our example of teenage pregnancy, the purpose of a programme might be to increase the proportion of sexually active teenagers who make use of the contraceptive services within a locality.

	Narrative summary	Verifiable indicators	Means of verification	Assumptions
Goal				
Purpose				
Outputs				
Activities				

Figure 4.4   A logical framework 4 × 4 matrix

The outputs are then identified. These are the immediate results, or deliverables, of the programme and could include material factors, organizational change or behavioural change. A number of outputs may be necessary to achieve the purpose. For example, running young people's contraceptive clinics that are user-friendly and scheduled for a time that most suits their needs along with raised awareness among young people of these services.

Finally, the activities that are required to bring about the outputs should be specified. These might include working with clinic managers to persuade them of the need to schedule sessions for young people, running focus groups with young people to establish how clinics could be made user-friendly and what times would be most appropriate for this age group and providing training for clinic staff to make them aware of the views of young people. Similarly, activities to raise awareness might include developing and pretesting posters, displaying posters in all schools in the locality and so on.

Bell (2001) summarizes the four vertical levels as:

Why do the thing? (goal)
What is the thing for? (purpose)
What are the outcomes of the thing? (outputs)
How to do the thing? (activities)

The vertical logic should then be verified by working backwards through these various stages and checking out, in principle, *if* one stage is in place, *then* the next will follow, as in Figure 4.5.

Such verification will reveal lapses in logic and identify both omissions and any redundancy. It will also make explicit any assumptions at each level. In our simple illustration, there are several major assumptions – for example, that the contraceptive service provider has both the capacity and resources to run designated young people's clinics, young people are well motivated regarding using contraceptives, schools will be willing to cooperate and

display posters, young people will read the posters and so on. Some consideration will need to be given to whether or not the assumptions are well founded or if they expose potentially fatal flaws in the vertical logic and overall design. Returning to our example, if sufficient resources are not available, then, however supportive clinic managers and staff are of the proposed changes, they will be unable to put them into practice. Obtaining funding could be included as an additional output, along with an appropriate cluster of activities. Work may also need to be done to gain the support of those in the position of gatekeeper with regard to displaying posters in schools. If, on the other hand, schools have been actively involved with the development of the project, it may be reasonable to assume that their cooperation will be forthcoming. Nancholas (1998) notes that the process is 'reitcrative' and each decision is reviewed and revised as necessary. The value of making explicit all assumptions is that it provides a check that all necessary conditions are in place to ensure the success of the project and that contingency plans exist for any problems that might be anticipated.

At this point it is worth emphasizing that participatory processes are central to LogFrame planning and decisions should be arrived at by achieving consensus among the stakeholders. Relevant literature and research evidence should also be consulted (Nancholas, 1998). Furthermore, plans should be based on sound preliminary analysis, which would include:

- **stakeholder analysis** to identify the key players, their influence (positive or negative) and level of participation
- **problem analysis** to identify the nature of the problem and its determinants using a 'problem tree' that progressively homes in on the root causes needing to be addressed
- **risk analysis** to identify major obstacles and risks.

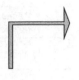

...*then* there will be a reduction in
teenage pregnancy.

If more young people use the clinics...

...*then* more young people who are
sexually active will use them.

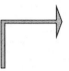

If we have Young People's Clinics
and they are appropriately scheduled
and young people are
aware of them...

...*then* we will have appropriately
scheduled user-friendly clinics for young
people and young people will be
aware of them.

If we run focus groups and establish what
the needs of young people are
and train staff
and persuade managers of the need for change
and have well-designed posters publicising
the Young People's Clinic
and posters are displayed in all schools...

Start here

Figure 4.5   LogFrames – checking the vertical logic

Objectively verifiable indictors (OVIs) need to be specified for each level of the vertical hierarchy and would answer the question 'How will you know that it has been achieved?' These are effectively the objectives of the programme and should be precise, including necessary detail, such as who, how much and when (for example, 80 per cent of school pupils aged fifteen to sixteen will be able to recall the name, location and opening times of at least one young people's contraceptive clinic in the locality within a month of coming into service). The evidence required to provide objective verification – the means of verification (MOV) – should then be considered. Again, returning to our example, this could be a written questionnaire survey of fifteen to sixteen-year-olds in all schools in the locality. Alternatively, in relation to the goal of reducing teenage pregnancy, an OVI might be a 10 per cent reduction in births to teenage mothers within two years of the introduction of the young people's contraceptive service and the MOV would be routinely collecting data on births. The means of monitoring activities and evaluating outcomes are therefore embedded within the planning process.

The final stages involve operational, management and financial issues. The inputs required for each of the activities should be identified, overall costs estimated and a budget prepared. A time plan, covering implementation of all activities and milestones, will also need to be produced.

Clearly, the preparation of a LogFrame can be demanding in relation to the level of detailed decision making required and the methodology is not without it critics. VSO Netherlands (undated) note two major criticisms of LogFrames in a position paper on the current status of the organization. First, predetermining objectives and indicators leaves no room for recording the often important, yet unanticipated, events that often arise. Second, the emphasis on consensus does not register differing views and diversity of opinion can be the source of innovation.

Broughton (2001) identifies the main weaknesses as being time-consuming, requiring sound understanding of the conventions used to complete LogFrames and, when completed, the danger of becoming 'frozen in time', hence limiting their applicability in rapidly evolving emergency situations. However, he also acknowledges their strength in bringing discipline to clarifying means, ends and assumptions and providing a framework for determining the way in which performance should be measured and for monitoring, evaluation and reporting. Furthermore, they contribute to collaborative working and consensus building.

Nancholas (1998) identifies similar advantages, along with some additional features. LogFrames have the capacity to combine the efficiency of rational planning models with flexibility. They also provide clear and concise summaries of whole programmes, which help to create overall visions of the programmes and communicate these to others.

Daniel and Dearden (2001: 2) note that LogFrames have been viewed as inflexible, restrictive and inappropriate for creative community projects and complex interventions. However, they suggest that the approach embraces the key elements of successful projects, notably:

- short- and long-term objectives have to be clarified and coherent
- risks have to be identified and strategies developed to meet them
- indicators for successful intervention need to be agreed at the outset
- methods of collecting and recording evidence of change also have to be set in place.

Daniel and Dearden report on the experience in the UK of using LogFrames for planning Health Action Zone (HAZ) Innovation Fund projects – innovative projects set up to demonstrate new ways of working towards the HAZ inequality and modernization agenda. The advantages of using a LogFrame for planning were identified as being:

- systematic, logical and thorough approach
- discipline and structure that it imposes
- identification of risks and assumptions
- provision of a framework for monitoring and evaluation
- encouragement of real partnerships
- flexibility and adaptability.

Conversely, disadvantages of the methodology included:

- conflict with other planning systems in place
- emphasis on quantitative rather than qualitative indicators
- assumption that partnerships exist
- time-consuming
- inflexible and controlling
- use of a lot of jargon
- appropriately timed training is required.

They (2001: 6) conclude that 'The logical framework works' in this context and quote one of the trainers:

> LogFrames really do take the mystery out of project planning for local people, they are simple and clear. The problem for professionals is that [working with LogFrames] they have to be transparent – something we have all learnt not to be in order to survive in bureaucracies! Managing that change is the biggest issue, not necessarily managing the LogFrame process...

The PABCAR model

In Chapter 1 we drew attention to the centrality of policy to definitions of health promotion. It follows, then, that development of healthy public policy should be of major concern for health promotion professionals and that advocacy is a legitimate part of their role – issues that will receive further attention in Chapters 6 and 8. Advocacy campaigns are, by their very nature, high profile and Maycock et al. (2001) suggest that there is frequently a dilemma about whether or not to become involved in such campaigns – not only are they time-consuming and costly, organisations risk damaging their reputation if they become publicly aligned with 'inappropriate' causes. Maycock et al. suggest that there is little in the literature to specifically guide decision making about advocacy campaigns. They propose the PABCAR model as a framework for deciding whether or not to support a public health issue. An overview of this model is presented in Figure 4.6.

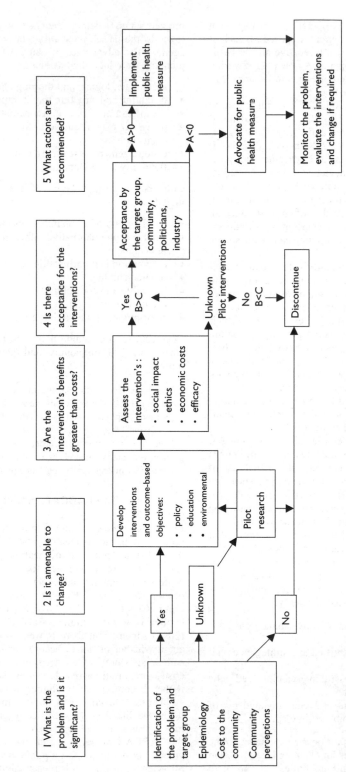

Figure 4.6 Public health decision-making model – PABCAR (after Maycock et al., 2001)

There are five mains stages:

1 identification of the problem and its significance for the community
2 assessment of whether or not the problem is amenable to change
3 analysis of the overall costs and benefits of intervening, which should be defined broadly and include social impact and ethical considerations, but, clearly, benefits should outweigh costs
4 assessment of the acceptability of intervening to the target group, community, politicians, industry
5 action and monitoring: if there is a high level of acceptability, it may be possible to proceed directly to implementing a public health intervention, but if, in contrast, acceptability is low, then advocacy on behalf of the public health measure will be required (such advocacy should be directed towards those who oppose the intervention as well as ensuring the continued support of those who are in favour of it).

Maycock et al. describe how an analysis using the PABCAR model was supportive of advocacy for the introduction of random breath testing in Western Australia. In short, alcohol-related road injuries were a significant problem. There was evidence that random breath testing offered considerable potential in relation to injury prevention and its sequelae, along with increased freedom for other road users. Over and above the actual cost of implementing random breath testing, other costs included the minor inconvenience of being tested, loss of freedom of the choice to drink and drive, loss of revenue for the alcohol industry and so on. There was a high level of acceptance of random breath testing among the community, but criticism from the alcohol industry, which attempted to gain the support of politicians by framing the argument in terms of the rights and freedom of individuals. Overall, there was a strong case for involvement in advocacy on behalf of the issue. Efforts were, in fact, successful, resulting in the introduction of legislation for random breath testing. Using a similar analysis, it was judged to be more feasible to advocate for a 0.05 per cent blood alcohol concentration than 0.0 per cent. Maycock et al. (2001: 64) conclude that the value of the model is that 'its use should help minimize the criticism that can result from advocating for measures that are inappropriate.'

A five-stage community organization model

Systematic planning is often aligned with top-down approaches and held to be inconsistent with community involvement. We would challenge this view and contend that strategies for involving communities are more likely to be effective if they are well planned. The key issue is that the planning process, in this instance, should explicitly address participation and draw on established principles of community development, together with relevant theory. Bracht et al. (1999), for example, describe a five-stage process for community organization, shown in Figure 4.7. Although the stages are represented as discrete in the model, the authors note that there is some overlap between the various stages.

Stage 1 is concerned with establishing the status quo and setting priorities. It involves:

• defining the community
• constructing a community profile, which includes health and demographic data and information on the community
• assessing the community's capacity by identifying ongoing activities and those organizations, groups or individuals who could offer support – this will also include feasibility and identification of the financial resources required
• assessing any barriers within the community
• assessing readiness for change.

Stage 2 involves designing activities and setting up an organizational structure to mobilize and coordinate community support and involvement. The key components of this stage are:

• setting up a core planning group and identifying a local coordinator
• choosing an organizational structure
• identifying and recruiting members
• defining the goals
• clarifying roles and responsibilities of members
• providing training and recognition.

Stage 3 focuses on implementing activities to achieve goals and includes:

• selecting and prioritizing intervention activities – particularly, assessing whether or not activities are appropriate and sufficiently comprehensive to achieve the goals
• developing a time plan to sequence activities to achieve maximum gains
• generating broader community participation
• planning media coverage
• obtaining financial and other support
• setting up intervention evaluation monitoring and intervention systems.

Stage 4 takes place when the programme is well under way and appraises the current position and future directions. It is concerned with:

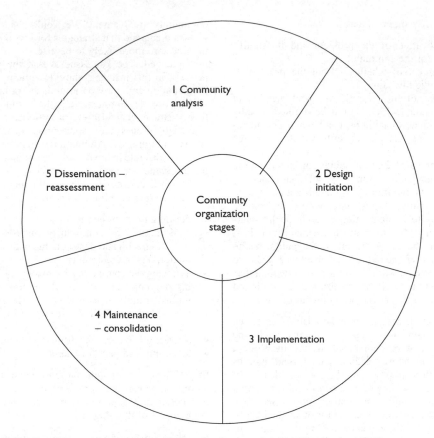

Figure 4.7 Bracht et al.'s community organization model (Bracht et al., 1999)

- sustainability by virtue of integrating activities into community structures
- establishing a positive organizational climate to encourage the retention of staff and volunteers
- having an ongoing recruitment plan for staff and volunteers
- acknowledging the contribution of volunteers.

Stage 5 involves dissemination and reassessment. Early dissemination of the evaluation findings in an appropriate manner will contribute to maintaining the visibility of the programme and provide a boost for those involved. Formative elements of evaluation will assist in shaping the development of the programme and a final summative evaluation will identify what has been achieved and lessons learned, which should inform future programmes. This stage includes:

- updating the community analysis to identify what changes have been achieved
- assessing the effectiveness of the interventions

- summarizing the findings in a suitable format for different constituencies and developing future plans.

Community empowerment

Empowerment, as we have noted, is a central tenet of health promotion. Yet, Laverack and Labonte (2000) assert that, in practice, although lip-service is paid to the discourse of empowerment, top-down programmes maintain unequal power structures in society. Such programmes address issues defined by professionals and empowerment, in this context, becomes a means of achieving predefined goals.

This contrasts with bottom-up approaches, which would involve the community in identifying and responding to its own needs. In such instances, empowerment would be a terminal goal – that is, an end in itself rather than a means.

COMMUNITY CAPACITY DOMAINS

1 Community participation.
2 Local leadership.
3 Empowering organizational structures.
4 Problem assessment capacities.
5 Ability to ask 'Why?'
6 Resource mobilization.
7 Links to others.
8 Equitable relationships, outside agents.
9 Community control over the programme.

Labonte and Laverack, 2001a, 2001b

Laverack and Labonte attribute the mismatch between discourse and practice to lack of clarity in how to operationalize empowerment within conventional top-down planning. They suggest that the two can be reconciled without empowerment being used instrumentally to achieve behaviour change goals, but that this requires consideration of empowerment at each stage of the planning process. They propose a model that pursues empowerment goals by means of a parallel track running alongside the conventional programme track, as illustrated in Figure 4.8, although it can also be used for bottom-up community development programmes.

At the design phase, sufficient time should be allowed for the often lengthy process of involving communities in an empowering way. Particular attention should be paid to the needs of marginalized populations who are least able to express their needs. Furthermore, programmes should begin with realistic aims and focus on relatively small-scale, achievable projects to generate early successes and build confidence. Programme planners need to question the ways in which planning processes and programme implementation will contribute to the nine domains of community capacity identified by Labonte and Laverack and listed in the box.

HEALTH PROMOTION PLANNING – REFLECTIONS

We have presented a number of planning models that differ from each other in relation to the levels of analysis that they include, the extent to which they specify the factors that should be considered at each level and the relative involvement of different stakeholders. Some models are more generic in

orientation than others and, hence, applicable to almost any situation or problem, while others, such as the PABCAR model, have been designed to suit more specific purposes. An interesting interchange between two groups of academics on the nature of planning models was sparked by an article by McLeroy et al. (1993: 307), which suggested that planning models (such as PATCH, precede–proceed, coalitions/partnerships, lay health adviser approaches, social change models, organizational change models):

> are largely a-theoretical and a-contextual [and further] they are largely independent of the specific health problem being addressed, they ignore what we know about the social production of disease, they are not connected to the field's collective wisdom about what works, with whom, under what conditions and they may lead to inappropriate interventions for the communities in which they are to be used.

They called for an ecological planning approach involving three stages:

1 **theory of the problem** which involves analysis of problems and the intrapersonal, interpersonal, organizational, community, cultural and public policy factors that produce and maintain them
2 **theory of intervention** which provides a state-of-the-art view of the relative effectiveness of different interventions
3 **understanding the context of practice** which allows interventions to be matched to the local community or organizational context.

The riposte to this article by Green et al. (1994) highlights some key issues concerning planning models. They put forward a strong argument that they are, in fact, grounded in theory and are consistent

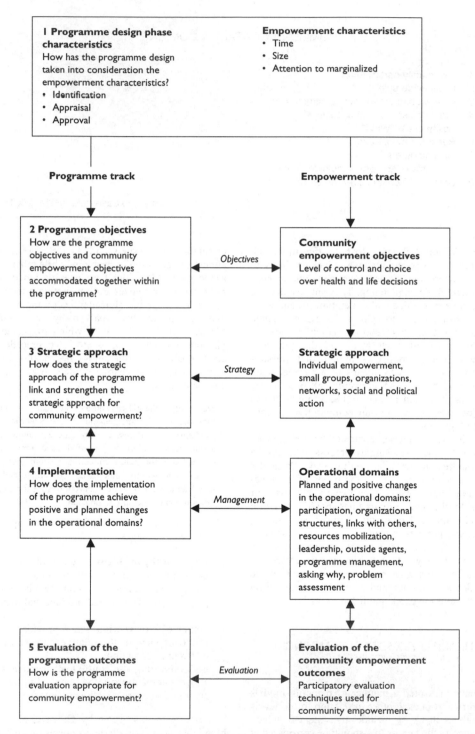

Figure 4.8   A planning framework for incorporating community empowerment into top-down health promotion programmes (Laverack and Labonte, 2000)

with a multilevel, multisector analysis – that is, an ecological approach to health promotion. Furthermore, we noted above that a precede–proceed analysis should incorporate a range of theoretical perspectives into the various stages.

Green at al. acknowledge that no planning model is immune from misuse, but inappropriate interventions arise from lack of rigour in the detailed application of models rather than from the model itself. Models such as precede–proceed provide a guide through the causal logic underpinning the development of health or health problems and impose a framework for considering all pertinent variables – exposing any omissions and assumptions. Rigorous application of planning models should therefore reduce the probability of interventions being inappropriate. Moreover, some planning models specifically incorporate consideration of contextual factors by means of, for example, a community diagnosis or analysis. Green et al. also suggest that the step-by-step procedure of planning models such as precede–proceed leads to the selection of an appropriate theory to suit both the context and the emergent requirements rather than imposing a theoretical structure at the outset. A sequential approach to planning should, therefore, ensure both relevance and rigour.

MacDonald and Green's (2001) analysis of the process of using a planning model to develop alcohol and drug prevention programmes in schools raises some interesting issues. The project was premised on the view that drug education would be more effective if it were based on local needs and context. Prevention workers were expected to work with schools using the precede–proceed model to guide the planning process. One of the dilemmas facing the workers was achieving a balance between the proactive planning demanded by the project and the tendency of the schools to respond to problems in a more reactive way. This raises questions about the suitability of rational planning models where there is a culture of reacting to problems and actions based on common sense and experience rather than analysis. A further issue was the variation in interpretation and application of the model by different workers. Training in the use of models and some assessment of the community's capacity to engage in the planning process will contribute to resolving these issues. However, the question still remains of whether or not fidelity in implementing the planning model is realistic or possible. MacDonald and Green suggest that successful implementation requires some flexibility to allow adaptation to local circumstances.

An additional consideration is whether or not the complex interplay of factors and alliances associated with health can be addressed by essentially linear planning models. French and Milner (1993) are critical of a simplistic linear view of causality and

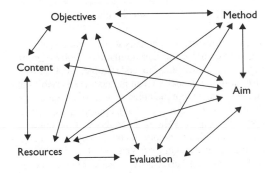

Figure 4.9 French and Milner's view of real planning (after French and Milner, 1993)

emphasise the need to consider the many interrelated variables that impact on health behaviour and health status. They also call for realism in relation to what can be achieved and suggest that there can be a number of different starting points from which programmes of work can emerge. For example, the availability of funding for particular streams of work could be the starting point. They suggest that real planning, as illustrated in Figure 4.9, is a systematic, although non-linear, process. Naidoo and Wills (1994: 221) also note that planning is often 'piecemeal or incremental. There is no grand design, but circumstances dictate many small reactive decisions.'

Notwithstanding this view, although we have presented the models in this chapter as a linear sequence, in practice it is not essential to start at the beginning – a point acknowledged by Green and Kreuter (1991). The planning process can, in principle, begin at some intermediate point, with the caveat that the preliminary stages should be worked through – as it were, retrospectively – to ensure logical and practical coherence. Furthermore, the possibility of including feedback loops between the various stages in the models provides opportunities for revisiting decisions in the light of emerging issues, thereby enhancing flexibility.

Writing from an evaluation perspective, Judge (2000) also highlights the problem of determining causality in complex social systems. We will provide a fuller discussion in Chapter 10, but this issue is also pertinent to a consideration of the inputs required to achieve change. Judge draws on the work of Pawson and Tilley (1997) to suggest that cause and effect are not 'discrete events', but mechanisms interact with context to produce outcomes. It is not simply a question of whether or not something works, but more with whom and under what circumstances. The following formula provides a simple summary:

Context + mechanism = outcome

The mechanism for change is seen as 'modifying the capacities, resources, constraints and choices facing participants and practitioners' (Judge, 2000: 2). A programme will seek to manipulate these variables to achieve change, but the outcome is also contingent on the context. Therefore, planning appropriate interventions will require a thorough analysis of the context. Judge notes that a 'theory of change approach' (originating from the work of Weiss et al. in the United States) can help to clarify exactly how proposed actions are expected to achieve intended outcomes. Using this approach, those involved in planning and implementing initiatives are encouraged to make explicit the ways in which they envisage the links between the various programme components and outcomes – that is, to articulate their theory of change or the assumptive logic underpinning the change that they are trying to achieve. In this context, theory is defined as 'the professional logic that underlies a programme' (Bauld and Judge, 2000).

A systems checklist for health promotion planning

Some years ago, Tones applied a systems approach to planning health education interventions (Tones, 1974). The systems approach had its origins in industrial processes, but, at the time, its relevance to education and programmed learning was receiving considerable attention. The purpose of the systems approach is to identify desired outcomes and all the factors that contribute materially to them. The inter-relationships between these factors are then examined so that they can be manipulated to achieve the outcomes with maximum efficiency. The advantages of this approach for education, and specifically health education, are that it demands precision in the formulation of objectives, a clear structure to programmes, the rational selection of methods and specification of the conditions for learning, both within the learner and the learning situation. With the benefit of hindsight, it is questionable whether or not educational processes can, or indeed should, be viewed in quite the same way as production-line manufacturing processes. We have already noted

the importance of context and the need for participation and stakeholder support.

There are several concerns about health promotion programme planning being driven by rational processes and governed by formal planning frameworks rather than being allowed to evolve in a more organic way. This is particularly evident in relation to community participation. However, to set rationality and systematic processes against participation, flexibility and context specificity is to impose a false dichotomy. Planning models provide an ordered structure that ensures all relevant variables are considered. The way in which decision-making processes are handled and the information that is brought to bear on this can correspond to a number of different ideological positions. Similarly, goals can be framed in relation to disease prevention, behaviour change, empowerment or community development. The advantages of rational planning may be summarized as:

- making explicit the anticipated causal mechanisms underpinning desired change
- identifying all the necessary conditions for change
- scheduling the various components of an intervention appropriately
- ensuring that all conditions are in place to maximize effectiveness.

Furthermore, the process of planning can serve as a vehicle for bringing together the various stakeholders.

Figure 4.10 provides a checklist of the key issues that need to be considered when developing health promotion programmes. The starting point involves establishing needs and stating the programme's aims or goals. Needs, as we will note in Chapter 5, may be defined in a number of different ways. The ideologies and values of those involved in planning and their conceptualization of health will not only inform the ways in which needs are defined and prioritized, but will also permeate each stage of the planning process. It is worth reiterating that the use of planning models does not in itself impose values on the planning process, but, rather, provides a vehicle for making explicit the values, rationale and assumptions underpinning any decisions. It also exposes those situations where rationality would dictate one course of action and political pressures another (see, for example, the box and the discussion of the 'Heroin Screws You Up' campaign on page 128).

COMPETING PRESSURES

Sell DRUGS to *adults* and you go to jail.
Sell CIGARETTES to *children* and you get fined.
Cigarettes kill 700 times those who die from illegal drugs.

ASH poster

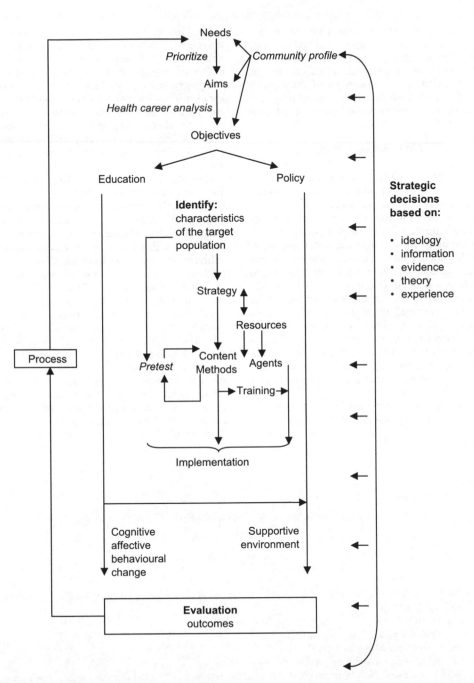

Figure 4.10   A systems checklist for health promotion

Needs, then, could be professionally or lay defined and focus on positive health states or disease or their various determinants, either environmental or behavioural. Prioritization involves a number of considerations – not least the contextual factors revealed by community profiling. These include the:

- extent and severity of the problem – clearly, life-threatening problems will rate higher than those causing minor inconvenience
- urgency of the problem
- number of people affected
- power and influence of those affected

- possibility of achieving change/improvement
- level of concern, support and commitment among the major groups of stakeholders
- feasibility of taking action in the current context, based on an assessment of the capacity within the organization and/or community
- consistency with the ethics and values of those involved.

Aims and objectives

Once priorities have been agreed, then a consensus should be achieved on the overall goal or aim of the programme. Not only does this provide a formal statement of intent as a point of reference to guide future action, but it also ensures that all those involved have a common understanding of what they are trying to achieve. Aims are general, global statements about what the programme intends to achieve (Dignan and Carr, 1992). However, vague, aspirational statements of intent, such as 'improving the quality of life' – while perhaps serving a motivational purpose and acting as a rallying call – offer little in the way of establishing a common purpose. It therefore goes without saying that, although aims are expressed in broad terms, some precision is still required (see box).

Aims may be either long- or short-term and framed in a number of different ways, as shown in Table 4.1.

Establishing the best way in which to achieve these aims demands a thorough analysis of the determinants of any problem or issue being addressed, along with the context. A health career analysis (referred to in Chapter 2) is a useful device for identifying the major influences on health status and locating possible intervention points. It also helps to identify appropriate target groups and agencies with which to develop collaborative working links. The characteristics of target groups will also need to be assessed.

Consideration of this information, along with relevant theory and empirical evidence of effectiveness, should enable a planning group to establish exactly what change needs to happen to achieve its goal. The broad vision encompassed within the stated aim can then be translated into more precise objectives. Whereas *aims* are, as we have noted, broad and relatively general statements of intent, *objectives* define goals in more specific terms. Thus one aim may generate a number of subordinate objectives.

Following our earlier discussion of health promotion as the synergistic interaction of policy and education, it should be possible to distinguish *policy* objectives from *educational* objectives. The former would be the specific goals to be attained in the development and implementation of policy, while the latter would be the specific learning outcomes that would result if the health education components of programmes were to be successful. The Health Promotion Authority Wales (1992)

THE IMPORTANCE OF CLEAR AIMS

Once upon a time a Sea Horse gathered up his seven pieces of eight and cantered out to find his fortune …
eventually
… he came upon a Shark, who said,
'Psst. Hey bud. Where ya goin'?'
'I'm going to find my fortune', replied the Sea Horse.
'You're in luck. If you'll take this short cut,' said the Shark, pointing to his open mouth, 'you'll save yourself a lot of time.'
'Gee, thanks', said the Sea Horse, and zoomed off into the interior of the Shark, and was never heard from again.

 The moral of this fable is that if you're not sure where you're going, you're liable to end up someplace else.

Mager, 1975: Preface

Table 4.1 *Examples of aims*

Focus	Example
Individuals or groups	Increase levels of empowerment among teenage girls in a locality
	Build social capital within a community
Disease	Reduce the level of coronary heart disease within a community
	Reduce the injuries from falls in the over sixties in a locality
Health status	Increase the levels of cardiovascular fitness in the senior citizens in a locality
	Reduce inequalities in health
Health behaviour	Reduce the level of smoking in a community
	Increase the uptake of physical activity within a community
Environment	Improve the safety of the community
Organizations	Introduce a health-promoting school initiative

EXAMPLES OF OBJECTIVES

Policy objectives

- Increase to over 95 per cent the proportion of people who have access to a variety of healthy foods in the staff canteen.
- Increase to over 90 per cent the population of Wales' residents who have local access to sporting and exercise facilities (including school facilities).

Educational objectives

- Increase to over 90 per cent those who eat green vegetables or salads most days (a behavioural outcome).
- Increase to over 95 per cent those who consider that physical exercise should be a normal part of life (a cognitive belief).

Health Promotion Authority Wales, 1992

identified both policy and educational objectives in its health strategy that would contribute to the overall aim of coronary heart disease reduction. These are listed in the above box.

The precise formulation of objectives is fundamental to the planning process for a number of different reasons. First, they indicate what strands of activity should be put in place and give structure to the programme. Second, the range of objectives should be sufficiently comprehensive to ensure that all the necessary conditions are achieved in pursuit of the overall aim. Third, as we will note in Chapter 10, they provide a means of evaluating the outcomes of the programme.

Objectives are highly specific and should be measurable. The acronym SMART is often used to describe the essentials of a clear objective (see the box).

SMART OBJECTIVES

Specific
Measurable
Achievable
Realistic
Time limited

Objectives should focus on outcomes rather than the process of achieving them. While objectives should be achievable, they should also be sufficiently challenging to attain worthwhile outcomes. The examples of policy and educational objectives given in the box earlier specify the levels of outcomes expected in percentage terms. These should not, of course, be arbitrary, but derived from consideration of baseline data and existing time trends. One of the oldest political devices for guaranteeing success is to set objectives that will be achieved automatically if existing time trends continue, independently of any intervention. However, such subterfuge is clearly anathema to the achievement of *worthwhile* goals!

There is typically some variation in the specificity of objectives – the most rigorous objectives are held to be behavioural objectives. Wherever possible, therefore, objectives should be expressed as behavioural objectives that conform to the pattern:

who will be able to do *what* to *what extent* and *when*.

For example, 90 per cent of mothers of children under three in locality Z will have had their children immunized against measles, mumps and rubella within three years of beginning the programme.

Alternatively, if we are focusing on policy and environmental rather than behavioural change, an example would be, Y town council will have introduced traffic-calming measures in 10 per cent of the residential streets in locality X within five years of beginning the programme.

Establishing such objectives presupposes that information is available on the levels of behaviour in question prior to beginning any intervention in order to set achievable, yet challenging, targets. For example, raising the uptake of immunization from 85 to 90 per cent would offer a completely different challenge than from 30 to 90 per cent. Moreover, it is not just a question of the magnitude of the change required. Reference to communication of innovations theory (Rogers and Shoemaker, 1971) in Chapter 3 would indicate that the early introduction of an innovation takes time (and, ipso facto, much health promotion effort) as the innovators and, subsequently, the early adopters accept the innovation. There follows a period of more rapid adoption and then the rate of uptake slows considerably as the laggards become involved. Increasing the uptake of behaviour from 5 to 10 per cent is therefore likely to require more effort than from 50 to 55 per cent, and the final 95 to 100 per cent can be particularly

problematic as laggards are notoriously difficult to change.

The most rigorous way of expressing behavioural objectives would (in addition to specifying what the learner should be able to do) also define the conditions and acceptable levels of performance. These three components are defined by Mager (1975: 21) as:

1 **Performance** An objective always says what a learner is able to do.
2 **Conditions** An objective always describes what the important conditions (if any) are under which the performance is to occur.
3 **Criterion** Wherever possible, an objective describes the criterion of acceptable performance by describing how well the learner must perform in order to be considered acceptable.

While, at first sight, it could appear that behavioural objectives might be more appropriate and easier to formulate when the focus of an intervention explicitly addresses behaviour change, they are readily applied to educational goals. Indeed, their origins are within education and the pursuit of behavioural objectives became a major driving force in the USA in the 1960s and 1970s and the subject of fierce debate (see, for example, Stenhouse, 1975, and Popham, 1978). Advocates of behavioural objectives claim that it is possible – and desirable – to develop appropriate behavioural objectives for all cognitive and affective learning outcomes.

One advantage of using behavioural objectives in an educational context is that this acknowledges the active role of the learner. It focuses attention on what we expect the *learner* to be able to do in the specification of outcomes rather than the teacher or health educator. The role of the 'educator' then becomes instrumental and involves putting the conditions in place to *enable* the learner to achieve the behavioural objectives. In that health promotion, by its very nature, is action-orientated, behavioural objectives are particularly relevant. Using behavioural objectives therefore specifies the target group and what we expect them to be able to do, along with how this would contribute to achieving the overall goal. However, we should emphasize that behaviour in this context is merely *indicative* of learning – it should not be taken to imply that the overall goal of the programme is necessarily concerned with behaviour change. For example, in pursuit of a safer environment, an appropriate objective might be, 'A majority of local councillors will vote in favour of the introduction of traffic-calming measures in locality X on Y date.'

Achievement of this objective may require a series of subsidiary objectives, such as '90 per cent of local councillors will respond accurately, when interviewed, that locality X has the highest rate of pedestrian injuries in the town within six months of starting the programme.'

Similarly, if participatory approaches are used, it could be phrased thus: 'Using participatory techniques, residents will produce a map identifying the high-risk areas within the locality within three months of starting the programme.'

Although we will return to this at greater length in Chapters 6 and 8, it is worth noting briefly at this point that programmes focusing on policy and environmental change require learning of some sort. This might include greater awareness of an issue, increased motivation to take action or the development of skills in advocacy and lobbying.

Clearly, the overall approach and the relative emphasis on environmental and behavioural factors will be fundamental to shaping objectives. A number of other key decisions will also influence the ways in which they are formulated – whether the programme is horizontal or vertical, the level of operation (individual, family, community, region and so on), the target groups and the timescale.

Listing the programme objectives provides an opportunity to check that consideration has been given to all the necessary elements required for the achievement of the programme's goal and identifies any omissions that may undermine the whole effort. Conversely, in the interests of economy, any overlap or redundancy can also be identified. Furthermore, it encourages articulation of the anticipated mechanism by means of which the change will be achieved – the so-called theory of change referred to above.

From objectives to action

Once programme objectives have been specified, the actual methods to be used – and combinations – can be considered. Clearly these are many and various and so will be discussed more fully in Chapters 6, 7, 8 and 9. The selection of methods will, again, be based on the intended purpose, local context and characteristics of any target group, theory and evidence of effectiveness – the art of health promotion practice lies in achieving the best fit in relation to all these. Attaching subsidiary objectives to the various activities clarifies their intended purpose. Any preconditions should also be identified. For example, effort may need to be directed towards building a sense of community before community action to improve safety can begin or, alternatively, school staff may need to be trained before a sex education programme can be provided for teenagers. Furthermore, materials and content should be pretested with the target group. Partnerships with other agencies may need to be consolidated and methods of achieving this will also need to be considered.

The so-called 'Penrith Paradox' (Adams and Armstrong, 1995) was born at a symposium to discuss the current state of health promotion theory and practice in the UK. It drew attention to the mismatch that often exists between the type of health promotion practice that might be expected based on theoretical principles and the dominant models seen in everyday practice. Of particular concern was the emphasis on individualism in practice when evidence and theory point to the greater effectiveness of community development approaches. The paradox is summed up in the box.

The solution to the paradox was held *not* to involve new models, nor was there a need to test current theories further. What was judged to be needed was a broad disciplinary alliance in both health promotion training and practice and more collaboration between academics and practitioners. Evidence of change is beginning to emerge in the UK with the development of initiatives such as 'Health Action Zones', 'Healthy Living Centres', 'SureStart' and

---

THE PENRITH PARADOX

We talk of a theory–practice gap. Maybe it is more complex and pervasive than this. Some models of health promotion are well supported by theory, quality of theoretical debate and quantity of papers published (e.g. community development/social action). Others (e.g. individualism) are starkly unsupported; in fact greater volume of debate is focused upon criticizing than supporting them. The paradox arises when examining practice in the UK today. The theoretically weak models are dominant in practice whereas theoretically based models to which many practitioners subscribe struggle to be maintained or developed in practice in the UK today.

Adams and Armstrong, 1995: 3

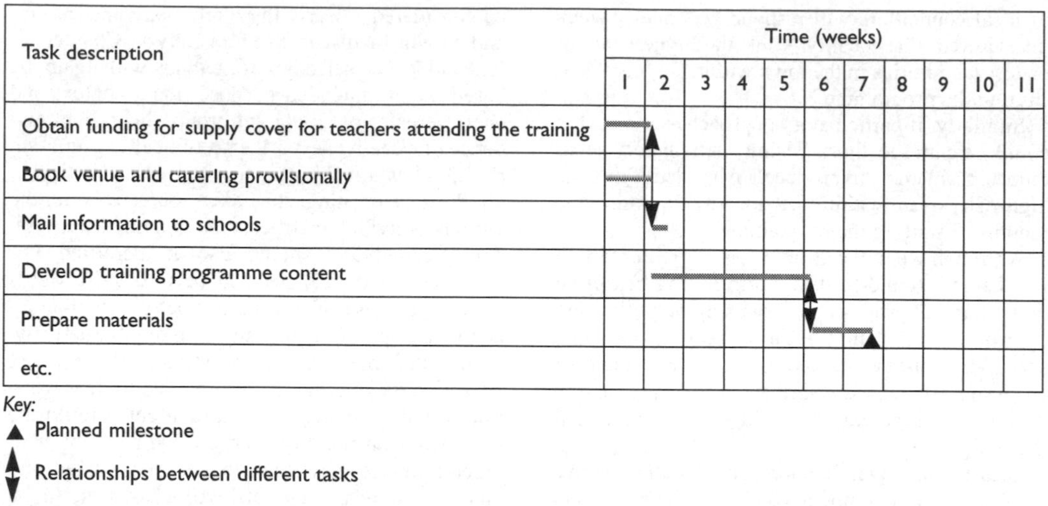

Task description	Time (weeks)										
	1	2	3	4	5	6	7	8	9	10	11
Obtain funding for supply cover for teachers attending the training											
Book venue and catering provisionally											
Mail information to schools											
Develop training programme content											
Prepare materials											
etc.											

Key:
▲ Planned milestone

↕ Relationships between different tasks

Figure 4.11 An extract from a Gantt chart for a sex education training programme for school staff

'New Deal', together with interest in social capital and urban renewal. There has also been some shift in the political pressures that have influenced practice. The top-down individualist approach that typified Thatcherism (it was Thatcher who famously said 'There is no such thing as Society. There are individual men and women, and there are families.') has given way to a greater emphasis on participation with the New Labour administration. The 'third way' concept at the heart of New Labour health policy involves a combination of state responsibility partnered with greater levels of public participation (Department of Health, 1997, and 1999).

As well as political influences shaping the overall climate within which health promotion activity takes place, political factors can be decisive in the selection of actual methods. The 'Heroin Screws You Up' campaign in the UK was a classic example of flying in the face of expert opinion by allocating considerable resources to funding a

high-profile mass media campaign (Tones, 1986). Conventional wisdom – and rational planning – would dictate that drug education for young people should involve a comprehensive programme of personal, social and health education. What the programme did achieve was a demonstration to 'Middle England' that the government was taking action regarding the drug problem, albeit inappropriately.

Returning to the systems checklist, at the implementation level, the 5WH formula (outlined in the box) is a well-known acronym for identifying which key issues to address.

Clearly, with complex, multilevel interventions, all the activities need to be orchestrated so that everything is in the right place at the right time to maximize the effects of the programme and, indeed, minimize the risk of programme failure. Administrative issues such as funding, staffing and deployment need to be managed efficiently. Devices such as Gantt charts are helpful to this end

5WH

- Who?
- What?
- Where?
- When?
- Why?
- How?

and for detailed operational planning. Gantt charts are essentially bar charts that can be used to visualize the relationships between the various tasks required to achieve the programme's goal. By way of illustration, a brief extract from a Gantt chart is provided in Figure 4.11.

Each task should be specified. Durfee and Chase (1999) suggest that they should also be expressed as an action with a duration. Milestones are important points in the development of the project or programmes and can be marked. They serve as a check that everything is proceeding according to schedule. Beginning some tasks is dependent on the completion of others and this relationship can also be indicated.

The final stages are monitoring and evaluation, which will be discussed at some length in Chapter 10. However, we should note some key points here. First, evaluation should be an integral part of the planning process and considered at all stages. Second, precision in formulating plans and objectives provides a clear focus for monitoring what has been done and evaluating what has been achieved. Finally, plans are not set in stone. Formative evaluation, which would include the pretesting of materials, aims to identify what is working well and what is working less well in order to make necessary modifications. Feedback loops in the planning cycle encourage such reflection and adaptation.

QUALITY HEALTH PROMOTION

Generally, the drive for greater efficiency within the health service has placed greater emphasis on value for money and cost improvements, yet the primary concern of the public – and indeed an overriding ethical imperative – is with the effectiveness and quality of the care they receive (Catford, 1993). Rather than focusing exclusively on cost-effectiveness, health promotion should also be concerned with quality and conforming to principles of good practice. The principles of the Ottawa Charter have been a guiding force within the health promotion movement. Evans et al. (1994) suggest that the following core principles should be considered in relation to quality assurance:

- equity
- effectiveness
- efficiency
- accessibility
- appropriateness
- acceptability
- responsiveness.

Catford (1993) also proposes that there should be a common set of criteria to assess performance and quality organized around a number of themes – see the box.

Quality assurance has been defined as:

a systematic process through which achievable and desirable levels of quality are described, the extent to which these levels are achieved is assessed, and action is taken following assessment to enable them to be reached.

Wright and Whittington, in Evans et al., 1994: 20

and

the work that takes place within any work unit, so as to follow up and improve the unit's own activities and to prevent mistakes or defects from arising.

Berensson et al., 2001: 188

THEMES FOR ASSESSING QUALITY

- Understanding and responding to people's needs fairly.
- Building on sound theoretical principles and understanding.
- Demonstrating a sense of direction and coherence.
- Collecting, analysing and using information.
- Reorientating key decisionmakers upstream.
- Connecting with all sectors and settings.
- Using complementary approaches at both individual and environmental levels.
- Encouraging participation and ownership.
- Providing technical and managerial training and support.
- Undertaking specific actions and programmes.

After Catford, 1993

Haglund et al. (1998) note the importance of establishing the purpose of quality assessment and whether it is concerned with checking if standards have been met (that is, providing a borderline between 'good enough' and 'not good enough') or a stimulus for continuous improvement. Speller et al. (1998) describe two main approaches to quality assurance that reflect this distinction . External standards inspection (ESI), where external standards are set in relation to a work process and monitored so that action can be taken if there is any failure to meet standards, and, in contrast, total quality management (TQM), which involves setting internal standards. TQM is also dynamic in approach and is concerned with continuous growth and improvement rather than just ensuring that minimum standards are met, which is typical of the more static approach of ESI. A survey of specialist health promotion services in England (Royle and Speller, 1996) revealed greatest support for internal peer review as being the best way in which to monitor standards. Opinion was mixed about whether or not there should be a set of national standards and criteria for assuring quality. A 'standard' has been defined as 'a statement that defines an agreed level of excellence' and 'criteria' as 'descriptive statements which are measurable, that relate to a standard' (Evans et al., 1994: 103–4). Speller at al. also distinguish between 'quality assurance programmes', which aim to ensure the quality of all aspects of a service, and 'quality initiatives', in which standards for a particular project or intervention may be agreed.

Quality has been described (British Standards Institute, 1978: BS 4778) as:

> the totality of the features and characteristics of a product or service that bear on its ability to satisfy stated or implied needs.

Speller notes that the assessment of the quality of interventions is often based, inappropriately, on outcomes rather than quality criteria. A consensus definition of quality assurance for health promotion was achieved by a European Commission-sponsored project in 1996:

> Quality assurance in health promotion is the process of assessment of a programme or intervention in order to ensure performance against agreed standards, which are subject to continuous improvement and set within the framework and principles of the Ottawa Charter.
>
> Speller, 1998: 79

The principle concern of quality assurance, therefore, is with what is done and whether or not this conforms with agreed standards of practice rather than what is achieved – neatly encapsulated as 'Doing things right is not enough if the right things are not done correctly' (Haglund et al., 1990: 100). The focus is therefore on *inputs* rather than *outcomes*. However, there is inevitably a reciprocal relationship between the two – quality health promotion should draw on evidence of effectiveness and be more effective.

The argument that runs through this book is that health promotion should be planned well and that planning should draw on sound evidence at all stages and be informed by principles of good practice. The characteristics of good practice in health promotion are listed in the box.

CHARACTERISTICS OF GOOD PRACTICE

- An agreed philosophy.
- A clear vision of health.
- Decisions based on needs.
- A planned approach.
- Working in partnerships.
- Strategic leadership.
- Realistic aims and claims.
- Use of effective methods.
- Consumer involvement.
- Disseminating results.
- Reflection.
- Motivated and skilled staff.

After Evans et al., 1994

Speller at al. (1998: 145) emphasize that quality assurance can ensure that interventions are 'acceptable, and applicable to the setting, and based on current best evidence'. They contend that only quality-assured programmes should be evaluated and, further, if they prove to be effective, clear guidance on what standards are expected in relation to implementation should be a necessary element of subsequent dissemination. As we will note in Chapter 10, such attention to quality would contribute to avoiding Type 3 errors in evaluation – that is, the inability to detect any effect when interventions were predestined to fail because of poor design and/or implementation.

Haglund et al. (1998) identify a number of tensions in applying models of quality assessment – largely deriving from the commercial and manufacturing sectors – to health promotion. First, quality production standards have generally been developed for routine and repetitive procedures, whereas health promotion interventions are usually unique. Second, quality standards are usually set by the consumer who, in the context of health promotion, may be difficult to define (is it the commissioning agency or the target group?) and also lack a clear voice. Third, health promotion is a multidisciplinary endeavour and views about quality may be influenced by the philosophies to which

practitioners subscribe. Furthermore, quality assessment instruments are generally designed for analysing the activities of a single organization and do not adapt well to assessing the cooperation between them.

The Society of Health Promotion Specialists in the UK has produced a manual on developing quality in health promotion services that identifies a number of core functions of a health promotion service (listed in the box). At service level, the essential issues to consider in relation to quality are considered to be (Totten, 1992):

- guidelines on service provision and practice
- professional development by means of education and training
- recruitment and selection
- principles of professional practice
- measuring and monitoring standards of practice.

Audits are seen as the means of assessing the quality of service provision. The Society has also produced a code of conduct (Society of Health Education and Promotion Specialists, 1997), which is based on a social model of health and methods of working that are participatory and foster equity, empowerment and autonomy.

CORE FUNCTIONS OF A HEALTH PROMOTION SERVICE

1 Determining health education/promotion priorities:

    (a) translating national health education/promotion guidelines to ensure that they meet local circumstances and planning needs and are implemented accordingly

    (b) assessing local health needs together with other professionals.

2 Providing input to the formulation of health education/promotion policies, plans and service agreements. This will include contributing to strategic and operational planning which relies on the identification of priorities, setting targets, and identifying the means of achieving these targets...

3 Managing health education/promotion programmes:

    (a) within agreed plans and priorities taking a significant lead in the design, implementation and management of health education/promotion programmes...

    (b) leading research on health education and health promotion issues, monitoring and evaluation of health education/promotion programmes.

4 Advice and consultancy.

Totten, 1992: 1.3

Evans et al. (1994: 103) note that the term 'audit' is interpreted in a number of different ways, but that it can be defined as 'the systematic critical analysis of the quality of a health promotion programme' and taken to be synonymous with quality assurance. They propose a quality assurance cycle based on six stages:

1 identifying/reviewing key areas for quality assurance
2 setting standards
3 selecting criteria with which to measure standards
4 comparing practice with standards
5 taking action
6 reviewing the previous stages.

The outcome of the final review stage should feed back into stage one of a new cycle.

Health promotion, by its very nature, is wideranging and services are organized in a number of different ways. Speller et al. (1997) argue that quality assurance should be applied to what might be considered the generic key functions of health promotion. Following a consultation exercise that reflected concern that quality assessment should be grounded in the reality of health promotion practice, they identified six key functions:

• strategic planning
• programme management
• monitoring and evaluation
• education and training
• resources and information
• advice and consultancy.

Strategic planning – particularly intersectoral planning – with a focus on health needs and healthy

public policy was seen to be a fundamental part of health promotion. Examples of standards that might be applied to some of these key functions are provided in the box. However, these can equally be developed by individual organizations, along with appropriate criteria.

Berensson et al. (2001) approached the task of identifying the key areas of importance for quality assurance rather differently. They conducted a meta study to search for the common elements deemed to be essential or important to health promotion and derived a number of key indicators grouped in relation to structure, process and outcome:

• structure:
  – goals
  – target groups design
  – responsibility
  – resources
  – organization

• process:
  – network
  – amount of exposure
  – commitment
  – participation

• outcome:
  – knowledge and behavioural changes
  – environmental changes
  – epidemiological changes
  – maintenance.

The various indicators were then operationalized by framing them as questions, with a negative response

---

EXAMPLES OF STANDARDS FOR SELECTED KEY FUNCTIONS

1 Strategic planning

1.1 There is a group which addresses strategic planning issues in health promotion.
1.2 The health promotion service makes an important contribution to this group.
1.3 A health promotion strategy is produced and/or health promotion figures prominently within other strategy documents.
1.4 The health promotion department's plan relates to the health strategies.

2 Programme management

2.1 A group exists for the planning, implementation and review of each programme area.
2.2 A range of health promotion methods and activities is considered for each programme area in order to determine action plans.

Speller et al., 1997

> # EXAMPLES OF INDICATORS OF QUALITY
>
> **Target group**
>
> Does the project have a defined target group?
>
> **Participation**
>
> Have organizations, groups and individuals concerned been given the opportunity to participate?
>
> **Changes in knowledge and behaviour**
>
> Are there surveillance methods to follow up possible knowledge, attitude and behavioural changes in the target group?

being indicative of a shortfall in quality. We noted earlier the tendency to confuse measures of quality with outcomes. It may seem somewhat paradoxical, therefore, to see outcomes figure in the above list. However, the concern here is not with measuring outcomes per se, but quality issues associated with incorporating an evaluation of outcomes into routine practice and the way in which this is achieved. Reference to the examples in the box should help to clarify this.

Haglund et al. (1990) contend that quality assurance can only be built into the planning phase of interventions. Rather than adopting the flexible TQM approach described above, they focus on the design and planning of interventions to ensure that all the necessary conditions for success are in place. The use of a standardized instrument enables the experiences of local projects to be collected and shared. The twenty-item questionnaire used to systematize 'telling the story' of different projects at the Sundsvall Conference (Haglund et al., 1993) was subsequently found to have a role in improving planning. The key issues that were identified for reporting purposes were also the key issues that should inform the development of projects. This interconnectedness should not be altogether surprising. The questionnaire has been revised and now includes six dimensions that relate to the various stages of the supportive environments action model (SESAME) (Haglund et al., 1998), as shown in Figure 4.12.

The approach to quality assurance adopted in the Netherlands is very similar, combining research and evaluation evidence with planning. Two key instruments are used to guide professional practice and achieve 'systematic and continuous improvement in health promotion'(Keijsers and Saan, 1998: 117). One of these is the PREFFI (health promotion effectiveness fostering instrument). The second is the Analys instrument for reporting and analysing research. This systematizes the collection of information on methodological quality, the effects of an intervention and the process by which the effect was achieved. The detailed information collected using this standard format is better suited to the needs of practitioners than traditional reviews and can then be fed back into the planning processes.

In essence, our discussion of quality has come full circle, returning us to the assertion that the process of planning is fundamental to the quality of health promotion, along with the contribution of planning models. Haglund et al. (1998) suggest that improving the quality of health promotion rests on three cornerstones:

- user-friendly instruments for practitioners
- quality assessment instruments that reflect the reality of health promotion practice
- professional training for health promoters.

ALLIANCES AND PARTNERSHIPS FOR HEALTH

Recognition that health is determined by a wide range of factors automatically leads to the view that efforts to promote health demand the coordinated action of a number of different sectors and agencies. Hagard (2000: 2) contends that a successful strategy requires:

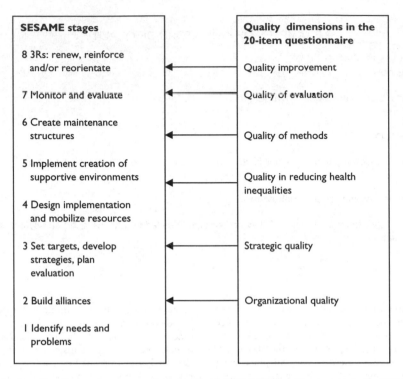

Figure 4.12   Quality dimensions associated with SESAME (after Haglund et al., 1998)

concerted action by a number of different players, including government at all levels, many sectors of society, such as social services, education, environmental protection and healthcare, the media and non-governmental organizations, and all public and private bodies that variously contribute to economic activity, social cohesion, justice and human rights.

This notion was recognized by the Ottawa Charter. It has been at the heart of the health promotion and 'Health for All' movements and is integral to settings approaches such as 'Healthy Cities' and the 'Health Promoting School' – indeed, Kickbush has identified partnerships as the 'key to successfully promoting health' (WHO, 1998b). The Jakarta Declaration (WHO, 1997) identified the current challenge as that of releasing the potential for health promotion in different sectors and at all levels of society. Breaking down barriers between sectors and creating partnerships for health were seen as essential. In addition to reaffirming the importance of involving communities and families, the Jakarta Declaration also introduced the issue of investment and public/private partnerships. Overall, the priorities for the twenty-first century were listed as being to:

- promote social responsibility for health
- increase investment in health development
- consolidate and expand partnerships for health
- increase community capacity and empower the individual
- secure an infrastructure for health promotion.

In line with this thinking, the World Health Assembly Resolution on Health Promotion urged all member states to 'consolidate and expand partnerships for health' (WHO, 1998c: 1(3)).

Within the UK, the importance of healthy alliances was recognized in the 'Health of the Nation' strategy (Department of Health, 1992) and it is integral to the more recent health strategy 'Saving Lives: Our Healthier Nation' (Department of Health, 1999). The need for the National Health Service to work in partnership and forge stronger links with local authorities was also recognized by the white paper *The New NHS: Modern Dependable* (Department of Health, 1997). Indeed, partnership between government, individuals and local communities is seen as the way forward in improving health. Government commitment to partnership working as a vehicle for improving local planning also underpins the development of 'Local Strategic Partnerships' (LSPs) (DETR, 2001). These are intended to bring together the various parts of the public, private and voluntary sectors and the community within local government areas to make strategic decisions on issues such as health, education, employment, housing and crime. Local people will have a voice in decision making and services can be more responsive to the community's needs. LSPs are also a mechanism for developing a coordinated local response to the major issues of social exclusion and neighbourhood renewal.

Over the years, there have been some changes in terminology concerning collaborative approaches to working – 'inter-agency working', 'intersectoral working', 'joint working', 'intersectoral collaboration', 'healthy alliances', 'coalitions' and, most recently, 'partnerships'. While it would be easy to dismiss these changes as merely rebadging a familiar concept, they do signal a subtle shift in emphasis. Sindall (1997: 5) notes that 'strategic alliances' are one of the defining characteristics of modern organizational relationships and quotes the Australian Institute of Management's Roundtable definition:

> a long-term partnership involving two or more organizations formed to benefit from the synergy of working together in an environment of trust, sharing information and resources to achieve a common objective.

The move away from using 'intersectoral collaboration' to 'alliances' and 'coalitions' is perhaps indicative of a more explicit concern to involve members of the community, rather than assuming their implicit representation as a result of the involvement of organizations. A 'coalition' has been defined (Feigherty et al., 1992, in Bracht, 1999: 95) as 'an organization of individuals representing diverse organizations, factions or constituencies who agree to work together to achieve a common goal.'

Furthermore, the notion of 'partnership' draws attention to the issue of power and implies participation on an equal footing with the sharing of power. Given the current emphasis on partnerships and alliances, we should consider the implications for planning health promotion before concluding this chapter. We will begin by looking briefly at alliances and intersectoral collaboration before moving on to partnerships.

Delaney (1994b) identifies four key features of organizations that contribute to effective collaboration. Similarity of structure and function is important, but there also needs to be agreement on respective remits and areas of responsibility, along with

awareness of interdependence and the collaboration serving to meet needs. Bloxham (1997), for example, provides a case study of inter-agency collaboration between teachers, community health practitioners, health promotion staff, and youth and community workers to develop a sexual health initiative for young people. It demonstrates that the work of each agency was enhanced by collaboration and it enabled a comprehensive response to be developed to meet young people's needs.

Dependence on resources is a further stimulus for collaboration. Delaney (1994b: 219) notes Hudson's (1987) assertion that the 'absence of alternative sources of resources is a "prerequisite" for successful collaboration.' Resources are not necessarily financial – they can include human resources, services and information.

Collaboration is clearly facilitated by formal commitment and structural arrangements for meetings and joint working. Formally ratified strategies and committee structures are a feature of the 'Healthy Cities' initiative. However, networking and the informal working arrangements that develop among people who share the same broad goals are also important. Reticulist (networking) skills that support strategic thinking and crossing boundaries therefore contribute to effective collaboration. Delaney (1994b: 221) cautions against seeing collaboration as 'a purely technical matter to be resolved by the right administrative arrangements' – it also involves negotiation and bargaining. Furthermore, drawing on the work of Lukes (see Chapter 3), she observes that the power relationships within alliances may be unequal and maintained in a variety of subtle ways so that particular organizations and values may come to dominate. At a very basic level, control may be exercised in the ways in which meetings are chaired and agendas constructed. Not only should the interactions within a collaboration be fair in themselves, but they must also be perceived to be fair. The optimal arrangement would appear to be formal structures coupled with informal networking within an overall climate of positive mutual awareness.

Delaney's (1994a) qualitative study of the factors perceived to influence intersectoral collaboration identified the following barriers to success:

- lack of vision and shared commitment
- lack of time
- competition:
  - between individuals and organizations
  - within and between professional networks and dominant or influential professional groups
- conflicting mechanisms and timescales

- different channels of accountability and communication.

In contrast, a summary of the key features of *successful* collaboration is provided in the box. The review of the 'Health of the Nation' strategy

(Department of Health, 1998) also proposed factors external to organizations that would encourage partnerships – notably, a statutory framework that would require local agencies to work together and incentives for developing partnerships for health.

KEY FEATURES OF SUCCESSFUL COLLABORATION

Identified by Tones and Delaney (1995: 22)

- Domain awareness and similarity of functions between agencies.
- Shared vision.
- Compromise and bargaining.
- Needs of all parties should be met.
- Resources exchange and commitment.
- Formal recognition.
- Organizational and communication structure, but also flexibility and opportunities to network.
- Reticulist skills.
- The interpersonal element.
- 'Flat', less hierarchical structures rather than authoritarian organizational forms.

Identified by Ansari (1998: 18)

- Early vision and understanding.
- Clarity of roles, rules, procedures and responsibilities.
- Wide representation of stakeholders and a strong membership.
- Leadership skills.
- Communication between the diverse parties.
- Human resource development.
- Build on the identified strengths and assets of the partners.
- Realistic timeframes and funding cycles.

Features of effective partnerships and coalitions identified by Bracht et al. (1999)

- Leadership.
- Management.
- Communication.
- Conflict resolution.
- Perception of fairness.
- Shared decision making.
- Perceived benefits versus costs.

Features of successful partnerships (*Saving Lives: Our Healthier Nation*, Department of Health, 1999: 10.13)

Successful partnership working is built on organizations moving together to address common goals; on developing in their staff the skills necessary to work in an entirely new way – across

(Continued)

(Continued)

boundaries, in multidisciplinary teams, and in a culture in which learning and good practice are shared. It also means:

- clarifying the common purpose of the partnership
- recognizing and resolving potential areas of conflict
- agreeing a shared approach to partnership
- strong leadership based on a clear vision and drive, with well-developed influencing and net-working skills
- continuously adapting to reflect the lessons learned from experience
- promoting awareness and understanding of partner organizations through joint training pro-grammes and incentives to reward effective working across organizational boundaries.

The Department of the Environment, Transport and the Regions (DETR) guidance on good prac-tice in partnership working refers to the stages in the development of a partnership from its initial setting up to maturity, and the need to balance structure and stability in relation to membership, rationale, mode of operation and activities with the opportunity to be flexible and evolve in an organic way in order to respond to specific cir-cumstances internal and external to the partnership (DETR, 2001). The guidance also draws attention to the lack of clarity that often exists in distin-guishing between the responsibilities of the part-nership and those of individual partners, and also between strategic and operational decision mak-ing. Individual partners may hold multiple – and conflicting – roles, for example, as a member of the community, representative of the community, service provider and strategic partner. A clear understanding of roles, and responsibilities *vis-à-vis* the partnership is therefore fundamental to success and provides a basis for ensuring account-ability. Indeed, the DETR recommends setting up formal systems for monitoring and reporting out-comes and a framework of accountability.

Gillies (1998: 101), commenting on a review of the literature on the effectiveness of partnerships, notes that those reported fell into two broad groups:

Micro-level – alliances or partnerships which involve one or more collaborators among individuals or groups or organizations in the public, private or non-governmental sectors in the promotion of health, but which do not seek to affect the underlying systems or structures or architecture for health promotion.

Macro-level – alliances or partnerships which involve one or more collaborators among institutions, organizations or groups in the public, private or non-governmental

sector which seek to affect the structural determinants of health.

While the published micro-level studies tended to focus on behavioural outcomes in assessing gains, Gillies notes that they could equally have focused on the wider environmental determinants. What emerged clearly from the review was that the stronger the representation from the community and the higher the level of involvement in practical activities, the greater and more sustainable were the gains. Mechanisms should therefore be put in place to involve local people in planning and practical health promotion activities. Furthermore, lay involvement should be based on power sharing and not mere tokenism. This view endorses that of Labonte (1993), who makes a clear distinction between consultation and participation. Central to participation is shared decision making, negotiated relationships and openness to identifying problems and issues. Furthermore, he suggests that less powerful groups may need support so that they can participate on an equal footing.

A review of the examples of best practice in alliances or partnerships for health collected from around the world (Gillies, 1998: 104) iden-tified the key elements of good partnership to include:

a relevant needs assessment combined with the setting up of committees crossing professional and lay bound-aries to steer, guide and account for the activities and programmes implemented.

It was also noted that non-industrialized countries are leading the way in relation to partnerships and community-based health promotion. These examples of good practice placed less emphasis on behavioural outcomes than the published studies and were more concerned with their impact on the

PROCESS INDICATORS FOR ALLIANCES

- Commitment:
    - group purpose
    - resources.
- Community participation:
    - liaison
    - empowerment.
- Communication:
    - shared information
    - accessibility.
- Joint working:
    - strategies and action plans
    - flexibility.
- Accountability:
    - responsibility
    - evaluation.

Funnell et al., 1995

broad environmental conditions and process of change. Key outcomes in relation to process (Gillies, 1998: 112) were:

> getting agencies to work together; engaging local people; training and supporting volunteers and networks; creating committees; capturing politicians' interest and sustaining political visibility; resource allocation; reorientating organizations and services; promoting flexibility in working practices; and undertaking needs assessment as a way of identifying priorities and galvanizing interest...

Open communication and trust are essential ingredients of partnership working and are dependent on good networks for sharing information and establishing common values and goals. However, partners may be drawn from diverse professional, cultural and social backgrounds. The management of this diversity will also be integral to success. On the one hand, any conflict that would be a barrier to joint decision making needs to be avoided – especially so when it is associated with an imbalance of power. On the other hand, the DETR (2001) cautions against the 'lowest common denominator' approach, which tends to reduce these differences and stifles creativity and innovation.

Funnell et al. (1995) propose five categories of process indicators that can be used to assess the ways in which alliances are functioning. Each category has two main components and these are listed in the box.

Clearly, developing partnerships that function well demands time and commitment. This style of working also requires supportive organizational structures and appropriate skills among those involved. Individuals might need to develop their skills in order to engage constructively in intersectoral activity and organizations might need to change their internal ways of working. Capacity building might be required in relation to individuals, communities and organizations before effective partnerships can be established.

Notwithstanding the challenges, partnerships offer great potential for developing a coordinated response to the multiple factors that influence health status and achieving health gains. There are also potential gains for partner agencies that might be motivated to enter into such partnerships for reasons not necessarily related to health (see the box).

Investment for health

We noted in Chapter 2 that social and economic factors are the single major determinant of health status. Ziglio et al. (2000) contend that health, as an essential personal and social resource, requires investment and, indeed, health promotion should be considered as an investment strategy. Clearly

GENERAL BENEFITS OF PARTNERSHIP WORKING

- Achievement of organizational objectives and enhanced efficiency and effectiveness.
- Improved coordination of policy, programmes and service delivery.
- Broadening the scope of influence to include other services and activities.
- Greater economy.
- Less bureaucracy and regulation.
- Business and commercial opportunities.
- Access to data and information.
- Access to a range of skills and competencies.
- Opportunity for innovation and learning.
- More involvement of local communities.

After DETR, 2001: Annex E

there is an inextricable link between health and social and economic development in that social and economic development leads to health improvement and, conversely, health supports social and economic development. Levin and Ziglio (1997: 363) note that, in many societies, the immediate priorities are 'economic competitiveness and fiscal soundness' rather than health priorities. The 'Investment for Health' (IFH) approach, which received considerable attention towards the turn of the twenty-first century, focused on integrating health promotion into mainstream social and economic development. This raises some questions about ends and means – is the emphasis on the promotion of health or is health merely instrumental to achieving wealth? The expropriation of health to service the needs of capitalist economies has been the subject of fierce criticism by authors such as Doyal and Pennell (1979). However, the IFH approach acknowledges that priority social and economic policy areas, such as education, employment, transport and housing, have a major influence on health. Policy decisions and initiatives by governments – and the private sector – have the potential to improve or harm health. The major concern of IFH, therefore, is to ensure that efforts to improve social and economic standing also improve health status and are equitable, empowering and sustainable (Ziglio et al., 2000a).

Kickbush (1997) has identified three key questions that should inform the development of a sound health promotion strategy:

Where is health promoted and maintained in a given population?

Which investment strategies produce the largest population health gains?

Which investment strategies help reduce health inequities and are in line with human rights?

Ziglio et al. (2000a: 4) add a fourth:

Which investments contribute to economic and social development in an equitable and sustainable manner and result in high health returns for the overall population?

In the post Ottawa era, there has been widespread acceptance of the importance of environmental influences on health, both directly and via their effect on behavioural choices. Latterly, there has been increased awareness of the complexity of environmental factors and the contribution of social networks, social capital and social inclusion to health. Ziglio et al. (2000) suggest that, notwithstanding the widespread commitment to a socio-ecological model of health, the health promotion response has been oversimplified. Most change has been 'first-order change', achieving some minor adjustment but without affecting the major determinants of health. They call for a more radical approach in order to achieve 'second-order change' (2000: 145), which involves new structures and processes – an approach whereby concern for health is interwoven into social systems and the focus is on the creation of health rather than disease prevention.

Organizational policies and activities tend to be sector-based, with little emphasis on intersectoral relationships. Watson et al. (2000: 17) refer to a 'silo model of governance', where different sectors, such as health, education and housing, traditionally have separate structures, funding, channels of accountability and professional 'domains' and there are few opportunities for links. In contrast, 'holistic governance' would be more flexible and involve 'shared objectives, a common understanding of what needs to be done and what others can contribute'. Similar arguments could also be put forward in relation to community involvement.

The issue of partnerships is therefore central to the IFH approach, along with accountability for health impact.

> The IFH approach therefore calls for a new form of partnership. In today's complex world, action for the promotion of health cannot come from the health-care sector alone. It needs to be built on strong cross-sector alliances between health and healthcare, social development and equitable and sustainable economic development.
>
> Ziglio et al., 2000a: 4

It also involves policy at all levels, from national to local, and this will be considered more fully in Chapter 6. The core principles of IFH (Ziglio et al., 2001) are:

1 A focus on health.
2 Full public engagement.
3 Genuine intersectoral work.
4 Equity.
5 Sustainability.
6 A broad knowledge base.

The Verona Benchmark was developed as a tool with which to assess the systems that would need to be in place at national, regional or local level in order to implement an IFH approach. The notion of benchmarking derives from the business practice of improving performance by studying the practices of competitors (Mittelmark et al., 2000). It involves learning from what others do and what is regarded as best practice in order to improve the performance of organizations. Watson et al. (2000) see the Verona Benchmark as a means of improving the quality of partnership working and the capacity to influence systems and the policy environment. The Verona Benchmark I set out seven key system characteristics and the assessment of each was guided by a series of questions. These seven themes are listed in the box.

THE VERONA BENCHMARK

Verona Benchmark I: Themes

- A high priority for health.
- Social capital for health.
- Public engagement.
- Accountablity.
- Sustained policy commitment.
- The investment process.
- Monitoring.

Revised Verona Benchmark

Enablers:

- leadership
- people
- policy and strategy
- resources
- programmes
- processes.

Results:

- targets
- economic impact
- social impact
- environmental impact
- health impact.

The tool has been extensively piloted. Although it was found to be complicated to use, the Verona Benchmark provided insight into the ways in which partnerships were functioning and was found to be a useful tool for improving the quality of community alliances for health (Perry and Markwell, 2000, and Watson et al., 2000).

A Delphi study among the European members of the International Union for Health Promotion and Education (Garcia et al., 1999) explored the skills needed by an IFH approach. The key skills were found to include:

- communication
- advocacy
- working with others.

Additional skills identified were training for IFH, empowerment, incorporating research and evidence into practice and using appropriate planning methods. Barriers to IFH included lack of political will and the dominance of the medical model with little awareness among health professionals of the socio-economic determinants of health.

Over and above the emphasis on partnerships and policy to address the structural determinants of health, the IFH approach draws attention to the capacity of systems to respond appropriately in order to foster health improvement. Ziglio et al. (2001) refer to the importance of maximizing the health assets in a community as well as identifying and responding to the community's health needs. Indeed, the primary focus of IFH is on strengthening health assets. These assets, they found, include:

- policy investments
- regulatory changes
- nurturing of non-governmental resources and programme initiatives

- strengthening of health promotion infrastructures and decision making
- refocusing education
- investing in research
- training in the requisite health promotion skills
- environmental improvement.

The principles of IFH offer a means of breaking down traditional barriers to partnership working and spreading accountability for health beyond the narrow confines of the health sector. Hancock (1998) suggests that the involvement of the private sector offers particular challenges, given that the primary motivation is profit and this may well conflict with health interests. He does, however, recognize the potential benefits of working with the private sector, provided partners and their subcontractors meet agreed ethical criteria. The proposed criteria are listed in the box.

SUMMARY AND CONCLUSIONS

We have argued in this chapter that effective health promotion is based on a systematic approach to planning. Indeed, planning is fundamental to the quality of health promotion. We have provided examples of a range of different planning models. While they differ to some extent in their orientation, there are several common features. They require the assessment and prioritization of needs and identification of objectives as a basis for appraising possible solutions and selecting the most appropriate courses of action. They also incorporate monitoring and evaluation elements. Perhaps the most important feature is that they provide a framework for integrating theory and empirical evidence into the various stages of the planning process. It is worth

---

ETHICAL PRINCIPLES FOR PARTNERSHIP WITH THE PRIVATE SECTOR

- The activities of the corporation are increasingly environmentally sustainable.
- Safe and healthy working conditions are provided for the workforce.
- Pay is fair with reasonable benefits, there is a right to collective bargaining and lay-offs are minimized.
- Taxes are paid fairly and economic activities do not increase poverty.
- Their activities do not pose a danger to consumers or the communities in which they operate and the public is fully informed about any potential hazards.
- There is respect for human rights.

After Hancock, 1998

emphasizing that theory can be concerned with community participation and policy development as well as behaviour change.

Resistance to using planning models often derives from an association with reductionism and top-down styles of working. We would contend the reverse to be the case. When used appropriately, they can serve to open up the entire range of health promotion options and avoid any tendency towards being blinkered by custom and practice. Many health promotion programmes are destined to fail because they focus on too narrow a range of factors or are based on unsubstantiated assumptions. Rational planning processes will serve to expose such weaknesses and ensure that programmes address all relevant variables. Furthermore, the process of planning can be a vehicle for involving all stakeholders ensuring wide ownership of plans.

The complex interplay of factors that influence health demands a coordinated response across a number of different sectors and at a number of different levels, from local to national and even supranational. The IFH approach is premised on the interrelationship between health and social and economic development and seeks to strengthen the assets for health within communities by means of partnerships and policy.

Partnerships are seen to be the 'key mechanism for pulling together effective local planning and action' (Watson et al., 2000: 17). The involvement of communities and creating opportunities for participation on an equal footing are also instrumental to success. Building effective partnerships is undoubtedly challenging, but offers huge potential for developing whole systems approaches to promoting health, rather than reacting in a piecemeal fashion. However, this requires commitment from partners and new ways of working.

By way of conclusion, we would draw attention to the proverb about the elephant in the box. This has been used as an analogy for taking a whole systems approach to tackling health issues (Newcastle Healthy City Project, 1997). It draws attention to the fact that there are a number of different perspectives on complex systems – all of which may be true, but, equally, none represents a complete view. Understanding how the whole system operates depends on sharing knowledge. Members of the community concerned are more likely to interface with more components of the system and, hence, have a more complete picture than professionals, whose awareness may be confined to the remit of a particular agency.

Furthermore, within complex systems, although all components could make a contribution to health and there are knock-on effects between the activities of different agencies, there is no single agency controlling and coordinating activity. Developing an intersectoral response to health issues and partnership working calls for a shift in emphasis away from the functioning of the 'parts' and towards their interrelationship and the functioning of the whole. The key to this is good communication, shared vision and clear strategic and operational objectives.

WHOLE SYSTEMS AND ELEPHANTS

There is an old Indian proverb about three blind people describing an elephant. One holds the trunk and says, 'This is a snake.' One holds the tail and says, 'No, it's a rope.' The third grabs a leg and says, 'You're both wrong. It is a tree trunk.'

Each person has offered their perception of the truth, but they have failed to describe the elephant. Even putting all three descriptions together would not make a recognizable elephant.

After Newcastle Healthy City Project, 1997

5

Information Needs

Out of the air a voice without a face
Proved by statistics that some cause was just
In tones as dry and level as the place.

W.H. Auden, 'The Shield of Achilles', 1955

INTRODUCTION

The first stage of systematic programme planning involves establishing what the problem is and determining what the causes are, along with any other contributory factors. Some understanding of the nature of the community, its members and the context in which they live is also needed before appropriate courses of action can be identified. Nutbeam (1998a) refers to this first stage as 'problem definition' and suggests that the research requirements include epidemiological and demographic analysis, along with a community needs analysis. The next phase of 'solution generation' on the other hand, draws on theory and models, evidence of effectiveness and practitioner experience. Nutbeam (1998a: 33) provides a useful summary of the key questions that should be addressed at each stage of programme planning and implementation.

- **Problem definition** What is the problem?
- **Solution generation** How might it be solved?

- **Innovation testing** Did the solution work?
- **Intervention demonstration** Can the programme be repeated/refined?
- **Intervention dissemination** Can the programme be widely reproduced?
- **Programme management** Can the programme be sustained?

In Chapter 2 we examined issues associated with the measurement of health status and the broad determinants of health and, in Chapter 3, the factors influencing behaviour and action. The purpose of this chapter is to apply these ideas more specifically to identifying the information needed for making decisions about possible interventions. We will begin by considering definitions of health needs before looking at different approaches to assessing needs and profiling the community. We will then focus on the development of possible solutions and, particularly, the application of theory and evidence to the rational selection of intervention strategies.

Advances in information technology in recent years, together with the development of new

> ## THE MAIN TASKS OF THE PUBLIC
> ## HEALTH OBSERVATORIES
>
> - Monitoring health and disease trends and highlighting areas for action.
> - Identifying gaps in health information.
> - Advising on methods for health and health inequality impact assessment.
> - Drawing together information from different sources in new ways to improve health.
> - Carrying out projects to highlight particular health issues.
> - Evaluating progress by local agencies in improving health and cutting inequality.
> - Looking ahead to give early warning of future public health problems.
>
> Association of Public Health
> Observatories, 2002

information systems and sources of data have done much to improve access to health information. The establishment of Public Health Observatories in each of the NHS regions of the UK in 2000 is an example of an attempt to make information available to support efforts to improve health generally, but specifically the health of the worst off in society. The tasks of the Observatories are summarized in the box. However, it is still pertinent to note that, all too often, the information that is most readily available is not necessarily the most useful or revealing – a situation pithily summed up in Murphy's Law of Information (Williams and Wright, 1998):

The information we have is not what we want.

The information we want is not the information we need.

The information we need is too expensive to collect.

NEEDS ASSESSMENT

The nature of health needs

The growing interest in health needs assessment has been attributed to the increasingly consumerist nature of society, economic concerns and the general squeeze on public funds, together with the current emphasis on effectiveness (Gillam and Murray, 1996). Within the UK, the restructuring of the NHS in the 1990s based on the notional 'internal market', focused attention on the identification of needs as a basis for commissioning services. This has been given further impetus – and a broader perspective – within the modernization agenda (Department of Health, 1997), which required health authorities and,

more latterly, primary care trusts to work collaboratively with local authorities and the voluntary sector to identify needs and develop health improvement programmes. It also has relevance to the emphasis on urban regeneration and neighbourhood renewal.

Given the debate about the nature of health and its determinants, the absence of a precise definition of health needs and the lack of a consensus about the means of assessing needs should come as no surprise. The interpretations of the term 'health needs' range from a narrow focus on heath service provision, through inclusion of a preventive element, to addressing social needs. There is an important distinction between health needs and healthcare needs. It will be clear from our earlier discussion that the broad remit of health promotion requires an analysis of needs that includes social and environmental concerns and also addresses wellbeing. However, in considering definitions of need, we will also draw briefly on interpretations of healthcare needs.

The traditional public health approach to assessing health needs has been to draw on epidemiological information to measure the disease burden or levels of ill health in communities and equates with a conceptualization of health as the absence of disease. Robinson and Elkan (1996) are critical of this problem-focused approach, which they feel ignores needs that are unrelated to narrowly defined problems – the need to stay well, for example. They further challenge it on the grounds that it does not immediately suggest strategies to respond to any deficiencies identified. Liss (1990) raises the issue of how, on what basis and by whom any deficiencies are identified and prioritized. Pickin and St Leger's (1993) lifecycle framework for assessing health needs is a development of this approach. It includes three main elements:

- measurement of health status, including both epidemiological and sociological analyses
- assessment of the resources available
- identification of ways of achieving maximum health gain.

Recognizing that needs will vary throughout a lifespan, the lifecycle framework also divides the population into a number of age groups with similar characteristics.

An alternative conceptualization of need – one that addresses the issue of what can be done – is based on the capacity to benefit. Culyer (1977) considers a need for healthcare to exist when there is potential to improve health status or avoid reduction in it, but only if an intervention exists that can achieve positive outcomes. This thinking is integral to Buchan et al.'s (1990) view that:

> people in need of a health service are defined as those for whom an intervention produces a benefit at reasonable risk and acceptable cost. The benefit may not necessarily be improved outcome. It may relate to information or reassurance or some other aspect of the care process.

A need is therefore determined not by the scale of the health problem, but the ability to benefit. These two approaches should not necessarily be seen as incompatible. The criteria used for identifying the key areas that should be addressed in the first health strategy document for England (Department of Health, 1991) included both the magnitude of the health problem (as assessed by its contribution to premature death and avoidable ill health) and availability of effective interventions.

Robinson and Elkan (1996) recognize the advantage of focusing on the capacity to benefit in that it encourages practitioners to specify what outcomes they are seeking to achieve. However, the ways in which these are framed will inevitably be influenced by value positions. Although in principle they could go beyond biomedical goals to include quality of life issues, in practice they are often defined rather narrowly as improved life expectancy. They are also critical of needs being defined by association with the effectiveness of an intervention – a view that overlooks the severity of problems to the individual. However they acknowledge Culyer's (1977) suggestion that, where no effective treatment exists, what is needed is research. We might also note the lack of precision about 'reasonable risk' and 'acceptable cost' and whether or not these should be defined in humanitarian or economic terms.

An emphasis on the capacity to benefit acknowledges that some interventions offer greater potential for gain than others. A key issue for health economists is the notion of 'allocative efficiency', which is concerned with achieving maximum benefits from available resources. Comparison of the respective gains from spending on different interventions is viewed as essential if resources are to be deployed to achieve the greatest good. Needs identified in this way will clearly be relative and heavily influenced by judgements, not least in relation to how benefits are defined and measured. The measures frequently used in this context include QALYs and DALYs, which, as we noted in Chapter 2, have been the subject of controversy.

Liss (1990) notes that the interpretations of 'needs' referred to above include matters of judgement in relation to what constitutes ill health, which health states *require* care and the services that *ought* to be provided. He suggests that there are two categories of assessors of need – the patient and the provider – that is, the doctor, but we might equally include the health economist or the planner. The identity of an assessor is clearly germane to any assessment of needs and Liss suggests that this should be included within the concept of need. Liss' (1990: 39) normative notion of a healthcare need is based on 'an "assessor" believ[ing] that healthcare ought to be provided'.

A further interpretation of healthcare needs derives from an instrumental perspective. Rather than focusing on deficiency states, needs are identified in terms of what needs to be done or what conditions need to be in place to maintain or improve health. Within the broader context of health promotion, a useful example is provided by the list of prerequisites for health identified in the Ottawa Charter (WHO, 1986) – peace, shelter, education, food, income, a stable eco-system, sustainable resources, social justice and equity – and updated in the Jakarta Declaration (WHO, 1997) to also include social security, social relations, the empowerment of women, respect for human rights and, above all, alleviation of poverty.

Liss' (1990) characterization of different views about healthcare needs provides a useful summary, one that could be applied more generally to health needs.

- **The ill-health notion** which equates a need for healthcare with a deficiency in health that requires healthcare.
- **The supply notion** which requires that acceptable treatment should also be available to respond to a deficiency.
- **The normative notion** which acknowledges that opinions about needs may vary and is based on an assessor believing that healthcare should be provided.

- **The instrumental notion** is based on the identification of care required to achieve certain states.

Bradshaw (1972) defined four types of social need, enshrined in his well-known taxonomy.

- **Normative need** is defined by experts or professionals often on the basis of a 'desirable standard' against which individuals or groups can be compared. However, normative needs may be defined differently by different professional groups and change over time. They cannot therefore be seen as absolute needs.
- **Felt need** is defined by lay people and equated with wants. It is limited as a measure of *real* need by people's perceptions, which may fail to recognize actual needs or else misrepresent wants as needs.
- **Expressed need** consists of felt need turned into action by seeking treatment or care.
- **Comparative need** is concerned with ensuring that people with similar characteristics receive equivalent levels of care and, if there is a shortfall, then individuals are in need.

Bradshaw (1994) acknowledges that there may be alternative views about normative needs and that comparative needs may themselves derive from normative judgements. Felt and expressed needs may differ widely, as illustrated in Figure 5.1.

As we noted in Chapter 2, even what purport to be objective assessments of needs based on disease burden remain essentially ideologically driven. A number of tensions exist in identifying health needs and derive both from the ways in which health and its determinants are conceptualized and where the focus of attention lies. These are summarized in the box.

Although Bradshaw's taxonomy provides a useful way in which to analyse different perspectives and, indeed, ensure that they are represented in any assessment of social needs, it offers little insight into the actual nature of need. Indeed, his assertion that 'real' need is likely to exist when all four types of need are present at the same time may be taken to imply that the individual 'types' are not sufficient in themselves as indicators of 'real' needs.

Two key issues remain unresolved – the distinction between needs and wants and whether needs are absolute or, ultimately, subjectively defined. Doyal and Gough's theory of human need sheds some light here.

Doyal and Gough's theory of human need

Doyal and Gough (1991: 9), in their meticulously constructed defence of the concept of objective and universal human need recognize critics on both sides of the political spectrum:

> Many argue that it is morally safer and intellectually more coherent to equate needs with subjective preferences – that only individuals or selected groups of individuals can decide the goals to which they are going to attach enough priority to deem them needs.

Critics from the New Right are concerned about state collectivism and the intrusion of the 'nanny' state into matters of individual choice. In the absence of an agreed basis for identifying need they advocate relying on individual preferences and market forces. Concerns on the Left and among minority and oppressed groups have their origins in the unequal power structure in society and the dominance of particular groups. The contention here is that needs are culturally determined and can only be

---

TENSIONS IN HEALTH NEEDS ASSESSMENT

View of health:

- positive or negative view of health
- holistic or atomistic view of health
- biomedical or social interpretation of determinants
- professional or lay perspective.

Focus of attention:

- upstream (prevention) or downstream (treatment)
- individual or community.

ct both absolute minimum standards and
dards. Instead, they advocate an optimum
r basic needs and propose a 'minimum
' level for intermediate needs – that is, the
evel of input of intermediate need satis-
chieve optimal basic needs satisfaction.
aining question concerns how needs will
. Doyal and Gough support the notion of
articipation by those whose needs are
ssed, although they caution that this can
se already in privileged positions who
ore influential than others without such
. They suggest that the development of
f intermediate needs will be fed, in an
ay, by the development of new codified
ential knowledge. They (1991: 169)
that both qualitative and quantitative
will be needed, but place considerable
n the latter:

both basic and intermediate indicators we
uire social indicators which are valid, distribu-
itative and aggregated, but which are open to
These indicators should be open to disaggre-
ween groups. In this way profiles of the need-
n of nations, cultural groups and other
s can be compiled.

rences arise between the views of needs
by expert-led approaches, which draw
d knowledge, and community-based
, which are grounded in experience, dia-
oposed as a mechanism for resolving the

eeds, wants and demands

cognized as being one of the fundamen-
f health promotion. Principles of social
uld presuppose that health resources
distributed in relation to needs. However,
apparent, access to services and wider
es to promote health are not necessarily
by needs. Some time ago, Hart (1971)
tion of the 'inverse care law' to describe
ly poorer provision of services in those
are most deprived and have the greatest
ill health. An emphasis on needs rather
s or demands is therefore integral to
tbeam (1998b: 7) captures this idea

eans fairness. Equity in health means that
needs guide the distribution of opportunities
eing.

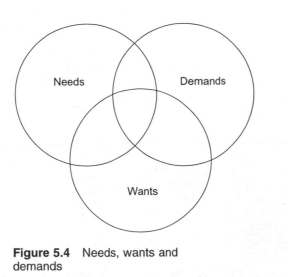

Figure 5.4 Needs, wants and demands

The management of public services on market or
quasi-market principles is necessarily demand-led.
In contrast, a needs-led approach will be more
consistent with a focus on social justice.

The defining characteristic of need in Doyal and
Gough's theory of need is its instrumentality in
achieving universal human goals. Wants, in contrast, are personal preferences and equate with what
Bradshaw might term felt need. These subjective,
personal preferences may overlap with an objective
view of need or be completely different, as summarized in Figure 5.4.

In general economic terms, a demand is associated with the consumer's willingness to pay for
desired goods or services (Bowling, 1997b).
However, the complexity of the health and healthcare market calls for a broader interpretation.
Mooney and Leeder (1997) describe demands as
being based on wants, but also involving action
directed at fulfilling the wants. There is a clear
parallel here with Bradshaw's expressed need.
Again, demands will overlap, to a greater or lesser
extent, with wants and needs. Foreman (1996) suggests that health professionals effectively 'ratify'
expressed needs or demands by providing services.

Clearly those with most power will be better
placed to articulate their wants and ensure that their
demands are met – regardless of whether or not this
is in the interests of the collective. Responding to
demands may also ultimately conflict with the
needs and longer-term interests of the individual.
Robinson and Elkan (1996) offer the example of an
individual demanding antibiotic treatment for a
viral infection. Prescribing an antibiotic would
serve no useful clinical purpose. Moreover, such
unnecessary prescribing would contribute to the

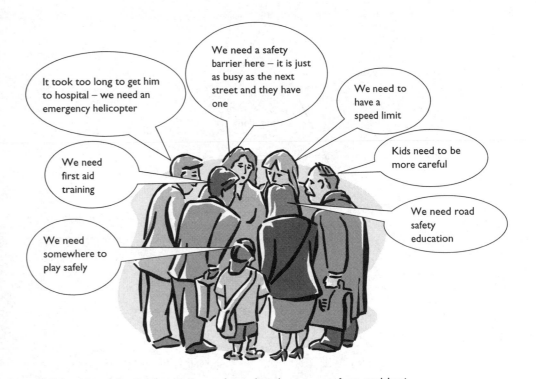

Figure 5.1 Alternative interpretations of need at the scene of an accident

fully understood by members of a group. They are
therefore subjectively defined, but at the group collective, rather than the individual, level. Doyal and
Gough challenge both these positions, along with
economic, sociological and postmodern interpretations of needs as relative and contend that objective
need does indeed exist. Furthermore, demonstrating
that there are objective universal needs creates a
moral imperative to meet those needs and effectively establishes them as fundamental rights.

The term 'need' has been used to refer to drives
or motivational forces that arise from some disequilibrium – for example, the need for sleep when tired
or food when hungry. Maslow (1954) identifies a
number of such needs that can be ordered into a
hierarchy premised on the requirement to satisfy
basic needs, such as hunger and warmth, before
higher-order needs can be addressed. The needs
identified are felt to be common to different
cultures. The hierarchy is conventionally represented as in Figure 5.2.

Each level in the hierarchy is assumed to be necessary for the achievement of the next level,
although there is no requirement for 100 per cent
satisfaction before moving on to the next level.
Maslow himself acknowledged that the hierarchy

was not fixed. For example, in those who gain
satisfaction from high-risk activities, such as mountaineering or hang-gliding, self-actualization needs
may take precedence over safety needs.

Doyal and Gough reject the interpretation of
needs as drives on the basis that needs and drives
can exist independently of each other. For example, individuals may have a drive to consume alcohol that cannot be construed as a need and,
conversely, they may have a need to take more
exercise, although they may not feel driven to do
so. While recognizing that choices are constrained
by biological factors, Doyal and Gough are wary
of placing too great an emphasis on biological
determinism.

An alternative way of looking at need is as a
means of achieving a goal. Liss (1990) suggests that
a goal therefore becomes a necessary precondition
to there being a need. Hence, statements about need
must conform to the pattern:

A needs X in order to G.

Wants would be distinguished from needs on the
basis that wants can be expressed merely as preferences with no requirement to specify the relationship

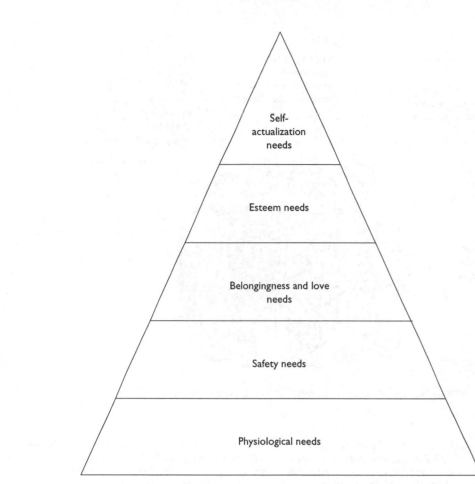

Figure 5.2   A representation of Maslow's hierarchy of needs (after Maslow, 1954)

to goals. A further distinction between needs and wants can be made based on the nature of the goal. Doyal and Gough suggest that needs would only apply in relation to *universalizable* goals – that is, goals that are in everyone's interests to achieve. Wants, in contrast, would vary from person to person, reflecting personal preferences. Such wants would be guided by individual perceptions, whereas needs draw on a shared understanding about the avoidance of harm. For example, an individual may say that they *need* a cigarette, but, from a *universalizable* goal perspective, they *want* a cigarette and *need* to give up smoking.

Doyal and Gough's analysis of universalizable goals identifies two key elements: the avoidance of serious harm and the ability to participate in a social form of life. They propose that the universal prerequisites for achieving these goals and participating

fully in society constitute basic human needs, which are identified as:

• physical health
• autonomy.

Autonomy is seen as including mental health, cognitive skills and opportunities to participate in society. In order to meet these basic needs, eleven categories of intermediate needs are identified, as seen in the outline of Doyal and Gough's theory of need in Figure 5.3. While basic and intermediate needs are universalizable, the ways in which these needs can be met may well vary.

Needs assessment will be concerned with assessing how well these basic and intermediate needs are being met. This raises the issue of what standard should be set concerning the satisfaction of needs. In relation to basic needs satisfaction, Doyal and

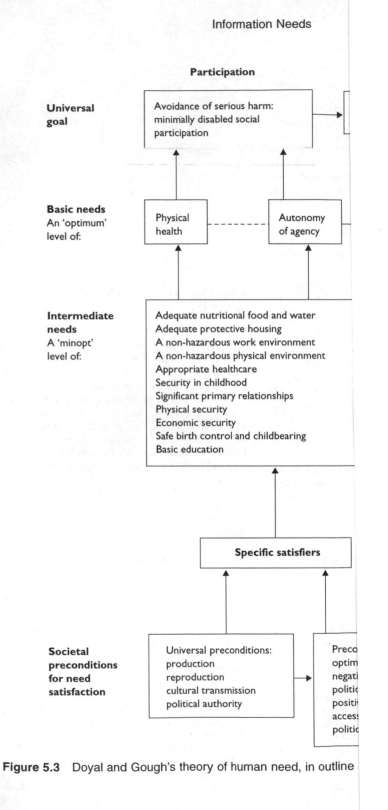

Figure 5.3   Doyal and Gough's theory of human need, in outline

THE TRAGEDY OF THE COMMONS

Hardin (1968) used the following analogy, first described in a pamphlet by the mathematician William Forster Lloyd in 1833, to exemplify the problem of overpopulation.

People graze their cattle on common land. So long as they do not, in total, exceed the 'carrying capacity' of the land, it is in the interests of everyone to graze as many cattle as possible. However, once the carrying capacity has been reached, there becomes a notional limit. From the individual's perspective, adding one more animal over the limit is an advantage because they get all the proceeds from selling the animal. The negative consequences of overgrazing are shared by everyone. While there is an imperative, therefore, for everyone to continue to graze as many cattle as possible to maximize personal gain, ultimately this will backfire as the number of animals increases to a level at which they all succumb. Everyone then loses. 'Freedom of the commons brings ruin to all.'

development of antibiotic-resistant strains of bacteria and, therefore, be against the longer-term interests of both the individual concerned and the wider population. There is an important distinction, therefore, between individual and collective interpretations of needs, wants and demands, as exemplified in the notion of the 'tragedy of the commons' outlined in the box.

Whether or not we accept that there are objective needs, decisions about the best ways in which to achieve them will inevitably involve a degree of subjectivity. For some, the very nature of needs remains subjectively determined. Therefore, the issue of values – both personal and professional – cannot be ignored. At the most fundamental level, the distinction between needs, wants and demands is value-laden. There is also the related question of who should arbitrate when there are conflicting views (Bartholomew et al., 2001).

A reductionist approach to needs assessment

The pursuit of the lowest-level causes of phenomena is referred to as 'reductionism'. Bringing a reductionist perspective to bear on the identification of needs would involve identifying the main health problems and constructing a causal chain that progressively homes in on factors that might be modified – that is, those factors that need to be changed to improve health status. Such a diagnostic approach would be very much in tune with the biomedical model of health promotion discussed in Chapter 1 and the public health approach to identifying needs referred to above. It could take either quality of life or disease as its starting point. This way of identifying needs would also equate with

Bartholomew et al.'s view that a need is 'a difference between what currently exists and a more desirable state' (2001: 16). It typically draws heavily on epidemiological analyses and, by way of example, Figure 5.5 shows how it might apply to coronary heart disease.

The emphasis is on identifying modifiable risk factors. This approach has been criticized for attaching undue importance to behavioural risk factors. However, it could equally implicate social and environmental risk factors as the major determinants of problems. A further area of interest is the existence of any high-risk groups, defined as (Bartholomew, 2001: 17), 'a group with a definable boundary and shared characteristics that have, or are at risk for, certain health and quality-of-life problems.'

As we will note below, reference can be made to major empirical studies and theoretical models to establish a framework for this type of enquiry. Such frameworks can be used to direct research at the local level towards identifying the key causative or contributory factors that should be considered when planning interventions. Analysis at the local level can then focus on identifying which of the generally recognized risk factors are the most pertinent in a specific context. Green and Kreuter (1991) suggest that one advantage of this approach is that it allows workers to direct their efforts at achieving maximum gains. However, it does not formally acknowledge the value of community insights or gaining the active involvement of members of the community.

Participation in needs assessment

The importance of community participation was recognized in the Ottawa Charter (WHO, 1986) and

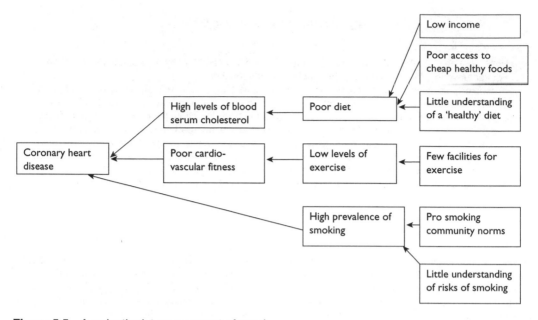

Figure 5.5 A reductionist assessment of need

reaffirmed in the Jakarta Declaration (WHO, 1997): 'People have to be at the centre of health promotion action and decision-making processes for them to be effective.'

Arguments supporting public participation in needs assessment can be based on the rights of individuals to have a voice and also, more pragmatically, on the premise that participation fosters higher levels of motivation and enhances the effectiveness of interventions (Watson, 2002). Participation can be a means of bridging the gap between planners and the community. As we noted in Chapter 3, when a community recognizes the existence of a problem and identifies its own solution, then adoption of an innovation is likely to be much more rapid than when an external agency prescribes a solution for a problem the community was not aware of or does not consider to be a priority.

Freire (1972) uses the term 'cultural invasion' for this latter approach, which involves external agents bringing their own value systems to bear in the analysis of problems. The limitations of a top-down assessment of need are summed up by Gough (1992: 12):

> Experts and professionals can put their own interest before the wellbeing of their clients or research subjects. Often too they will be so ignorant of the reality of life for ordinary people that their proposals can be counterproductive or just plain stupid.

Knowledge held within the community must therefore become an integral part of any needs assessment. It offers a complementary insight that should be considered alongside epidemiological and economic approaches. However, this raises the issue of the weight attached to the views of the public in contrast to those of so-called professionals (Foreman, 1996) and how to deal with any differences. Comparison of the professionals' views of priorities within an area with the actual priorities of the community that emerged from a rapid assessment exercise (Ong and Humphris, 1994) demonstrates only too clearly how professional assessments can differ markedly from those of the communities concerned, as shown in Table 5.1.

Stacey (1994) prefers the term 'people knowledge to 'lay knowledge' as the term 'lay' often carries connotations of having less competence or worth. People knowledge is often informal, experiential and mostly unwritten. It offers insights into the constellation of factors particular to specific situations from the perspective of those who are most familiar with them. The professional perspective, in contrast, draws on codified and systematized knowledge, often operating at a more general level.

Stacey is critical of the pressure to express lay understanding in official language and use acceptable research methods – that is, to operate within professionally defined parameters – and draws a number of lessons about participation:

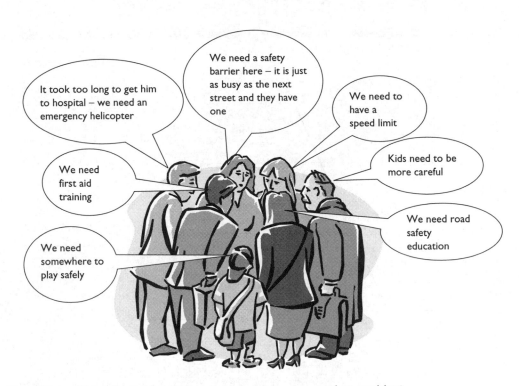

Figure 5.1   Alternative interpretations of need at the scene of an accident

fully understood by members of a group. They are therefore subjectively defined, but at the group collective, rather than the individual, level. Doyal and Gough challenge both these positions, along with economic, sociological and postmodern interpretations of needs as relative and contend that objective need does indeed exist. Furthermore, demonstrating that there are objective universal needs creates a moral imperative to meet those needs and effectively establishes them as fundamental rights.

The term 'need' has been used to refer to drives or motivational forces that arise from some disequilibrium – for example, the need for sleep when tired or food when hungry. Maslow (1954) identifies a number of such needs that can be ordered into a hierarchy premised on the requirement to satisfy basic needs, such as hunger and warmth, before higher-order needs can be addressed. The needs identified are felt to be common to different cultures. The hierarchy is conventionally represented as in Figure 5.2.

Each level in the hierarchy is assumed to be necessary for the achievement of the next level, although there is no requirement for 100 per cent satisfaction before moving on to the next level. Maslow himself acknowledged that the hierarchy

was not fixed. For example, in those who gain satisfaction from high-risk activities, such as mountaineering or hang-gliding, self-actualization needs may take precedence over safety needs.

Doyal and Gough reject the interpretation of needs as drives on the basis that needs and drives can exist independently of each other. For example, individuals may have a drive to consume alcohol that cannot be construed as a need and, conversely, they may have a need to take more exercise, although they may not feel driven to do so. While recognizing that choices are constrained by biological factors, Doyal and Gough are wary of placing too great an emphasis on biological determinism.

An alternative way of looking at need is as a means of achieving a goal. Liss (1990) suggests that a goal therefore becomes a necessary precondition to there being a need. Hence, statements about need must conform to the pattern:

A needs X in order to G.

Wants would be distinguished from needs on the basis that wants can be expressed merely as preferences with no requirement to specify the relationship

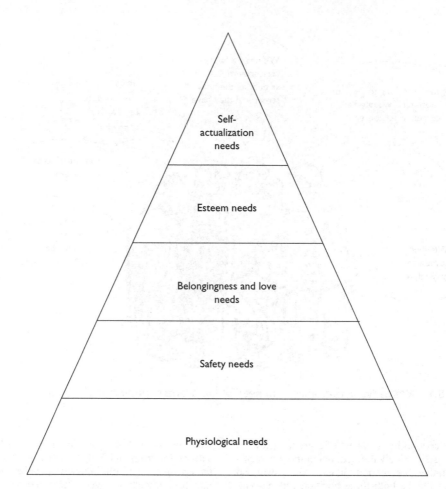

Figure 5.2 A representation of Maslow's hierarchy of needs (after Maslow, 1954)

to goals. A further distinction between needs and wants can be made based on the nature of the goal. Doyal and Gough suggest that needs would only apply in relation to *universalizable* goals – that is, goals that are in everyone's interests to achieve. Wants, in contrast, would vary from person to person, reflecting personal preferences. Such wants would be guided by individual perceptions, whereas needs draw on a shared understanding about the avoidance of harm. For example, an individual may say that they *need* a cigarette, but, from a *universalizable* goal perspective, they *want* a cigarette and *need* to give up smoking.

Doyal and Gough's analysis of universalizable goals identifies two key elements: the avoidance of serious harm and the ability to participate in a social form of life. They propose that the universal prerequisites for achieving these goals and participating fully in society constitute basic human needs, which are identified as:

- physical health
- autonomy.

Autonomy is seen as including mental health, cognitive skills and opportunities to participate in society. In order to meet these basic needs, eleven categories of intermediate needs are identified, as seen in the outline of Doyal and Gough's theory of need in Figure 5.3. While basic and intermediate needs are universalizable, the ways in which these needs can be met may well vary.

Needs assessment will be concerned with assessing how well these basic and intermediate needs are being met. This raises the issue of what standard should be set concerning the satisfaction of needs. In relation to basic needs satisfaction, Doyal and

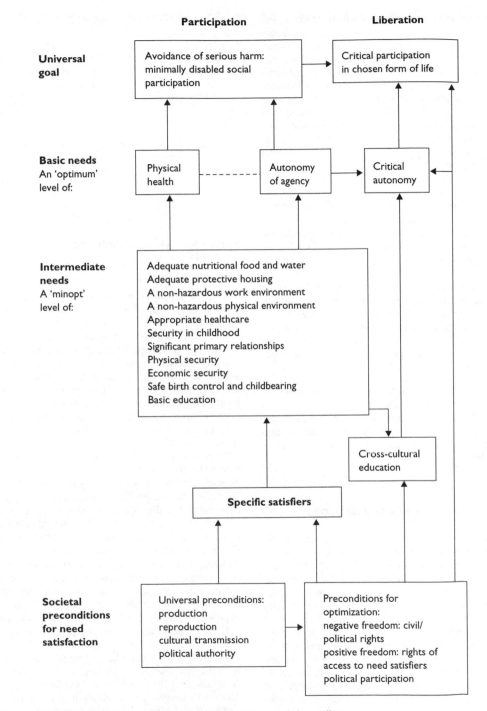

Figure 5.3 Doyal and Gough's theory of human need, in outline

Gough reject both absolute minimum standards and relative standards. Instead, they advocate an optimum standard for basic needs and propose a 'minimum optimorum' level for intermediate needs – that is, the minimum level of input of intermediate need satisfaction to achieve optimal basic needs satisfaction.

The remaining question concerns how needs will be assessed. Doyal and Gough support the notion of informed participation by those whose needs are being assessed, although they caution that this can favour those already in privileged positions who may be more influential than others without such advantages. They suggest that the development of indicators of intermediate needs will be fed, in an iterative way, by the development of new codified and experiential knowledge. They (1991: 169) recognize that both qualitative and quantitative indicators will be needed, but place considerable emphasis on the latter:

> To chart both basic and intermediate indicators we ideally require social indicators which are valid, distributive, quantitative and aggregated, but which are open to revision. These indicators should be open to disaggregation between groups. In this way profiles of the need-satisfaction of nations, cultural groups and other collectives can be compiled.

When differences arise between the views of needs established by expert-led approaches, which draw on codified knowledge, and community-based approaches, which are grounded in experience, dialogue is proposed as a mechanism for resolving the situation.

Needs, wants and demands

Equity is recognized as being one of the fundamental tenets of health promotion. Principles of social justice would presuppose that health resources should be distributed in relation to needs. However, as is all too apparent, access to services and wider opportunities to promote health are not necessarily governed by needs. Some time ago, Hart (1971) used the notion of the 'inverse care law' to describe the generally poorer provision of services in those areas that are most deprived and have the greatest burden of ill health. An emphasis on needs rather than wants or demands is therefore integral to equity. Nutbeam (1998b: 7) captures this idea perfectly:

> Equity means fairness. Equity in health means that people's needs guide the distribution of opportunities for wellbeing.

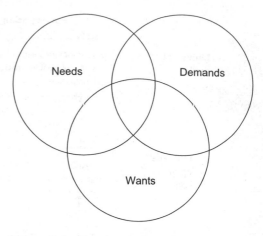

Figure 5.4   Needs, wants and demands

The management of public services on market or quasi-market principles is necessarily demand-led. In contrast, a needs-led approach will be more consistent with a focus on social justice.

The defining characteristic of need in Doyal and Gough's theory of need is its instrumentality in achieving universal human goals. Wants, in contrast, are personal preferences and equate with what Bradshaw might term felt need. These subjective, personal preferences may overlap with an objective view of need or be completely different, as summarized in Figure 5.4.

In general economic terms, a demand is associated with the consumer's willingness to pay for desired goods or services (Bowling, 1997b). However, the complexity of the health and healthcare market calls for a broader interpretation. Mooney and Leeder (1997) describe demands as being based on wants, but also involving action directed at fulfilling the wants. There is a clear parallel here with Bradshaw's expressed need. Again, demands will overlap, to a greater or lesser extent, with wants and needs. Foreman (1996) suggests that health professionals effectively 'ratify' expressed needs or demands by providing services.

Clearly those with most power will be better placed to articulate their wants and ensure that their demands are met – regardless of whether or not this is in the interests of the collective. Responding to demands may also ultimately conflict with the needs and longer-term interests of the individual. Robinson and Elkan (1996) offer the example of an individual demanding antibiotic treatment for a viral infection. Prescribing an antibiotic would serve no useful clinical purpose. Moreover, such unnecessary prescribing would contribute to the

THE TRAGEDY OF THE COMMONS

Hardin (1968) used the following analogy, first described in a pamphlet by the mathematician William Forster Lloyd in 1833, to exemplify the problem of overpopulation.

People graze their cattle on common land. So long as they do not, in total, exceed the 'carrying capacity' of the land, it is in the interests of everyone to graze as many cattle as possible. However, once the carrying capacity has been reached, there becomes a notional limit. From the individual's perspective, adding one more animal over the limit is an advantage because they get all the proceeds from selling the animal. The negative consequences of overgrazing are shared by everyone. While there is an imperative, therefore, for everyone to continue to graze as many cattle as possible to maximize personal gain, ultimately this will backfire as the number of animals increases to a level at which they all succumb. Everyone then loses. 'Freedom of the commons brings ruin to all.'

development of antibiotic-resistant strains of bacteria and, therefore, be against the longer-term interests of both the individual concerned and the wider population. There is an important distinction, therefore, between individual and collective interpretations of needs, wants and demands, as exemplified in the notion of the 'tragedy of the commons' outlined in the box.

Whether or not we accept that there are objective needs, decisions about the best ways in which to achieve them will inevitably involve a degree of subjectivity. For some, the very nature of needs remains subjectively determined. Therefore, the issue of values – both personal and professional – cannot be ignored. At the most fundamental level, the distinction between needs, wants and demands is value-laden. There is also the related question of who should arbitrate when there are conflicting views (Bartholomew et al., 2001).

A reductionist approach to needs assessment

The pursuit of the lowest-level causes of phenomena is referred to as 'reductionism'. Bringing a reductionist perspective to bear on the identification of needs would involve identifying the main health problems and constructing a causal chain that progressively homes in on factors that might be modified – that is, those factors that need to be changed to improve health status. Such a diagnostic approach would be very much in tune with the biomedical model of health promotion discussed in Chapter 1 and the public health approach to identifying needs referred to above. It could take either quality of life or disease as its starting point. This way of identifying needs would also equate with

Bartholomew et al.'s view that a need is 'a difference between what currently exists and a more desirable state' (2001: 16). It typically draws heavily on epidemiological analyses and, by way of example, Figure 5.5 shows how it might apply to coronary heart disease.

The emphasis is on identifying modifiable risk factors. This approach has been criticized for attaching undue importance to behavioural risk factors. However, it could equally implicate social and environmental risk factors as the major determinants of problems. A further area of interest is the existence of any high-risk groups, defined as (Bartholomew, 2001: 17), 'a group with a definable boundary and shared characteristics that have, or are at risk for, certain health and quality-of-life problems.'

As we will note below, reference can be made to major empirical studies and theoretical models to establish a framework for this type of enquiry. Such frameworks can be used to direct research at the local level towards identifying the key causative or contributory factors that should be considered when planning interventions. Analysis at the local level can then focus on identifying which of the generally recognized risk factors are the most pertinent in a specific context. Green and Kreuter (1991) suggest that one advantage of this approach is that it allows workers to direct their efforts at achieving maximum gains. However, it does not formally acknowledge the value of community insights or gaining the active involvement of members of the community.

Participation in needs assessment

The importance of community participation was recognized in the Ottawa Charter (WHO, 1986) and

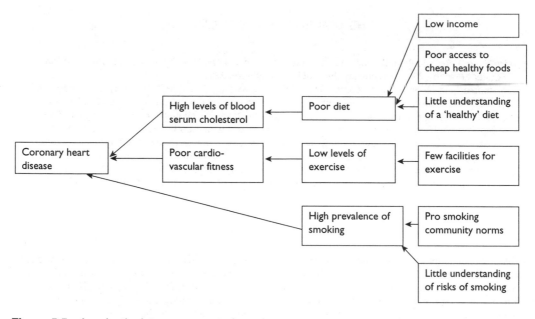

Figure 5.5   A reductionist assessment of need

reaffirmed in the Jakarta Declaration (WHO, 1997): 'People have to be at the centre of health promotion action and decision-making processes for them to be effective.'

Arguments supporting public participation in needs assessment can be based on the rights of individuals to have a voice and also, more pragmatically, on the premise that participation fosters higher levels of motivation and enhances the effectiveness of interventions (Watson, 2002). Participation can be a means of bridging the gap between planners and the community. As we noted in Chapter 3, when a community recognizes the existence of a problem and identifies its own solution, then adoption of an innovation is likely to be much more rapid than when an external agency prescribes a solution for a problem the community was not aware of or does not consider to be a priority.

Freire (1972) uses the term 'cultural invasion' for this latter approach, which involves external agents bringing their own value systems to bear in the analysis of problems. The limitations of a top-down assessment of need are summed up by Gough (1992: 12):

> Experts and professionals can put their own interest before the wellbeing of their clients or research subjects. Often too they will be so ignorant of the reality of life for ordinary people that their proposals can be counterproductive or just plain stupid.

Knowledge held within the community must therefore become an integral part of any needs assessment. It offers a complementary insight that should be considered alongside epidemiological and economic approaches. However, this raises the issue of the weight attached to the views of the public in contrast to those of so-called professionals (Foreman, 1996) and how to deal with any differences. Comparison of the professionals' views of priorities within an area with the actual priorities of the community that emerged from a rapid assessment exercise (Ong and Humphris, 1994) demonstrates only too clearly how professional assessments can differ markedly from those of the communities concerned, as shown in Table 5.1.

Stacey (1994) prefers the term 'people knowledge to 'lay knowledge' as the term 'lay' often carries connotations of having less competence or worth. People knowledge is often informal, experiential and mostly unwritten. It offers insights into the constellation of factors particular to specific situations from the perspective of those who are most familiar with them. The professional perspective, in contrast, draws on codified and systematized knowledge, often operating at a more general level.

Stacey is critical of the pressure to express lay understanding in official language and use acceptable research methods – that is, to operate within professionally defined parameters – and draws a number of lessons about participation:

Table 5.1 *Views of the community and professionals compared – community priorities, Linacre ward, 1989 (derived from Ong and Humphris, 1994)*

Concerns	Community priorities	Professional team's view of priorities
Physical environment		
Rubbish in the street	1	4
Poor-quality housing	2	1
Air pollution	3	2/3
Disposal of syringes in public places	4	5
Lack of recreational space	5	2/3
Disease and disability		
Depression and anxiety	1	2
Drinking, tobacco, tranquillizers, hard drugs	2	4
Respiratory problems	3	1
Poor diet	4	3
Health services		
Lack of overall preventive children's services	1	2
GPs appear 'too busy'	2	3
Lack of home support after hospital discharge	3	1
Lack of 'Well Woman' services	4	4
Lack of chiropody services	5	5

Degrees of actual power	{	Control
		Delegated power
		Partnership
Degrees of tokenism	{	Placation
		Consultation
		Informing
Non-participation	{	Therapy
		Manipulation

Figure 5.6 Arnstein's ladder of participation (after Arnstein, 1971)

- people's points of view should be understood in their own terms
- the distinction between *people* and *professional* is not rigid
- people knowledge is consistent and rational
- people are producers of health as well as consumers of healthcare
- lack of real influence in decisions alienates people from participation.

The Freirean notion of 'cultural synthesis' describes a situation in which professionals or external agents attempt to learn *with* the people about their experiences of the world.

Public participation in needs assessment can range from tokenistic consultation to having a controlling influence in arriving at what the needs are and how they should be prioritized. Arnstein's (1971) ladder of participation (see Figure 5.6) is a well-known device for distinguishing between genuine participation, mere tokenism and, indeed, attempts to manipulate. The degree of active participation increases progressively from none at the bottom to genuine control at the top.

Brager and Specht (1973) provide a similar analysis of the spectrum of participation (see Figure 5.7). Their depiction of the various levels is particularly pertinent to health promotion planning and needs assessment.

A further consideration – over and above the actual level of participation – is the motivation underpinning attempts to involve communities. Clearly the chief beneficiary of participation in needs assessment and planning processes should be the community itself. Participation should not be a covert means of furthering professional or organizational interests – a situation graphically encapsulated in a French student poster from the 1960s (see box).

Health Promotion

Degree	Participants' action	Illustrative mode
High	Has control	The organization asks the community to identify the problems and make all the decisions regarding goals and means. It is willing to help the community at each step to accomplish its own goals, even to the extent of administrative control of the programme
	Has delegated authority	The organization identifies and presents a problem to the community, defines the limits and asks the community to make a series of decisions that can be embodied in a plan it will accept
	Plans jointly	The organization presents a tentative plan subject to change and invites recommendations from those affected
	Advises	The organization presents a plan and invites questions. It is prepared to modify the plan only if absolutely necessary
	Is consulted	The organization tries to promote a plan and develop the support to facilitate acceptance of, or give sufficient sanction to, the plan so administrative compliance can be expected
	Receives information	The organization makes a plan and announces it. The community is convened for informational purposes; compliance is expected
Low	None	The community is told nothing

Figure 5.7 A spectrum of participation (after Brager and Specht, 1973)

COMMUNITY PARTICIPATION: DECLINING THE VERB

Je participe
Tu participes
Il/elle participe
Nous participons
Vous participez
Ils profitent

A number of different vehicles have been used for consultation. These include citizens' juries, postal panels, face-to-face panels, local user and carer groups and surveys and opinion polls. Oregon Health Decisions is a widely known example of an attempt to give people a voice and involve them in the development of health policy (see the box below). Jordan et al. (1998) suggest that consultation methods can be classified on the basis of whether or not:

- respondents are provided with any information
- respondents are involved in discussion or deliberation before recording their views.

OREGON HEALTH DECISIONS

Oregon Health Decisions originally started in 1982 as an outreach effort by the Oregon Health Council. Eventually Oregon Health Decisions evolved into an independent civic organization dedicated to bringing the general public into the process of shaping health policy... The organization is most well known for its role in organizing community meetings for the Oregon Health Services Commission in its work of creating a prioritized list of health services, a central feature of the innovative Oregon Health Plan.

Website: www.oregonhealthdecisions.org/index.htm#welcome

Citizens' juries, for example, would be presented with information and involved in deliberation before reaching their decisions. In contrast, opinion polls would collect information from individuals on the spot.

A further issue relates to the representativeness of the various groups. Clearly, surveys can explicitly attempt to obtain representative samples. In contrast, the selection of jury members is usually more purposive and, despite membership generally rotating at intervals, cannot be regarded as being truly representative. There are similar concerns about the composition of user and care consultation groups and panels.

Another pertinent issue is whether individuals are commenting on behalf of themselves or the group that they purport to represent – especially when there may be conflict between individual and community needs.

Furthermore, within any community, the more articulate will inevitably be better placed to make their concerns known, so a conscious effort may be needed to secure the participation of marginalized groups.

The key aspects of the 'informed citizen process', which takes account of these concerns are summarized by Blackwell and Kosky (2000):

- **information** people must be presented with accurate, unbiased information
- **time** sufficient time must be allowed to be informed and to be able to reflect
- **scrutiny** opportunity must be provided to ask questions before making preferences
- **deliberation** there must be a chance to reflect on information given
- **independence** participants must have some control over how their findings are presented and to whom
- **authority** participants must feel assured that their findings will be listened to.

Rapid assessment and appraisal

Rapid assessment techniques have their origin in the broad move towards community participation and recognition of the need for local knowledge. They emerged in so-called developing countries as a response to inappropriate research by outside agencies – typified by overconfidence, lack of communication and consultation with the community or other professional groups, the use of theoretically rigorous, but time-consuming, methods and failure to translate research findings into action within a reasonable timescale (Vlassoff and Tanner, 1992).

Rapid assessment and appraisal attempts to overcome professional dominance and works towards developing a joint understanding of the needs of the community by bringing together the views of key stakeholders. It places emphasis on knowledge indigenous to a community and acknowledges the importance of qualitative research methods. However, it does not preclude the need for quantitative data, such as epidemiological information (Foreman, 1996).

A variety of terminology is used in relation to rapid assessment and appraisal, as summarized in the box below. In the literature, a clear distinction has not always been made – indeed, some authors have used the terms interchangeably. Rifkin (1992), however, identifies two broad strands, which helps to resolve the semantic confusion. One emerged from epidemiology and is concerned with collecting information on ill health and disease – usually referred to as 'rapid assessment' or 'rapid epidemiological assessment'. It draws on all forms of local data, including routinely collected data and the views of the community, but the role of the community members is generally as informants only.

The second strand originated in the 'rapid rural appraisal' techniques developed for use in agriculture and rural development and the move from extractive

DIFFERENT TERMINOLOGY FOR RAPID INFORMATION COLLECTION APPROACHES

REA   Rapid epidemiological assessment
RA   Rapid appraisal
RRA   Rapid rural appraisal
PRA   Participatory rural appraisal
PA   Participatory appraisal
PNA   Participatory needs assessment
RPA   Rapid participatory appraisal
REA   Rapid ethnographic assessment

to participative methods of research. It gives greater attention to the *process* of gathering data and involving communities in data collection and analysis. This latter approach is referred to as 'rapid appraisal'. The terms 'participatory rural appraisal' and 'participatory appraisal' are also used and, as these names imply, they place particular emphasis on community participation.

The distinction between the two broad strands revolves around the level and nature of participation and the emphasis on particular methodologies. Is the assessment merely community *based* or is it community *led*, taking its direction from issues raised by the community?

Notwithstanding this difference, there is some overlap between the two schools. Both take a holistic view of health and aim to collect information quickly and at low cost to inform planning at the local level.

The use of the term 'rapid' should not be taken to imply any sacrifice of rigour or attention to quality. Speed is achieved by using a battery of research methods and involving a range of professionals and lay people. Accuracy is also a major concern and triangulation is an important feature in relation to cross-checking the validity of findings (triangulation is considered more fully in Chapter 10). Rapid assessment and appraisal strategies usually incorporate opportunities, while still in the field, to reflect on findings and redefine data collection requirements in the light of any emergent conclusions or hunches. While there is considerable attention to validity, it should also be noted that rapid assessment and appraisal takes a realistic view of the level of precision required to meet the research objectives (Vlassoff and Tanner, 1992) and acknowledges that

there are limits to what actually needs to be known (Heaver, 1992: 14):

> The principles apply here of optimal ignorance – not trying to find out more than is needed; and of appropriate imprecision – not trying to measure what does not need to be measured, or not measuring more accurately than is needed for practical purposes.

Ong et al. (1991) note that this approach goes beyond attempting to objectively assess the magnitude of a problem to address the strength of feeling in the community about the issue, which will inevitably be influenced by its wider ramifications. For example, although the actual number of people using hard drugs within a community may be small, drug use may have consequences for a much wider group and, therefore, be perceived to be a major problem.

Heaver (1992) identifies a number of advantages of these approaches over and above speed and economy:

- the information generated is accurate and context-specific as it draws on people's in-depth understanding of the local situation and provides opportunities for cross-checking
- plans drawn up by insiders are more likely to work than ones created by those outside the community because they take account of the local context
- the process is empowering – it enhances people's understanding of problems and enables them to have a voice in decisions made about the most appropriate course of action.

Annett and Rifkin (1990) represent the key information needs of a community as a pyramid (see Figure 5.8). Data can be collected from a number of

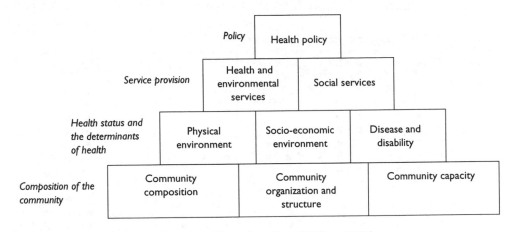

Figure 5.8 Information profile (derived from Annett and Rifkin, 1990)

different sources and using a range of different methods for each of the levels.

The data collection methods used in rapid appraisal are many and varied. An example of the development of a food calendar by members of a coastal community in Guinea is provided in the box (below). The use of visual and oral methods is particularly appropriate where there are low levels of literacy. A selection of methods used in participatory appraisal is provided in the next box, but such lists are limited only by the creativity of individuals involved in the process.

Professionals may well require training in the use of these methods. Moreover if they are to operate within a true spirit of participation they will also need to abandon their expert role and go into a community prepared to learn from the people – communication and listening skills are therefore particularly important. Similarly, if members of the community are to be more than just informants they will also need to develop skills in data collection methods and interpretation.

AN EXAMPLE OF USING A FOOD CALENDAR

Extract from notes of a food and nutrition PRA:

Having heard about a 'hungry season' during the focused walk we decided to investigate the general diet and seasonal variation...

... a team member drew out a six-season calendar framework in the sand as the women talked about their main staple food, rice; marked the top line with a grass frond to represent the rice; and allocated palm-nuts in each of the six sections according to the women's remarks on availability...discussion ensued...and they insisted that one season be left empty, not because they have nothing to eat then, but because their own rice has been eaten or sold off to repay debts. They buy 'foreign' rice for that period...

... the conversation about fish livened up. 'Give me those nuts' said a lady in red 'we can do this kind of writing'.

(Continued)

(*Continued*)
Calendar of Main Elements of Household Budget

Season	Mist and fog D J F	Hot and dry M A	Early rains M J	Rains J A S O	Late rains S O	Clear skies N
Own rice to eat	• • • / • • • • / • • • • / • • • • / • • • •	• • • / • • • • / • • • • / • • • • / • • • •	• • / • •	• / • • / • •		• • / • • / • • / • • • • / • • • •
Fish for smoking	• • • • / • • • •	• • / • • • • / • • • •	• / • • • •	• / • • • • / • • • • / • • • •	• • • / • • • •	• • / • • • • / • • • • / • • • •
Cash in	• • • / • • • • / • • • •	• • • / • • • • / • • • •	• • • • / • • • •	• • • / • • • • / • • • •	• • • / • • • •	• • / • • • • / • • • •
Cash out	• / • • • •	• • • •	• / • •	• / • • / • • / • • • / • • • • / • • • •	• • / • • •	• / • • / • • •
Debt cycle	Repayments			Highest debts		Repayment

Subsequent discussion of the calendar with other members of the community resulted in a decision to explore the possibility of setting up a rice store.

Appleton, 1992:79

A SELECTION OF METHODS USED IN PARTICIPATORY APPRAISAL

- Mapping
- Transects
- Social mapping
- Body mapping
- Timelines and trends, including seasonal trends
- Historical transects
- Photography
- Ranking and scoring exercises
- Sequence matrices
- Causal and flow diagramming
- Chapatti (Venn) diagramming
- Case histories
- Life histories
- Diaries
- Focus groups
- Observations

An important practical issue is the selection of key informants and ensuring that they are representative of the community. How this should best be tackled will require consideration of local contextual factors. Ong et al.'s (1991) rapid appraisal in an area in the North West of England identified three groups of key informants:

- people with knowledge of the community because of their professional roles (such as health visitors, police, social workers)
- community 'leaders' (such as 'leaders' of voluntary associations, self-help groups, political groups)
- people centrally placed within the community (such as postal workers, local shopkeepers, school crossing patrols).

The data generated can be fed into any stage of the planning cycle (Vlassoff and Tanner, 1992) and, as we earlier noted, the approach is particularly useful in motivating communities. However, Rifkin's (1992) discussion generates some fundamental questions.

- Is participation viewed as a means or an end?
- Is participation active or passive?
- Does the community have control over the way in which the findings are used?
- Does the community have a say in planning processes?

The principles of participatory appraisal would require that the community should not merely be used as providers of information to slot into a conceptual framework already established by the researchers. True participation would involve the community members in developing the conceptual framework. It would also view them as equal partners in decision making – especially if the tokenism referred to by Arnstein (1971) is to be avoided.

It will be clear from our earlier discussion of empowerment in Chapter 3 that community involvement in rapid appraisal and participatory appraisal can be empowering. There can be formal acknowledgment of the value of community members' knowledge and experience and they can exercise power and control in decision making and planning. However, there is always the risk of raising expectations that cannot be met and the consequent negative repercussions.

Here are the key features of rapid and participatory appraisal:

- the community is involved in information collection and analysis – that is, they are done in/with/and by the community
- action-orientated
- attempts to include all perspectives

- use of multidisciplinary teams and interactive methods
- emphasis on communication and listening skills
- use of a range of data collection methods and triangulation
- analysis is carried out while still 'in the field'
- iterative
- incorporates critical reflection and self-criticism
- flexible – the direction of research may be reoriented as new information becomes available
- holistic view of health and its determinants
- optimal ignorance and appropriate imprecision.

While developing countries have paved the way in the use of these methods, there has also been increasing interest in the developed world. Indeed, Manderson and Aaby (1992) refer to an 'epidemic' in the use of rapid assessment procedures and Cornwall et al. (2001: iii) describe the spread of PRA through Kenya as being 'like a bushfire'. The approach has been particularly relevant when involving members of deprived and marginalized communities in identifying their needs and making them known. Often the technique has been used in geographically discrete areas, but it is equally applicable to more diffuse communities, such as refugees and asylum seekers (Vallely et al., 1999). It has also been used with young people as a means of giving them a voice. Morrow (2001), for example, adopted this approach with school pupils to build up a picture of how they see their social networks and communities.

Critical reflections on participatory appraisal

Participatory appraisal has grown rapidly in popularity. Cornwall et al. (2001) reflect on the consequences of the extensive use of PRA in Kenya and it having become almost a routine requirement of development organizations – many of which have done little to accommodate this participatory style of working within their own modes of operation. They feel that the range of meanings of participatory appraisal, different conceptualizations of what it involves and the variety of practices carried out under its name threaten its quality and create difficulties in establishing quality standards. A concern is that people may subscribe to the rhetoric without fully embracing the principles. The 'Pathways to Participation Project' aims to consolidate the use of PRA by reflecting on the experiences of practitioners and addressing the issues raised (working papers are available from the Institute of Development Studies' website at: www.ids.ac.uk).

CHANGES RECORDED AFTER USE
OF A PRA IN EDINBURGH

- Local bus route altered to go into a council estate with 30 per cent increase in passengers.
- Fenced-off play areas provided by the local council.
- Use of community room for community education classes, residents' association and councillors' meetings.
- Three companies tendering to build a local supermarket.
- Improvements to medical facilities – additional telephone line, toys in the waiting area, ramp, patients spoken to with more respect.

Murray and Graham, 1995

While recognizing the potential offered by rapid appraisal and the rewarding nature of working in this way, Murray (1999) draws on the experience of five projects in the UK to identify a number of practical limitations. It tends to work best when there is a clearly defined, homogeneous community. Bias may occur if the informants selected have similar backgrounds and there is no conscious attempt to seek out any contradictory viewpoints. There may also be professional bias unless a multidisciplinary team is used and, in any event, there may be a degree of subjectivity in interpreting what people say. Any statistics generated may need to be interpreted with caution because of the rapid and highly focused nature of data collection.

The use of this approach requires training at the local level and the coordination of the various layers of activity can be demanding. Butcher and Kievelitz (1997) comment on the particular difficulty of developing analytical skills. Using the analogy of a jigsaw, Murray (1999: 444) suggests that rapid appraisal can provide 'key pieces of the jigsaw but not the complete picture' and that postal surveys and primary care data could help to complete the picture.

However, RPA appears to have a greater capacity to bring about change than the other methods. The changes documented after the technique was used in Edinburgh are listed in the box above.

The London Health Economics Consortium (1996) carried out a review of practice in community needs assessments in four test-bed sites in the London area. It noted the lack of explicit attention to validity and practical problems with triangulation – particularly that of finding truly independent sources of information. There was concern about bias introduced by the selection of key informants. It also commented on a tendency to confuse causation with mere association and suggested that a more critical approach to causality was needed. The report noted that the findings of community needs assessments are often very similar, regardless of the areas in which they are carried out. The findings that commonly emerge are listed in the box below.

COMMON FINDINGS OF NEEDS ASSESSMENT EXERCISES

- Pollution and the environment.
- Housing.
- Employment.
- Poor education and recreational facilities.
- Vandalism and crime.
- Transport.
- Loneliness, stress and mental health.
- Other diseases and disability.
- Information on, and availability of, general practitioner and social services.

London Health Economics Consortium, 1996

The chief concern that emerged from the study was the issue of priority setting. Particular problems concerned having too many options and the lack of criteria or appropriate mechanisms for choosing between them, the non-comparability of options, a reluctance to make decisions about rationing and a preference to view recommendations as *additional to* rather than *in place of* existing provisions – that is, incrementalism without loss.

Participatory appraisal techniques have both their critics and advocates. Some of the criticism centres on specific practical and methodological issues, in contrast to other more fundamental ideological concerns. The approach tends to work best when it conforms to a true spirit of participation and follows an agenda established by the community – a position that requires considerable skills in listening and facilitation on the part of those involved in the process. Problems tend to arise when the findings have to be slotted into a pre-existing agenda, which can lead to a mismatch between what the community is saying and what planners want to hear. As a method of working, it goes beyond merely providing a technical response to the issues of problem definition and solution generation to contributing to empowering communities by virtue of the value it places on individuals' contributions.

COMMUNITY PROFILES

Whichever way problems and needs are defined, additional information about the population or community is needed before decisions can be made about health promotion interventions and how they will be implemented. Bartholomew et al. (2001) emphasize the importance of getting to know the community as well as analysing its problems. A community profile will include information

relevant to the assessment of needs, together with this wider contextual information.

Haglund et al. (1990: 91) define a community profile as:

> blending quantitative health and illness statistics and demographic indicators with qualitative information on political and socio-cultural factors. The profile includes a community's image of itself and its goals, its past history and recent civic changes, and its current resources, readiness and capacity for health promotion activities.

It provides a basis for setting priorities and planning. 'It should define community strengths as well as potential problem areas' (Rissel and Bracht, 1999: 59) and help to ensure that there is a good match between the characteristics of a community and any proposed intervention (see the box). The profile is the product of a process of community analysis. The term 'community diagnosis' has also been used, particularly in the North American context. Comparing community diagnosis with needs assessment, Stuart (in Quinn, 1999: 685) stated that:

> Diagnosis is much broader and aims to understand many facets of the community including culture, values and norms, leadership and power structure, means of communication, helping patterns, important community institutions and history. A good diagnosis suggests what it is like to live in a community, what the important health problems are, what interventions are likely to be most efficacious, and how the program would be best evaluated.

Although the two terms are synonymous, our preference here is to use 'community analysis', which we feel gives a better sense of the broad remit of the process and an emphasis on the positive aspects of a community. It reduces the risk of misinterpretation arising from associating the word, 'diagnosis' with a narrow focus on the identification of problems.

DIFFERENT COMMUNITIES, DIFFERENT INTERVENTIONS

Community A:

- traditional
- homogeneous
- family ties and hierarchies within families important
- religious
- church leaders respected
- school curriculum controlled at national level – no provision for sex education
- general reluctance to talk about sex
- media are tightly controlled
- strong censorship laws
- strong sense of community.

(Continued)

(Continued)

Community B:

- progressive
- heterogeneous
- variety of different family structures and ties
- few members of the community belong to any religion
- schools are required to provide sex education, although the quality varies between schools
- young people laugh and joke among themselves about sex, but feel uncomfortable talking to their parents or teachers about it
- little control over the media
- censorship is very liberal and there is a considerable amount of sexually explicit material in the media
- no real sense of community.

Responding to the problem of HIV/AIDS would demand completely different intervention strategies in these two communities.

As with the assessment of needs, a community analysis may be undertaken from a biomedical perspective or adopt community development principles and a more participative approach. It will include both quantitative and qualitative information derived from a variety of different sources, both primary and secondary.

Haglund et al. (1990) identify four main features of a community that would require consideration:

- specification of geographical boundaries
- assessment of social institutions – health, education and so on
- identification of social interaction patterns
- examination of social control mechanisms and norms, both formal, via institutions such as the police, school and church, and informal, via values, norms and customs in the community.

While establishing geographical boundaries is important in delimiting the area of enquiry, it should be noted that communities are not necessarily defined in geographical terms – they can be based on shared characteristics, such as ethnicity, gender,

sexual orientation and disability. The concept of 'community' will be discussed further in Chapter 8.

Bartholomew et al. (2001) comment on the importance of assessing community competence, capacity and social capital because of their relevance as:

- **inputs** factors that contribute directly to health promotion intervention
- **throughputs** factors that will affect successful programme implementation
- **outputs** the products of programmes.

'Community competence' focuses on how a community is currently functioning. The concept of 'community capacity' is closely related. It includes the notion of current competence, but also the potential within the community to respond to issues of common concern. Smith et al. (2001) note that, although there has been increasing emphasis on the concept of community capacity, there has been relatively little attempt to define it. The box provides an overview of some of the definitions used.

SOME DEFINITIONS OF 'COMMUNITY CAPACITY'

... a wholistic representation of capabilities (those with which the community is endowed and those to which the community has access) plus the facilitators and barriers to realization of those capabilities in the broader social environment.

Jackson et al., 1997, in Smith et al., 2001: 33

(Continued)

(Continued)

... the characteristics of communities that affect their ability to identify, mobilize and address social and public health problems.

McLeroy, 1996, in Bartholomew et al., 2001: 26

... the degree to which a community can develop, implement and sustain actions for strengthening community health.

Smith et al., 2001: 33

The National Civic League (2002) in the United States has developed a Civic Index to assist communities in assessing their capacity to deal with issues of concern. It covers ten broad areas:

- citizen participation
- community leadership
- government performance
- volunteerism and philanthropy
- inter-group and intra-group relationships
- civic education
- community information sharing
- capacity for cooperation and consensus building
- community vision and pride
- regional cooperation

Reference to our earlier discussion of social capital in Chapter 1 will confirm the considerable overlap between it and community capacity. However, social capital tends to focus on the networks, relationships and structural conditions rather than the resources that can be tapped into, material or otherwise (Smith et al., 2001). Eight verifiable domains of social capital have been identified and are listed in the box. The notion of social cohesion is also closely related and refers to the bonds within communities based on shared social and cultural commitments. The Home Office's Community Cohesion Review Team (2001) draws on the work of Ferlander and Timms to identify the principal characteristics of community cohesion:

- commitment to common norms and values
- interdependence as a result of shared interests
- identification with the community.

The domains of community cohesion are listed in the box, along with the domains of social capital.

THE DOMAINS OF SOCIAL CAPITAL AND COMMUNITY COHESION

Social capital

Domain	Description
Empowerment	People feel that they have a voice that is listened to, are involved in processes that affect them, can themselves take action to initiate changes
Participation	People take part in social and community activities. Local events occur and are well attended
Associational activity and common purpose	People cooperate with one another by forming formal and informal groups to further their interests
Supporting networks and reciprocity	Individuals cooperate to support one another for either mutual or one-sided gain. An expectation that help would be given to, or received from, others when needed
Collective norms and values	People share common values and norms of behaviour
Trust	People feel that they can trust their co-residents and local organizations responsible for governing or serving their area

(Continued)

(Continued)	
Safety	People feel safe in their neighbourhood and are not restricted in their use of public space by fear
Belonging	People feel connected to their co-residents, their home area, have a sense of belonging to the place and its people

Community cohesion

Domain	Description
Common values and a civic culture	Common aims and objectives, common moral principles and codes of behaviour, support for political institutions and participation in politics
Social order and social control	Absence of general conflict and threats to the existing order, absence of incivility, effective informal social control, tolerance, respect for differences, intergroup cooperation
Social solidarity and reductions in wealth disparities	Harmonious economic and social development and common standards, redistribution of public finances and opportunities, equal access to services and welfare benefits, ready acknowledgement of social obligations and willingness to assist others
Social networks and social capital	High degree of social interaction within communities and families, civic engagement and associational activity, easy resolution of collective action problems
Place attachment and identity	Strong attachment to place, intertwining of personal and place identity

Source: Forrest and Kearns, 2000, in Community Cohesion Review Team, 2001

It would be invidious to even attempt to draw up a generic checklist of all the issues that need to be considered before the detailed planning of interventions to improve the health status of a population can begin. However, they fall into five broad categories that are applicable regardless of whether there is a professional or community-led approach to data collection and whichever ideological position underpins the endeavour:

- the health status of the population – identification of problems and any groups particularly 'at risk'
- the key determinants of health status and disease – behavioural and environmental micro meso and macro levels.
- motivation and capacity to respond – individually and collectively
- channels of communication and patterns of influence

- characteristics of the community and power structures within it and wider society.

SOLUTION GENERATION

Following on from establishing what the priority health needs are and analysing the characteristics of a community, the principal dilemma for those involved in health promotion planning is the selection of an appropriate intervention or combination of interventions. To an extent, the options considered will be constrained by ideological commitments. As we have noted in Chapter 1, those who subscribe to the ideology of empowerment will opt to work in participative ways. In contrast, more authoritarian, top-down approaches would be consistent with a preventive model. The range of options can be represented

ICONIC AND ANALOGIC MODELS

- **Iconic models** are descriptors or characterizations that offer a simplified view of a recognized aspect of reality.
- **Analogic models** provide a framework to assist understanding of reality and use analogies or metaphors that need not necessarily currently exist (Rawson, 1992).

using either iconic or analogic models (see the box). Beattie (1991) provides a useful analogic taxonomy of the range of different health promotion approaches.

Beattie's model, as represented in Figure 5.9, incorporates two fundamental dimensions – the mode of intervention, which ranges from authoritative to negotiated, and the focus of intervention, which is either on the individual or the collective. An individual's personal and professional values will have a bearing on the preferred mode of operation. Furthermore, imperatives within the workplace may direct the activities of practitioners – regardless of whether or not the implicit values are consistent with their own.

Rawson notes that the advantage of analogic models over iconic models is that they have a theoretical structure, which can assimilate new forms of practice. However, the disadvantage is that 'they may seem remote from the detail of reality' (1992: 211). Clearly the demarcation between authoritative and negotiated approaches is not absolute. Rather, they represent polar extremes, with some possible gradation between the two. For example, we have already observed that community participation can range from a minimum, tokenistic consultation to the community having genuine control and a recognized decision-making role. Similarly, there is the possibility of differing levels of authoritarian control. Indeed, we might postulate that this could even include the instrumental use of participative methods – not because of any commitment to negotiated styles of working, but because it is the best way to achieve predefined goals. The focus of intervention will also be subject to parallel variation. A collective approach could involve change at the group, setting, community or population level.

Notwithstanding an ideological commitment to broad styles of working, the rational selection of specific methods will be based on a combination of:

- theory
- evidence about effective practice
- context
- professional judgement based on experience.

The role of theory

Recourse to theory will be useful both in pursuing the cause of health problems and identifying what should be done to tackle them – referred to respectively by the National Cancer Institute (1997) in the USA as the 'theory of the problem' and 'theory of action'. In short, theory supports the identification of key relevant variables.

The theory of the problem draws on explanatory theory that will guide the search for modifiable risk factors. For example, if the proportion of young people taking up smoking has been implicated as the problem, a HAM analysis would direct attention towards exploring the principal determinants of young people's behavioural intention concerning smoking – that is, their belief, motivation and normative systems and self concept. Furthermore, investigation of any factors that facilitate or act as a barrier to their translating intentions into practice would also be required.

In contrast, the theory of action draws on change theory and will inform decisions about the most appropriate strategy. It will make clear any assumptions underpinning the chosen strategy and also check that all the necessary elements of the intervention are in place (see the box).

A VIEW OF THEORY AND PROFESSIONAL PRACTICE

Like an expert chef, a theoretically grounded health education professional does not blindly follow a cookbook recipe, but constantly creates it anew, depending on the circumstances. Without a theory, she or he has only the skills of a cafeteria line worker.

National Cancer Institute, 1997

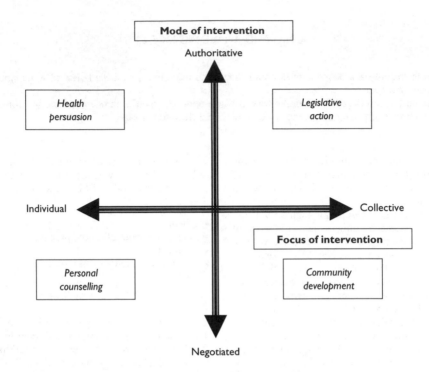

Figure 5.9　Beattie's model of health promotion (Beattie, 1991)

Unless a full, rational appraisal of the problem and possible solutions is undertaken, interventions might easily:

- address wrong or inappropriate variables – that is, miss the target completely
- tackle only a proportion of the variables required to have the desired effect – that is, hit only a few of the total possible targets and not enough to achieve any meaningful change (Green, 2000).

Theory, then, can make an important contribution to solution generation by virtue of its explanatory and predictive capabilities. Indeed, Eiser and Eiser's (1996: 43) review of the effectiveness of video for health education is adamant on this point:

> Interventions without a clear theoretical rationale almost always fail or achieve only a semblance of success that disappears when submitted to critical examination.

However, this type of theoretical analysis of problems and possible solutions is not without its critics.

It has been aligned with authoritarian, individualistic approaches and the preventive model discussed in Chapter 1. A particular concern is that it objectifies human experience and is therefore inconsistent with the central tenets of health promotion – holism and empowerment. Buchanan (1994) attributes scepticism about the relevance of theory to health promotion practice to a narrow view of theory equated with the natural sciences and positivism. This interpretation of theory would see it as establishing the relationships between factors (independent variables) and some outcome (dependent variable). It should also be possible to predict the changes in outcome that would be caused by manipulation of the independent variable/s and, indeed, verify this by testing. The role of the health promoter would therefore simply be to identify and change the relevant independent variables to achieve the desired outcome. Failure to achieve success would demand a more thorough and detailed analysis of the variables and ever more precise targeting and tailoring of interventions. 'Targeting' involves designing interventions to suit the characteristics of particular subgroups (such as age, gender, ethnicity, social

HUMAN AGENCY AND REALITY

Human beings are not 'things' to be studied in the way one studies ants, plants or rocks, but are valuing, meaning attributing beings to be understood as subjects and known as subjects... To impose positivistic meanings upon the realm of social phenomena is to distort the fundamental nature of human existence.

Hughes, 1976: 25

class, occupational group) whereas 'tailoring' adapts interventions to meet the specific requirements of individuals. Kreuter and Skinner (2000: 1) offer the following definition of tailoring:

Any combination of information or change strategies *intended to reach one specific person,* based on characteristics that are unique to that person, related to the outcome of interest, and have been *derived from an individual assessment.*

Buchanan contends that human action is not governed in the same law-like way as natural processes and, hence, the methods used to study natural phenomena cannot be applied to human behaviour. The role of human agency in constructing reality is well recognized in this regard (see the box for an example).

Buchanan (1994: 274) does not reject the need for theory per se, but calls for a broader conceptualization of theory that recognizes that 'knowledge is contingent and contextual rather than universal, determinate and invariable.' The purpose of theory, then, is not to offer universal explanations or predictions, but to clarify understanding of complex situations. It therefore needs to interplay with a range of contextual factors. Buchanan proposes Aristotle's notion of 'phronesis' or 'practical reason' as a means of understanding the unique features of each situation. This contrasts with '*episteme*' or 'theoretical knowledge' based on universal laws that Aristotle himself recognized could not capture the complexity of the social world. Practical reason (Buchanan, 1994: 279) is the:

ability to recognize, acknowledge, pick out and respond to the singular salient features of a complex and unique situation. It is not deduction from abstract generalizations. ...Practical reason is the thinking process involved in deciding what to say or how to do that which best suits the particular situation at hand. Practical reason is involved in weighing which of the available courses of action is more appropriate given the specific circumstances.

Theory, then, can provide important insights into the nature of problems and the strategies that could be adopted. As Kurt Lewin is famously noted to have said, 'there is nothing so practical as a good theory' (Marrow, 1969). However, an abstract analysis alone is insufficient. A complementary understanding of specific contextual factors is also required before a decision can be made about the most appropriate course of action, as noted in our consideration of community profiles above.

Health promotion has a plethora of theories to draw on. A key issue concerns the selection of appropriate theory for the task in hand. The factors that influence health status range from micro-level individual factors to macro-level policy and environmental issues. The various levels of an ecological approach identified by the National Cancer Institute (1997) are:

- intra-personal factors
- interpersonal factors
- institutional or organizational factors
- community factors
- public policy.

Clearly, each level will have its own repertoire of theory to draw on. Relevant theory at the interpersonal level might, for example, include the HBM and theory of planned behaviour and, at the organizational level, diffusion of innovations. Some theories will bridge different levels – for example the HAM. Comprehensive multilevel approaches will therefore need to combine different theories from the different levels of analysis. McLeroy et al. (1993: 305) contend that *'no single theory,* certainly no psychological theory, is adequate for developing truly effective and comprehensive health education programmes'. They also note that there are no guidelines for selecting individual theories, let alone combinations of theories. The National Cancer Institute (1997) cautions against attempting to fit a square peg into a round hole! The box below lists some key questions to consider when assessing how well a theory is suited to the task.

WHICH THEORY?

- Does it include all relevant variables?
- Is it parsimonious (does not include any redundant variables)?
- Does its use make logical sense in the particular situation?
- Has it been used by others for similar purposes?
- Are there any published studies that use the theory for similar purposes?
- Is it consistent with the values integral to the work?

The choice of theory will clearly be influenced by ideological perspectives. By way of illustration, let us pursue the example of high levels of heart disease in a socially disadvantaged community, where it is recognized to be a problem by both professionals and the community itself.

A major risk factor is the diet of many members of the community, which is known to be high in saturated fats and refined carbohydrates. An authoritarian or preventive approach would search for the key variables to address by means of the application of cognitive behavioural or psycho-social theory – for example, the HAM would identify the main factors associated with dietary practice and the stages of change model would assess the readiness of the community to change. A two-pronged strategy might be adopted. One strand would focus on attempting to change behavioural intention concerning a healthy diet and develop skills in preparing healthy meals at low cost. The selection of actual methods should also be informed by a range of relevant theories – learning theory, diffusion of innovations theory and communication theory. The other strand would be concerned with making healthy foods available at lower cost – for example, by working with local shops to gain their cooperation. The selection of methods to achieve this would be enhanced by reference to diffusion of innovations theory and organizational change theories. Should the remit of the programme be more ambitious and attempt to influence food policy more generally, then recourse to policy theory would be needed.

In contrast, a negotiated approach would draw on community development theory to identify ways of working with the community to enable it to identify the main causes of the problems it is experiencing and the most feasible solutions. These might include the need to empower people to achieve a healthy diet on a low income, either individually or by working collectively to reduce food costs by setting up food cooperatives. Both may require some form of learning and, again, communication and learning theory will be important as will community organization theory. Should any environmental change and political action be needed – for example, getting the council to set aside land for allotments so that people can grow their own food, then additional lobbying and advocacy skills will be needed, together with an understanding of how to influence political processes derived from policy theory.

An overview of both these approaches is presented in Figure 5.10 on page 170.

Evidence-based practice

The latter part of the twentieth century witnessed a move towards evidence-based practice in health and social care generally, but also in health promotion. Indeed, the Fifty-first World Health Assembly (WHO, 1998c) urged all member states to, 'adopt an evidence-based approach to health promotion policy and practice, using the full range of quantitative and qualitative methodologies.'

While evaluation has been recognized as being integral to good practice in health promotion, there is now even greater emphasis on the *utilization* of evaluation evidence in practice. The need for such evidence of effectiveness has been a major driver for the production of systematic reviews, and groups such as the Cochrane Collaboration have played a leading role. Some of the major sources of systematic reviews and other evidence to be found online are listed in the box.

SELECTED ONLINE SOURCES OF EVIDENCE AND SYSTEMATIC REVIEWS

NHS Centre for Reviews and Dissemination
Website: www.york.ac.uk/inst/crd

HDA Evidence Base
Website: http://194.83.94.80/hda/docs/evidence/ eb2000/corehtml/intro.htm

Evidence from systematic reviews of research relevant to implementing the 'wider public health' agenda
Website: www.york.ac.uk/inst/crd/wph.htm

The Evidence for Policy and Practice Information and Coordinating Centre (EPPI-Centre)
Website: http://eppi.ioe.ac.uk/EPPIWeb/home. aspx

National Health Promotion Website for Wales
Website: www.hpw.wales.gov.uk

Health Education Board for Scotland (HEBS)
Website: www.hebs.scot.nhs.uk

Health Technology Assessment Database (HTA)
Website: http://nhscrd.york.ac.uk/htahp.htm

NHS Economic Evaluation Database (NHS EED)
Website: http://nhscrd.york.ac.uk/nhsdhp.htm

International Union for Health Promotion and Education (IUHPE)
Website: www.iuhpe.org

Reviews of health promotion and education online (RHP&EO)
Website: http://rhpeo.org

The Cochrane Collaboration
Website: www.cochrane.org

This site includes access to Abstracts of Cochrane Reviews and the Cochrane Library, which provides access to a number of databases, such as The Cochrane Database of Systematic Reviews and The Database of Abstracts of Reviews of Effectiveness.

Cochrane Health Promotion and Public Health Field
Website: www.vichealth.vic.gov.au/cochrane

Campbell Collaboration
Website: www.campbellcollaboration.org

WHO Reproductive Health Library
Website: www.update-software.com/RHL

Much of the discussion about evidence-based practice in the past has focused on ways of measuring effectiveness. A particular concern has been the emphasis on positivist methodology and the use of randomized controlled trials (RCTs). We will focus on the issue of evaluation and the generation of evidence in Chapter 10. However, we should note, in passing, that there is a developing consensus – endorsed by

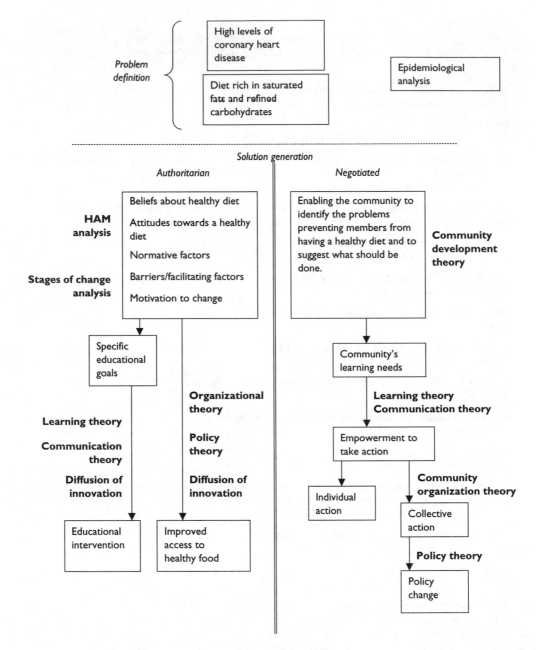

Figure 5.10 Choice of intervention – the contribution of theories

WHO (1998a) – on the value of methodological pluralism for health promotion evaluation.

Notwithstanding these concerns and the ongoing debate, it is still the case that most of the evidence included in systematic reviews to date derives from experimental or quasi-experimental studies – see, for example, the hierarchy of evidence given in the box.

AN EXAMPLE OF A HIERARCHY OF EVIDENCE

I   Well-designed randomized controlled trials
II.i   Well-designed controlled trials with pseudo-randomization or no randomization
II.ii   Well-designed cohort studies
II.iii Well-designed case control (retrospective) studies
III   Large differences in comparisons between times and/or places, with or without interventions
IV   Opinions of respected authorities, based on clinical experience, descriptive studies or reports
       of expert committees.

After NHS Centre for Reviews and Dissemination, 1996

Furthermore, some of the central concerns of health promotion – participation, empowerment, policy development and environmental change – present a greater challenge for robust evaluation than individually orientated behaviour change. It is perhaps not surprising, therefore, that there is less evidence to draw on in relation to these areas than is the case for others. Tilford (2000) notes that, as health promotion has evolved from health education, there has been a time-lag in evaluations focusing on the social rather than the individual determinants of health. However, there is considerable interest in developing appropriate indicators for complex concepts, such as social capital (Cooper et al., 1999, Campbell et al., 1999, Community Cohesion Review Team, 2001, Coulthard et al., 2001) and the application of theoretical frameworks to evaluation of comprehensive multilevel interventions (see, for example, Pawson and Tilley, 1997).

Comparatively little attention has been given to the ways in which practitioners use evidence in planning health promotion interventions. Ideological commitments will, again, influence views about the credibility and utility of different types of evidence and its appeal to practitioners. However, over and above the issues associated with evaluation methodology, systematic reviews (and, indeed, published evaluations more generally) are recognized as having a number of limitations for the end-users. These are summarized by Tilford (2000) as being:

- insufficient attention to the quality of interventions
- the theoretical basis of interventions is not always made clear
- insufficient information on the process of implementation of interventions
- tendency for reviews to focus on health education rather than the broader sphere of health promotion
- the short-term follow-up time of many studies
- dominance of studies from the USA.

She notes that the mismatch between the types of interventions that have been rigorously evaluated and those commonly used in practice further limits the relevance of the evidence base for practitioners. It is self-evident that innovative approaches will have little, if any, evidence to draw on.

South and Tilford's (2000) study of the use of research by health promotion specialists in England found two different interpretations of evidence-based practice among practitioners. On the one hand, it was associated with using sound empirical research and, on the other, it was conceptualized more broadly as additionally drawing on theory, principles of good practice, the academic literature and national policy. Some practitioners used a systematic approach to retrieve and appraise evidence, whereas, for others, this was done on a rather more ad hoc basis or, alternatively, seen as falling within the general context of keeping up to date. Practitioners also used their professional judgement to make decisions about the appropriate level of evidence required. The valuable contribution of research to planning interventions was recognized, but only as one element alongside theory and professional expertise.

Nutbeam (1996) identifies three levels of practice that differ in the extent to which they are based on research evidence – planned , responsive and reactive. *Planned* health promotion is based on a rational and systematic review of evidence concerning health needs, effectiveness of interventions and contextual factors. *Responsive* health promotion involves addressing the expressed needs of the community in ways it sees as most appropriate – the use of research evidence is only one factor in the decision-making process. Although this style of working is consistent with the rhetoric of the Ottawa Charter, Nutbeam (1996: 321) cautions that:

the interventions chosen may not be effective or efficient, and not tackle fundamental problems even though they are strongly supported by the community.

Reactive health promotion takes the form of a rapid and often high-profile response to a problem or crisis. Political imperatives may drive both the pace and type of response – for example, the early public awareness campaigns about HIV. The short timescale of this knee-jerk type of response does not allow sufficient time for evidence-based planning.

Although evidence-based practice had been narrowly equated with evaluation research, a broader interpretation will provide a more secure base for practice. This view, as we have noted, is reflected in the field, where there is some concern that other forms of evidence may be omitted from decisions about interventions (South and Tilford, 2000). Green (2000) has argued for a greater emphasis on the contribution of theory to evidence-based practice. Furthermore, empirical evidence and theory are not alternatives, but should be inextricably linked. In short, research evidence about the effectiveness of interventions should contribute to the development of intervention theory, which will itself shape subsequent interventions and the ways in which they are evaluated. Sackett et al. (1996: 71) also draw attention to the importance of professional expertise in their definition of evidence-based medical practice as, 'integrating individual clinical expertise with the best available external clinical evidence from systematic research.'

A combination of these elements should allow state-of-the-art solutions or interventions to be identified and an appropriate selection made. McLeroy et al. (1993) refer to this as 'theory of intervention' – statements or summaries of what we know about the relative effectiveness of different intervention strategies with particular populations.

Professional judgement and context

We have already noted the importance of the professional perspective in our discussion of the contribution of both theory and evidence-based practice to solution generation. At grass roots level, this derives from experience and is grounded in familiarity with particular contexts and specific groups, which enables the most appropriate course, of action to be identified. Adherence to the professional values of health promotion will also make some approaches more acceptable and preclude others. These values have been discussed at length in Chapter 1 and are integral to statements on the principles of good practice, such as those developed by, for example, the Care Sector Consortium (1997), the Society of Health Education and Health Promotion Specialists (1997) and the Society of Public Health Educators (SOPHE, 2001).

Realist approaches to evaluation are attracting considerable attention and will be discussed more fully in Chapter 10. Unlike other approaches, they focus particularly on attempting to understand the contexts and mechanisms underpinning observed outcomes (Pawson and Tilley, 1997). However, much of the research evidence about effectiveness and theoretical analyses remain largely context-free. Health promotion, though, does not operate within a vacuum. Effective health promotion interventions must be designed to have a good fit with contextual factors and local circumstances. For example, any attempt to bring about organizational change will need to give due regard to the culture and norms within the organization. Similar attention should be given to the range of relevant contextual factors, regardless of the level of the proposed intervention – be it individual, group, community, organization, environmental or policy change.

We noted above the broad range of factors included within a community profile that are relevant both to understanding needs and the contextual factors that will influence the response. McLeroy et al. (1993) emphasize that this understanding should include the capacity of families, social networks, communities and organizations to address the needs of their members and that health promotion interventions should take a form that strengthens this. Otherwise, health promotion interventions risk becoming a substitute for these local mechanisms, reducing the community's capacity to cope independently – effectively becoming a de-powering, rather than an empowering, influence.

Over and above contributing to strategic decisions, contextual information also informs operational planning. It identifies who the most appropriate target groups are and what channels are most appropriate for reaching them. It also identifies any gatekeepers. Indeed, it may be more appropriate to target gatekeepers than those it is hoped will ultimately benefit. For example, attempts to improve the nutrition of young children will need to target families, particularly mothers. In patriarchal societies, improving women's access to contraception may require working with men to gain their support. Similarly, if access to interventions is controlled by gatekeepers, their cooperation will be needed. For example, schoolteachers have an important gatekeeper function in relation to young people's access to health education materials. If there are important opinion leaders or referent groups, then it is also wise to work with them.

Understanding what channels of communication exist will increase the potential for success. This might be something as obvious as access to radio or

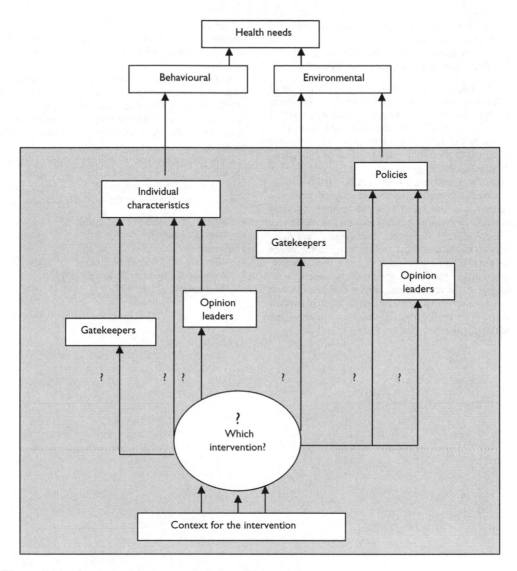

Figure 5.11 Contextual factors and choice of intervention

television and details of listening audiences at particular times of day, if a mass media campaign is being planned, or details of social interaction networks, if a peer education programme is being developed. Larkey at al. (1999), for example, used systematic network measurement techniques to identify individuals who were most centrally and socially connected before offering them the opportunity to train as peer health educators for their worksite dietary change intervention. Similarly, effective lobbying and advocacy is dependent on being able to identify and target those with most political power

and influence. An overview of how these various strands fit together is provided in Figure 5.11.

SUMMARY

This chapter has focused on identifying the information needed to plan interventions. A theme running through the chapter has been the tension between different approaches to defining needs and proposing solutions – particularly between:

- participative, bottom-up and professionally led top-down approaches
- subjective and objective interpretations
- reductionist and interpretive perspectives.

This will inevitably influence the ways in which health needs are defined and prioritized. Different interpretations of the concept of need and ways of assessing it have been discussed and alternative approaches to solutions. Ideologies and values are influential in shaping the approach to problem definition and solution generation.

Health promotion, by its very nature, is action-orientated towards improving health status – whether this is viewed as addressing specific problems or creating conditions that are supportive of health. Health promotion interventions are more likely to be successful if they respond to the needs recognized by individuals or a community. Furthermore, interventions should be based on an analysis of environmental, social and behavioural determinants. The application of theoretical models can help to ensure that all relevant variables are included within such an analysis.

Community profiling will provide some of the information required for needs assessments, along with contextual information relevant to solution generation.

A systematic approach to solution generation will draw on a combination of theory, research evidence of effectiveness, contextual factors and professional judgement to identify the range of possible solutions. Then, the most appropriate solution for the particular context can be selected.

Participative approaches will draw on the practical knowledge and experience of the community. However, whichever approach is adopted, information is needed to answer the following key questions.

- What is the nature of the problem?
- Who is affected?
- What are the causes?
- What are the contextual factors?
- What do we need to do to tackle it?
- How should we do it?

6

Healthy Public Policy

We know what happens to people who stay in the middle of the road. They get run down.

Aneurin Bevan, *The Observer*, 6 December 1953

INTRODUCTION

Recognition that the major influences on health status are outside the immediate control of individuals has focused attention on the role of the environment and healthy public policy. Indeed, the defining feature of health promotion has been an emphasis on the environmental determinants of health rather than individual behaviour. Healthy public policy has been seen as the vehicle for 'creating supportive environments to enable people to lead healthy lives' (WHO, 1988: 1).

The use of public policy measures to protect health is not new. Many of the health improvements in the nineteenth century were achieved by public policy, such as the Public Health Acts of 1848 and 1875, which attempted to control aspects of the environment – water supply, sewage disposal, slaughtering of animals, parks and open spaces, isolation hospitals and the beginnings of housing control (McKeown and Lowe, 1974, and Jones and Sidell, 1997).

The rediscovery of the importance of environmental influences on health underpinned the emergence of health promotion and the 'New Public Health' movements in the latter part of the twentieth century. However contemporary conceptualizations of the environment have broadened to include social and economic as well as physical aspects. Furthermore, simple causal sequences linking environment and disease have been replaced by complex causal webs of factors affecting health status. The policy response required is similarly more complex and wideranging. Jones and Sidell (1997) trace three main strands that have influenced the development of healthy public policy:

- public health, the 'New Public Health' and, alongside these, health education and health promotion

THE OTTAWA CHARTER'S PRIORITY ACTION AREAS

- Build healthy public policy.
- Create supportive environments.
- Strengthen community action.
- Develop personal skills.
- Reorientate health services.

WHO, 1986

- social welfare reforms and the welfare state
- new social movements, such as women's and civil rights movements and the environmental movement.

We will begin this chapter by examining the WHO position on healthy public policy. We will then define healthy public policy and consider the process of policy making to identify ways of bringing influence to bear. The issue of power will be discussed, along with the role of advocacy and lobbying as means of influencing policy processes.

The role of policy in influencing health will be viewed in two broad ways. First, the development of policy explicitly to tackle health issues – policy here is seen as the solution and health concerns are the primary focus. Second, the effects on health of policy designed for other purposes. The chapter will conclude with a consideration of the growing field of health impact assessment, which aims to identify any potential negative impacts of policy. The combination of these two perspectives can, therefore, contribute to maximizing health gain and minimizing harm. There are clear links between this chapter and the sections on media advocacy and community activism in Chapter 8 and persuasive communication in Chapter 7.

HEALTHY PUBLIC POLICY – THE WHO POSITION

The central role of healthy public policy has been a consistent theme running through major WHO documents on health promotion. The Ottawa Charter (WHO, 1986) – which has been a constant source of reference in the development of health promotion and the 'New Public Health' – identified building healthy public policy and the creation of supportive environments as two of the five priority action areas, listed in the box.

Health promotion action was seen to involve (WHO, 1986):

- **advocacy** to secure favourable conditions for health
- **mediation** between the different interests in society
- **enabling** people to achieve their health potential by having control over the factors that influence their health.

The importance of the Ottawa Charter's action areas was reaffirmed by the Jakarta Declaration (WHO, 1997), which identified additional priorities for the twenty-first century – see the box below.

THE JAKARTA DECLARATION'S PRIORITIES FOR HEALTH PROMOTION IN THE TWENTY-FIRST CENTURY

- Promote social responsibility for health.
- Increase investments for health development.
- Consolidate and expand partnerships for health.
- Increase community capacity and empower the individual.
- Secure an infrastructure for health promotion.

WHO, 1997

Multisectoral and partnership working were seen to underpin all these priorities, together with a commitment to healthy public policy. The pursuit of social responsibility for health involves decisionmakers in the public and private sectors adopting polices and practices that:

- avoid harming the health of individuals
- protect the environment and ensure the use of sustainable resources
- restrict the production of, and trade in, inherently harmful goods and substances, such as tobacco and armaments, as well as discourage unhealthy marketing practices
- safeguard both the citizen in the marketplace and the individual in the workplace
- include equity-focused health impact assessments as an integral part of policy development (WHO, 1997: 3).

Healthy public policy was the specific focus of the second International Conference on Health Promotion held in Adelaide, which defined it as, 'characterized by an explicit concern for health and equity in all areas of policy and accountability for health impact'. (WHO, 1988: 1).

The recommendations of the Adelaide Conference formally recognized that the activities of a number of different government sectors influence health status and that there should be accountability for health impacts. This would include effects on the social and physical environments, which may influence the possibility and ease of making healthy choices or, alternatively, effects that are directly health-enhancing or damaging. Health was also seen as a fundamental right and sound social investment.

A central concern was equity and narrowing the health gap in society by means of policies that attach high priority to disadvantaged and vulnerable groups. Furthermore, developed countries were considered to have an obligation to ensure that their own health policies impacted positively on developing nations.

Healthy public policy was seen to be important at all levels of government, from national to local, and 'public accountability for health ... an essential nutrient for the growth of healthy public policy'(WHO, 1988: 2). Community action can therefore provide the motive force for policy development. The other side of the coin is that governments should assess and report the impact of policies in a way that can be understood by all groups in society.

Although government was seen to have a key role, other groups – such as the private and business sectors, non-governmental and community organizations – were also identified as important influences that could be harnessed for health promotion.

The Fifth Global Conference on Health Promotion held in Mexico in 2000 focused on 'Bridging the Equity Gap'. Unlike the previous international conferences, it included a ministerial programme and issued a ministerial statement, which was signed by some eighty-seven countries, including the United Kingdom (WHO, 2000a). The statement acknowledged that 'the promotion of health and social development is a central duty and responsibility of governments that all sectors of society share' and concluded that 'health promotion must be a fundamental component of public policies and programmes in all countries in the pursuit of equity and health for all.'

A strong theme to emerge from the Mexico conference was the need to 'work with and through existing political systems and structures to ensure healthy public policy, adequate investment in health and facilitation of an infrastructure for health promotion' (WHO, 2000b: 21). This would require:

- democratic processes
- social and political activism
- a system of equity-orientated health impact assessment
- reorientation of health services
- improved interaction between politicians, policymakers, researchers and practitioners
- strengthening existing capacity for implementing health promotion strategies and supporting synergy between different levels – local, national and international.

Recognition of the importance of policy also emerges in the 'Health for All' literature. *Health for All in the 21st century*, 'guides action and policy for health at all levels (international, regional national and local), and identifies global priorities and targets for the first two decades of the twenty-first century' (WHO, 1998: 2). International and national policies and actions are seen as the means of securing the right to health (WHO, 1998: 20):

through adoption of international and national human rights instruments Member States assume specific responsibilities and duties to promote and protect the health of their populations by:

- ensuring that sustainable health systems are accessible to all people
- promoting intersectoral action to address the determinants and prerequisites of health.

It could be argued that all of the regional targets identified by 'Health for All 2000' ('HFA 2000'),

(WHO, 1985) and latterly *Health for All in the 21st century* ('Health21') (WHO, Regional Committee for Europe, 1998) demand a policy response. For example, achieving Target 10 below will be dependent on environmental policy.

European Health21 Target 10 – A Healthy And Safe Physical Environment: By the year 2015, people in the Region should live in a safer physical environment, with exposure to contaminants hazardous to health at levels not exceeding internationally agreed standards.

Similarly, let us briefly consider:

European Health21 Target 12 – Reducing Harm From Alcohol, Drugs And Tobacco: By the year 2015, the adverse health effects from the consumption of addictive substances such as tobacco, alcohol and psychoactive drugs should have been significantly reduced in all Member States.

Achieving this target, to an extent, involves behavioural choices. However, it will also be influenced by tobacco, alcohol and drug policies. At a more general level, poverty and social inequality are known to be associated with substance misuse and so addressing this requires consideration of broader areas of policy, such as employment, economic and social policy.

More specifically, European Health21 Target 21 states:

By the year 2010, all Member States should have and be implementing policies for health at country, regional and local levels, supported by appropriate institutional infrastructures, managerial processes and innovative leadership.

One of the keys to successful implementation of 'Health21' has been identified as strengthening the capacity for policy making. Governments are expected to take a lead in developing policy based on sound research and evidence and have an obligation 'to ensure that health is explicitly considered in the development of public policy' (WHO, 1998: 42). Policy analysis is also required to ensure that the policies and activities across different sectors are aligned in relation to achieving health goals. International and foreign policy should also consider health impact.

The key issues to emerge are:

- the centrality of healthy public policy to health promotion at all levels, from international to local
- the link between healthy public policy and supportive environments
- the multisectoral scope
- the need for public participation

- governmental responsibility and accountability for considering health in the development of public policy – national and international.

HEALTHY PUBLIC POLICY – MEANINGS AND SCOPE

Health, as we noted in Chapter 1, is both a relative and contested concept. The notion of policy is equally nebulous, as encapsulated in the metaphor, 'Policy is rather like the elephant – you recognize it when you see it, but cannot easily define it' (Cunningham, 1963: 229).

The term 'policy' is subject to variation in meaning and usage in different contexts. Hogwood and Gunn (1984), for example, suggest that policy can be characterized as:

- a label for a field of activity
- a statement of aspiration or purpose
- specific proposals
- (government) decisions
- formal authorization
- a programme
- output(s)
- outcome(s)
- a theory or model
- a process.

Another view of policy that emerged from a qualitative study (Green, 1995: 108) of the development of sex education policy by schools is that it is a written document, which may or may not guide practice, 'We don't actually look at [the policy] in school ... Basically we've got a piece of paper if anybody asks and I think that is the bottom line.'

This illustrates the point that, while policy is often associated with government activity, it also exists outside of government circles and is developed at the local as well as regional and national levels.

Colebatch (1998) identifies three key elements of policy:

- **authority** the implication that there is official endorsement
- **expertise** applied to a problem area and identifying what should be done about it
- **order** decisions are not arbitrary but consistent and structured.

Jenkins (1978: 15) provides a useful definition that focuses on the instrumentality of policy and emphasizes that it should not merely be aspirational, but also within the control of those responsible for making policy:

A set of interrelated decisions taken by a political actor or group of actors concerning the selection of goals and the means of achieving them within a specified situation where these decisions should, in principle, be within the power of these actors to achieve.

While the implication of this definition is that policy is concerned with action, it can equally involve inaction – deciding what *not* to do. Ignatieff (1992, in Walt, 1994: 40) draws attention to the longer-term view of policy in his acerbic commentary on short-term economic policy:

A policy ought to be something more than a galvanic twitch. It ought to have legs for distances longer than those implied in a 'dash for growth'. It ought to have some end in view larger than seeing an addled government through the next month ... policy is not about surviving till Friday. Nor is policy to be confused with strategy, which is about getting through to Christmas. Policy is the selection of non-contradictory means to achieve non-contradictory ends over the medium to long term.

What, then, is healthy public policy?

There is a clear distinction between 'public health policy', which focuses narrowly on healthcare and, frequently, illness management, and 'healthy public policy', which has a much broader remit (Hancock, 1982). Healthy public policy is concerned with the role of government and the public sector in creating the conditions that support health. Milio (1988: 26), who has played an influential role in shifting the emphasis from health policy to healthy public policy and raising its profile within WHO, offers the following definition of public policy:

Simply put, public policy – the guide to government action – sets the range of possibilities for choices made by public and private organizations, commercial and voluntary enterprises, and individuals. In virtually every facet of living, the creation and use of goods, services, information and environments are affected by government policies – fiscal, regulatory, service provision, research and education, and procedural.

Further, she contends that healthy public policy should be:

- ecological in perspective
- multisectoral in scope
- collaborative in strategy.

Draper (1988: 217) has defined the goal of healthy public policy as being:

to make government activity across the board contribute as much as possible to health development, while recognizing the tradeoffs that are an inevitable and necessary part of the policy process.

The key characteristics of healthy public policy are listed in the box.

Given the plethora of factors that influence health status (discussed in Chapter 2), the scope of healthy public policy is necessarily wideranging. Some indication of that breadth is provided by Terris (in Tesh et al., 1988) in an editorial submitted to the Yale Symposium on Healthy Public Policy.

The logic of our discipline makes it necessary to support a healthful standard of living through full employment and adequate family income; improved working conditions; decent housing ...; effective protection from environmental discomforts ...; good nutrition that will foster optimal physical and mental development; increased financial support to public education and elimination of financial barriers to higher education; improved opportunities for rest, recreation, and cultural development; greater participation in community activities and decision making; an end to discrimination against minority groups based on race, gender, age, social class, religious belief, national background or sexual preference; and freedom from the pervasive fear of violence, war and nuclear annihilation.

CHARACTERISTICS OF HEALTHY PUBLIC POLICY

- Commitment to social equity.
- Recognition of the important influence of economic, social and physical environments on health.
- Facilitation of public participation.
- Cooperation between health and other sectors of government.

After Draper, 1988

INDEPENDENT INQUIRY INTO INEQUALITIES IN HEALTH (THE ACHESON REPORT): RECOMMENDATIONS

General recommendations

1   We recommend that, as part of health impact assessment, all policies likely to have a direct or indirect effect on health should be evaluated in terms of their impact on health inequalities, and should be formulated in such a way that by favouring the less well off they will, wherever possible, reduce such inequalities.
2   We recommend a high priority is given to policies aimed at improving health and reducing health inequalities in women of childbearing age, expectant mothers and young children.

Specific recommendations are also made about the following twelve areas:

- poverty, income, tax and benefits
- education
- employment
- housing and environment
- mobility, transport and pollution
- nutrition and the Common Agricultural Policy
- mothers, children and families
- young people and adults of working age
- older people
- ethnicity
- gender
- equity within the National Health Service.

Acheson, 1998

Policy can support health in a number of different ways (Milio, 1986, in Abel-Smith, 1994):

- fiscal/monetary – incomes and incentives
- regulation – economic and environmental
- provision of goods and services
- supporting participation
- research, development, information, education.

In the UK, the 'Independent Inquiry into Inequalities in Health' chaired by Sir Donald Acheson (1998) made thirty-nine detailed recommendation about future policy development to tackle inequalities in health linked to socio-economic status, gender and ethnicity, and variations throughout the lifecycle. These are summarized in the box.

The specific areas identified include both upstream and downstream policies. The former would include, for example, the development of preschool education to meet the needs of disadvantaged families or reducing the fear of crime and violence and creating a safe environment. In contrast, the latter would focus on policies intended to prevent disease, such as fluoridation of drinking water or ensuring equitable access to healthcare. Furthermore, because of the synergistic effect between many of the recommendations, the report advises policy development across a broad front rather than 'cherry picking' those areas that are most amenable to change.

Tesh et al. (1988) welcome the growing acceptance within the policy field that health has little to do with medical care, together with the move away from monocausal models and reductionist analyses and towards recognition of the complex interplay of factors that impact on health. However, they have a number of concerns about the adoption of multifactorial models of causality. First, they offer little insight into exactly how to prevent disease. Because everything is interlinked, any one action may appear insignificant, yet it is unlikely that sufficient resources will be available to tackle everything. The enormity of the task can become a reason (excuse) for not taking action and thus lead to inertia.

Second, because all elements of a multicausal web appear equally weighted, policymakers are provided with an opportunity to appear to be responding to a problem while at the same time opting for interventions that are less socially disruptive or costly and may well be less effective than some other course of action. For example, providing smoking cessation clinics rather than tackling poverty or encouraging people to improve their diet rather than addressing the issue of whether or not those on low incomes or receiving state benefits can afford a healthy diet.

This also provides the opportunity to effectively opt out of responsibility for a health issue by attributing major responsibility elsewhere. For example, there would be no need to address the activities of the food industry if the major influences on a healthy diet were perceived to be acceptable minimum levels of income and awareness of what constitutes a healthy diet.

The third point is that an emphasis on cause overlooks those who are more likely to experience ill health – notably those of lower socio-economic status. Recognition of the 'primacy of poverty' (Tesh et al., 1988: 258) presupposes that all elements of the web are not equal, but that some have more fundamental significance. Therefore, constructing a hierarchy of causes may be necessary to target those that are likely to have the greatest impact on health.

Clearly, when considering policy options there will be a need to make tradeoffs in choosing one course of action rather than another and between those groups that benefit and those that bear the costs – a distinction that is frequently not clear-cut (Draper, 1988, and Tesh et al., 1988). Tuohy (in Tesh et al., 1988) contends that the criteria and processes used to make these tradeoffs should be made explicit and proposes the common themes emerging at the Yale Symposium on Healthy Public Policy as a starting point:

- importance of ensuring healthy minimum standards of living – internationally as well as intra-nationally
- establishment of participatory decision-making structures – but these need the support of a balanced structure of interests and power.

Christoffel (in Tesh et al., 1988: 259) asserts that 'Knowing how to solve a public health problem is not enough when powerful interests are threatened by the solution, which seems to be the case most of the time'. He sees the major problem for health as not being an overall shortage of resources, but an uneven distribution of them. The redistribution of resources would require that some (albeit a minority) lose and these are, in general, those who hold 'critical political power' (in Tesh et al., 1988: 260). Christoffel concludes that the main barrier to

healthy public policy is the concentration of wealth and power among those who stand to lose.

While the role of the state has been at the forefront of thinking about healthy public policy, it is important to also recognize the importance of non-governmental policy on health, at all levels. Bunton (1992: 130) writes:

> The concept anticipates a new culture of public policy that is pluralistic and looks beyond state administrative planning structures to develop and implement policy, calling for multisectoral, multilevel, and participatory initiatives.

The table in the box on page 182 from the UK health strategy 'Saving Lives: Our Healthier Nation' (Department of Health, 1999) provides an example of local and national policy responses.

Delaney (1994c) makes the distinction between policy as *problematic* for health promotion and policy as the *solution*. The former focuses on identifying the negative impacts of policies on health status. The growing field of health impact assessment is concerned with analysing the potential health impact of policies (we will return to this below). The latter is concerned with the use of policy to tackle the problems and create conditions that are supportive of health.

Choice and control

Recognition of the duty of governments to create conditions that support health and enable community participation is a core principle of health promotion. Individuals are also seen as having a responsibility individually and collectively to contribute to health. A key question is, what should be the respective roles and responsibilities of the individual and the state for controlling the determinants of health?

As we observed in Chapter 1, one of the fundamental ethical principles of health education has been a commitment to voluntarism, or, free choice. This was aptly summarized in the North American Society of Public Health Educators Code of Ethics, 'change by choice not coercion' (Society of Health Education and Promotion Specialists, 1997). Milio (1981: 277) contends that, 'There is no "free choice" but only "choice" within a limited number of options …'. The key issue is what options will be made available and how health-promoting or damaging those options are.

The concern of healthy public policy should be to ensure that the environment does not damage health and that there is an equitable distribution of 'health-important resources'. Furthermore, it should make 'health-damaging choices the more

A NATIONAL CONTRACT FOR CANCER – THE ROLES OF NATIONAL AND LOCAL PLAYERS

	Local players and communities can:	Government and national players can:
Social and economic	Tackle social exclusion in the community to make it easier for people to make healthy decisions	Increase the tax on cigarettes by 5 per cent in real terms each year
	Work with deprived communities and businesses to ensure a more varied and affordable choice of food (including fruit and vegetables)	End advertising and promotion of cigarettes
		Prohibit sale of cigarettes to youngsters and ensure enforcement
		Seek to ensure cheaper supplies of fruit and vegetables
		Tackle joblessness, social exclusion, low educational standards and other factors that make it harder to live a healthier life
Environmental	Through local employers, make smoke-free environments the norm, with adequate separate provision for smokers and availability of smoke extractors where possible	Encourage employers and others to provide a smoke-free environment for non-smokers
	Tackle radon in the home (for example, by ensuring that direct advice from local authorities is given to affected householders)	Encourage local action to tackle radon in the home and eliminate risk factors in the workplace (such as enforcing regulations on asbestos and encouraging provision of non-smoking areas) and the environment (such as air pollutants) Continue to press for international action to restore the ozone layer

Source: Department of Health, 1999: Appendix 1

costly ones, and health-improving choices less costly, to both organizations and individuals' (Milio, 1981: 303).

Healthy public policy is generally seen, therefore, as a vehicle for tackling structural and environmental threats to health – as both protective and opening up healthy choices by removing constraints to action. However, we should also note that, over and above making the healthy choice the easy choice, policies can make it the *only* choice (Tones and Tilford, 1994). Beattie (1991) sees legislation and policy as an authoritative approach directed at the collective (see Figure 6.1).

Curtailing individual choice can clearly be defended when exercising that choice may put others at risk. For example, it would be difficult to

uphold the rights of individuals to choose to drive through residential areas at excessive speed or while intoxicated or subject others to inhaling tobacco smoke.

However, control takes on a more coercive complexion when applied to behaviour that only places the individual concerned at risk. Such an approach equates with a narrow, preventive model of health education and leaves health promoters open to accusations of health fascism. The anti-health lobby has been quick to pick up on this element of coercion and frequently uses arguments about liberty and civil rights in its activities. For example, the home page of FOREST (The Freedom Organization for the Right to Enjoy Smoking Tobacco, 2002) describes itself as:

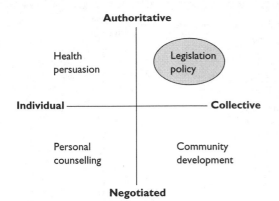

Authoritative

Health
persuasion

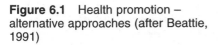
Legislation
policy

Personal
counselling

Community
development

Individual ——————————— **Collective**

Negotiated

Figure 6.1 Health promotion –
alternative approaches (after Beattie,
1991)

founded in 1979 to defend the rights of adults who
smoke tobacco. We take the civil liberties standpoint
and provide advice on how the needs of smokers and
non-smokers may be met. Our aim is to fight the growing intolerance of some sectors of society towards
smokers and the increasing efforts to prohibit smoking,
or to make it illegal.

The pro-gun lobby in the United States and the
opponents of pool fencing in Australia take a similar
stance.

Health education and health promotion – lifestyle and structure

Healthy public policy is generally associated with
attempts to influence the structural determinants of
health. Health education, in contrast, is seen as a
means of influencing lifestyle. However, this representation is overly simplistic and ignores the complexity of the interplay between these various
elements.

As we have noted earlier, structural factors can
have a major influence on lifestyle and behaviour –
and vice versa. Similarly, a major goal of policy
may be to widen access to education, as evidenced
by, for example, efforts to secure universal primary
education. Education policy will influence the content of education generally and, more specifically,
the opportunities afforded for health education.

Within England and Wales, educational
policy on sex education has been instrumental in
shaping schools' response (Green, 1997 and 1998).
Furthermore, the introduction of health promoting
schools initiatives has policy implications from the
national level down to individual schools (see

Chapter 9). Conversely (as we will discuss in more
detail in Chapters 8 and 9), health education is the
means of raising awareness of issues that need to be
addressed and getting them onto the political
agenda.

Critical consciousness raising, as we note in
Chapter 7, is at the heart of Freirian approaches to
education. Furthermore, health education can
develop the skills required for political activism,
including lobbying and advocacy skills.

Thus, it can be seen that representing health
education and healthy public policy as competing
options for promoting health is to create a false
dichotomy. As Figure 6.2 illustrates, health education is a major driver in the process of policy
development.

DEVELOPING POLICY – FROM RHETORIC TO REALITY

The potential for organizations and communities to
influence public policy will inevitably be dependent
on the structure of the state. Walt (1994) notes that,
in contrast to more authoritarian regimes, liberal
democracies will, at least in theory, encourage participation and that participation can be both direct
and indirect.

Direct participation involves explicit attempts to
shape the development of policy by means of
involvement in the policy-making process or lobbying and advocacy. Alternatively, indirect participation consists of exercising influence via electoral
processes. Walt also notes that opportunities for
participation may be limited in relation to 'high
politics' where consideration of major issues may
be dominated by small 'élites'. High politics has
been defined as, 'the maintenance of core values –
including national self-preservation – and the long-
term objectives of the state' (Evans and Newnham,
1992, in Walt, 1994: 42).

In contrast, there may be greater opportunity for
participation in more run-of-the-mill issues of
policy – that is, 'low politics'. Generally individuals have little direct influence on the role of policy
making and their voice is more likely to be heard as
part of a collective or via organizations. However,
public opinion can be an important contextual
factor (Milio, 1988) and, in particular, in terms of
the political risk of alienating public opinion.

Walt (1994) identifies a number of other contextual factors that influence policy development and,
following Leichter (1979), categorizes these as being:

• **situational factors** temporary conditions or
situations

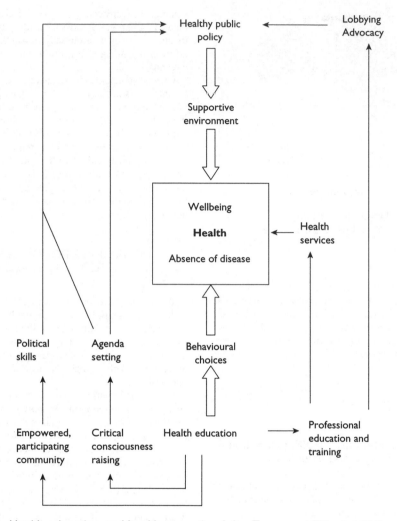

Figure 6.2   Health education and health promotion (after Tones and Tilford, 1994)

- **structural factors** relatively stable elements of society polity
- **cultural factors** the values within communities and society
- **environmental factors** factors external to the political system or international factors, such as international trade agreements, international aid and the activities of transnational corporations.

Understanding the machinery of government and the relative roles of local, national and supra-national organizations is clearly a necessary pre-condition for those seeking to influence policy. However, Delaney (1994c) contends that this is insufficient in itself. Healthy public policy is

essentially a political undertaking (Draper, 1988, Tesh et al., 1988, and Signal, 1998) and analysis of the location of political power and influence is of critical importance to the process of policy development. Yet Signal (1998) comments that the politics of health promotion receive comparatively little attention.

There are several different perspectives on the politics of policy making. Walt (1994) distinguishes between pluralist and élitist views. 'Pluralist interest group theory' presupposes that power is distributed among a number of different interest groups within the policy arena and that no single group dominates. The alternative position is that 'the political arena is dominated by "ruling élites"' and that the state acts 'in the interests of capital accumulation or that major interests are incorporated into a "corporate" non-competitive network' (Delaney, 1994c: 7). The former is consistent with neo-Marxist interpretations and the latter with the new institutionalism.

Hogwood and Gunn (1984: 71) note that the concentration of power in élite groups is seen as deriving from 'office-holding, political power, or the way the state is structured to favour the interests of the dominant class'. Norsigian (Tesh et al., 1988), writing from a feminist perspective, contends that women have a major role in supporting health by their childrearing, caregiving, homemaking and food production and preparation roles, yet have a very limited role in policy making.

Signal (1998) applies these three perspectives to the politics of health promotion. 'Pluralist interest group theory' is seen as offering a micro-level analysis of the interest groups within the policy arena and their influences on public policy. Identifying the key players and the location of support and opposition is necessary for building alliances to achieve desired policy changes and tackling any opposition.

Signal uses 'the new institutionalism' as a meso-level theory to explore the effects of institutional characteristics in shaping the process of policy making – focusing on the effects of organizational structure, together with the ways in which organizations operate, the rules that guide their operation and the ideas integral to their functioning. Clearly there will be a stronger impetus to address issues of healthy public policy among those organizations that have a 'health promotion mandate' or those that perceive health issues as falling within their legitimate sphere of activity. Furthermore, wider recognition of health being part of an organization's accepted remit will lend authority to its voice within the policy arena. Key issues to consider in assessing the potential of different interest groups are summarized in the box.

We noted in Chapter 4 that institutions vary considerably in their degree of openness and the extent to which they interlink with other institutions and involve communities. This will inevitably impact on alliance building and responsiveness to the community's needs.

Finally, Signal draws on neo-Marxist theory to analyse macro-level political and economic factors that set the broad context for policy. She refers to two traditions within neo-Marxist analysis – the functional perspective and the political class perspective.

The former is concerned with the organization of the state in relation to capital accumulation and emphasizes the importance of locating health promotion policy development within the broader economic and social policy context.

The political class perspective focuses on power and the capacity to take collective action among the three main political class groupings – organized capital, organized labour and political parties. In particular, it draws attention to the need to harness the forces of business, labour (and the trades unions) and political parties in the interests of healthy public policy.

We might summarise the key points as follows:

- know your potential allies and adversaries
- know the structures with which you are working
- know the context within which you are working.

Rational and incremental approaches

There are two broad schools of thought about the process of policy making – the 'rational' and the 'incremental'. The former conforms with the principles of rational decision making discussed in Chapter 7 and assumes:

- clear explication of goals
- identification of all the alternatives for addressing the issue
- rational and objective appraisal of each alternative
- selection of the most appropriate alternative.

ASSESSING THE POTENTIAL OF DIFFERENT INTEREST GROUPS

- How well organized is the group?
- What resources are available – financial, time, skills, experience?
- What strategies are used to influence the political process?

After Signal, 1998

The view that policy is the product of such rational processes is considered to be overly idealized. A more realistic interpretation is offered by incrementalism, which describes policy as evolving gradually 'on the basis of previous decisions and pragmatic considerations' (Delaney, 1994b: 219).

Lindblom (1987) – one of the main proponents of incrementalism – suggests that the complexity of many problems is such that analysis is beyond the capacity of our small minds. As Lindblom and Woodhouse (1993: 66) state,

> It is impossible to unambiguously calculate even how a single complex policy will interact with another, much less how it will interact with all others. Nor does anyone really ever attempt such a task.

The choice is therefore between inaction in the face of the enormity of the task of ensuring that the right course of action is being taken or at least making some headway. The notion of 'bounded rationality' accepts that rational decision making will inevitably be constrained by factors such as cost and practicability. A further factor limiting the practical feasibility of purely rational approaches is that policymakers are not value-free (Walt, 1994). Indeed, we have identified the core values of health promotion in Chapter 1 and, clearly, health promotion policy should be consistent with these core values.

Incrementalism is characterized by:

• lack of a clear distinction between goals and the means of achieving them
• consideration of a restricted number of alternatives
• identification of the major consequences rather than all consequences
• no ideal policy option – the best option is the one that policymakers agree is the most appropriate
• achieving small changes to existing policy rather than major change (after Walt, 1994).

Incrementalism is also typical of pluralist, democratic approaches. Decisions about policy are arrived at by means of bargaining and compromise between different interest groups – referred to as 'partisan interaction' and 'mutual adjustment' (Lindblom, 1979, and Lindblom and Woodhouse, 1993). Each attempts to pursue its own interests, but, to accommodate the interests of other groups, may be prepared to fall back to a compromise position (Janis and Mann, 1977: 34):

> Whenever power is distributed among a variety of influential executive leaders, political parties, legislative factions, and other interest groups, one centre of power

can rarely impose its preferences on another and policies are likely to be the outcome of give and take among numerous partisans. The constraints of bureaucratic politics, with their shifting compromises and coalitions, constitute a major reason for the disjointed and incremental nature of the policies that gradually evolve.

Small changes are held to be more feasible than radical ones. Incrementalism, therefore tends to maintain the status quo (Delaney, 1994c) or support gradual change and so has been challenged on account of its inherent conservatism. The incrementalist view is that small changes can be made quickly and a series of small changes can, when judged as a whole, achieve major change. It is, therefore, associated with serial policymaking – that is, revisiting and readjusting policy (Walt, 1994). It is also consistent with the environmental maxim attributed to Dubos 'think globally, act locally'.

The notion of mixed scanning (Etzioni, 1967) adopts a middle ground position and attempts to capitalize on the strengths of both rational and incremental approaches. It involves developing a broad overview of the policy field as a basis for distinguishing between those areas that can be approached incrementally and those requiring a more thorough analysis of options before making major strategic decisions.

Conflict and consensus models

'Conflict models' see groups as having their own interests and competing to ensure that they achieve their own goals. The issue of tobacco control offers a clear illustration in which the interests of the transnational tobacco conglomerates cannot be reconciled with those of public health or, indeed, the consumer when, as Action on Smoking and Health (ASH, undated) reminds us, 'Tobacco is unique: the only product that kills when used normally'. British American Tobacco (BAT), as part of its strategy to be seen as a responsible company, has initiated a process of social reporting based on the company's audit of its social and ethical performance. The stakeholder dialogue that was set up to contribute to this was met with the following response from ASH (2002a):

> [There is] no public health benefit to justify the time and cost. We see little benefit coming from it in public health terms, and that is our objective. There are virtually no areas where BAT and ASH can find common cause – we characterize BAT's relationship with public health as a zero sum game. Our efforts and limited resources are best spent in pressing for meaningful public policy measures at national, European and

international level that control the activities of tobacco companies and reduce smoking. An invitation to a stakeholder dialogue, is an invitation to spend our funds on BAT's initiative, when we believe we can spend our money and time better in other ways. Where we do believe there is potential common ground we retain the option to meet with tobacco companies on a case-by-case basis.

While ASH was prepared to provide information, it defended its reluctance to engage in a fuller dialogue on the grounds of the unethical activity of the tobacco industry, summarized in its own report on the social impacts of the activities of the tobacco industry (ASH, 2002a).

Bunton (1992) sees the state as having an important role when major corporations bring power to bear to thwart public health interests. Equally, the state must balance economic and other interests with public health concerns. By way of example, let us briefly consider the issue of sports sponsorship. The UK, under a Conservative administration, had been one of the countries blocking the introduction of a European directive on banning tobacco advertising. Subsequent to the election of the Labour government in 1997, support was more forthcoming, with the caveat that time would be needed for sports to find alternative sponsors and the Directive was adopted in 1998. However, there were still concerns about the effect on Formula One racing – variously reported to receive between £35 million (Department of Health, 1998) and £70 million (ASH, 2002b) in sponsorship from the tobacco industry in the UK – together with the knock-on effects on employment. The UK White Paper on Tobacco (Department of Health, 1998), which required sports sponsorship to be phased out by 30 July 2003, extended the time period for Formula One racing until 30 July 2006, in line with the maximum period allowed under the European Directive.

As well as conflict arising from different sectional interests *vis-à-vis* an issue or problem, Bunton (1992) also suggests that it can arise from the reactions to change and forces for innovation competing with forces of inertia. Furthermore, conflict theorists contend that power may be exercised in framing the political agenda. Powerful insider groups may effect closure to confine debate to their own areas of concern, excluding other issues and, indeed, interest groups (Jones and Sidell, 1997).

Clearly, conflict models are marked by a power struggle that results in some groups 'winning' or an impasse. The power strategies that are used in groups and organizations to exert control are summarized in the box. Variations between different groups in their access to resources will influence the pressure that they can bring to bear. The structure of the policy environment may be such that some groups are excluded and, where there are steep social gradients, the most disadvantaged will have greatest difficulty in making their voices heard (Bunton, 1992).

Lindblom and Woodhouse (1993: 128) identify three methods for conflict resolution:

- non-rational and irrational persuasion, as via propaganda campaigns or symbolic rhetoric
- logrolling – that is, steam rollering – vetoes, bribery or other interpersonal means for inducing acquiescence without actually persuading on the merits
- informed and reasoned persuasion.

Profound differences in ideological commitments between different groups make it unlikely that reasoned persuasion will be effective and it may therefore be necessary to resort to less rational and more persuasive – or, indeed, coercive – strategies.

POWER STRATEGIES

- **Physical power** coercive power, either real or threatened.
- **Resource power** (also referred to as reward power) deriving from possession of valued resources that may or may not be material.
- **Position power** (also referred to as legitimate power) associated with position or status.
- **Expert power** attributed to individuals on account of acknowledged expertise.
- **Personal power** emanates from the personality and is associated with charisma.
- **Negative power** the inappropriate use of power outside the recognized domain of interaction. Its intention is subversive, for example not passing on information.

After Handy, 1993

A 'consensus model' is premised on the view that it is possible to reach agreement and is consistent with pluralism and the 'muddling through' notion of incrementalism.

Bunton (1992) contends that the development of healthy public policy can be built on cooperation and collaboration. Agreements are reached by means of negotiation and bargaining – partisan mutual adjustment. The role of health promotion is to influence the process to maximize health gain via persuasion techniques, such as 'information dissemination, incentives and sanctions' (Bunton, 1992: 146). Hogwood and Gunn (1984) note Dror's criticism that, while approaches emphasizing consensus may be acceptable during periods of relative stability, they are unlikely to achieve major innovation or offer solutions to complicated problems.

Lindblom and Woodhouse (1993: 120) contend that, overall, the level of fundamental disagreement in society is surprisingly small:

Instead, politics normally proceed on the basis of what some call the 'underlying consensus' in a society. Is this agreement brought about by reasoned persuasion, or does much of it evolve through social indoctrination processes …? Who has the capacity and incentive to use schooling and other socializing institutions to bring about widespread agreements?

Their views draw attention to the narrowness of contemporary debates and raise the question, why has there not been a greater challenge to issues such as inequality? Furthermore, any attempts to do so have, to date, been relatively modest and have avoided tackling root causes.

The players – terminology

'Policy actors' are those individuals, groups or organizations involved in policy making. Their level of involvement may well vary at different stages of the policy development process. For example, groups that are at the forefront of lobbying activity may have a less prominent role in the formulation and implementation of policy. However, an important consideration at each stage is not only who is included, but, equally, who is left out. 'Stakeholders' are all those who stand to be affected, in whatever way, by the introduction of a policy and who may be, but are not necessarily, involved in policy making.

The 'policy keeper' is the agency that, either by mandate or its own initiative, holds a policy and moves the policy forwards during any phase of policy making (Milio, 1988). The identity of the policy keeper may change during these different phases. Milio provides the example of the non-governmental

National Nutrition Council in Norway acting as policy keeper in advocating a national food and nutrition policy, but, once this became part of the government agenda, a ministerial office assumed the role of policy keeper.

There are various different groups that seek to influence policy. The term 'interest or pressure group' is generally used for groups that exist outside government. Walt (1994) identifies the common feature of interest groups to be aiming to achieve goals without becoming part of the formal mechanism of government – that is, attempting to influence from outside rather than inside government. If they do gain formal political power, then they cease to be an interest group and become part of the institutional process of government.

Lindblom and Woodhouse (1993) note the lack of precision in the term 'interest group'. They suggest that business interest, for example, cannot be seen as a 'group' in the conventional sense, but that businesses are organized bureaucracies dominated by a small number of executives. Some of the so-called interest groups may, in fact, be highly influential individuals who take on interest group activity to influence the direction of policy. Somewhat unusually, Lindblom and Woodhouse also suggest that government departments and officials may seek to shape the development of policy by lobbying on behalf of their own interests – operating in substantially the same way as private interest groups. For example, the ministry of health trying to influence fiscal policy on tobacco or transport policy. They (1993: 75) therefore define 'interest group activity' rather more broadly to include the activity of government officials that falls outside the usual channels of authority and spheres of activity:

interactions through which individuals and private groups not holding government authority seek to influence policy, together with those policy-influencing interactions of government officials that go well beyond the direct use of their authority.

Milio (1988: 266) subscribes to this broader view and refers to the major players as interest groups:

any organized groups or parts of groups whose resources, authority, status, influence or survival is affected by a policy. Such groups include political parties; parliamentary committees, ministerial offices and bureaucratic units; commercial enterprises; and voluntary, professional, religious, communications or minority organizations.

Interest groups fall into two broad divisions – those concerned with protecting the interests of their members, such as Trades Unions, Disability Rights groups and Gay Rights groups, and those coming together around a specific issue, such as abortion, pollution or opposition groups to local planning developments. It follows that membership of the former will be restricted to particular groups, whereas in the latter it will be open to anyone with an interest in the issue.

The terminology for these groups varies – Walt (1994) suggests 'sectional' and 'cause groups'. She also notes a further distinction between 'insider' and 'outsider groups'. Insider groups are respected by policymakers, there are often close working relationships and, because of their recognized legitimacy, these groups tend to be consulted on policy issues and invited to participate in policy making. Outsider groups, in contrast, have greater difficulty in gaining access to the policy process and may resort to direct action to make their voices heard. Walt cites the activities of Greenpeace, drawing attention to the pollution generated by industry, or anti-abortion groups demonstrating outside clinics. Less extreme activity would involve advocacy and lobbying on behalf of a cause.

An alternative strategy would be to move from outsider to insider status. Walt notes that groups such as the Family Planning Association in the UK and HIV activist groups in a number of countries have achieved insider status by providing services and building up acknowledged expertise in particular areas. Walt also draws attention to the important role of non-governmental organizations (NGOs) in developing countries and Constantino-David's witty categorization (see the box). While not formally recognized as interest groups, NGOs may consciously seek to influence policy or ensure the public accountability of the state.

Generally, members of the public do not, as individuals, engage directly with policy-making processes. Their influence is more usually via action groups or contributing to creating a collective opinion, such that adoption of a particular policy becomes the most prudent course of action for politicians seeking to maintain their popularity with the electorate. There are notable exceptions and committed individuals have managed to secure policy change. A well-known example is the case of Victoria Gillick, who challenged a Department of Health circular stating that young people under the legal age of consent could receive confidential contraceptive advice and treatment. She succeeded in 1984 in winning an appeal court ruling that girls under sixteen should not be given contraceptives without their parents' consent, although this was subsequently overturned by a House of Lords decision in Gillick v West Norfolk and Wisbech Area Health Authority and another [1986] 1 AC 112. More recently, Laura Ahearn is known for her work in attempting to change policy on the prevention of child sexual abuse and the introduction of 'Megan's Law' in the United States.

A 'policy network' is the 'collection of actors and organizations which influences decision making in a policy sector' (John, 1998: 205). A network is made up of a number of 'policy communities'. John (1998: 83) suggests that this term implies that 'the participants know each other well and ... share the same values and policy goals' and defines it (1998: 204) as 'a restricted set of actors and organizations which influence decisions on a policy sector'.

Walt (1994) contends that policy communities are characterized by an ongoing interchange of information and ideas.

Smith (1997) distinguishes between 'policy communities' and 'issues networks'. The former have limited membership (possibly with the conscious exclusion of some groups), regular and frequent contact, common values and a relationship based on exchanges of resources. Issues networks tend to be larger and more variable in their composition and the interests of members and arrangements for contact may be more ad hoc. Access to, and sharing of, resources will also vary, along with the power that different members command. Several government departments may be included within an issues network. For example, some fourteen government departments have been identified by the White

---

NON-GOVERNMENTAL ORGANIZATIONS (NGOs)

BINGOs	big NGOs
GRINGOs	government run or inspired NGOs
BONGOs	business-oriented NGOs
COME'NGOs	NGOs set up opportunistically and which do not last long

Constantino-David, 1992, in Walt, 1994: 116

Paper on Tobacco (Department of Health, 1998a) as contributing to tackling smoking, plus all those reviewing their internal smoking policies.

In that networks include different public, private and commercial organizations, it is likely that a range of different viewpoints will be represented. 'Coalitions' may, therefore, develop between groupings sharing similar values. They can become a major force within the policy arena. Coalitions have been defined (Feighery and Rogers, 1989, in Butterfoss et al., 1993: 316) as:

> an organization of individuals representing diverse organizations, factions or constituencies who agree to work together to achieve a common goal.

and (Brown, 1984, in Butterfoss et al., 1993: 316):

> an organization of diverse interest groups that combine human and material resources to effect a specific change the members are unable to bring about independently.

The key elements can be summarized as:

- unity in working towards a common goal
- pooling of resources
- increased capacity to achieve the goal.

Butterfoss et al.'s (1993) review of the literature on coalitions identifies three types of coalition, based on Feighery and Rogers (1989):

- **grassroots coalitions** generally set up by volunteers to respond to a crisis, such as closure of a local hospital
- **professional coalitions** formed by professional organizations
- **community-based coalitions** usually initiated by an agency, but involving professionals and grass roots leaders.

The review also identifies a number of factors associated with the importance of coalitions and these are summarized in the box.

Herman et al. (1993) draw attention to the issue of recruitment. Their study of the development of a coalition among a number of organizations to address inadequate state-subsidized family planning found that recruitment relied heavily on existing interpersonal and interorganizational networks. While, on the one hand, this supported the rapid mobilization of an effective coalition, it also resulted in gaps in representation and the exclusion of some groups. Rogers et al. (1993) also note the lack of representation from key community constituencies in local tobacco control coalitions.

We have already considered the issue of intersectoral working and healthy alliances in Chapter 4. However, we should note here some of the factors associated with the success of coalitions. Butterfoss et al.'s (1993) analysis indicates that one of the key elements in coalition formation is the development of a clear goal to which all members can subscribe. Individual interests then become subsumed within a collective purpose. Indeed, development of a spirit of cooperation is fundamental to cohesive, effective coalitions. While a whole range of factors related to structure, leadership and interpersonal factors will affect the maintenance of the coalition, member satisfaction is important – members need to perceive the coalition as beneficial Achieving some short-term success will increase motivation and the credibility of the coalition. However, this should not detract from a focus on the overall goal. Clearly, evaluation of outcomes is essential in demonstrating progress and sustaining momentum. Feighery and Rogers

THE IMPORTANCE OF COALITIONS

- Coalitions spread responsibility across a number of organizations and enable them to become involved in a broader range of issues.
- Coalitions both demonstrate and mobilize public support for an issue.
- Coalitions can maximize the power brought to bear on an issue and achieve a 'critical mass'.
- Coalitions can minimize duplication of effort.
- Coalitions provide access to a wider range of talent and resources – human and material – and can 'enhance the leverage' of groups.
- Coalitions are a vehicle for recruiting additional groups – across a range of constituencies – to a cause.
- The flexibility of coalitions enables them to draw on new resources as situations change.

After Butterfoss et al., 1993

(1989) found that the following influenced members' satisfaction with the coalition:

- it is managed effectively
- good communication among membership
- low costs of, and barriers to, participation.

Gottlieb et al. (1993) recommend:

- formalization of agreements, mission statements and goals and objectives
- attention to the process of group formation
- clarification of expectations.

POLICY MAKING

The main stages in policy making are problem identification, policy formulation, implementation and evaluation. While this may be taken to imply a chronological sequence, in reality the process may be more iterative and complex. Milio (1988: 266) suggests that it is a 'continuous, but not necessarily linear, social and political process'. Springett (1998) also notes that, in practice, there is often no clear distinction between policy development and implementation and the two strands frequently develop in parallel.

Delaney (1994c: 7) cites the questions posed by Anderson (1975) as a means of identifying key issues at each stage and proposes adding 'Why?' and 'Why not?' to expose more fundamental concerns – particularly the location and operation of political power:

1 Problem formation. What is a policy problem? How does it get on the agenda of government?

2 Formulation. How are the alternatives for dealing with the problem developed? Who participates?
3 Adoption. How is a policy alternative adopted or enacted? Who adopts?
4 Implementation. What is done, if anything, to carry a policy into effect? What impact does this have on policy content?
5 Evaluation. How is effectiveness measured? Who evaluates? What are the consequences?

Milio (1988) also offers a series of generic issues to consider in relation to policy making and these are set out in the box.

Milio (1988: 265) contends that those seeking to influence policy making need to identify 'points of entry into policy-making processes, sources of support, and strategies to enhance the feasibility of specific health promotion policy options in any given policy sector'. In the same way that healthy public policy should make the healthy choice the easy choice, efforts to influence policy should make the healthy policy option the most attractive option. Clearly, both insiders and outsiders will need political skills and acumen to effectively exert influence within the policy arena.

Ideally, policy should be based on sound evidence and there is clearly a need to produce relevant information to inform the policy-making process. De Leeuw (1993) notes that epidemiological research findings are often not translated into effective policies. Discussion tends to centre on:

- what information is needed by policymakers
- how can information be used to influence the development of policy.

However, she contends that it is naïve to suppose that information will automatically be assimilated

---

POLICY MAKING – ISSUES TO CONSIDER

- Agenda setting – whether or not a given public issue is an appropriate problem for public policy.
- Problem framing – determining the definition and scope of the problem.
- Priority setting.
- Option setting – finding possible optional solutions, including goals and strategies.
- Criteria selection – by what criteria options should be chosen.
- Policy selection – who bears the responsibility to decide.
- Means choice – how, and by whom, the policy should be implemented.
- Success indicators – determining the criteria and sources of evaluation.
- Changing goals or means – how the policy should be reformulated.

After Milio, 1988: 266

into policy making and achieve change by means of rational processes. The reality is that policy making is heavily influenced by assumptions, vested interests and power positions. Bearing in mind our various earlier discussions, it will be apparent that the relative power of the key groups of players is of paramount importance. At a government level, conflict between ministers is a well-known phenomenon. Powles' (1988) analysis of the development of a food and nutrition policy in Victoria, Australia, provides an example of attempts to reconcile the conflicting interests of different groups and, in particular, to address the concerns of the Victorian Employers Federation, which represented the interests of food processing companies. Crucial elements in achieving a resolution (albeit at the expense of protracting the process and considerably lengthening the document) were the tenacity of individuals and clarity about where it might be possible to make concessions to alternative positions and where not – for example, refusal to negotiate on the concept of dietary guidelines.

Key assumptions in the policy-making process concern 'cause and effect' and 'intervention effect' – that is, if we do X then Y will follow. While data can be collected to establish the nature of a problem and predictions can be made about the effects of policy change (see the box opposite for an example – estimating what will happen if the price of cigarettes is increased), the challenge is to convert research findings into a form that conveys a powerful message that appeals to dominant values. It is also important to understand the power structures within the policy arena and how to manipulate them. As Milio (1988: 265) suggests, the development of 'policy relevant' information requires consideration of the following issues:

- how to extrapolate the policy implications of data
- how to propose feasible policy options
- how to judge the social and political responses to issues and proposals
- who to contact, when and how.

The notion of 'creative epidemiology' is concerned with making research findings and epidemiological data more accessible: 'It is particularly concerned with placing unfamiliar or complicated data in perspective against data that are more familiar to people' (Chapman and Lupton, 1994: 160). For example, expressing death rates from smoking-related diseases in conventional epidemiological terms as rates per 100,000 or as relative risk – while undoubtedly essential in establishing evidence of the effects of smoking on health – has little impact outside professional circles. The statement that, in the UK, 120,000 smokers will die each year as a result of their smoking habit (ASH, 2002) is easier to visualize and more attention-grabbing. The information becomes even more dramatic when converted to a toll of 328 lives *per day* – equivalent to a major air crash. This instantly raises the profile of smoking-related deaths from hidden daily occurrences to a major national tragedy.

Other strategies for gaining attention include comparison with issues that already stimulate public concern, such as smoking kills around six times more people in the UK than road traffic accidents (3391), other accidents (8933), poisoning and overdose (3157), murder and manslaughter (495), suicide (4485) and HIV infection (180) *all put together* (20,641 in total – 1999 figures) (ASH, 2002).

Similarly, information can be manipulated to emphasize the potential risk for individuals – for example, half of all teenagers smoking today will die of tobacco-related causes if they continue to do so (ASH, 2001).

Chapman and Lupton (1994) provide a detailed account of the various strategies that might be used and cite an example of the use of creative epidemiology that convinced politicians of the effects of tobacco sponsorship on children and led to the Federal Government in Australia supporting a ban on tobacco sponsorship. Data were collected on cigarette brand preferences in four states in Australia and were found to correspond with the major football sponsors in each state. Steve Woodward, the then Australian Director of ASH, converted the data into visually appealing graphs that were distributed to all politicians and the media.

Agenda setting

The 'policy agenda' has been defined (Kingdon, 1984, in Walt, 1994: 53) as:

the list of subjects or problems to which government officials and people outside of government closely associated with those officials are paying serious attention at any given time.

A key question concerns how issues get on to – or fail to get on to – the policy agenda. Jones and Sidell (1997) refer to the well-known UK example of the effective 'burying' of Sir Douglas Black's report, *Inequalities in Health* (Department of Health and Social Security, 1980) by tactics such as producing a limited number of copies and its publication on an August bank holiday, which ensured minimum publicity. Whitehead's update on inequality, *The Health Divide* (1987), suffered a similar fate and there was only tacit reference to

ESTIMATED EFFECT OF AN INCREASE
IN THE PRICE OF CIGARETTES

	Scenarios			
	1 euro increase in price		10 per cent increase in price	
Proportional increase in the price of a packet of 20 cigarettes				
The Netherlands	39.4		10	
England and Wales	26.0		10	
Denmark	22.1		10	
Sweden	26.6		10	
Decrease in the prevalence of smoking (percentage)				
	15–24-year-olds and light smokers[1]	Over 25-year-olds and heavy smokers[2]	15–24-year-olds and light smokers[1]	Over 25-year-olds and heavy smokers[2]
The Netherlands	28	16	7	4
England and Wales	18	10	7	4
Denmark	16	9	7	4
Sweden	19	11	7	4

[1]Calculated on the basis of 0.7 price elasticity, assuming greater sensitivity to changing prices among younger and light smokers.
[2]Calculated on the basis of 0.4 price elasticity, assuming greater tolerance among older and heavier smokers.
Source: After Baan et al., 1999

inequality in the first national health strategy 'Health of the Nation' (Department of Health, 1992).

Notwithstanding the lack of national political attention, sound research evidence demonstrating inequality to be a major public health issue generated a groundswell of opinion at local and national levels, including public health professionals, academics, pressure groups and the public. Against this backdrop, inequality has received progressively increasing government attention – initially with the 'variations' agenda (Department of Health, 1995a) and more latterly with the response to the publication of the *Independent Inquiry into Inequalities in Health* (Acheson, 1998). Tackling inequality and

social exclusion now forms a central plank of the national health strategy *Saving Lives: Our Healthier Nation* (Department of Health, 1999).

Hogwood and Gunn (1984) suggest that an issue is most likely to get on the policy agenda if any of the following apply:

- it has reached crisis proportions
- it has achieved particularity – that is, it exemplifies a larger issue
- it has an emotive aspect
- it is likely to have wide impact
- it raises questions about power and legitimacy in society
- it is currently 'fashionable'.

However, the influence of 'agenda setters' (see the box) can also be pivotal. As we have already noted, the élitist viewpoint (Hogwood and Gunn would also include anything other than the most naïve pluralist interpretation) acknowledges that there may be unequal access to the policy agenda. John (1998: 147) suggests that:

> the distribution of power is the underlying factor, but it is more normal in radical accounts to stress the salience of ideas and political language which marginalizes certain interests and ideas. Power is expressed through the hegemony of certain ideas. Created by the middle or upper classes and by economic interests, ruling ideologies ensure that certain issues are off the agenda and others are on it.

The notion of 'bounded pluralism' has been applied to gaining access to the policy agenda. Elite groups may have dominant influence over major issues, of high politics, whereas there may be much more open debate on more minor and less politically sensitive issues. In addition to what gets on to the policy agenda, an important consideration is what is kept off. Elite groups may take on a gatekeeper function in relation to major – potentially politically damaging – issues (Walt, 1994, and Jones and Sidell, 1997). Efforts to confine the agenda to safe issues can simply involve filtering out more contentious ones, but also, and perhaps rather more sinisterly, implicitly or explicitly shape people's perceptions of what they want and need (Lukes, 1974).

Reich (2002) maintains that policy change is dependent on the political will of leaders. The role of policy advocates, therefore, is to create that political will. This requires political analysis to identify the key stakeholders, their intentions, potential losers and winners and where support and opposition will lie. It also requires the adoption of appropriate political strategies.

ADVOCACY

Healthy public policy depends on political vision and leadership and Draper (1988: 218) contends that leadership 'must begin with the people who have a strong professional responsibility for public health'. It also requires an effective advocacy function and strengthening of the advocacy role of health professionals.

Defining advocacy

Advocacy was identified as a key strategy by the Ottawa Charter (WHO, 1986). The term 'advocacy' has traditionally been used to describe activity on behalf of those in a less powerful position. The International Union for Health Education (1992) identified three main areas in which advocates can operate:

- influencing government to develop healthy polices and legislation
- influencing commercial and other organizations to consider the health impact of their activities and exert pressure on governments and citizens
- influencing individuals and groups to make healthy choices and support initiatives to promote health.

The Advocacy Institute (2001) defines advocacy as the:

> pursuit of influencing outcomes – including public policy and resource allocation decisions within political, economic, and social systems and institutions – that directly affect people's lives.
>
> Advocacy consists of organized efforts and actions based on the reality of 'what is'. These organized actions seek to highlight critical issues that have been

---

AGENDA SETTERS

- Organized interests
- Protest groups
- Political party leaders
- Senior government officials and advisers
- Informed opinion
- Mass media

After Hogwood and Gunn, 1984

ignored and submerged, to influence public attitudes, and to enact and implement laws and public policies so that visions of 'what should be' in a just, decent society become a reality.

Wallack et al. (1993: 27) suggest that:

Advocacy is a catch-all word for the set of skills used to create a shift in public opinion and mobilize the necessary resources and forces to support an issue, policy, or constituency. Advocacy involves much more than lobbying in support of a certain piece of legislation. Health professionals routinely engage in a wide array of advocacy activities, including patient advocacy, client advocacy, and policy advocacy, all designed to make the system function better to meet health and safety goals...

They draw on Amidei (1991, in Wallack et al., 1993: 28) to identify several characteristics of advocacy:

- Advocacy assumes that people have rights, and those rights are enforceable.
- Advocacy works best when focused on something specific.
- Advocacy is primarily concerned with rights and benefits to which someone or some community is already entitled.
- Policy advocacy is concerned with ensuring that institutions work the way they should.

Patient and client advocacy are concerned with ensuring that individuals obtain their rights. Our concern here is with the broader area of policy advocacy – specifically, healthy public policy advocacy and issues affecting collective rights. The related activity of lobbying is taken to apply narrowly to attempts to persuade members of government to take up a cause.

Walt (1994) distinguishes between 'commercial lobbyists', who will take on any cause, and 'cause lobbyists', who are seeking to further the specific cause to which they subscribe. Both may adopt similar tactics and seek close relationships with civil servants as well as elected representatives.

In contrast, the target of advocacy may range wider than government circles to generate support among interest groups, the media and the general public. Based on the premise that democratic governments tend to act in line with major public opinion – or at least not risk alienating it – the overall intention of public health advocacy is to create a climate of support for healthy policy options (see the box). As Milio (1981: 304) argues:

The development of organized advocacy for the public's health may well be necessary to demand that government use its resources for health-making purposes. If so, advocacy must go far beyond the usual voicing of discontent, or of admonitions to individuals to change their ways. The message must be conveyed in ways that create widespread and informed public debate. Usable translations of the message are necessary. Explanations are needed of the complexities of the health problem, of alternate health strategies, and of their costs and gains. The true costs of not preventing illness must be addressed, as well as the protections that are possible for those whose livelihoods might be harmed during transitions. Workable formats for presenting the message and convenient forums for discussion are needed for the general public and for its subgroups, for the mass media and specialized professional media, for policymakers, and for scientists and methodologists. Such groundwork seems essential to effective policy-influencing action. Its ultimate strategic purpose is to make health-promoting policy decisions easier for policymakers to choose.

Chapman and Lupton's (1994: 6) influential text defines public health advocacy as:

the process of overcoming major structural (as opposed to individual or behavioural) barriers to public health goals. Numbered among such barriers are some of the most formidable political, economic and cultural forces imaginable. Theses forces include political philosophies that devalue health and quality of life at the expense of economic outcomes; political and bureaucratic opposition or inertia to health-promoting legislative or regulatory provisions and policies, and to the participation of consumers in healthcare planning; the marketing of unsafe and unhealthy products, often by transnational

EDUCATION: THE ADVOCACY FUNCTION

Public discontent can ... be a potent influence – perhaps the most potent influence – in securing progress in community care. No parliamentary indifference, no political chicanery, no administrative difficulties can in the long run obstruct the sustained will of the people.

Irvine, 1948

corporations of immense influence and wealth; and the pervasiveness of major cultural values such as racism and sexism, which find expression in institutional values and personal attitudes and behaviours relevant to public health issues.

Wise (2001) contends that, although the overall aim may be to change the legislative, fiscal, physical and social environment, advocacy is fundamentally a political process that aims to influence political decisions. She draws on Wallack (1998) to distinguish between advocacy and public education or social marketing. Although they may use the same media to communicate their messages, the latter are predicated on the assumption that problems are due to lack of information and focus on filling the information gap. Advocacy, on the other hand, focuses on the *power* gap and problems are seen to be due to lack of sufficient power to achieve social change. Advocacy, therefore, attempts to mobilize support and political involvement.

Strategies

Effective advocacy involves identifying and assessing the power of opposition groups and supporters as a basis for targeting action to build support and develop coalitions, along with undermining the opposition. It relies on the tactical use of persuasive communication. It also involves framing issues to convey their fundamental essence and constructing arguments to appeal to potential supporters. The various players present what is in the best interests of their group by filtering information from factual reality. Their stated reason for their stance on policy is the 'publicly acceptable justification of their material or political interests' (Milio, 1988: 267).

Given that there is no objective reality, public health policy initiatives are open to a range of interpretations (Chapman and Lupton, 1994). These will inevitably be influenced by values and ideological commitments. Milio suggests that we need to understand how a policy will affect major stakeholders and how they frame their support or opposition. For example, the Acheson inquiry (1998) noted strong evidence that fluoridation of water improves dental health in children and significantly reduces inequality in dental health. However, notwithstanding the sound supportive evidence, attempts in the UK to add fluoride to drinking water have been variously interpreted as:

- offering all children the benefits of protection from dental caries
- offering particular benefits for disadvantaged children who are more vulnerable to caries
- compensating for a deficiency in the drinking water in some geographic areas and restoring it to normal levels
- contaminating drinking water
- mass medication
- an infringement of liberty
- state interference
- placing children at risk of toxic effects.

Effective advocacy requires careful framing of arguments and, conversely, understanding of the way the opposition is framing its own arguments so that an appropriate response can be mounted. By way of example, see the box, which contains a brief extract from a guide for members of the hospitality trade on developing a smoking policy for their premises.

SMOKING POLICIES – CONVINCING THE HOSPITALITY TRADE

Extract from the 'ASH Guide for Proprietors and Managers'.

There is a belief amongst many owners and proprietors that imposing smoking policies will lead to losing custom and that any ban would be difficult to enforce. Obviously the health benefits are the reason why smoking policies exist. A smoking policy also offers customers choice to drink or eat in the environment they wish. Offering customers the choice is important, but all the proprietors featured in this booklet who have implemented a smoking policy have done so because, above all, it makes sound business sense.

'Since we have introduced smoke-free areas customers have complimented us and business has increased', New Inn, Salisbury.

ASH, 1999

SYMBOLIC REPRESENTATION OF A CAUSE

The red ribbon – a powerful symbol of HIV awareness.

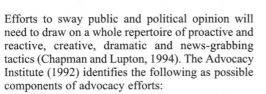

Efforts to sway public and political opinion will need to draw on a whole repertoire of proactive and reactive, creative, dramatic and news-grabbing tactics (Chapman and Lupton, 1994). The Advocacy Institute (1992) identifies the following as possible components of advocacy efforts:

- coalition and alliance building
- media advocacy
- using symbols (the red ribbon symbol in the box, for example)
- lobbying
- information dissemination and communication
- grass roots organization
- strategies for countering opposition.

It also offers examples of case studies of advocacy initiatives (see the box).

ADVOCACY IN ACTION

The Utica COMMIT (COMMunity Intervention Trial) project mounted a successful protest against the Philip Morris tobacco company's attempts to gain social legitimacy by sponsorship of the arts. One of the overall goals of the project was to reframe the community's perception of tobacco companies as 'merchants of death'.

A pamphlet was developed to distribute to the audience as they entered the theatre on the night of the performance. The message was carefully constructed to reframe Philip Morris from a 'patron of the arts' to a 'merchant of death' by rephrasing the advertising slogan, 'Philip Morris brings you the arts' to 'Philip Morris brings you more than art ... they also bring you cancer, emphysema, heart disease, stroke, bronchitis, 135,972 deaths every year.' Rather than state the total number of deaths in the USA, using a creative epidemiological approach, the figure used was calculated to reflect Philip Morris' market share.

The expenditure on sponsorship was put into perspective by pointing out that the company's profits in 1988 amounted to $190,000 per hour.

The leaflet explained the purpose and consequences of tobacco sponsorship and asked parents to talk to their children about the dangers of smoking and the tactics used by tobacco companies in sponsoring arts events. The leaflet concluded with a request to give a donation to the dance company being sponsored at the event to break its dependence on tobacco sponsorship. This also served to frame the dance company as a victim of the tobacco industry and maintained the focus on Philip Morris as the 'enemy'.

Press releases were circulated in advance of the event and considerable media attention was generated.

Advocacy Institute, 1992

Table 6.1 *Framing the debate – arguments of supporters and opponents of pool fencing*

Supporters	Opponents
Expert opinion favours pool fencing	Expert opinion discredits pool fencing arguments
Community support for pool fencing revealed by survey	Community support discredited
Personalizing the issue by presenting the human face of infant drowning	State intrusion into the home
Parents as fallible	Supervisory negligence responsible for drowning
	Drowning as a consequence of trespass
	Fencing swimming pools is arbitrary when there are many unfenced water sources
Aesthetics versus saving a child's life	Hysteria and emotional claptrap
Need to ensure consistency with other safety standards	Overkill to fence all pools even in households where there are no children
Vocal selfish minority are opposed to pool fencing	Opponents portrayed as ordinary citizens and proponents as paid civil servants
Votes versus children's lives	
Defenders of the innocent and helpless	

Source: After Chapman and Lupton, 1994

The media can be particularly effective in bringing issues to public attention and influencing opinion. Chapman and Lupton (1994: 19) note that relatively few key decisionmakers need to be convinced before action is taken and that highly placed individuals – politicians, senior bureaucrats and heads of non-governmental organizations – are 'often highly sensitive to the ways in which the media are framing issues and setting public expectations about the roles they should perform'. Furthermore, where there is dispute, the media can become the 'battlegrounds on which each side seeks to secure the most powerful connotations for its cause, and to attribute to its adversaries the most negative associations' (Chapman and Lupton, 1994: 99). They contend that the success of an advocacy campaign can hinge on the way in which issues are framed in the media and how they are reframed to respond strategically to the efforts of the opposition. Chapman and Lupton's analysis of the themes emerging in press reports of the debate

about fencing domestic swimming pools in New South Wales is summarized in Table 6.1 (see also the box).

Given that many – if not most – public health pressure groups have insufficient funds to buy advertising space in the media to publicize their causes, maximizing free media coverage becomes essential. Like the well-known acronym for giving information to politicians – KISS (keep it short and simple) – gaining access to the media demands brevity rather than protracted rational argument. Presenting the human side of an issue is both powerful and emotive. Witness, for example, the moving address to the thirteenth International AIDS Conference in 2000 by Nkosi Johnson given in the box on the facing page. At the age of eleven, he was South Africa's longest-surviving child with HIV. His words were televised worldwide and were influential in changing the attitudes of individuals, companies and governments to people with AIDS.

ALTERNATIVE FRAMES FOR CHARITABLE ACTION

Archbishop Helder Camara of Brazil said, 'When I feed the hungry, they call me a saint. When I ask why they have no food, they call me a Communist.'

Cited by Wallack et al., 1993

NKOSI JOHNSON'S SPEECH TO THE THIRTEENTH INTERNATIONAL AIDS CONFERENCE

Care for us and accept us – we are all human beings.
We are normal.
We have hands.
We have feet.
We can walk, we can talk, we have needs just like everyone else.
Don't be afraid of us – we are the same.

Nkosi Johnson AIDS Foundation, undated

The association of a celebrity with an issue or cause can attract considerable publicity. Well-known individuals, such as Arthur Ashe, Rock Hudson, Ervin (Magic) Johnson and Freddie Mercury, brought the issue of HIV and AIDS to the forefront of public attention by generating substantial media coverage. Similarly, the association of Diana, Princess of Wales with the landmine issue gave it considerable international prominence.

Chapman and Lupton (1994: 99) note that:

> newsworthiness requires that issues be framed through the transformation of facts and arguments into metaphors, labels and symbols, to allow them to be told as news 'stories'.

We will consider the issue of media advocacy more fully in Chapter 8. The box provides a set of tips for gaining media coverage (see also Chapman, 1994). While the media may be very effective in raising awareness of issues, Walt (1994) notes that policy-makers are unlikely to be influenced by a single account and poses the question of how long media coverage has to be sustained before an issue is put on to the policy agenda. Finnegan and Viswanath (1999: 123) also refer to the need for sustained action on the part of community groups:

> The mass media can be highly effective in building the community agenda for public policy change on behalf of public health, but media attention alone is seldom sufficient without sustained efforts by empowered community groups and coalitions.

Campaign groups will therefore need to consider strategies for maintaining the visibility of issues over a protracted period. Furthermore, Walt raises the issue of what controls the media agenda. In some parts of the world, state control of the media casts doubt on its impartial reporting. Similarly, economic interests may dictate what gains coverage. Newspaper editors and radio and television producers occupy a key gatekeeping role. Over and above dominant ideological frameworks shaping the content of the media, there may also be more conscious filtering of information. Walt refers to the 'propaganda model' of Herman and Chomsky, which is based on the view that the media are

TIPS FOR GETTING ITEMS INTO THE MEDIA

- Get to know the media – know what types of stories they publish.
- Develop good relationships with local journalists and local radio and television.
- Build up a list of contacts of people who handle your sort of story.
- Be realistic about the amount of interest your story will attract.
- Find a local angle.
- Use concrete examples rather than abstract ideas.
- Find a human interest angle.
- Think visual and use a good picture.
- Involve celebrities.

Teenage Pregnancy Unit, 2000

controlled to further the interests of the state and powerful groups. Factors that may affect the filtering of news coverage include ownership, profit orientation, advertising and sources of information.

Returning to the more general issues of advocacy, Baum (2001: 107) suggests that successful advocacy strategies should:

- set an agenda
- frame the issue for public consumption
- advocate specific solutions.

The 'A' Frame for Advocacy developed by the Johns Hopkins Center for Communication Programs (undated) identifies six stages in the advocacy process.

1 **Analysis** of the problem, the need for policy change, stakeholders and, specifically, supporters, opponents, decisionmakers and vote swingers, policy-making structures and processes and means of influencing decisionmakers.
2 **Strategy** based on clear objectives suited to the context.
3 **Mobilization** of potential partners and coalition building to maximize collective resources and power.
4 **Action** achieving maximum visibility for the cause using credible messages and appropriate channels, including the media.
5 **Evaluation** to identify what has been achieved and what still needs to be done.
6 **Continuity** planning for the longer term, keeping coalitions together, keeping arguments fresh and adapting them to current circumstances.

Having clear objectives is a key factor in coordinating activity during the various stages. Furthermore, advocacy efforts are more likely to be successful if decisions about the most appropriate courses of action are based on an analysis of contextual factors and the location of power and influence. Chapman and Lupton (1994: 130) also caution that those involved in advocacy should be clear about their goals and not lose sight of 'the big picture'. Moreover, advocacy should not become an end in itself, but a means of achieving public health goals.

ADOPTION AND IMPLEMENTATION

Whether polices are adopted or not will depend on a range of factors. Bunton (1992: 137) suggests that these would include:

> how the policies are conceived, how they are introduced, the group's commitment to them, the local resources available to assist their introduction, and a range of other socio-economic factors.

Furthermore, he notes that policies may be modified and considerably watered down during the process of development and implementation. This may be the product of powerful interests bringing their weight to bear or, alternatively, the decisions and routines established by what Lipsky (1997) terms 'street-level bureaucrats' – workers in public services, such as welfare departments, schools, health services and so on.

Walt (1994: 165) also sees that the implementation of policy requires the cooperation of many different groups and that 'policy formulation, even in the form of a legal statute, is not a sufficient condition for implementation'. Hogwood and Gunn (1997) contend that the perfect implementation of policy is extremely unlikely and specify the conditions that would need to exist for this to happen:

- circumstances external to the implementing agency not imposing crippling constraints
- adequate time and sufficient resources being made available
- the required combination of resources being available
- the policy being based on a valid theory of cause and effect
- the relationship between cause and effect being direct and few, if any, intervening links
- dependency relationships being minimal
- understanding of, and agreement on, objectives
- tasks being fully specified, in the right sequence
- perfect communication and coordination
- those in authority being able to demand and obtain perfect compliance.

Springett (1998) notes that intersectoral policy is notorious for failure during implementation. Clearly, ensuring that the conditions specified are met is particularly problematic when a number of different agencies and sectors are involved. Colebatch (1998: 56) states that there is held to be a problem in implementation when 'the outcome was likely to be quite different to the originally stated intentions'. By way of illustration, he quotes the title of the seminal work by Pressman and Wildavsky (1973) – *Implementation: How Great Expectations in Washington are Dashed in Oakland: or, Why It's Amazing that Federal Programmes Work at All, This Being a Saga of the Economic Development Administration as Told by Two Sympathetic Observers Who Seek to Build Morals on a Foundation of Ruined Hopes*. The problems identified by Pressman and Wildavsky include having a large number of participants and diversity of goals, such that approval needed to be obtained at a number of different points.

Colebatch provides a useful overview of the ways in which implementation problems are perceived. The vertical perspective assumes a top-down approach and sees implementation as requiring compliance with the directives of those in authority. In contrast, a horizontal perspective recognizes that participants have their own agendas and interpretations of policy. It also acknowledges that the flow of influence is not only vertically within organizations, but that there is negotiation with people external to them.

The horizontal perspective views the implementation of policy rather more flexibly than the vertical. It would see implementation as a collective action that evolves to be compatible with the policy goals and the perspectives of participants rather than a strict adherence to top-down directives.

A further distinction is between normative frameworks, which are concerned with what 'ought to be', and empirical frameworks, which are concerned with 'what is'.

Colebatch equates the vertical perspective on implementation with normative frameworks and the horizontal with empirical frameworks. He notes, too, that there can be two coexisting accounts of the implementation process – the *sacred*, which presents the ideal, and the *profane*, which is a more realistic account of what actually happened.

The means of securing policy implementation will inevitably vary according to the perspective. The vertical perspective will focus on policy goals and compliance, whereas the horizontal will pay greater attention to processes and the people involved.

HEALTH IMPACT ASSESSMENT

We turn our attention now to the wider issue of health impact assessment (HIA). As we noted earlier, the notion of healthy public policy is not just concerned with the development of policies to tackle health issues, but also requires an appraisal of the health impact of all policies.

Kemm (2001) suggests that healthy public policy is dependent on predicting the health consequences of different policy options and ensuring that the policy process gives consideration to these potential consequences at all stages. The Gothenburg consensus paper on HIA (European Centre for Health Policy, 1999: 1) sees the purpose of HIA as being to:

> improve knowledge about the potential impact of a policy or a programme, inform decisionmakers and affected people, and facilitate adjustment of the

proposed policy in order to mitigate the negative and maximize the positive effects.

HIA therefore leads to informed policy making and provides the opportunity to adapt decisions to avoid potential harm. It is considered to add value to policy and decision-making processes (National Assembly for Wales, 1999).

The move towards a more integrated approach to health and development has focused the attention of governments and international organizations, such as WHO and the World Bank, on HIA. Within the European Community, Article 152 of the Amsterdam Treaty (Regional Office for Europe, 2002a) states that:

> A high level of human health protection shall be ensured in the definition and implementation of all Community policies and the Council resolution of June 1999 calls for the establishment of procedures to monitor the impact of Community policies and activities on public health and healthcare.

Within the UK, the importance of assessing the impact of government policy on health and inequality was recognized in the health strategy 'Saving Lives: Our Healthier Nation' (Department of Health, 1999) and the recommendations of the Acheson report, referred to in the box on page 180. The National Assembly for Wales (2002) demonstrated its commitment to developing the use of HIA by setting up a series of pilot projects and the publication of *Developing Health Impact Assessment in Wales* (National Assembly for Wales, 1999).

Identifying the potential health impact of policy is necessarily complex – given the plethora of factors that interact to influence health status, both directly and indirectly. Indirect effects are seen to operate 'through intermediate factors that influence the determinants of health of the population' (European Centre for Health Policy, 1999: 4). Furthermore, policy development in one sector may have a knock-on effect in another – for example, education policy on sex education may well have repercussions for the Department of Health meeting its targets for reducing teenage pregnancy and the rate of sexually transmitted infection (Green, 1998). The Social Exclusion Unit (1999) identifies twenty-eight government programmes that impact on teenage parenthood.

HIA has been defined (European Centre for Health Policy, 1999: 4) simply as:

> a combination of procedures, methods and tools by which a policy, programme or project may be judged as to its potential effects on the health of a population, and the distribution of those effects within a population.

KEY QUESTIONS CONCERNING HIA

What   ... policies will be screened and what are the criteria for deciding?
              ... impacts will be assessed? Will these include health outcomes, determinants, risks and equity?
How   ... will HIA happen? Will it be integrated or conducted separately? Will it be a voluntary or legal
              requirement?
              ... can we infer causality between policy and outcome?
When   ... will HIA be introduced into the policy process?
Who   ... does the assessment? Will this be the policy proponent or an external agency?
              ... pays?
Where   ... at international, national or local levels?

After European Centre for Health Policy, 1999: 8

Kemm refers to Morgan's (1998, in Kemm, 2001: 80) more detailed definition:

a methodology which enables the identification, prediction and evaluation of the likely changes in health risks, both positive and negative (single or collective) of a policy programme, plan or development action on a defined population. These changes may be direct and immediate or indirect and delayed.

HIA can apply to policy, programmes or projects, but, for simplicity, we will just use the term policy. Some of the key questions concerning HIA are listed in the box.

There is general agreement that HIA should be carried out early enough for there to be sufficient fluidity in the decision-making process to respond to the findings. Although, optimally, HIA will be predictive in order to enable remedial action to be taken, the National Assembly for Wales (1999) identifies three types of assessment:

- **prospective**   predicts the effects of policy before it is implemented
- **retrospective** identifies the consequences of a policy already implemented (such evidence may inform future prospective assessments – see, for example, the box about HIA of the Common Agricultural Policy)
- **concurrent**   aims to identify consequences as policies are implemented, particularly when negative impacts are anticipated and there is some uncertainty about them, and allows prompt action to be taken should any negative consequences arise.

To have maximum influence, HIA will need to be integrated into the various stages of policy making.

EXTRACT FROM THE HIA OF THE EU COMMON AGRICULTURAL POLICY (CAP)

Overall assessment

The impact of the Common Agricultural Policy (CAP) on public health is complex. As the case studies have shown, the link between the CAP and health varies from sector to sector. Its main positive contribution to health has been to ensure security of supply in Europe, but the re-emergence of food poverty suggests that, in a modern economy, having plentiful supplies does not automatically mean that these are available and accessible to everyone at reasonable cost. Equity issues need to be brought to the fore once more to refocus debates on the original CAP objectives of ensuring availability and reasonable prices for all ...

Dahlgren et al., 1996: 16

(Continued)

(Continued)

CAP regime for fruit and vegetables

The European Union Common Agricultural Policy rules on fruit and vegetables are a barrier to increased fruit and vegetable consumption. This has a damaging effect on health and imposes unnecessary health costs. Since the CAP fruit and vegetable regime particularly penalizes low-income consumers, it may be regarded as a significant obstacle to equity. Under the current rules, sometimes 50 per cent of the 1.5 billion Ecu spent on the fruit and vegetable sector goes on withdrawing perfectly good produce simply to keep consumer prices high …

Dahlgren et al., 1996: 22

Banken (2001) identifies two conceptual streams that have informed the development of HIA – namely, environmental impact assessment, which focused on the environmental consequences of projects, and the public health emphasis on the social and environmental determinants of health.

Lerer (1999) notes that the current focus tends to be on identifying health hazards and health-risk management, but there is clearly scope to broaden this. Although HIA is usually concerned with policies in the non-health sector, Kemm (2001) suggests that it also has a role in identifying the indirect and unanticipated consequences of health-sector policy.

The potential remit, then, is enormous and this raises questions about the feasibility of assessing the health impact of all policies. There are two responses to this. The first is to filter out for scrutiny only those policy areas that are likely to have health consequences. The second, more radical approach, is to make HIA an integral part of all public policy development and part of the mindset of those involved (Barnes and Scott-Samuel, 2000: 2):

> In the longer term it [HIA] has the potential to make concern for improving public health the norm and a routine part of all public policy development.

This latter approach undoubtedly has the advantage of institutionalizing concern for health. Kemm (2001) sees ownership of HIA by the policy proponent as the ideal state – one that supports shared understanding of values and, at a more practical level, allows HIA to be embedded in all stages of policy development. This is in marked contrast to the situation in environmental impact assessment, where there is usually an external regulatory authority.

Banken (2001) is also supportive of institutionalization of HIA, but cautions that raising health to superordinate status may be perceived by other players in the policy arena as health imperialism, resulting in some resistance. She (2001: 30) emphasizes that the aim should not be to increase the power of public health actors, but to 'add health awareness to policy making' by enabling those in non-health sectors to 'produce public health knowledge for use by decisionmakers'. Clearly, this may require the development of skill and awareness among those involved. She also suggests that enabling non-health actors to produce this kind of information needs to be followed through with quality control to ensure rigour and avoid tokenism. As Bartlett (1989, in Banken, 2001: 31) notes:

> the politics of bureaucracy provide an environment in which the effectiveness of impact assessment can be tempered, subverted, and broken in the absence of adequate provisions for external accountability.

It has been suggested that the use of an alternative term to HIA might advance the cause more effectively. Kemm (2001) suggests 'overall policy appraisal' and Banken (2001) 'human impact assessment'.

Drawing on the principles of economic appraisal, the Department of Health (1996: 1) identifies the following stages:

- define the objectives
- identify the [policy] options
- identify and measure the [health] costs and benefits associated with each option, where possible in monetary terms
- identify and assess the uncertainties of each option
- assess the balance between the options
- present the results
- set up any monitoring that may be necessary to gauge the effects of the policy, and evaluate the policy at a later stage.

Within this framework, all significant health impacts should be identified and the implications of each should be considered in relation to quantity and quality of life and resource costs in the health-care and other sectors. It is unlikely, however, that sufficient information is available to allow this to be done in monetary terms (National Assembly for Wales, 1999). The various impacts identified may well have contradictory effects on health or, indeed, on different groups and, in principle, this could be reduced to an overall net effect. However, it is more useful to maintain an overview of the various pathways that might improve or harm health.

Table 6.2 *Health impacts on different population groups under transport scenario 1 (low spend) and scenario 3 (high spend)*

	Accidents		Pollution		Physical activity		Access to goods and services		Community network	
	1	3	1	3	1	3	1	3	1	3
Young children										
Affluent	+	+	—	+	−	+	−	+	−	++
Deprived	—	+	−	+	—	+	—	+	−	++
Adolescents										
Affluent	−	++	—	+	−	+	—	++	−	++
Deprived	—	+	−	+	−	++	—	++	−	++
Elderly										
Affluent	−	++	−	+	—	++	−	+	−	++
Deprived	—	+	−	+	−	++	—	++	−	++
Working people										
Affluent	0	+	—	+	−	+	−	++	−	+
Deprived	−	+	−	+	−	++	—	++	−	++
Unemployed										
Deprived	−	+	−	+	−	+	—	++	—	++

Key:
++ very positive impact   0 no impact   — very negative impact
+ positive impact   − negative impact

Source: After Douglas et al., 2001

Kemm (2001) also emphazises the importance of differentiating between winners and losers by including consideration of which groups are affected as well as the nature and magnitude of health impacts. For example, in the development context, the construction of a dam may secure a supply of potable water, support irrigation schemes to increase agricultural yields and increase health and prosperity for some, but may require others to relocate, losing homes and farmland, and shift the distribution of diseases such as schistosomiasis. Douglas et al.'s (2001) case study of three possible scenarios for developing transport policy in Edinburgh differentiated the effects on various subgroups of the population, as shown in Table 6.2.

It is axiomatic that HIA should be based on sound evidence. Kemm (2001) distinguishes two main approaches to assessment. One is characterized by a 'tight focus', based on an epidemiological model of exposure and dose–response relationships. Outcomes are usually defined in terms of death and disability, but could potentially be extended to include additional dimensions. The other 'broad focus' adopts a more wideranging approach and draws on informed opinion and local knowledge. A combination of the two is held to be most likely to

generate a complete picture. HIA, therefore relies on both qualitative and quantitative information and a multidisciplinary input. Kemm (2001: 82) suggests that this multidisciplinary input is particularly relevant to:

situational validation will the policy objectives be relevant to the problem
societal vindication will the policy have instrumental value for the health of society as a whole
social choice will the fundamental ideology of the policy be compatible with health.

While acknowledging the persuasiveness of quantitative data and providing guidance on the production of robust quantitative HIA, Mindell et al. (2001) express a number of reservations:

- not everything that can be quantified is important
- not everything that is being quantified at the moment should be
- not everything that is important can be quantified.

Communities may well have different perceptions of risks and benefits than professionals. The National Assembly for Wales (1999: 6) considers community participation to be essential:

THE GOTHENBURG STATEMENT'S VALUES GOVERNING HIA

- Democracy
- Equity
- Sustainable development
- Ethical use of evidence

European Centre for Health Policy, 1999

The involvement of the public is particularly important as many judgements within Health Impact Assessment are value judgements rather than scientific judgements.

Lerer (1999) also advises including communities and an ongoing iterative consultation with major stakeholders. The Gothenburg statement (European Centre for Health Policy, 1999: 5) proposes that HIA should include:

- consideration of *evidence* about the anticipated relationships between a policy, programme or project and the health of the population
- consideration of the *opinions*, experience and expectations of those who may be *affected* by the proposed policy, programme or project.

Careful consideration will need to be given to ways in which to involve the public. Mittelmark (2001) notes that the trend towards more technical and complex methods of assessment, along with the use of inaccessible jargon, makes it difficult for the average citizen to participate. He calls for an approach to HIA that is user-friendly and inclusive and cites the example of the People Assessing Their Health (PATH) project in Eastern Nova Scotia. This involved members of the community in developing local HIA tools suited to the needs of the community. As we have noted, commitment to participation is a central concern of health promotion and is supported by the Gothenburg statement's list of values governing HIA (see the box). Furthermore, there are clear links with health advocacy and ensuring that there are opportunities for individuals who stand to be affected by policy to have a say in shaping its development.

While decisionmakers need to be confident that the conclusions of HIA are robust (Mindell et al., 2001), predicting the consequences of policy will inevitably be associated with some uncertainty. In some instances, there will be evidence on which to draw, whereas in others predictions may need to be based on informed opinion, experience of similar situations and theory. Examples of evidence and data collection methods are provided in the box. Identifying indirect effects may be particularly problematic, especially if they operate via complex systems. It may be possible to extrapolate precise figures and attach confidence intervals to these, but, equally, predictions are often expressed as crude ordinal scales from very certain to very uncertain (Kemm, 2001) or very positive impact to very negative impact, as shown in Table 6.2. The National Assembly for Wales (1999: 6) recognizes this and suggests that those involved:

should make the best assessment they can using the information and skills available to them and by accepting that some degree of uncertainty may be unavoidable.

EXAMPLES OF EVIDENCE AND DATA COLLECTION METHODS

- Depth/key informant interviews
- Focus group discussions
- Equity audits
- Surveys/questionnaires
- Secondary analysis of existing data
- Community profiling
- Health needs assessment
- Expert opinion
- Documentary sources

Taylor and Blair-Stevens, 2002

Stages in HIA

The key principles that underpin HIA are summarized in the box. The main stages in the process of HIA identified by the technical briefing for the World Health Organization Regional Committee for Europe (2002) are:

1 **Screening** to quickly establish whether a particular policy, programme or project is relevant to health. This assessment may involve the use of checklists or other tools. It will flag up if there is a need for a more detailed assessment.

2 **Scoping** to identify the relevant health issues and public concerns that need to be addressed during appraisal. It generates questions, maps out possible connections, sets the boundaries and the terms of reference for the appraisal.

3 **Appraisal** to identify, and when possible quantify, the potential impacts on health and wellbeing in the context of available evidence and the knowledge, experience and opinions of stakeholders. It can be a *rapid* or an *in-depth appraisal*, depending on the level of detail and quantification needed to inform the policy decision, and may include mitigation and health-promoting measures.

4 **Reporting** that is, communicating with stakeholders about the expected impacts on health and about how the policy, programme or other development could be modified to minimize negative and maximize positive impacts.

5 **Monitoring** of compliance with recommendations and of expected health impacts following the implementation of the policy or programme. This allows the existing evidence base to be expanded.

The main stages identified by the National Assembly for Wales (1999) and the Gothenburg Consensus (European Centre for Health Policy, 1999) are broadly similar to these, although more explicit at stage 4 about decision making rather than communication. Although the stages are presented sequentially, the process is essentially iterative.

The Gothenburg Consensus (European Centre for Health Policy, 1999) emphasizes the importance of taking into account the values and goals within a given society and suggests that the process of HIA should be informed by the core values identified in its Statement, given in the box on page 205. Furthermore, it identifies three categories of HIA that can be instigated following the scoping exercise:

- **rapid health impact appraisal** based on existing knowledge and the exchange of information between experts, decisionmakers and representatives of those affected by the proposed policy
- **health impact analysis** involves a more in-depth analysis based on existing evidence and, if necessary, the generation of new data
- **health impact review** used when policies are very broad, it aims to produce a convincing estimation of the major impacts of a policy on health without disentangling the detailed impacts of the various policy components and is more concerned with broad relationships than precise cause-and-effect ones.

While it is not possible here to pursue in detail the actual process of conducting risk assessment, guidance and checklists are available – see, for example, European Centre for Health Policy (1999), National Assembly for Wales (1999), Barnes and Scott-Samuel (2000), and National Assembly for Wales (2002). However, we will conclude with the list of recommendations developed by Douglas et al. (2001: 152):

- screen to select policies for HIA
- negotiate
- share ownership
- be timely
- define and analyse the policy

KEY PRINCIPLES OF HIA

- A social model of health and wellbeing.
- An explicit focus on equity and social justice.
- A multidisciplinary, participatory approach.
- The use of qualitative as well as quantitative evidence.
- Explicit values and openness to public scrutiny.

Barnes and Scott-Samuel, 2000: 2

- define and profile the population
- use an explicit model of health
- be aware of underlying values
- be systematic
- think broadly
- use appropriate evidence
- involve the community
- take into account local factors
- recognize differences within communities
- monitor impacts continuously following an initial prospective HIA
- make practical recommendations.

CONCLUSION

We have established that healthy public policy is a central concern of health promotion. It is a means of upholding the rights of individuals to health by creating a supportive environment – one that:

- does not threaten health
- provides the conditions to:
  - make the healthy choice the easy choice
  - encourage the participation of citizens.

While policy can be explicitly developed to further health goals, the contention is that all policy should consider potential impacts on health – direct and indirect.

We have considered definitions of policy and the process of policy development. Furthermore, we have contrasted incremental and rational approaches to policy development. A key theme running through this discussion has been the location and exercise of power. Advocacy and participation in HIA has been identified as a means of influencing policy development.

Health education and healthy public policy have been seen by some as competing options – the former associated with individual behaviour change and victim-blaming and the latter with an emphasis on structural factors and enabling. However, making healthy public policy a reality is dependent on the skills and awareness of those involved. Health education, viewed more broadly, can therefore be a major driver in developing healthy public policy by virtue of its contribution at a number of different levels – from consciousness raising and the development of the skills needed for advocacy and community activism through to professional training and lobbying.

Education for Health – the Conditions of Learning

To *propagandize* is to spread particular systematized doctrines; to *advertise* is to proclaim desirable qualities in order to arouse a desire to purchase or invest; to *campaign* is to conduct a series of operations to bring about a desired result; to work at *public relations* is to seek to win public goodwill for an organization; to inform is to give news or factual data; to *publicize* is to spread information designed, or slanted, to advance special interest; to *interpret* is to bring out the real meaning; to *teach* or to *educate* is to cause, or facilitate, learning; and to *learn* is to find out about, and to gain knowledge and understanding.

National Health Assembly, 1949, cited by Brown and Margo, 1978

CONTENT OF CHAPTER 7

IDEOLOGICAL AND TECHNICAL DIMENSIONS

In Chapter 1 we provided a succinct and technical definition of 'health education' as a planned process designed to achieve health- and illness-related learning. A good deal of discussion centred on philosophical and ideological dimensions – in other words, attempts to answer the question as to what education *ought* to be about – rather than the technical aspects of what is involved in achieving educational goals. In this chapter, the focus is, in fact, on these technical aspects. We are, therefore, concerned here with the nature and dynamics of the learning process.

In Chapter 1 reference was made to a number of different kinds of learning-related influences on individuals. These were arranged on a spectrum of coercion. At one end of this spectrum was the

A SELECTION OF PROCEDURES DESIGNED TO PROMOTE LEARNING

Education	Indoctrination	Advising
Teaching	Propaganda	Social marketing
Instruction	Conditioning	Lobbying
Training	Facilitating	Brainwashing
Persuasion	Counselling	Advocating

ethically correct process of empowerment, which fulfils the requirement of voluntarism that characterizes true education and the model of health promotion that is espoused in this book. Other more coercive activities, such as persuasion and brainwashing, were also represented on the spectrum. However, they were merely indicative of a much wider range of potential interventions. Some may be ideologically neutral; others may be more or less acceptable in the context of our empowerment imperative. They are all concerned with promoting learning.

The negative connotations of at least some of the activities listed in the box will doubtless be obvious. These connotations are typically associated with coercion and/or with the methods used to coerce. Some of the terms lack clear definitions. It is interesting, for instance, to consider the meaning of 'propaganda', which currently has negative associations but this was not always so. For instance, in the early days of health education, 'health propaganda' was considered perfectly acceptable. Doubtless using it to refer to the activities of politicians and dictators – particularly in wartime – has tarnished its image. Perhaps, on the other hand, its etymological derivation determines in part its acceptability. If it is viewed as 'converting the pagan', the coercive force of zealotry may render it politically incorrect. On the other hand, if it is conceived in horticultural terms – as an exhortation to propagate ideas by 'pegging out shoots' – it might be considered as a legitimate (and effective) stratagem for creating social action. Especially so if that action is designed to challenge repressive political systems that perpetuate inequity!

In all events, the various activities listed in the box are often used in 'health education' despite the ethical and ideological difficulties this poses. They all have, by definition, one thing in common – learning. Even learning, though, involved in the policy-based 'environmental coercion' that parallels

psychological coercion. For instance, individuals must learn that certain actions may result in sanctions if the preventive objectives of the coercive measures are to be effective and efficient. Again, in accordance with our empowerment model, a different kind of learning is involved when communities respond to critical consciousness raising by taking political action that may ultimately lead to the introduction of coercive environmental measures.

In this chapter, we will be considering health education's function of providing the conditions necessary to generate different varieties of health- or illness-related learning. In line with the emphasis we are placing on empowerment, we will give particular attention to health education's radical imperative and its concern to create social change. We use the term 'critical health education' to describe this function. We will, however, start by examining a process that is a prerequisite for *all* kinds of learning. That process is communication.

THE COMMUNICATION PROCESS

The word 'communication' is sometimes used to refer to the whole educational process. For instance, Fletcher (1973: 2), who played a major part in presenting medical matters to the public via the medium of television, viewed communication as synonymous with learning, as the first of his principles of communication demonstrates:

> The purpose of communication is not just to deliver a message but to effect a change in the recipient in respect of his knowledge, his attitude or, eventually, in his behaviour.

Our view differs from Fletcher's formulation. We consider that, whereas communication is a necessary prerequisite for learning, it is learning per se that is responsible for change. The communication

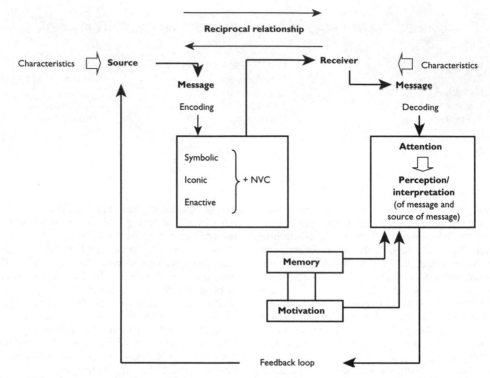

Figure 7.1 A communication model

process is essentially concerned with the transmission and reception of messages and these may or may not result in learning.

The model shown in Figure 7.1 developed out of work in telecommunications. An information source sends a message via a transmitter and this, hopefully, reaches its destination and is decoded by a receiver. Inevitably the process is afflicted to a greater or lesser extent by noise. This is not just technical interference, but may refer to psychological as well as physical 'noise'. It would thus include any distortions resulting from individuals' beliefs and attitudes, as well as defects or limitations of their sensory systems.

Key features of the communication process

The communication process involves three components:

- a sender
- a message
- a receiver.

Terminology may differ. For instance, the sender may merely be described as the 'communicator'.

More commonly, the originator of the message may be called the 'source' – in which case, the receiver is likely to be defined as the 'audience' (even if it is an audience of one). The source constructs or, more accurately, *encodes* the message and it is the task of the receiver to decode it.

The key features of the process are summarized below.

- The source may be personal or 'mediated' – that is, it may be in the form of a poster or leaflet or any other variety of mass media.
- The coded message may take three forms – frequently described as 'symbolic', 'iconic' and 'enactive'. 'Symbolic' refers to spoken or written language (or, of course, mathematical and scientific symbols). 'Iconic' refers to pictorial or diagrammatic presentations. 'Enactive' describes situations where communication (and learning) takes place as a result of the active involvement of the receiver or audience. The relative merits of these three communication formats have been embodied in an epigrammatic piece of advice to teachers:

I hear and I forget
I see and I remember
I do and I understand.

Like many such aphorisms, this contains half-truths, as does the assertion that 'one picture is worth a thousand words'. It may be true that one picture may have much greater emotional force than the same information presented verbally and thus be 'worth a thousand words'. However, conversely, it could be argued that one word, embodying an abstract concept, might encapsulate a thousand simple pictures in terms of information content. However, the aphorism doubtless refers to the affective impact of pictorial presentation.

- Whenever the source is present in person, non-verbal communication (NVC) will accompany the message.
- It is the task of the receiver to decode the message. The decoding process happens as follows:

  - first of all, the message must reach the receiver's senses (if this does not happen, communication and learning fails at this earliest of stages in the process – it is obviously the responsibility of the communicator to ensure that this does not happen)
  - second, the receiver must pay attention to the message for as long as it takes to achieve the goals of the communication
  - third, the processes of perception are brought into play – the message must be correctly interpreted.

- Attention and accurate perception will be determined by past experience (stored in the memory) and current motivation (also partly determined by past experience).
- The nature and success of the communication process will be influenced by the characteristics of the source and the receiver. The source (and his or her non-verbal communication – NVC) is an integral part of the procedures involved in coding and transmitting messages. For instance, the receiver's perception of the source may influence whether or not he or she pays attention or interprets the message appropriately. As we will note later, the credibility of the source will also have a major effect – not only on communication, but on learning. Indeed, identification and manipulation of source characteristics are two of the main concerns in devising 'persuasive communication'. Clearly, receiver characteristics are all-important in the decoding process – cultural beliefs, language skills, intellectual capabilities and personality traits will influence attention and, in particular, perception and interpretation of messages.

- Figure 7.1 includes an 'immediate feedback loop', which defines the reciprocal relationship between communicator and receiver, between source and audience. (Note also the 'long-term' feedback system in Figure 7.2 on page 214.) As has frequently been remarked, communication is (or should be) a two-way process. More accurately effective communication involves a constant shifting of roles, with the source becoming the audience and the audience becoming the source. A critically important part of this reciprocity is the (immediate) feedback loop, which should be an integral and continuing part of the interaction. The only way in which communication can be maximized is when the source of the message constantly checks the reactions of the receiver (often by accurately perceiving his or her NVC).
- Successful communication occurs when the receiver's interpretation of the message exactly matches the communicator's interpretation.

Reflections on literacy

Symbolic communications – readability

Written communications constitute one of the most common forms of symbolic coding and a good deal of effort has been directed at trying to ensure that written materials are intelligible to the target audience. Quite clearly, if the target audience is illiterate, written communication is out of the question. However, to the extent that the audience possesses some competence in reading, communicators have to ensure that their written materials match the audience's level of competence. Accordingly, a plethora of tests of readability – or 'reading ease' – have been developed to assess the degree of difficulty of written communications. This makes it possible for material to be assessed and appropriate modifications made until the leaflet or booklet appears to be suitable for the abilities of the intended recipients of the message.

A detailed review of the construction of readability tests is not appropriate here. We will merely note that several techniques are available for assessing 'reading ease', such as assessing the proportion of commonly used words incorporated in the communication. However, by far the most popular tests have gauged readability by means of a combined measure of sentence length and the number of polysyllabic words contained in each sentence. It so happens, 'linguistically', that longer words tend to be more difficult. Unsurprisingly, longer sentences are likely to contain more information, so more likely to overload individual 'channel capacity' and be generally more daunting than short sentences. Probably the most frequently used tests of this kind have used some version of the 'Flesch formula' (Flesch, 1948). A simpler version has the appropriate acronym 'FOG' (frequency of gobbledegook, Harrison, 1980) and the US Office of Cancer Communications has recourse to 'SMOG' (subjective measures of gobbledegook, McLaughlin, 1969).

As most computer programmes now assess the numbers of words, syllables and so on in a given piece of writing at the touch of a button, the Flesch and related formulae are simple to use. A cautionary note is necessary, though. All such measures of reading ease infer intelligibility indirectly. None of them measure the *actual* level of understanding of target groups or individuals. Only a direct test of people's understanding of a particular communication will do that. Moreover, as communicators need to be aware of the cultural interpretations and emotional reactions of their audience to written communications, it makes sense to do a comprehensive pretest of communications (a key principle of social marketing – see Chapter 8). This might involve, for example, the use of 'copy editing' – a technique employed in pretesting printed information. This typically consists of asking a representative sample of the intended audience to underline words that they find difficult and write comments about pictures or expressions that are confusing or offensive.

Making print materials easier to read

Despite some uncertainty about the validity of reading ease measures, a useful body of knowledge that is applicable to the practical task of writing intelligible communications has been accumulated over recent years. Text should be:

- introduced, stating the purpose to orientate the reader
- summarized at the end to review major points
- presented in short sentences within short paragraphs
- 'broken up' with visuals placed to emphasize key points and text
- 'bullets' and titles or subtitles to reinforce important points
- written in the active, not passive, voice
- underlined, in bold or 'boxed' for reinforcement
- clarified with the use of examples

- tested for readability
- tested with audience
- explained, if necessary, in a glossary (with key words defined within the sentence).

Try to avoid:

- jargon and technical terms or phrases
- abbreviations and acronyms.

Just as necessary as clear writing are text that is easy to read and graphics that help the reader to understand and remember the text.

Graphics should be:

- immediately identifiable
- relevant to the subject matter and reader
- simple, uncluttered
- used to reinforce, not compete with the text.

Try to avoid:

- small type (less than 10 point)
- lines of type that are too long or too short
- large blocks of print
- 'justified' right margins
- photographs that won't reproduce well
- less than professional-quality drawings (they may make your text appear less credible).

Adapted from 'Making Health Communication Programs Work: A Planner's Guide' (National Cancer Institute, 1998).

Communication and learning

Before moving on to consider the nature of learning and the conditions necessary for success, it is important to make some further brief observations about communication. At first sight, it might appear that, as communication is a kind of precursor to all kinds of learning, it is a relatively neutral process. This interpretation is doubtless responsible for the American Society of Public Health Education (SOPHE) including 'communication' in its list of voluntaristic, therefore ethical, interventions (see the discussion of coercion in Chapter 1). People have a right to information and communication supplies information.

There is, of course, some truth in this, but the mere selection and manipulation of symbols may reflect cultural assumptions and the source–audience relationship frequently involves an imbalance of power. Indeed, it could be said that one of the goals of an empowerment model of health promotion is to enhance the assertiveness skills of the audience so that they can question and challenge the sources of the messages directed at them. More generally, it seeks to shift the power balance between certain communicators and audiences.

Again, although it is important to be able to separately identify key features of the communication process, it is unduly simplistic to imply that this process is completely separate from the more extensive and complicated system involved in attempts at influencing audiences – such as education, teaching, persuasion. Indeed, it is very difficult to envisage a communication situation where no learning takes place. It is *possible* to identify such scenarios – for instance, a green traffic light may communicate a clear message that involves little learning but merely signals the fact that the driver may proceed. The fact that the driver correctly interprets the message is, of course, based on prior learning. On the other hand, a poster vividly depicting the horrific results of anti-personnel mines will not merely communicate an iconic message, it may produce a relatively permanent change of attitude to landmines and even to war itself. Such a case *does* represent learning and, as the learning is the result of a deliberate attempt to influence an audience, it also represents *persuasion*.

Involvement of people in the enactive process of a role play could be defined as a form of communication embodying a number of messages, but the purpose of the exercise would inevitably be to influence the participants in some way – for instance, to provide them with skills. Moreover, the participants in the role play will engage in communication as well as the teacher who devised the role play in the first place. In other words, the communication process is converted into a quite complicated teaching/learning process as the messages delivered by the source (symbolic, iconic and enactive) are designed to provide the conditions necessary to create some relatively permanent change in disposition and/or capability in the role players, as well as in the audience observing the role play.

By way of a further example, a dental health education project used an enactive form of communication to convey the message that there were different kinds of teeth. They were provided with plastic incisors, canines, molars and premolars and had to place these teeth in a modelling clay bed in a U-shaped tray that mimicked the shape of a lower jaw. They checked each other's mouths so that they were in the right order. While this clearly communicated the message and ensured that attention was paid to it, the students actually acquired information that they did not already possess and, provided that they remembered this, then learning had taken place.

Figure 7.2 (on page 214) shows the frequently seamless link between communication and learning.

EDUCATION – CREATING THE CONDITIONS FOR LEARNING

Two diverse and often conflicting approaches to health promotion were discussed in Chapter 1 and a preventive medical model was contrasted with an empowerment model. The contribution of health education to these models was characterized, respectively, as follows.

- **Health education as persuasion** Associated with 'coercing' people into adopting health, illness and sick role behaviours in order to prevent disease at primary, secondary and tertiary levels. Often seen as complementary to environmental interventions, such as legislation, economic and fiscal measures, social and environmental engineering. Various attitude-change strategies are used to achieve the preventive goals.
- **Health education as empowerment** Concerned to strengthen individual capacity (*self-empowerment*) and achieve social and political change in order to provide supportive, empowering environments by influencing healthy public policy.

It is also useful to note a radical variation on an empowerment model of health promotion/education that is primarily concerned with creating social and political change in the interests of promoting public health. While this approach is an integral part of the empowerment model described in this book, we will follow contemporary practice by labelling this as 'critical health education'.

It is also important to note an additional variation on the health education theme. For many years, patient education has been located under the general health education umbrella. However, perhaps because of its association with the medical model, it tends to be marginalized by mainstream health promotion. This is unfortunate. Not only is the education of patients a task of major importance, it can be comfortably accommodated within the general empowerment model of health promotion. Indeed, empowering strategies typically result in more effective preventive outcomes than so-called victim-blaming approaches. In fact, the only real logical distinction between patient education and other varieties of health education is the fact that it is, by definition, concerned to promote the health of people who have been defined as patients!

All three varieties of health education involve health- or illness-related learning and the task of the health educator is to marshal methods that provide the conditions needed to ensure efficient learning.

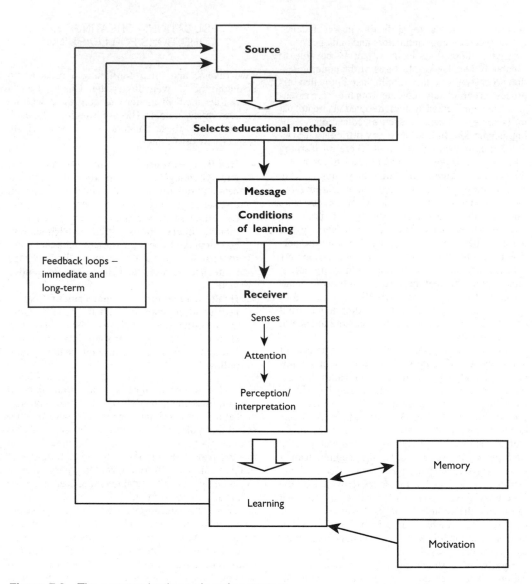

Figure 7.2 The communication to learning process

A taxonomy of types of health learning

It has long been recognized that there are different types of learning and, although there may be common factors, it is important to take account of the differences. The simplest typology has been mentioned in Chapter 3, which categorizes learning into cognitive, affective and conative. However, a more refined and comprehensive typology is possible and necessary for the design of effective interventions (see, for instance, the theory developed over many years in the seminal work of Gagne, (1985)). Four key principles may be identified:

- there are various different and separately identified types of learning and learning outcome
- learning is hierarchical – typically 'lower-order' learning outcomes must be fulfilled before higher levels of learning can be attained
- successful learning requires that learning-specific *internal* and *external* conditions be supplied – where internal conditions relate to

previously acquired capabilities and dispositions and external conditions are provided by the deliberate organization of external events to facilitate learning

- those who seek to influence learning – via persuasion, training, education and so on – must check that the necessary internal conditions have been met and then provide the appropriate external conditions by using the right educational methods for the situation.

The cognitive domain

A detailed technical analysis of cognitive learning is beyond the scope of this chapter. At a common-sense level, it is clear that a distinction may be made between the rote learning of facts and acquiring deeper levels of understanding (typically defined by such terms as 'concepts' and 'principles'). While factual data may be useful, understanding is necessary for the transfer of learning and problem solving. As we noted in Chapter 3, beliefs are best conceptualized as cognitive constructs and, as we demonstrated in our detailed discussion of the HAM, perhaps the most important goal of health education is to create or modify health-related beliefs.

Cognitive skills – problem solving

The term 'skill' is often used in a general sense merely to indicate a high level of competence. Learning theory has, however, identified particular and more precisely defined types of skill. Three kinds of skill are of interest to us here and to the practice of health promotion. These are: psycho-motor, social interaction and problem-solving or decision-making skills.

Problem solving is usually categorized as a cognitive skill. For instance, Gagne (1985) defines it primarily as a 'cognitive strategy' that 'enables the learner to select appropriate information and skills and to decide when and how to apply them in attempting to solve the problem.' However, as health-related decision making is typically considered to be inextricably linked with values, it inevitably involves the affective domain.

Problem solving can be viewed as a heuristic device to achieve decision making. It is worth noting that it does not necessarily involve 'meaningful' learning. Indeed, the algorithm is one of the most effective devices for making accurate decisions. It merely requires a series of step-wise discriminations resulting in yes or no answers until the final solution is reached.

Memorizing a series of guidelines for solving problems does not guarantee understanding – it is mere rote learning, which is not as efficient as using an algorithm. On the other hand, where problem solving does involve understanding, it is, by definition, meaningful and can result in higher-order learning.

Two kinds of learning may result in this latter situation – namely, the learner can acquire new principles and associated concepts or the learner can acquire some generalizable problem-solving skill. For instance, consider the case of diabetic labourers working on building sites. Two problems they face are finding ways to inject themselves at work and eating small snacks between meals. A solution might result from learning that the privacy of the lunch hut could be used for injections, but only at certain times of day. Furthermore, a thorough understanding of the function of insulin, the causes of comas and their association with diet and an awareness that insulin should be adjusted to take account of the balance between exercise and dietary intake may result in their changing their way of life at weekends, too, without any further specific instruction. Consequently, they might make appropriate choices when eating in pubs and on picnics.

However, a cautionary note is necessary – transfer of learning is only likely to occur where there is a good deal of similarity and common ground between the different types of problem to be solved.

Psycho-motor skills

The relevance of psycho-motor (or motor) skills to health education is doubtless self-evident. They range from simple to complicated and the following examples will serve to illustrate this particular kind of learning:

- competence in cardio-pulmonary resuscitation
- use of a toothbrush for the efficient removal of plaque
- removing a condom from its packet, squeezing the teat to eject air, placing it on the tip of an erect penis and unrolling it.

The techniques needed to supply the conditions for efficient psycho-motor learning have been subjected to considerable research and a more detailed review is not possible here. We will, however, devote rather more space to considering social interaction skills learning – largely because of the potential importance of their contribution to empowerment.

Social interaction skills

At one level, it might be argued that socially skilled interaction is a feature of social health itself.

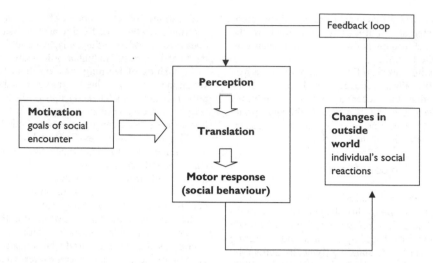

Figure 7.3   Motor skills model of social interaction (after Argyle and Kendon, 1967)

Defective social skills are, of course, one aspect of recognized mental disorders and dysfunctions (see, for instance, Trower et al., 1978). However, as we have already intimated, capabilities such as assertiveness are of special importance in empowering individuals and groups and increasing the likelihood of their gaining control over their lives and the political systems that govern them. The essential elements of these capabilities are the skills involved in interacting with other people. There is an important parallel with psycho-motor skills learning – as the late Michael Argyle, one of the key authorities in researching social interaction, has amply demonstrated. Indeed, in the 1960s, he made particular reference to a 'motor skills model' of social interaction (Argyle, 1978), shown in Figure 7.3.

As with any other kind of learning, the essential conditions for effective performance must be supplied by appropriate teaching and training. The acquisition of social interaction skills, for example, requires the learner to accurately perceive both environmental and proprioceptive cues. In learning to drive a car, the learner must respond appropriately to those muscular sensations involved in turning the steering wheel and resulting from depressing the clutch. In a similar way, socially skilled communicators will accurately interpret the non-verbal cues provided by other people – such as facial expressions – and, at the same time, will be in control of their own non-verbal responses, such as gesture and tone of voice. A skilled person also makes an appropriate choice from a wide repertoire of potential responses on the basis of incoming interpersonal information, then he or she reacts in

the most appropriate way. For instance, an interviewer might deduce that an interviewee's eye contact and facial expression indicates hesitancy in the face of a particular question. The researcher might then encourage the client's participation by the various techniques of 'active listening', such as, affirmative head nodding, appropriate eye contact and posture. The skilled interviewer will then note any 'change in the outside world' – that is, the client's reactions – interpret those reactions correctly and continue to respond to those cues in a flexible and appropriate manner.

Reference was made to the importance of non-verbal communication (NVC) in our earlier analysis of the communication process. It will be apparent from our comments above that it is also of central importance to the acquisition of social interaction skills. For instance, respect, empathy and genuineness have been described as the 'holy trinity' of counselling. It is relatively easy to *say* the right things, but a lack of genuineness is readily revealed by what has been called 'non-verbal leakage'.

NVC is of paramount importance in communicating feeling and attitudes. Numerous studies have demonstrated, for example, that when there is a contradiction between verbal and non-verbal, non-verbal is more powerful. If someone comments that a friend's holiday photographs are really interesting and does so with impassive face, dreary tone of voice and while looking out of the window, she does not also have to stifle a yawn in order to cast doubt on the genuineness of her expressed interest!

Table 7.1 sets out some of the key features of NVC that the effective health educator or advocate

Table 7.1   *Key features of NVC*

Channel	Examples
Proxemics	Personal space, territory, body orientation, seating arrangement, body angle
Haptics (touch)	Playful, ritualistic, aggressive, affection
Chronemics (time)	Waiting time, punctuality, duration, urgency
Kinesics	Direction of gaze, facial expression, smiling, gestures, head movements, posture, gait
Physical appearance	Body shape, weight, height, hair and skin colour, clothing, cosmetics, adornments
Vocalics	Tempo, pitch, loudness, dialect, fluency, pauses, articulation, breathiness
Artifacts	Volume of space, size, ventilation, furniture arrangement, décor, lighting, temperature

Behaviour   **Client/learner in control**

Listening
Drawing out
Reflecting back
Clarifying
Questioning
Summarizing
Suggesting
Advising   **Educator in control**
Prescribing
Insisting
Ordering

Figure 7.4   Empowering or de-powering educator behaviour

will be capable of interpreting and using to good effect.

It is also worth noting, in the context of our concern with empowerment, that a skilful educator or counsellor can contribute to clients' or learners' self-efficacy beliefs and self-esteem. Figure 7.4 reveals how the use of particular verbal and non-verbal behaviour might empower or, conversely, de-power clients. A comparison might also usefully be made with our earlier discussions about the distribution of power in medical consultations.

As we noted above, the conditions necessary for the efficient acquisition of social interaction skills are virtually identical with those required for psycho-motor skills learning.

Detailed task analysis and the identification and provision of component skills, such as training in listening, would be followed by repetition and practice – probably using a role play. Also, detailed monitoring and analysis of performance, with the provision of immediate knowledge of results to indicate when the micro components of performance were appropriate or inappropriate. The use of video feedback in this task is of particular importance.

For a more complete review of social skills training, readers are advised to consult Trower et al. (1978) and particularly, Dickson et al. (1989).

Decision-making skills

As mentioned above, it is difficult in practice to distinguish between problem-solving skills, social interaction skills and decision-making skills. They all tend to be viewed as part and parcel of 'life skills' (or 'action competences') that form an integral part of education for empowerment (see Chapter 9). It is, however, worth mentioning the important contribution of Janis and Mann (1977) in popularizing and applying decision-making theory to real-life scenarios. A more complete discussion of their valuable analysis of defective individual and group decision making cannot be undertaken here. We might, however, note the application of one form of (arguably) defective decision making typically applied to the development and implementation of policy. Janis and Mann (1977: 34) refer to this – rather picturesquely – as plain 'muddling through' and draw on the work of Lindblom (1959, 1980) and Braybrooke and Lindblom (1963):

Since the term muddling through evokes images of incompetence and aimlessness, it is tempting to conclude that it could be the preferred technique only of lazy or third-rate minds. But Braybrooke and Lindblom view it as the method by which societal decision-making bodies, acting as coalitions of interest groups, can effectively make cumulative decisions and arrive at workable compromises. Whenever power is distributed among a variety of influential executive leaders, political parties, legislative factions, and interest groups, one centre of power can rarely impose its preferences on another and policies are likely to be the outcome of give and take among numerous partisans. The constraints of bureaucratic politics, with its shifting compromises and coalitions, constitute a major reason for the disjointed and incremental nature of the policies that gradually evolve.

AFFECTIVE LEARNING – INFLUENCING EMOTIONS, VALUES AND ATTITUDES

Reference was made at the beginning of this chapter to the ideological basis of education and learning. Moreover, in line with our advocacy of the empowerment philosophy, we have challenged the ethics of using coercion to achieve the goals of health promotion. We now turn our attention to affective learning in general and, in particular, the use of techniques that have traditionally been associated with coercion. These techniques are usually described in terms of 'persuasion' and 'attitude change'.

In discussing the ethical dimension for health promotion, we should first of all note the importance, on the one hand, of distinguishing between *deliberate* attempts to persuade and coerce by generating emotional responses and, on the other, those situations in which emotional responses occur as an almost *incidental* effect of learning. For instance, to the extent that people come to understand and accept the reality of personal risk or realize the ways in which social injustice creates squalor and ill health, it is quite probable that emotions will be roused. In the first instance, it may involve anxiety or concern over personal vulnerability. In the second instance, it may result in feelings of indignation and commitment to take political action. Moreover, while the deliberate use of attitude-change techniques are most closely associated with attempts to manipulate rather than empower – and, thus, are ethically dubious – there is, paradoxically perhaps, a situation where persuasion rather than empowerment is justified. In short, as the use of persuasion is standard practice for lobbyists and other political activists seeking to bring about changes in health-related policy, it is presumably

acceptable for health promotion activists to become skilled in the use of attitude-change techniques. There may, of course, be a difference in degree between, say, a community health worker utilizing persuasive techniques with a local politician and advertisers' use of persuasive messages to persuade young children to pester their parents to buy them unhealthy products. The principles, however, are fundamentally similar. Accordingly, we will select from the vast literature on attitude change a number of these principles.

Conditioning and related interventions

The different aspects of affective learning that are addressed here are encapsulated in the motivation system of the HAM, discussed in Chapter 3. More particularly, values and attitudes are specified – and these are the main concern of the persuasive attempts described as 'attitude change'. Emotional states are also of interest, together with associated drives. For instance, the fear drive has figured quite prominently in research and theory. Returning to the HAM, it should be recalled that two inputs have been identified. The first of these affects motivation via the mediation of the belief system, while the second provides a direct input into the motivation system itself – for instance, by using emotive imagery to generate anxiety or other feelings directly.

Conditioning – classical and symbolic

Classical (or Pavlovian) conditioning was probably the earliest form of affective learning subjected to 'scientific' research. While, the classical variety makes little contribution to the attitude research tradition, the terms 'vicarious' and 'symbolic' conditioning have been used to describe some kinds of persuasive influences. For instance, advertising has been viewed as a form of symbolic conditioning (see the box).

USING SYMBOLIC CONDITIONING IN MARKETING

Find some common desire, some widespread unconscious fear or anxiety; think out some way to relate this wish or fear to the product you have to sell; then build a bridge of verbal or pictorial symbols over which your customer can pass from fact to compensatory dream, and from the dream to the illusion that your product, when purchased, will make the dream true.

Aldous Huxley (1932) *Brave New World*

Although the iconic message format is typically used in persuasive communication, the *enactive* format may be used for educational and persuasive purposes in a variety of ways. For instance, it has been employed as a device to achieve affective learning, and Janis and Mann (1964) provided a classic demonstration of the use of role play in attitude change.

Heavy smokers played the parts of patients in a clinic or adopted the role of a doctor who informed the patients that they had lung cancer. A number of role-playing sessions were held that involved the 'actors' interacting with doctors, other patients, viewing X-rays and so on. The role-playing group's reactions were compared with those of two other groups some six months later. First, a group who listened to a tape recording of the role plays and, second, a sample of smokers who were not involved in either experimental situation, but had been exposed to the publication of the Surgeon General's report on smoking and health. The experimental group members were smoking an average of twelve cigarettes a day (compared with twenty-four before the intervention), the passive 'listeners' were smoking sixteen a day compared with twenty-two initially, while the third group (merely exposed to the Surgeon General's report) had not changed their smoking habits.

The main type of learning involved in this persuasive exercise may be described as 'vicarious' conditioning.

Primary socialization as brain washing?

In the context of our earlier discussion of a 'spectrum of coercion', it is worth emphasizing that the typical techniques involved in the primary socialization of children (namely modelling and various forms of conditioning) are probably more powerful than the excoriated techniques of brainwashing. Accordingly, those involved, directly or indirectly, in childrearing and who are committed to voluntaristic principles,

should perhaps give careful thought to developing empowering socialization strategies!

PERSUASION AND ATTITUDE CHANGE

The theory and practice of attitude change has been a centrepiece of social psychology for decades, so it has been very extensively researched. It is also true to say that attitude change has occupied a prominent part in traditional health education as health educators have eagerly searched for ways in which to persuade individuals to adopt healthy practices.

A comprehensive review of the field is neither possible nor desirable here. However, although empowerment rather than persuasion should be the main concern of health promotion, attitude-change techniques figure prominently in interventions associated with lobbying and advocacy in the imperative to build healthy public policy.

Affective hierarchies and attitude change

We noted earlier the existence of four interrelated motivational constructs featured in the HAM – drives, emotional states, values and attitudes. Attitudes were conceptualized as specific rather than general and deriving from 'higher-order' motives. Emotional states can result from basic drives, such as fear, while attitudes emerge from values. Both values and emotional states may influence attitudes – that is, determine the importance attached to certain objects, people or courses of action. Rokeach (in Sills, 1965: 80) emphasizes the importance of hierarchy:

> A grown person probably has tens of thousands of beliefs, hundreds of attitudes, but only dozens of values. A value system is an hierarchical organization – a rank ordering – of ideals or values in terms of importance. To one person truth, beauty and freedom may be at the

---

LAW OF PRIMACY – EARLY CHILDHOOD BRAINWASHING?

Give me a child for the first seven years, and you may do what you like with him afterwards.

Jesuit maxim, cited by the UK National Child Development Survey (Davie et al., 1972)

Apparently the Communist regime in the USSR required an additional year.

Give us the child for eight years, and it will be a Bolshevist forever.

Lenin, speech to the commissars of education, Moscow, 1923 (Lenin, 1969)

Level of difficulty in achieving each stage	Communication characteristics				
	Communication and learning outcomes	Source	Message	Channel	Audience
LOW ↑	Exposure to message				
	Attention: • attract • sustain				
	Perception/interpretation				
	Recall of essential information				
	Understanding of message*				
	Beliefs: accept truth of message				
	Positive attititude to recommended action				
	Acquisition of skills**				
↓	Adopt approved action				
HIGH	Sustain approved action				

Key:
*In-depth understanding is rarely needed – it may even be a disadvantage!
**The acquisition of skills would be incidental to an attitude-change programme

Figure 7.5   Relationship of major communication variables to the communication to learning process (adapted from McGuire, 1989)

top of the list, and thrift, order and cleanliness at the bottom: to another person, the order may be reversed.

The significance of the hierarchical dimension for health education is doubtless obvious. Given the enduring power of values, attempts to change attitudes may be ineffectual or counterproductive *unless* these underlying values are acknowledged and, where possible, the association between value(s) and attitude(s) are severed.

THE YALE APPROACH TO ATTITUDE CHANGE

From the plethora of theories, the particular approach adopted by the Yale University Communication Research Program has been selected as a framework for this relatively brief analysis of attitude change.

Its approach – sometimes called the Yale-Hovland model after its director, Carl Hovland – was explicitly designed to develop efficient ways in which to

influence public attitudes. An early concern, for example, was with finding the best way to convince American servicemen – in the middle of a general euphoria over victory in Europe in World War II – that they faced a long and difficult struggle with Japan.

The general framework of the approach derived from Lasswell's (1948) recommendation to examine, 'who says what to whom via what medium and with what effect?' Hovland et al., therefore, researched the relative contributions of the message, the source of the message, the characteristics of the audience for whom the message was intended and the nature of the action resulting from the process of attitude change (for a more complete review of the early work, see Hovland et al., 1953).

Figure 7.5 has been adapted from McGuire and colleagues (McGuire, 1989) who have made a major contribution to the development of the Yale-Hovland model and its evaluation. Our adaptation aims to accommodate the model to the analysis of communication and learning presented at the beginning of this chapter and to our subsequent discussions of mass media and methods. The figure provides a matrix relating source, message and audience factors to the various key stages in the communication and learning processes. The idea of a 'channel' has also been included and allows us to consider and contrast the relative roles of mass media and interpersonal methods.

Figure 7.5 not only shows the various stages in the communication to learning process, but gives an indication of the relative ease or difficulty in achieving the necessary change. Certain of the stages would be of greater or lesser importance to typical attitude-change initiatives. For instance, although it would be essential to understand and remember information associated with attitude change and the actions ensuing from that, the learning of principles and concepts would not normally be of concern – indeed, genuine understanding might militate against persuasive pressure! The cells in the matrix (following McGuire's formulation) can be used as a convenient evaluation device in the form of a checklist to assess to what extent various intermediate, process and outcome objectives have been achieved.

Before proceeding further, a cautionary note should be introduced. Psychology is replete with studies that have demonstrated statistically significant effects of particular approaches to attitude change. These are most commonly achieved in the laboratory. The effect is real, but their applicability to real life may be limited, insignificant or completely irrelevant. This is typically due to the fact that minor effects revealed in the laboratory are completely submerged by much more powerful real-life influences – often in combination with other equally powerful influences. As a full discussion of the complicated field of attitude theory is beyond the scope of this book, a selection of effects that do seem to be relevant to real concerns for health promoters will be outlined below.

Source factors

Reference was made earlier in this chapter to the role of the communicator or 'source' in the communication process. We noted the obvious point that communicator skills were central to effective communication, but also emphasized that this involved not only audience perception and interpretation of the message, but also perception of the source's intentions and characteristics. We also emphasized in Chapter 1 the centrality of personal power in achieving actual compliance as well as influencing beliefs and attitudes. The real and perceived characteristics of the source are thus considered to be pivotal in the attitude-change endeavour and have been extensively researched.

We must content ourselves here with merely listing the most important features identified by research:

- power and leadership
- source credibility:

  - legitimate and expert authority
  - perceived trustworthiness
  - source attractiveness

- homophily and referent authority
- group pressure.

Message factors

Considerable research effort has been devoted to the relative effectiveness of different ways of presenting persuasive messages in producing changes in attitudes and behaviour. Again, only relatively brief comments are possible here.

Five message factors have received special attention:

- repetition, primacy and recency
- sidedness
- the use of positive effect
- fear appeal
- arousal.

Repetition, primacy and recency

One of the most common assumptions is that, generally speaking, the more frequently a message is

---

COMMUNICATOR CHARACTERISTICS

... nothing is so apt to restrain an excited multitude as the reverence inspired by some grave and dignified man of authority who opposes them ... therefore whoever is at the head of an army, or whoever happens to be a magistrate in a city where sedition lies broken out, should present himself before the multitude with all possible grace and dignity and attired with all the insignia of this rank, so as to inspire the more respect.

Machiavelli, 1950: 251, cited by Zimbardo et al., 1977: 32

repeated, the more effective it will be. By contrast, a good deal of laboratory evidence has been accumulated to demonstrate that a message delivered first or last in a sequence of different persuasive attempts is more likely to be influential.

Drawing implicit v. explicit conclusions

One of the subjects that occupied attitude theoreticians was whether or not greater attitude change would result when conclusions were explicitly drawn for the audience or that the inclusion of 'implicit conclusions' in the construction of the message would have a greater effect. The most likely answer to this query is that it depends on the audience. In brief, a more expert or intelligent audience would demonstrate a greater shift in opinion and attitude with implicit conclusions, whereas less experienced or less intelligent people might need to be told much more directly what they should believe!

Sidedness

Another interesting message factor having practical implications has been identified by psychological research. The subject in question has been labelled 'sidedness'.

The question addressed by the researchers was whether greater atttitude change would result when a one-sided persuasive argument was presented or when both sides were presented. Again, it would seem as if the outcome would depend on the audience. If the audience is well educated, intelligent or both, a two-sided approach should be dopted. If the audience is uneducated/intelligent or it could be guaranteed that it would never be exposed to the counter-arguments, the one-sided approach might be used.

Inoculation and refutational preemption

One of the findings to emerge from the work on sidedness was that people exposed to two-sided messages who already favoured the advocated measure (such as fluoridation), maintained their support, even when exposed to attempts to change their commitment. This phenomenon provoked not only further research, but also, ultimately, resulted in deliberate measures designed to 'inoculate' individuals against attempts to persuade them to adopt unhealthy activities, such as smoking. McGuire (1970: 37, cited by Pfau, 1995: 100) played a substantial role in this research and his position is clear:

We can develop belief resistance in people as we develop disease resistance in biologically overprotected man or animal, by exposing the person to a weak dose of the attacking material strong enough to stimulate his defences but not strong enough to overwhelm him.

The analogy with biological immunization is quite appropriate. The essence of the technique involves, 'threat and refutational preemption'. The threat might be an anticipated challenge to existing attitudes, such as a threat to existing negative feelings about smoking. Pfau (1995: 103–4) summarizes the situation as follows:

adolescents commence the transition from the primary to middle grades with strong attitudes opposing smoking. 'They have *already been persuaded* that smoking is bad (Pfau and Van Bockern, 1994: 420)... these attitudes often do not persist during the two years following the transition from elementary school to junior high school. The large majority of adolescents began this transition with negative attitudes toward smoking, but those attitudes deteriorated during the next two years. Adolescents grew more positive towards smoking, more positive towards peer smoking, and less likely to overtly resist smoking (Pfau and Van Bockern, 1994) ... at the point of transition from the primary to middle school grades, adolescents possess reasonably established attitudes opposing smoking. What is needed at this point is a strategy to protect these antismoking attitudes from deterioration during the turbulent middle school years.

'Refutational preemption' is the proposed strategy. The threat component centres on the possibility that they may unwillingly become smokers – probably due to peer pressure. The attitude change method or channel might be a video employing an attractive source in the form of a young teacher.

Pfau distinguishes inoculation 'proper' from 'social inoculation'. He defines this latter as an approach that uses a combination of strategies designed to anticipate future anti-health arguments and pressures. Typically, these have involved peer-leadership (see Chapter 9), peer modelling and videos. In practice, it is social inoculation that has been used most frequently in the context of the prevention of young people's recruitment to smoking – for instance, the so-called Minnesota Model (Evans, 1976, and Murray, 1984).

Interestingly, the analogy of immunization can be further extended to include the use of 'booster' doses of education to maintain immunity. Botvin (1984) added these to his successful 'life skills training model', which demonstrated a reduction of 50 per cent or more in school students' recruitment to smoking.

Positive and negative affect

The majority of communications will produce an affective reaction of some kind in the audience, whether this be revulsion, humour or just interest. However, in this section, we are concerned with *deliberate* attempts to create a message designed to produce affective responses that will lead to attitude and behaviour change.

Two important situations merit discussion. These relate to generating *positive* affect – that is, creating positive emotional responses in the audience – and, by contrast, the use of negative affect – an approach more usually described as 'fear appeal'.

Although there is some evidence for the success of approaches seeking to generate positive affect (see, for instance, Monahan, 1995, Zajonc, 1980, and Murphy and Zajonc, 1993), most research has concentrated on the creation of negative affect in the form of fear appeal. Monahan's (1995) observation that there is little evidence to suggest that positive affect can change strongly held negative attitudes is most likely correct. However, her belief that positive emotional appeals can generate attitude change in those who have no great involvement in an issue and may change attitudes indirectly is rather less convincing. In all events, there can be no real objection to using positive messages as, quite clearly, they at least attract attention and are likely to be more memorable than dry, factual data. However, from an ethical standpoint, any message must not be economical with the truth and, of course, will make no contribution to health promotion's prime commitment to empowerment. On the other hand, there are fundamental objections to the use of negative affect in changing attitudes and behaviour, irrespective of the question of effectiveness.

Fear appeal – creating negative affect

Despite generations of research, the use of fear appeal in general – and for health promotion in particular – is still highly controversial, both regarding the ethics of its use and its relative effectiveness.

Research into the use of fear to bring about an attitude change was famously triggered by the work of Janis and Feshbach (1953). Their influential study into the use of different levels of fear appeal in persuading individuals to brush their teeth regularly seemed to demonstrate that there was actually an inverse relationship between level of fear and (reported) tooth-brushing behaviour. Those experiencing a very high level of fear were least likely of all to change their dental practices, while those experiencing a relatively neutral presentation were most likely to report an increase in dental hygiene. The results of those receiving the midlevel of arousal were, naturally, located somewhere in the middle!

Innumerable studies into the use of fear followed this counter-intuitive result, but none replicated Janis and Feshbach's results, though they did demonstrate the complexity of the situation. Indeed, Hale and Dillard (1995: 70, 78), in a review, appear to be convinced about the effectiveness of using negative affect.

> Three quantitative reviews (Boster and Mongeau, 1984; Mongeau, in press; Sutton, 1982) all show reliable and compelling evidence that fear is persuasive. [These] and several newer studies, perhaps the best of the lot, concluded that perceived fear and the attitude of the target were positively correlated, as were perceived fear and behavior... abandoning the use of fear would be to abandon an effective persuasive strategy...
>
> Fear appeals have enormous persuasive potential and can promote better health.

Hale and Dillard quite rightly observe that the use of fear and research into its effectiveness is complicated and excursions into attitude change that employ fear appeal are frequently poorly constructed. A complete account of this complicated arena is not possible here. We will however try to summarize the situation below.

Key questions for fear appeal   Any comprehensive theory of negative affect on behaviour must address the following key questions.

- What exactly do we mean by fear ? What level of arousal justifies using the word 'fear'? Why does one individual's perception of particular messages result in the experience of fear?
- What is the effect of given levels of fear on such individual responses as interest, attitude and compliance?
- How do audience factors influence perceptions of fear-arousing stimuli and reactions to these?
- How enduring is the effect of fear on an audience's attitudes and behaviour?

Leventhal and Cleary (1980) provided a comprehensive and succinct review of the complicated interactions of fear appeal variables in the context of discussing smoking prevention (see also Leventhal, 1980) and concluded that they could see little or no evidence that fear was a necessary, or even essential, ingredient for behaviour change.

How can we reconcile the two conflicting points of view described above? Some additional illumination may be provided by reference to the so-called 'Yerkes–Dodson law'.

Arousal, fear appeal and the Yerkes–Dodson effect

One of the questions posed above concerned the nature of fear. One of the problems with drawing conclusions about and, indeed manipulating, levels of fear is that this notion – as typically used in attitude theory – is rather vague. A more useful representation owes its origins to very early research into learning and resulted in the formulation of the Yerkes–Dodson law (Yerkes and Dodson, 1908). Later researchers applied this to the attitude change field, although some workers have questioned the generalizability of this phenomenon (Winton, 1987, for example). In short, the Yerkes–Dodson law demonstrated that both a very low level of arousal and a very high level of arousal resulted in poor learning. Moreover, more complicated and intricate learning tasks were disrupted by a lower level of arousal than simple tasks. This is entirely consistent with common sense – an individual who is totally disinterested will be motivated to neither learn nor to perform. An individual whose state of arousal has resulted in an attack of panic and is paralysed with terror will also not be in position to learn or act. A very simple task, such as running at high speed, will be achieved with a higher rather than a lower level of arousal (indeed people can deliver quite remarkable physical performances when very frightened). On the other hand, a task involving learning rather than just performance may be disrupted by relatively low levels of arousal. For instance, tasks involving mental arithmetic or fine psycho-motor performances will be most successfully performed at a moderate level of arousal.

The Yerkes–Dodson Law is often described in terms of an inverted 'U' curve where some optimal level of arousal figures at the top of the 'U'. While the effect of extreme levels of arousal is unchallengeable, it is more problematic finding evidence of a smooth curve – although a nicely constructed piece of research by Krisher et al. (1973) into uptake of mumps vaccination did produce results consistent with the curvilinear predictions of Yerkes–Dodson.

It also seems clear that the shape of the curve or the level of 'threshold arousal' will depend on the nature of the proposed actions. For example, presenting immediate action opportunities that are perceived to be attainable would increase the likelihood that a relatively high level of arousal might lead to action. Again, as noted above by Leventhal (1980), audience characteristics would also be important. High self-esteem and self-efficacy certainly tends to result in vigilance and people having such characteristics would be able to

cope with relatively high levels of arousal without resorting to defensive behaviour or succumbing to paralysis!

At the risk of being simplistic, we might draw a number of practical conclusions about using fear appeals. In short, they might be used in the following circumstances:

- when individuals felt vulnerable to a deadly disease
- when they enjoyed high levels of perceived internal locus of control together with high self-esteem
- when the action required of them was perceived as effective
- when it was perceived as simple and required an immediate response
- when an action plan was provided.

The sleeper effect   One final point is worth making about the use of fear appeal. There is some evidence that both the impact of an attractive/credible source and emotional responses – such as those resulting from fear appeal – diminish over time. It is as if the effect of message style – and the credibility or attractiveness of the source – decay, leaving only the informational content of the message. The message lingers on. This has been described as the 'sleeper effect' (Hovland and Weiss, 1951, and Gruder et al., 1978). To the extent that this is true, doubt must be cast on using fear appeal in the first place – especially given the difficulty of taking into account the complex of confounding factors that programme design would require and its potential for creating side-effects.

Audience factors

The final aspect of attitude change under consideration here is the contribution of the audience itself. As emphasized in Chapter 6, detailed information about the target group of a health promotion should be an essential part of effective planning. Attitude change theory, too, urges persuaders to know their audience. It is, self-evidently, important to know people's existing attitudes and the values from which they are derived.

At a macro level, there is evidence that there may be social class differences in reactions to persuasive messages (see our discussion of social marketing in Chapter 8). At the micro level, there also seems to be some variation in individuals' suggestibility, which can render them more amenable to persuasive influences. Moreover, reference has already been made to the importance of self-esteem in several contexts. It is generally accepted that individuals having high self-esteem (and belief in their capacity to control their lives) are better able to handle threat and threatening messages with vigilance and take action to minimize the source of the threat. Accordingly, an individual enjoying a good level of self-esteem, would be able to cope with a high fear communication when an individual having low esteem may resort to defensive avoidance and denial. Of course, the high self-esteem would probably result in vigilant action with or without the artificially generated fear! Self-esteem is also associated with an audience characteristic that has been much studied (and was briefly mentioned in Chapter 3).

Dissonance and reactance

In addition to 'personality' factors, such as the empowerment-related variables of perceived locus of control and self-esteem, it is worth mentioning two audience characteristics that have relevance for health promotion and have also been the subject of much research.

The first of these is the phenomenon known as 'cognitive dissonance'. Briefly, cognitive dissonance theory (Festinger, 1957) is one of a group of so-called 'balance theories' that contend that a state of imbalance between psychological components, such as belief, attitude and behaviour, creates pressure for change. Accordingly, an imbalance between one's beliefs and attitudes should result in a change of one or more of these in order to restore 'consistency' or 'congruence'.

Festinger indicated how an imbalance between cognitions about one's feelings and behaviour created an uncomfortable state of 'dissonance'. In Chapter 3, we located 'dissonance' in the motivation system of the HAM, equating it with with such emotional states as guilt and anxiety in terms of its capacity to influence intentions to act. For instance, a smoker who is health-conscious and concerned about his family's welfare is likely to experience a high degree of dissonance that could, of course, be readily resolved by following the advice of health workers. However, as this is frequently not possible – for many well-rehearsed reasons – smokers have to resolve their dissonance by resorting to alternative, less healthy measures!

Festinger and colleagues performed an ingenious series of experiments demonstrating the effects of dissonance and attempts to reduce it. Many of these were counter-intuitive. Again, a more comprehensive discussion is precluded here, so for a comprehensive account, see Aronson, 1976.

Many of the recorded research results have no substantial implication for practice – often because

the strength of the motivation from dissonance is much less powerful than competing values, attitudes or, in the case of smoking, drives. One example will suffice, however, to indicate a situation where dissonance was associated with quite dramatic actions, having major political implications. It is reported by Aronson, who was concerned to demonstrate how dissonance reduction was related to the justification of cruelty in the context of significant US policy decisions. He described a notorious situation at Kent State University when four students were shot and killed by the Ohio National Guard during a demonstration against the Vietnam War. According to Aronson (1976: 121, citing Michener, 1971) the guilt and dissonance experienced by the community in relation to respectable students could only be assuaged by modifying beliefs and attitudes so that the killing could be justified:

> several rumors quickly spread to the effect that: (1) both of the slain women were pregnant (and therefore, by implication, were oversexed and wanton); (2) the bodies of all four students were crawling with lice; and (3) the victims were so ridden with syphilis that they would have been dead in two weeks anyway.

Two of the more important generalizations from research are, first of all, that dissonance is proportional to the seriousness of the issue that creates the dissonance. Second, it seems clear that the level of dissonance is also proportional to the level of self-esteem. Someone having high self-esteem who 'acts out of character' or in contradiction to moral values that he or she has espoused is likely to experience such discomfort that the mere contemplation of the act is likely to result in its rejection. On the other hand, those having low self-esteem may well argue that the most recent inconsistency is yet another example of the individual's lack of integrity and weakness of will.

The second audience characteristic of relevance to health promotion is 'reactance'. One of the important facts of life is that most people do not like to be bludgeoned into taking action, even if they believe it is for their own good. Brehm (1966: 9), who studied this characteristic extensively, provides a key definition.

> Reactance is the motivational state experienced whenever any behaviour that the audience might have freely engaged in is either eliminated or threatened; its aim is to re-establish freedom of choice. Freedom will be re-established by changing attitude in a direction away from the advocated position.

Sutherland's (1979) commentary on the negative reaction to the establishment of the (English) General Board of Health in 1850 provides a commonsense example of reactance in the field of public health. In his (1979: 7) words:

> Many local 'interests', however, resented the central power of the Board, and particularly Chadwick's thrustful, tactless methods, and these probably led *The Times* to comment: 'We prefer to take the chance of cholera and the rest than to be bullied into health'.

The objections to healthy public policy illustrated above clearly involved a clash of political and economic interests. This, though, is not the same as the *psychological* phenomenon of reactance. The 'law of reactance' developed by Brehm and colleagues (Brehm, 1966, and Brehm and Brehm, 1981) makes the simple, but highly relevant, point that, whenever individuals feel that their freedom of action will be curtailed, they tend to react against the message and its source. The reactance may take the form of developing a negative attitude to the message (even if the individual was initially favourably disposed towards it) or physical action. An intriguing example of the latter response is provided by a 1978 report on reactance to attempts in the US to impose seatbelt legislation (see the box). It has especial relevance to health promotion for not only is car safety a health promotion concern, but, also, the use of legislation, and other forms of social engineering, is a key feature of healthy public policy.

A considerable amount of research contributed to the formulation of this 'law of bloody mindedness'. A full review is inappropriate here, but one interesting case study has implications for minimizing reactance in face-to-face settings. It centres on a technique that London (1973) describes as 'ingratiation' (Jones, 1964). The importance of source characteristics is also revealed in the research. London was concerned to identify the characteristics that discriminated between successful and unsuccessful advocates in a face-to-face legal encounter. Accordingly, ten pairs of trainee lawyers were asked to, first, read the essentials of a law case and register prediscussion verdicts individually. They were then paired on the basis of having different initial points of view and instructed to argue their cases until they reached unanimity. Those whose views prevailed were labelled 'persuaders' and those who yielded were 'persuadees'. The face-to-face encounters were tape-recorded and researchers looked for factors that might reveal which particular characteristics of the persuaders could account for their successful advocacy. One major feature emerged – that of 'expressed confidence'.

The researchers constructed a 'vector of persuasion' (representing persuasive force, resistance to pressure and the direction of the resulting force). The vector comprised the number of statements conveying self-confidence about the self and the other member of the pair and the number of statements expressing doubt and confidence about the other person. Expressed confidence was the only factor that significantly accounted for the successful persuasion attempt.

Although the sessions were tape-recorded, a measure of non-verbal (para-linguistic) communication was assessed and this was consistent with the verbal expressions.

This finding is perhaps not surprising. However, the encounters were divided into chronological

---

REACTANCE AND HEALTHY PUBLIC POLICY – A CASE OF CAR SAFETY

... all automobiles manufactured from January 1st 1972 to August 15th 1973 were equipped with a buzzer-light system in which a noise and a light displaying the words 'fasten seatbelts' were activated for at least one minute when the ignition switch was turned on. [Only 28 per cent of drivers used the seatbelts] ... presumably, the remaining 72 per cent of drivers had taken action to disconnect the buzzer-light system.

The ... system was replaced in 1974 ... with a federally mandated interlocking device designed to permit the automobile to start only when the driver's safety belt had been buckled ... [The venture was initially successful and] ... the total use rate was up to 59 per cent ... However, by spring 1975, the rate had dropped to 33 per cent. Not only did the interlocking device fail to effect any long-term increase in seatbelt usage, it also *prompted widespread negative public reaction.* [our emphasis]

[The following year the law was repealed since] ... at least 50 per cent of drivers had taken active, and fairly complicated steps to deactivate the interlock.

(Faden and Faden, 1978: 192–3)

segments – that is, each third of the discussion was plotted in terms of the vector of persuasion. Again, it is perhaps unsurprising that the level of confidence of the persuadees decreased over time. What did surprise the researchers, though, was the fact that the successful persuaders' statements of levels of confidence paralleled those of the persuadees. The authors' argued that their successful persuaders not only avoided expressions of overconfidence as they perceived that they were 'winning', but had employed a strategy of 'ingratiation'.

Further insights into the components of ingratiation are provided by Silberstein (1970) who used Bales' (1951) classic system for analysing social interaction by using the following categories in an analysis of ingratiation situations:

Category 1:   Shows solidarity, raises other's status, gives help, reward.
Category 2:   Shows tension release, jokes, laughs, shows satisfaction.
(Positive social and emotional)
...
Category 11: Shows tension, asks for help, withdraws from field.
Category 12: Shows antagonism, deflates other's status, defends or asserts self.
(Negative social and emotional)

Channels and methods for attitude change

Reference was made earlier to the importance of taking into account both the channel used to deliver persuasive messages and the particular methods used. We exemplified the specific method of role play earlier and mentioned in passing the use of group techniques. We will give further consideration to a number of different strategies and methods in Chapters 8 and 9, but, at this juncture, we will merely note that particular methods and strategies, or particular variations on those methods and strategies, may be intrinsically appropriate to changing attitudes. For instance, mass media are often deliberately employed to change attitudes by utilizing particular sources and messages that are deliberately tailored to specific audiences and take account of their characteristics.

We will complete this present chapter by considering education as a radical and emancipatory activity – arguably its most important function for health promotion. We use 'critical health education' as a generic term to describe this function.

CRITICAL HEALTH EDUCATION – STRATEGIES FOR SOCIAL AND POLITICAL CHANGE

The third variety of health education considered in this chapter derives from critical theory. Although critical education incorporates all of the categories of learning described in this chapter, its major concerns are essentially affective. It aims to motivate people to take action to achieve the various goals that characterize health promotion's ideological commitments. The key difference between critical education and the kinds of attitude change that we have discussed above is that the attitudes to be changed relate to achieving social and political outcomes that, in turn, address issues of equity and social justice. As will be clear from our discussions so for, an empowering approach to health promotion is essentially and fundamentally concerned with equity.

As Tones and Tilford (2001) point out, the critical theory tradition is complicated (see, for instance, Habermas, 1972, and Lyotard, 1984). In discussing the application of critical theory to research, they (2001: 164) cite Harvey (1990: 2), as follows:

> At the heart of critical social research is the idea that knowledge is structured by existing sets of social relations. The aim of a critical methodology is to provide knowledge which engages the prevailing social structures. These social structures are seen by critical social researchers as *oppressive* structures. [Our emphasis.]

HEALTH PROMOTION AS A POLITICAL ENTERPRISE

Health promotion is an inherently political enterprise. Not only is it largely funded by government, but the very nature of its activity suggests shifts in power. Its recognition that peace, shelter, food, income, a stable ecosystem, sustainable resources, social justice and equity are basic prerequisites for health implies major redistribution in power and wealth.

Signal, 1998: 257

Again, discussing implications of critical theory for health promotion research, Connelly (2001: 118) leaves no doubt about the social activist goals of health promotion.

> Reality is produced and reproduced by the causal powers of generative mechanisms whether these are our activities and attitudes or our encounters with social structures. Why we should want to strengthen some or undermine other generative mechanisms emerges from the inescapable reality of making ethical and political decisions in the light of our human interest in emancipation and enlightenment.

We have, on several occasions, noted the relationship between health education and healthy public policy. We have also asserted the primacy of education in achieving health promotion outcomes. Accordingly, as we demonstrated in the empowerment model of health promotion in Chapter 1, critical health education is viewed here as potentially the most powerful means of achieving the supportive environments needed to empower choice. Although, education aims to achieve individual empowerment, at this point, our focus is primarily on those empowering strategies that influence the physical, socio-economic and cultural environment. In other words, to build environments that facilitate healthy choices and remove the barriers that militate against these. There are five separately identifiable (but frequently overlapping) approaches to achieving this end:

- activism and social action
- critical consciousness raising
- providing 'life skills' and 'action competences'
- community organization
- media advocacy.

Only brief reference will be made here to the last two items in the above list as they will receive further consideration in Chapter 8.

Social action

Although it may not be especially important in practice, it is a matter of some theoretical importance to clarify our claims for the primacy of health education in the health promotion enterprise. It is also a matter of some political importance, as health education has been marginalized in recent years, and practical importance for the training of health promoters. As we explained earlier, health education is concerned with health- (or illness-) related learning. Moreover, we argued that education and policy development and implementation were mutually interdependent – it is rare to find examples where healthy public policy does not in fact involve – and,

indeed, depend on – health-related learning. For instance, persuasion and attitude-change strategies are intimately involved in such activities as lobbying and advocacy, which are typically associated with influencing policymakers. On the other hand, social action has not infrequently been contrasted with the pusillanimous efforts of 'traditional' health education and its focus on individuals. Our view is that *critical* health education is the major means for achieving social action. It is therefore opportune to give some thought at this point to the definition and dynamics of this well-established radical strategy for political change.

First of all, as we observed in the Introduction, the only clear instances of policy implementations that could occur without any education at all would be the decisions of omnipotent (benevolent) despots who used their power to introduce and implement healthy public policies. Apart from ethical considerations, it is difficult to conceive such a situation in reality – even if the policy were to be enforced by the deployment of large numbers of heavily armed health police.

Perhaps the closest approximation to education-free social change is provided by revolution and what Ross and Mico (1980) describe as 'violent disruption'. They contrast this with 'non-violent disruption', mentioning various historical examples, such as Gandhi's civil disobedience and Martin Luther King's civil rights movement. Clearly persuasion and other forms of education are central to these latter examples and we will not labour this point further. However, Ross and Mico applied this second category to the work of Saul Alinsky, whose radical approach is relevant to current conceptions of the social determinants of health. Alinsky's work (1969, 1972) is also of interest in the context of community development, as his approach is considered both ethical and appropriate to achieving radical health outcomes. Alinsky's main concerns were with alienation and social disadvantage. His procedures included the recruitment and training of a cadre of leaders and, in the words of Minkler and Wallerstein (1997: 243):

> This *social action organizing* emphasized redressing power imbalances by creating dissatisfaction with the status quo among the disenfranchised, building communitywide identification, and helping community members devise winnable goals and non-violent conflict strategies as means to bring about change.

For further discussion of Alinksy's approach, see Pruger and Specht (1972).

Freudenberg (1978, 1981, 1984) has been consistently associated with a radical approach. He (1984: 40) reminded us that radical action for health is not a recent phenomenon and described how, between 1910 and 1920, Dr Alice Hamilton investigated health conditions in the lead and mercury industries:

> When employers refused to allow her on their premises, she set up clinics in the back rooms of bars and social clubs. ... she also instructed them on how to protect themselves against toxic exposure and she lobbied forcefully for stricter regulations of these metals.

A flavour of activism in the field of health and safety is provided by a case study of the work of the Delaware Valley Toxics Coalition (DVTC). As Freudenberg (1984: 41) reports:

> Among their educational methods were demonstrations at polluting companies, testimony of victims of poisoning at public hearings, and written reports by scientists, physicians and epidemiologists. They developed a flair for using the media creatively. [See Chapters 6 and 8 on media advocacy.] At one city council hearing, a union member who was appearing in support of the bill sprayed an unmarked canister into the chamber. 'Stop that,' the legislators shouted, 'you're poisoning us.' The unionist replied, 'This can has only air, but everyday we have to work with chemicals we know nothing about.' His testimony made headlines in the local paper.

Critical consciousness raising – the Freirean perspective

Paulo Freire, who died in 1997, is probably the best-known advocate of a radical, libertarian approach to education for social change. His work originated with literacy programmes for impoverished cane-cutters in plantations near Recife in Brazil in 1958. He rapidly realized that de-powered individuals viewed reading and writing as virtually magical activities. The way to achieve literacy was therefore by developing a radical challenge to poverty and the social systems that created it. Only in this way could illiterate workers be empowered. Freire's emancipatory approach has inspired not only those concerned to promote social justice, but also those who seek to promote the health of the disadvantaged.

The libertarian philosophy

Freire's philosophical and ideological concerns and the associated values base are readily stated. They are essentially humanistic and concerned with human dignity. Freire sought to fight oppression and the poverty, helplessness and alienation that result from these social pathogens. The approach mirrors the empowerment model we propose in this book in that it not only seeks to liberate people from environmental barriers derived from oppressive power structures, but also free them from their perceptions of an 'external locus of control' revealed in 'magical thinking'. Oppression may be 'political' or 'religious'. In all events, in Freire's words, 'Sectarianism, fed by fanaticism, is always castrating.' He (1972: 132) illustrates the 'magical explanation' as follows:

> the oppressor is 'housed' within the people, and their resulting ambiguity makes them fearful of freedom. They resort (stimulated by the oppressor) to magical explanations or a false view of God, to whom they fatalistically transfer the responsibility for their oppressed state.

> [A Chilean priest of high intellectual and moral calibre visiting Recife in 1966 told him] a Pernambucan colleague and I went to see several families living in shanties in indescribable poverty. I asked them how they could bear to live like that, and the answer was always the same: 'What can I do? It is the will of God and I must accept it'.

Following our earlier discussions of the meaning of education, we can say that Freire is committed to 'true education' – that is, to voluntarism and depth of understanding rather than persuasion and propaganda. Indeed, he (1972: 43) criticizes the 'activism' of revolutionary leaders who fail to genuinely educate the populace:

> [Unless] one intends to carry out the transformation *for* the oppressed rather than *with* them ... the oppressed ... must intervene critically in the situation which surrounds them and marks them: propaganda cannot achieve this ... It is my belief that only this latter type of transformation is valid. The object in presenting these considerations is to defend the eminently pedagogical character of the revolution.

In justifying his educational approach, Freire (1972: 67) cites Mao Tse-tung:

> We should not make the change until, through our work, most of the masses have become conscious of the need and are willing and determined to carry it out ... There are two principles here: one is the actual needs of the masses rather than what we fancy they need, and the other is the wishes of the masses, who must make up their own minds instead of our making up their minds for them. (From the collected works of Mao Tse-tung, 1967.)

Unconditional positive regard – and the OK Corral

It is perhaps worth noting in passing that, irrespective of his radical concerns, Freire's humanistic

I'm OK A	I'm OK B
You're not OK	You're OK
I'm not OK C	I'm not OK D
You're not OK	You're OK

Key:
A Distrustful, B Optimistic, C Despairing, D Depressed

Figure 7.6 The OK Corral (Turner, 1978: 72)

approach to education frequently includes references to the intrinsic value of people. These are essentially similar to Rogerian notions of 'unconditional positive regard' – a mainstay of non-directive counselling, which affirms that, although individuals' behaviour may be a cause for condemnation, their essential humanity must be respected. Freirean observations are also often reminiscent of transactional analysis' notion of healthy 'life positions' (Berne, 1964, and Harris and Harris, 1986). It is argued that, as a result of early socialization and life experiences, individuals adopt basic attitudes to the self. There are four such positions, deriving from the extent to which people accept that they and other people are 'OK'. Turner (1978) adopted the term 'OK Corral' to describe the matrix shown in Figure 7.6.

As will probably be apparent, the 'healthy' state is depicted in the top right cell, indicating an individual belief that the people in question feel content with themselves and have good self-esteem, but also trust others and feel concern for them. In other words, we have a remarkably concise definition of mental and social health, having links to such concepts as a 'sense of coherence'.

The pedagogy – educational methods

A number of psychological factors are brought to bear on ideological goals as part of the process of planning any curriculum. The psychological factors contributing to an emancipatory curriculum such as Freire's are both cognitive and affective and the pedagogical methods employed take this into account. They are concerned with creating a level of critical awareness and translating that awareness into action. The method is primarily 'dialogical' and involves problem-solving approaches.

Critical consciousness raising Freirean ideology cannot be separated from its methodology. The purpose is '*conscientizacao*', or 'conscientization' – most readily translated as 'critical consciousness raising'. In the words of the translator of *Pedagogy of the Oppressed* (Freire, 1972: 16,

footnote), 'conscientization' 'refers to learning to perceive social, political, and economic contradictions, and to take action against the oppressive elements of reality.'

The link between consciousness raising and action is defined in terms of 'praxis'. Praxis is the interactive process of reflection and action. Action without reflection is mere 'activism'; reflection without action can involve mere detached intellectualism.

Problem posing v. banking Freire compared traditional educational approaches that treat learners as empty vessels to be filled by a teacher with a problem-posing approach that seeks to engage learners and put them in control of their learning. The traditional approach was described by Freire as 'banking' (traditional teachers/educators being 'bank-clerk educators'!) The distinction between 'banking' and 'problem-posing' is not new, as we noted earlier in our analysis of rote learning, problem solving and decision making. The novelty here lies in the purpose of education – that is, it is radical, political and essentially affective.

The banking approach is not viewed merely as a technical method of teaching, but has deep ideological connotations – namely, in respect of the emphasis on the inequality of the teacher–learner relationship and the consonance between 'banking' and political domination. Freire (1972: 102, citing Giddy, *Hansard*, Vol. ix, 798, 13 July, 1807) provided a revealing quotation from Niebuhr (1960) to illustrate the threat that problem-posing education is to the 'oppressor' and the establishment:

> However specious in theory the project might be of giving education to the labouring classes of the poor, it would be prejudicial to their morals and happiness; it would teach them to despise their lot in life instead of making them good servants in agriculture and other laborious employments; instead of teaching them subordination it would render them fractious and refractory as was evident in the manufacturing countries; it would enable them to read seditious pamphlets, vicious books and publications against Christianity; it would render them insolent to their superiors and in a few years the legislature would find it necessary to direct the strong arm of power against them.

In addition to clearly demonstrating the perceived threat of education to the social order, Giddy's observations are of particular interest for health education – an interest spiced with not a little irony. Barnard (1961) provides a more complete report of the affair and its background circumstances. It was initiated by a Samuel Whitbread who introduced a bill in the House of Commons (UK Parliament).

The bill sought to establish 'free' schools funded by local taxation. Whitbread was motivated by the alleged fact that (Barnard, 1961: 54):

> there has been discovered a plan for the instruction of youth which is now brought to a state of great perfection; happily combining rules by which the object of learning must be infallibly attained with expedition *and cheapness*. [Our emphasis]

The new plan was, in fact, the development of the 'monitorial system' by Bell (a clergyman) and Lancaster (a Quaker) and it generated international interest. In brief, the monitors were pupils in the school who acted as surrogate teachers under the command of the headmaster. Large numbers of children could be taught in this fashion – it was mass production in education and, above all, it was cheap! There was, of course, no question of problem posing or radical analysis of social conditions. In Barnard's words, 'The whole technique was mechanical; there was not opportunity for the asking of questions nor, of course, for the development of individuality.'

Apart from Giddy's objections, the proposal was vigorously opposed by the Archbishop of Canterbury in the House of Lords, who feared that it would challenge the monopoly of the Church in education and would, 'subvert the first principles of education in this country, which had hitherto been, and he trusted would continue to be, under the control and auspices of the Establishment' (*Hansard*, Vol. ix, 1178, 11 August, 1807).

Ironically, the monitorial system has been seen as one of the precursors to contemporary interest in the use of peer education and peer leadership (see later discussion in Chapter 9) Interestingly, such peer techniques can be used as part of a victim-blaming approach to attitude change or to empower peers and enhance their self-esteem. Returning to Freire's conceptualization of 'banking', the practice was considered to have the following ten main characteristics.

- The teacher teaches and the students are taught.
- The teacher knows everything and the students know nothing.
- The teacher thinks and the students are thought about.
- The teacher talks and the students listen – meekly.
- The teacher disciplines and the students are disciplined.
- The teacher acts and the students have the illusion of acting through the action of the teacher.
- The teacher chooses the programme content and the students (who were not consulted) adapt to it.

- The teacher confuses the authority of knowledge with his own professional authority, which he sets in opposition to the freedom of the students.
- The teacher is the subject of the learning process, while the pupils are mere objects.

The specific techniques employed by Freire in problem posing include the use of 'culture circles' – that is, informal group work. The culture circles explore their thematic universe, which is composed of a complex of generative themes that refer to key social and cultural issues. The culture circle (or 'thematic investigation circle') is presented with 'codifications of reality' – in other words, pictures or other triggers to discussion that incorporate major social issues, of which the participants are not yet conscious. The 'decoding' process works through dialogue and group members typically:

- reflect on aspects of their reality, such as poor housing
- search for a root cause of the problem
- consider implications and consequences
- devise a plan of action.

Because of its relevance to the important 'strategy' of community development – and personal and social education in schools – we will revisit Freirean methodology in Chapter 8. For the present, some examples of the deliberate application of Freire's approach to health promotion will be considered.

Applications of Freirean principles to health promotion As we noted above, the whole Freirean philosophy chimes with the ideological commitments of health promotion (as formulated by WHO and distilled in the empowerment model discussed in Chapter 1). Accordingly, any radical approach operating on Freirean principles could be said to be health-promoting. However, it is enlightening to consider a limited number of examples to illustrate both the direct and indirect application of Freirean principles to health.

As we will see, one of the characteristics of interventions inspired by the principles of consciousness raising, praxis, problem posing and the like is a tendency to adapt and modify those principles to meet particular needs. This would not be seen by Freire as a form of treason, but, rather, an appropriate development of his work. For instance, Macdonald and Warren (1991) amalgamated the Freirean approach with Frankena's (1970) model for analysing the philosophical basis of educational programmes and applied this to primary healthcare (as prescribed by WHO). Figure 7.7 outlines this amalgamation.

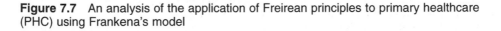

┌───┐   ┌───┐
│ **Basic normative premises**   │   │ **Basic factual premises**   │
│   │   │   │
│ PHC should be viewed as an educational   │   │ Most ill health has its roots in   │
│ process   │   │ socio-economic conditions often created by│
│ Education should be an act of liberation │   │ exploitation and its consequences in the │
│ Education should empower people   │   │ unjust distribution of health resources │
│   │   │ Human beings have the ability to overcome│
│   │   │ their oppression   │
└───┘   └───┘

┌───┐   ┌───┐
│ **Dispositions to be fostered**   │   │ **Methodological premises**   │
│   │   │   │
│ People should be motivated to discover   │   │ Education for health involves more than │
│ the causes and solutions of ill health   │   │ information transmission – it includes   │
│ rather than merely address symptoms   │   │ enhancing confidence in ability to improve│
│ An assertive, enquiring outlook should be│   │ own and community's health   │
│ fostered   │   │ Real learning involves *problem posing* │
│ An acceptance of learning as dialogue   │   │ and *praxis*   │
└───┘   └───┘

┌──┐
│ **Recommendations for practice**   │
│   │
│ The practice of education involves *dialogue* between *equals*   │
│ It should start from people's own knowledge and experience – the teacher is   │
│ a facilitator   │
│ PHC should be based on people's own knowledge and experience of health and   │
│ disease   │
│ The wider social and socio-economic context should be the prime consideration   │
│ for dialogic interaction between 'equal but different' stakeholders in relation to   │
│ health concerns   │
└──┘

Figure 7.7 An analysis of the application of Freirean principles to primary healthcare
(PHC) using Frankena's model

Critical consciousness and the healthcare setting – Honduras and Tenderloin

Minkler and Cox (1980) provide a detailed application of a Freirean system. Although the title of their article refers to the healthcare setting, the focus is substantially on health education and health promotion.

Two settings are described: rural Honduras and urban USA. The first of these documents the ways in which the Caritas Organization worked through local housewives' clubs to create and train a cadre of '*promotoras de salud*' (health promoters). Their role was to 'bridge the gap between healthcare and the *campesino*'. Although 50 per cent of the *promotoras* were functionally illiterate – some had never attended school and none had held responsibilities outside the home – they learned (Minkler and Cox, 1980: 315–6):

basic diagnostic and curative skills, first aid, nutrition, hygiene, midwifery, how to give injections, how to diagnose common health problems, and the criteria useful in deciding whether a patient should make the long, arduous trip to the hospital. They further learned to keep accurate records and how to order medicines. At the end of the course, each woman received a medicine kit, containing many of the drugs used in treating common health problems. Apart from its utilitarian function, the medicine kit was a status symbol.

Despite the medical trappings, the treatment role was secondary to the consciousness-raising function, which involved helping the population view health within the context of the 'total oppressive social structure' of Honduras.

The programme was evaluated over a two-year period. The *promotoras* themselves (who were quite evidently operating as 'homophilous' peer leaders) were substantially empowered, with consequent enhancements of their self-esteem. In addition, their work was associated with the following developments:

- a school was built
- a contribution was made to land reform by encouraging civil action, such as squatting on illegally owned land, and, after intervention by the army, 100,000 people marched on the capital
- a coalition was established, based on Freirean principles.

The second example described by Minkler and Cox, of a very different context, was a project to empower the elderly poor in the Tenderloin area of San Francisco. The following features are worth emphasizing. First, the goal of the critical consciousness raising and praxis here was broad-based, comprising a focus on the generally de-powered living conditions and social isolation of the elderly residents.

A health fair was located in various cheap hotels where the old people lived. This served as a trigger for developing the equivalent of Freire's culture circles in support groups established in twelve of the hotels led by twelve of the elderly people. The media proved to be inappropriate for 'coding' and resource people were used to stimulate dialogue. Poverty and powerlessness rapidly emerged as major factors.

How effective was the venture? The authors conceded that results were limited. For instance, they had hoped to generate 'power through the ballot box', using the potential voting power of the 14,000 Tenderloin residents, but this did not materialize – substantially due to curtailment of the project. Additional problems were ascribed by the authors to a lack of a 'sense of community' (clearly present in the Honduras venture) and, importantly, conflict with the 'existing aid power structure'. They emphasized the importance of avoiding a heavy reliance on 'volunteer conscienticizers' who would be subject to the uncertainties of funding. The authors also felt that it might have been beneficial to concentrate on a community development approach.

Application of Freirean principles to an alcohol and substance misuse prevention programme (ASAP) One of the most substantial and detailed analyses of the application of Freirean

notions to health promotion has been provided by Wallerstein and Bernstein (1988). It is particularly interesting because it could, at first glance, be seen as 'mainstream', preventive health promotion addressing the problems of substance misuse. It is also of interest as it links Freirean theory with an 'alternative' theoretical model that has frequently been applied to health education. Its emphasis throughout is on empowerment, which is linked with principles of community organization and the use of peer leaders.

The ASAP programme involved collaboration between an emergency centre and local schools in New Mexico. Its goal was, 'to reduce excess morbidity and mortality among multi-ethnic middle and high school students' by empowering youth 'from high-risk populations to make healthier choices in their own lives, to play active political and social roles in their communities and society, and, as community participants, to effect positive changes.' (Wallerstein and Bernstein, 1988)

Only a few details of the programme can be provided here, but it is interesting to note the deliberate attempt to utilize Freirean notions in the context of the groupwork handled by peer educators. For instance, the peer facilitators used a five-step questioning strategy that moved from the personal to the social and action levels. Using the 'coding' devices of trigger videos, participants were asked to:

- describe what they could see and feel
- as a group, define the many levels of the problem
- share similar experiences from their lives
- question why this problem exists
- develop action plans to address the problem.

This discussion was guided by the acronym 'SHOWED'. Thus, after a four-minute trigger film depicting the life of an Indian woman who came to the emergency centre drunk and who had been raped, the participants' discussion was guided as follows (Wallerstein and Bernstein, 1988: 386):

S   What do we **S**ee here?
H   What is really **H**appening?
O   How does her story relate to **O**ur lives?
W   **W**hy has she become an alcoholic?
E   How can we become **E**mpowered by our new social understanding?
D   What can we **D**o about these problems in our own lives?

Wallerstein and Sanchez-Merki (1994) provide an illuminating update on the progress of the ASAP programme and, as a result of their deliberations, give us an interesting theoretical model that combines the Freirean principles of 'listening, dialogue and action' with protection motivation theory

(Rogers, 1975) that emphasizes the interaction of threat appraisal (severity and susceptibility), coping appraisal (self and response efficacy) and protective behaviour.

The programme evaluation is thoughtful and focused on three 'self-identity changes'. Stage one was labelled 'action orientation of care' and there was evidence of changes in such measures as 'recognition (emotionally and cognitively) of one's personal connection and susceptibility to the problem'. Stage two – 'individual responsibility to act' – revealed, for example, 'evidence of increased self-efficacy to talk and help others and their own self-articulated behaviour changes reinforced their self-confidence and their own recognition of their personal changes in self perception and in perception of others.' Stage three – 'social responsibility to act' – indicated changes such as student involvement in peer education and 'tribal council presentations'.

Photo novella – photographs as policy Prior to offering a few final thoughts on Freire's radical approach, Wang and Burris' (1994) discussion of their use of the photo novella provides a significant illustration of how Freirean 'coding' can be extensively used as part of radical empowering education. In fact, the use of photography (rather than just photographs) might be seen as an empowering operation in its own right that fits remarkably well with the general dialogical process. The photo novella ('picture stories') gives just such a function for photographs, which are used not only to document people's lives and as a basis for consciousness raising, but also as a deliberate device to influence policy.

The authors used as a model for their project an empowerment project in Peru designed to encourage illiterate and semi-literate rural women to participate in local health and family planning initiatives. The project – *Asociacion Peru-Mujer* – used colouring books as a catalyst for stimulating group discussion. Women used crayons or coloured pencils to colour the booklets as a group activity or took the booklets home and, occasionally, coloured them in with their children and husbands. The coloured images were used in the group to 'decode' the associated 'generative themes'.

Wang and Burris' project was located in China's Yunnan province. The use of documentary photography has a long tradition in consciousness raising and Wang and Burris added an extra empowering dimension by providing intensive training in the use of the photo novella for sixty-two rural Chinese women (many of whom were illiterate) to use cameras to document their lives and circumstances. This technique proved to be especially effective in stimulating consciousness and praxis – doubtless

helped by the fact that, as the authors observe, many of their older women subjects were familiar with the 'culture circles' and 'study sessions' from the days of Mao Tse-tung.

In the authors' (1994: 185) words:

The photographs taken by the village women are an exquisite history of a place, a community, and a way of life that is unseen by most outsiders and that is undocumented by insiders and outsiders alike ... the rural Chinese women we worked with had little money, power, or status. For these ... women to photograph their lives evokes a double power: it records for future generations what is happening now, and it enables the village women to define for themselves and others, including policymakers, what is worthy to remember and where change must occur.

The Freirean perspective – problems and prospects

It is hopefully now apparent that the ideological approach intrinsic to Freire's pedagogy is entirely consistent with the commitments and concerns of empowering health promotion as revealed in WHO's many publications over some twenty-five years or so. However, there are problems to be addressed by those health promoters seeking to utilize Freirean enlightenment. For example, it has been argued that Freire's focus on overtly oppressive state control and class is not relevant to all societies and cultures. However, Freire himself argued that his approach could be adapted to fit all those situations in which there was oppression and a lack of empowerment. As some of the examples cited above have shown, the techniques can, and have, been applied to different contexts – for example, as a feminist challenge to male hegemony.

However, in accordance with the ever-present threat of false consciousness, a greater challenge to Freirean ideology and practice is the suggestion that Freire's ideas have been co-opted and thus emasculated (for example Zacharakis-Jutz, 1988, and Kidd and Kumar, 1981). Kidd and Kumar refer to the co-option threat in terms of the emergence of a 'pseudo-Freirean' perspective that appears, superficially, to have radical credentials, but, in fact, does not significantly challenge the status quo and its power structure. Referring to adult education (in all its many aspects), Kidd and Kumar (1981: 28) identify the following features of pseudoradical education:

- naming the central problem as 'poverty' rather than as 'oppression' (that is, ignoring the primacy of power)
- identifying the cause of poverty as the self-inflicted deficiency of the poor rather than

oppression (that is, the problems of the poor are acknowledged but considered to be due to a 'culture of poverty' created by the shortcomings of the poor themselves)

- proposing, as treatment, to change the behaviour of the poor by means of a transmission of information and skills
- converting Freire's method into a 'neutral', apolitical classroom technique (for example, the use of group discussion – *any* kind of group discussion – rather than true dialogue leading to praxis, and the conversion of 'problem posing' into 'discovery learning' where the learner is helped to 'discover' the correct, predetermined answer to the problem)
- defining 'action' as coping activity (that is, the acquisition of personal competences other than those associated with political challenges to authority).

Freirean practice – difficult and dangerous

It should be stated that the emancipatory practices associated with critical consciousness raising and praxis are difficult to achieve and there is clearly a temptation to follow 'pseudo practices'. In certain circumstances (as Freire himself acknowledged), the pedagogy of the oppressed can be physically dangerous to both educator and learner. We are reminded of a cartoon embodying advice to would-be radical educators, that showed an ostrich with its head in the sand. The novice educators are counselled not to ignore reality in that way, but an accompanying picture showing the ostrich on the receiving end of a fusillade of rifle fire also advises them not to stick their heads above the parapet!

In short, as some of the examples provided earlier have implied, Freirean approaches may benefit from additional techniques and approaches. More particularly, effectiveness may be increased and the risks reduced if the oppressed and powerless could enlist the support of an alliance of those who possess both goodwill and power – see the empowerment model, in Chapter 1. Moreover, the process of praxis may be facilitated and, again, the element of risk reduced if consciousness can be supplemented by the acquisition of key 'protective' skills and those that facilitate the attainment of power. We will now, therefore, examine this latter suggestion and consider the role of life skills and action competences as part of critical health education.

Life skills, action competences and health – education as a subversive activity

One of the more influential texts for those seeking to revolutionize the traditional values base of school education was Postman and Weingartner's (1969) book, which quoted, approvingly, Ernest Hemingway's rejoinder to the question of what it takes to be a great writer, 'In order to be a great writer a person must have a built-in shockproof crap detector.'

The authors point out that, 'One way of looking at the history of the human group is that it has been a continuing struggle against the veneration of crap.' This questioning of the relevance of the curriculum to important contemporary issues and problems was also the central theme of an influential parable by Benjamin (1971), who described the almost ineluctable tendency for schools systems and curricula to be out of touch with current realities. In Benjamin's words, schools are shackled by a 'Saber-toothed curriculum' – that is, a curriculum that is intrinsically outdated and always irrelevant to real, contemporary needs.

Postman and Weingartner's (1969: 19) critique mirrors Freire's beliefs about the hegemony of the ruling class and the 'stultifying influence' of religion – 'Religious indoctrination' is seen as 'domesticating', to use Freire's terminology:

> irrevocable commitment to any religion is not only intellectual suicide, it is positive unfaith because it closes the mind to any new vision of the world. Faith is, above all, openness – an act of trust in the unknown. (Acknowledgements made to Alan Watts)

Although reference has been made above to schools and the formal education system, as will have been apparent from the discussion of Freire's approach, radical education is equally relevant to informal contexts and adult audiences. In this particular section of the chapter, we shall concern ourselves with the application of life skills teaching and action competences to critical education – inside or outside the school sector. There is a good deal of overlap and congruence of purpose between life skills and action competences – although, arguably, the latter have been more directly derived from critical theory. Life skills teaching enjoyed a good deal of popularity in Great Britain originally for personal and social education in schools and, subsequently, for health education generally. The figures having the greatest influence on this development were Hopson and Scally (1981, 1980–2).

The values base of life skills teaching is interesting in the light of our various observations about the radical purpose of education. It is illustrated by debate in the UK at the time of government action to raise the school leaving age, which offered the prospect of those pupils who were eager to leave school at the earliest possible moment having to face a further year of what they perceived as generally irrelevant teaching.

Two opposing schools of thought emerged. The first of these argued that pupils should be taught only what they needed to cope with their existing circumstances. The alternative view to this restrictive process of 'dumbing down', was that all pupils were entitled to full and rich experiences of all that their culture could offer.

Life skills were certainly more relevant than the traditional curriculum, but were, accordingly, criticized as being a sanitized version of victim-blaming. Advocates of life skills argued vigorously that their major purpose was empowerment – and this was certainly congruent with their emphasis on the skills' application to real-life problems. Sprinthall (1980: 487), for instance, discussed the importance of empowerment:

the psychological domains of self-empowerment, ego-maturity, competence, efficiency, moral development and interpersonal conceptual growth need to be emphasized as the real goals of the educational enterprise.

Hopson and Scally (1981) summarized the key elements of life skills teaching in terms of providing a 'survival and growth kit for an age of future shock':

a school should provide a basic survival kit for young people … they need to be taught skills like values clarification, decision making, how to cope with crises, intellectual and emotional problem solving, helping, assertiveness, relationship building, how to find appropriate information and use personal and physical resources which are available in the community. They need to be made aware of themselves, others and the world around them, in order to become more self-empowered people.

The reference to *self*-empowerment is perhaps revealing. Critics of a radical persuasion saw the reference to self as evidence that the life skills approach was effectively blind to socio-economic circumstances. While it is true that many life skills do indeed refer to individual empowerment and sometimes to an acceptance of the social status quo (for example, skills such as how to present yourself at interview in order to get a job). The following points should, however, be noted.

- Many skills are indeed concerned with invidual growth and development and include, for example, preventive health skills, such as stress management.
- The armamentarium of life skills includes large numbers of transferable skills that may be applied to a wide variety of situations – both conformist and revolutionary! Indeed, we noted earlier that lack of literacy skills is essentially de-powering and intimately associated with

Freire's adult education approaches. Again, skills involved in working with groups could be used to manipulate committees designed to achieve changes in health policy or organize revolutionary freedom movements.
- A number of what might be called 'skills for radicals' are incorporated in Hopson and Scally's life skills menu.

Hopson and Scally separately identified four life skills scenarios:

- *me* skills – for example, literacy and numeracy, enhancing one's self-esteem
- *me and you* skills – such as effective communication and managing conflict
- *me and others* skills – for instance working in groups, assertiveness, influencing people and systems
- *me and specific situations* – including skills for education, skills at work, skills at home, skills at leisure, skills in the community.

Figure 7.8 shows the interrelationships between these scenarios.

It will be evident that the key skill of assertiveness has been incorporated into the skills shown in Figure 7.8. In the context of our discussion of emancipatory education, it is perhaps worth recalling that the etymology of the word 'assertive' is '*asserere*', which means to free a slave by a laying on of hands – a rather nice metaphor. We might also note that advocates of assertiveness training argue that its rationale was based on the UN Declaration of Human Rights (Barker, 1990).

We would also suggest that the consciousness-raising work in Freirean 'culture circles' should ideally be supplemented by life skills designed to translate intention into action. We will also argue in Chapter 8 that community development work, which frequently incorporates aspects of Freire's approach, would benefit from the support of 'coalitions' of the great and good.

Critical theory and action competences

Although Hopson and Scally's work is firmly committed to Freirean principles, the action competence approach is, on the face of it, somewhat more radical. This is doubtless due to its overt commitment to critical theory and, thus, critical education. The work on action competences is very much associated with Denmark and its emphasis on education for democracy in school and community. Indeed, the 'revolutionary' *The Little Red School Book* provided a 'toolbox' for oppressed schoolchildren, giving them guidelines for challenging authority!

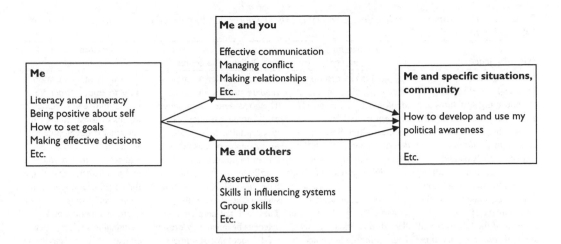

Figure 7.8   Life skills and community action (after Hopson and Scally, 1980)

THE LITTLE RED SCHOOL BOOK

Grown-ups do have a lot of power over you: they are real tigers. But in the long run they can never control you completely: they are paper tigers ... Children and grown-ups are not natural enemies. But grown-ups themselves have little real control over their lives. They often feel trapped by economic and political forces ... Cooperation is possible when grown-ups have realized this and have started to do something about it. If you discuss things among yourselves and actively try to get things changed, you can achieve a lot more than you think. We hope that this book will show you some of the ways in which you can influence your own lives ...

Hansen and Jensen, 1969

An example of one of the 'life skills' proposed in Chapter 8 of *The Little Red School Book* (English language edition) is provided by advice on 'How to make a complaint', which included collecting evidence, going to the teacher or to the school council, going to the headmaster, going to the authorities, consulting examples of a complaint and discussing factors associated with the sacking of a teacher.

Critical theory and environmental education

Education about the environment, its conservation and sustainability, is frequently incorporated into health education. For instance, the Danish School of Education has specialized in the application of action competences to health education generally and environmental education in particular. Fien

(1994) has adopted a similar approach and specifically applied the principles of critical education to the 'health of the environment'. He (in Gibson, 1986: 2) provides an illuminating definition of the application of critical theory:

Critical theory attempts to explain the origins of everyday practices and problems, but it goes further. It claims to offer replies to those awkward questions which ask what should be done. [About the organization and running of schools] Critical theory is not simply explanatory, but is committed to enabling change towards better relationships, towards a more just and rational society. In identifying the biases and distortions which prevent healthy personal and social growth, it helps teachers to free themselves and their pupils from those malforming constraints. In asserting that individuals and groups should be in control of their own lives, it has

Table 7.2   *Philosophical implications of a critical theory approach in environmental education (Huckle, 1993: 62, cited in Fien, 1994: 24).*

Type of science	Human interests served	Related ideologies	Environmental education
Seeks to explain the empirical world in terms of underlying structures and mechanisms and the events that set them in motion. This requires not only empirical analysis and hermeneutic understanding, but also theoretical accounts of the mechanisms. It is the development of valid theories of the 'abstract real' and their use in explaining concrete events and experiences that are the fundamental tasks of critical science	The goal is *emancipation* – freeing people from the ideological (and material) constraints to their understanding. Self-determination or the full development of human potential requires knowledge, not only of the empirical and hermeneutic kind – valuable though this is – but also of the critical sciences. These aim to expose people to exactly how and why their society operates, thereby allowing them to become fully involved in its transformation to the sort of society that they want. Radical, ecocentric environmentalism draws on critical science	The critical sciences are fundamentally radical. They oppose the domination of the empirical sciences in a capitalist society, for example, because these do not tackle, and so implicitly promote, the basic inequalities on which such societies are built. They fault the hermeneutic sciences because they present a false ideology of human self-determination. The critical sciences are potentially dangerous as they would unmask society's ideology and expose its role in the promotion of vested interests that continue to exploit both people and nature	Environmental education aims to empower people so that they can become agents of social change and sustainable development. It enables them to reflect, and act, on the structures and mechanisms that shape the social use of nature in ways prefiguring future democratic and sustainable society. Such education draws heavily on critical knowledge of the environment and education and can be termed 'education for sustainability'

as its goal that people should be able to determine their own destinies.

Wals and Jickling (2000) also support this view in their comprehensive discussion of the role of environmental education, which they consider should be essentially emancipatory with reference to social, political and economic matters and concerned with 'recognizing, evaluating and potentially transcending social norms.' (See also Fien and Trainer, 1993).

The philosophical implications of critical theory when applied to environmental education are listed in Table 7.2.

Critical thinking and praxis

Mogensen (1997) describes praxis and critical thinking in environmental education as a holistic combination of feeling and reason – a dialectical process of examining situations from multiple perspectives and 'constantly challenging, querying, criticizing, breaking down parts of existing practice with the aim of reconstructing a new and alternative practice.'

Jensen makes an interesting comparison between Freire's formulation of critical thinking and praxis

and political literacy. We have some reservations about the profligate use of the term 'literacy', but Crick and Lister's (1978: 41) use of the term (as cited by Fien, 1994: 43) explicates the notion of praxis as applied to the school curriculum:

> The ultimate test of political literacy lies in creating a proclivity to action, not in achieving more theoretical analysis. The politically literate person would be capable of active participation (or positive refusal to participate) … The highly politically literate person should be able to do more than merely imagine alternatives … The politically literate person must be able to devise strategies for influence and for achieving change.

Schnack (2000) provides a valid justification for adopting a critical educational approach to health and environmental issues. It provides an interesting parallel with Hopson and Scally's rationale that life skills teaching should provide an antidote to, or rather an inoculation against, 'future shock'. According to Schnack, critical thinking and praxis are essential in the context of what he calls 'the dissolution of tradition'. He also makes the point that action competence for health and environmental education should include the traits associated with C. Wright Mills' (1959) concept of 'sociological imagination' – that is, 'the capability of shifting perspective backwards and forwards between the individual, personal level, which is often seen as the purely private sphere, and the social, structural level.'

THE PRIMACY OF EDUCATION

In this chapter, we have reiterated and emphasized the point that, following the 'formula' health promotion = healthy public policy × health education, education is a sine qua non for contemporary health promotion. Indeed, it is challenging to find a situation in which education (following the definition embodied in the three approaches examined in this present chapter) cannot be identified as being a major component in health promotion.

Following the environmental theme that has formed part of the above discussion of action competences, we draw your attention to the following observation about the importance of health education in a UNESCO-EPD report (1997: 32, cited in Fien, 2000: 47):

> Ethical values are the principal factor in social cohesion and, at the same time, the most effective agent of change and transformation. Achieving sustainability ... will need to be motivated by a shift in values. Without change of this kind, even the most enlightened legislation, the cleanest technology, the most sophisticated research will not succeed in steering society towards the long-term goal of sustainability *Education in the broadest sense will by necessity play a pivotal role in bringing about the deep change required in both tangible and non-tangible ways.* [Our emphasis]

We next consider the relevance of particular strategies for achieving critical health education goals.

8

Mass Communication and Community Action

Nothing is easier than leading the people on a leash. I just hold up a dazzling campaign poster and they jump through it.

Joseph Goebbels, cited in Rhodes, 1976

INTRODUCTION

In this chapter, we give some critical consideration to two of the major strategies used in health promotion work. Both of these are, in their different ways, somewhat problematic and both have especial relevance to our commitment to empowerment and critical health education.

We first argue for a particular role for mass media and then proceed to examine the empowering dimensions of certain kinds of health promotion work in communities.

MASS COMMUNICATION AND HEALTH PROMOTION

The term 'mass communication' is often used interchangeably with 'mass media'. While both definitions coincide in the use of the word 'mass', in the interest of clarity, it is worth giving some brief consideration to the use of the terms 'communication' and 'media'.

Adhering to our earlier definition of 'communication' as the business of transmitting messages from a source to a receiver is to limit the scope of 'mass communication' in a way that is certainly not intended by those who use it. The intended meaning is almost certainly equivalent to 'education' – as we have used it in Chapter 7, but with an emphasis on its persuasive dimension. The educational messages are, however, mediated by the use of a range of electronic and print media. As we will observe later, the strengths and limitations of mass media are inherent in these two words. Their potential advantage derives from the possibility of contacting very large numbers of people at any one time. Their limitations derive from the fact that, as the messages are mediated, interpersonal contact is not possible. It is therefore very difficult to precisely tailor communications to the audience and impossible to react immediately to people's reactions to the mediated messages.

What exactly is a *mass* audience? It is meaningless to refer to precise numbers as it is not so much the actual numbers that are important but the feedback limitations. For instance, a typical 'block' lecture to the public or a student group has more in common with mass media than with interpersonal education, despite relatively small numbers. Lecturers must tailor their message to some notional average student and there is no significant immediate feedback potential – apart from that provided in obvious non-verbal responses signifying amusement or boredom!

This phenomenon has been emphasized by media researchers for many decades. For example, Schramm and Roberts (1972: 392, cited by Reardon, 1981: 195) refer to the 'latitude of interpretation and response' that characterizes mass media:

> Characteristics of the mass communication situation, such as the receiver's freedom from many of the social constraints which operate in interpersonal communication, greatly attenuated feedback, and lack of opportunity to tailor messages for specific people allow any individual receiver a good deal more latitude of interpretation and response than he has when speaking face-to-face with friend, colleague or acquaintance.

Issues for health promotion

There are four main areas of interest and debate for health promotion in respect of mass media.

- Mass media may be viewed as having a direct and unhealthy influence – for example, in relation to copy cat violence, promoting health-damaging behaviours, such as excessive alcohol consumption, and contributing to sloth and idleness, and even reducing the stock of social capital – see Putnam's, (1995) suggestion that the decline in social capital is substantially due to the increase in people's television viewing.
- The negative effects on health of marketing unhealthy products.
- The advisability of using mass media to promote health promotion goals by means of 'social marketing' and associated debate about their effectiveness in achieving these goals compared with alternative interpersonal approaches.
- A debate concerned with social marketing that centres on the use of persuasive messages to 'sell health' rather than empower choice.

Media varieties and learning resources

The variety of available media is substantial. However, despite the shared characteristics mentioned above, it is unwise to treat mass media as completely homogeneous. It is obvious that there are differences between, for example, media used in persuasive advertising, documentary programmes on radio and TV, posters, soap opera and 'edutainment'. It is also important to make a clear distinction between mass media and superficially similar devices, such as videos that are used to trigger discussion and involve interpersonal interaction with a teacher. A video endlessly repeated in a shopping mall is an example of mass media; the same video used as an aid to discussion and learning is a 'learning resource' or visual aid.

Furthermore, we should note a form of media that can be positioned somewhere between the two instances exemplified above. Computer-assisted learning and certain uses of the Internet can embody feedback to learner responses and, in some instances, tailor messages specifically to the learner's needs (Bernhard, 2001).

In this chapter we pose the question, what can we expect from mass media in health promotion? We question the value of a 'traditional' approach and assert that media advocacy should be central to the model of critical health promotion that we espouse in this book.

MASS MEDIA THEORY – CAPABILITIES AND FUNCTIONS

What, then, can we expect from mass media? Implicit in such a question when posed by politicians and practitioners is an expectation of mass behaviour change. While it is clearly the case that mass media can have quite dramatic and often unanticipated effects on populations, an expectation of producing behaviour change – either in pursuit of profit or social welfare and health goals – will typically fail to materialize. Mass media are not a 'magic bullet' that will generate dramatic and widespread success, despite the fact that decisionmakers still tend to ascribe magical qualities to mass communication. Although, doubtless, they are unaware of the fact, the model of mass media on which they base their optimistic expectations is now rather disparagingly described as the 'direct effects' model or 'hypodermic model'. The analogy with the hypodermic is revealing as it derives from the assumptions that:

- mass media have a direct effect on the audience
- mass media act like a hypodermic syringe – the message is like a vaccine, advertisers filling it with a powerful message and injecting it into the population at large
- if it does not actually achieve the desired result, a bigger syringe should be used (more intensive

media blitz) or a different kind medicine (new, more persuasive message)!

This view still prevails, despite the fact that evidence of the limitations of media has existed for decades. For example, Katz and Lazarsfeld (1955) described the influence of mass communications on the audience as a two-step process. Communications instigated by national leaders and transmitted via mass media (in those days, chiefly radio and the press) were 'intercepted' by opinion leaders (see the communication of innovations theory, Chapter 3). Opinion leaders were, almost by definition, more open to, and receptive of, mass media information. They also tended to be sought out for advice by what Katz and Lazarsfeld rather quaintly called the 'rank and file'.

This is not to say that mass media do not, on occasions, have dramatic repercussions (sometimes unintended!). For instance, Orson Welles' dramatic radio broadcast of H.G. Wells' *War of the Worlds* (Cantril, 1958) famously created widespread panic in America. Substantial numbers of people wrote their wills and said farewell to loved ones. Hillbillies, armed with shotguns, went hunting for Martians!

Mendelsohn (1968) also challenged the direct effects model, preferring to use the metaphor of an aerosol spray, arguing that, as the mass media message was sprayed on to the target population, only a small amount actually hit it, most of it 'drifted away' and only a very small proportion 'penetrated'. Klapper (1960, cited in Wallack, 1980: 15) made a similar point:

> Within a given audience exposed to particular communications, reinforcement, or at least constancy of opinion, is typically found to be the dominant effect, minor change as in intensity of opinion is found to be the next most common, and conversion is typically found to be the most rare.

It is also interesting to note that, some thirty years ago, Lazarsfeld and Merton (1955), in their challenge to simplistic views of mass communication effects, identified three conditions for mass media effectiveness.

- **Monopolization** the success of any given influence attempt was most likely where there was no opposition or counter-messages (and, arguably, where there was a limited overall volume of media activity).
- **Canalization** success was most likely to occur where persuasive messages were consistent with the audience's existing motivation and could be 'plugged in' to these existing prejudices, desires and wishes.

- **Supplementation** mass communication would be more likely to succeed when this supplemented, and was supported by, interpersonal influences.

These principles still hold true, but it is possible, as Klapper (1995) argued, to gain greater insights into, and exercise control over, media effects only when mass communication is viewed in the context of broader theories of the individual and society. For these reasons, a brief and selective review of normative and empirical theories is provided below.

The broader context of media effects – normative theory

The term 'normative theory' follows Morrow and Brown's (1994) terminology (see earlier discussion in Chapter 3). It seeks to define the elements essential to adopting a coherent values position and indicates what *ought* to be. In relation to our current concern, it has to do with how mass media ought or ought not to operate in a given social system. A simple instance of this has already been provided when we asserted that, within an empowerment model of health promotion, it is inappropriate to use the techniques associated with a persuasive/marketing model of mass media.

Analytical theories of mass media operation

Berger (1991) has provided one of the most succinct analyses of theories of mass communication. His classification separately identifies:

- a semiological analysis
- a Marxist analysis
- psychoanalytic criticism
- sociological analysis.

A full account of these is not feasible here, but a flavour of the application of psychoanalytical theory is provided in Packard's (1981: 76) classic analysis of the use of depth psychology on Madison Avenue in the following, somewhat exotic, example of marketing women's underwear.

> The most controversial of the eye stoppers … was the 'I Dreamed I Stopped Traffic in My Maidenform Bra' campaign. The situations varied but always the girl involved, dressed fully except that she wore only a bra above the waist, was wandering about among normally dressed people. The theory was that since she was dreaming, her undressed state was permissible. The ad men themselves argued about the wisdom of the ad and the deep-down effect it had on women seeing it. Some

were convinced, after talking with their psychological consultants, that the scene depicted would simply produce an anxiety state in women since it represented a common oneiric, or dream expression of the neurotic anxieties experienced by many women. Others in the trade, however, became convinced, after checking their psychologists, that the ad was sound because the wish to appear naked or scantily clad in a crowd is 'present in most of us' and 'represents a beautiful example of wish fulfilment'. This view evidently prevailed because the campaign was intensified and Maidenform began offering the public prizes up to $10,000 for ideas on dream situations that could be depicted.

Clearly, advertising agencies were convinced about the effectiveness of their use of depth psychology and evidence was produced to demonstrate that particular advertisements resulted in dramatic increases in sales. What, however, is not clear is just what particular aspects of the advertising were responsible for the effect and whether or not it was genuinely due to the application of psychoanalysis. For instance, the Maidenform campaign was allegedly extremely successful, but the novelty value of the presentation would certainly have attracted attention and, as women clearly wanted to buy underwear, the exposure (!) alone might have caused the effect.

When Packard reviewed the relevance of the first edition of his book to society in the 1980s, he acknowledged that in the 1950s, when the book was first published, society was dramatically different. For instance, explicit sexual imagery was quite commonplace in the 1980s and the Maidenform Bra advertisement would certainly lack the novelty value it enjoyed in the 1950s. There is, on the other hand, little doubt that advertisers continue to spend much time, effort and money on developing imagery designed to sell products. The interpretation of this imagery, however, is in our view better explained by semiological theory using discourse analysis techniques than by having recourse to psychoanalysis.

A Marxist perspective

Unlike the individualist focus of psychoanalysis, Marxist media theory demonstrates the ways in which capitalism exercises control over the proletariat by, among other means, use of mass media. Many of the key concepts of Marxism can be applied to the analysis of mass media. McQuail (1994) provides a very succinct summary:

- mass media are owned by the bourgeois class
- media are operated in the interest of the bourgeoisie

- media promote working-class false consciousness
- media access is denied to political opposition.

The notion of 'hegemony' is one of a number of key Marxist notions that Berger thought relevant to the role of mass media in society. Berger (1991: 49) defines hegemony as:

a complicated intermeshing of forces of a political, social, and cultural nature [that] transcends but also includes two other concepts – culture, which is how we shape our lives, and ideology, which, from a Marxist perspective, expresses and is a projection of specific class interest ... Ideology may be masked and camouflaged in films and television programmes and other works carried by mass media but the discerning Marxist can elicit these ideologies and point them out.

Unsurprisingly, mass media would provide an invaluable tool in the process of creating false consciousness and reducing potential threats to the status quo. Similarly, and in relation to the key notion of alienation, Berger (1991: 43–4) argues that:

the media play a crucial role. They provide momentary gratifications for the alienated spirit, they distract the alienated individual from his or her misery (and from consciousness of the objective facts of his or her situation) and, with the institution of advertising, they stimulate desire, leading people to work harder and harder. (Advertising has replaced the Puritan ethic in America as the chief means of motivating people to work hard.)

and, in respect of the consumer society:

people must be driven to consume, must be made crazy to consume, for it is consumption that maintains the economic system. Thus the alienation generated by a capitalist system is functional, for the anxieties and miseries generated by this system tend to be assuaged by impulsive consumption ... Advertising generates anxieties, creates dissatisfactions, and, in general, feeds on the alienation present in capitalist societies to maintain the consumer culture. There is nothing that advertising will not do, use, or co-opt in trying to achieve its goals, and if it has to debase sexuality, co-opt the women's rights movement, merchandise cancer (via cigarettes), seduce children, or terrorize the masses, all of these tactics and anything else will be attempted. One thing that advertising does is divert people's attention from social and political concerns into narcissistic and private concerns. Individual self-gratification becomes an obsession and, with this, alienation is strengthened and the sense of community weakened.

Bearing in mind our early comments on policy and WHO's imperative to deal with inequity in particular and social issues in general, the implication of the above analysis for fostering healthy public policy needs no further emphasis!

Insights from semiology

'Semiology' is the science of signs (from the Greek, *semeion*, which means sign) and derives originally from linguistics. Its founding father was Saussure (1915). Semiology is used virtually interchangeably with 'Semiotics' – a term devised by the American Pierce (1839–1914). Although language was the original sign system subjected to semiotic scrutiny and 'discourse analysis', the methods of study were increasingly applied to signs of all kinds.

One especially relevant application of discourse analysis to mass media is embodied in the concept of 'myth'. Despite the sense in which it is used in everyday parlance, 'myth' does not necessarily mean false beliefs. Chapman and Egger (1983: 167) define it as follows:

> any real or fictional story, recurring theme or character type that appeals to the consciousness of a group by embodying its cultural ideals or by giving expression to deep, commonly felt emotions.

They provide a revealing demonstration of the ways in which myth frequently figures in cigarette advertising in its embodiment of major interests and concerns in a given society. They offer a useful analytical framework for decoding cigarette advertisements and demonstrate how a particular Australian advertisement for Winfield Cigarettes (which enjoyed a 20 per cent share of the market) sought to create the myth of the Winfield smoker. Some key features of the campaign were as follows.

- It used Paul Hogan – a comedian who later enjoyed international fame for his movie portrayal of *Crocodile Dundee*. Hogan was originally a painter on the Sydney Harbour Bridge and was discovered in a talent show prior to becoming 'Winfield Man'. He personified the anti-hero 'rags-to-riches' myth of the working-class male who had made it to the top from humble beginnings without losing the common touch – and thus appealed to the market segment targeted by this particular brand of cigarettes.
- The word 'anyhow' was used in all Winfield advertising – ('Anyhow, Have a Winfield!') This word is allegedly associated in Australian minds with another expression 'she'll be right', which connotes a fatalistic outlook on life (and death), but with a touch of optimism in the face of adversity. As Chapman and Egger indicate, 'the word "anyhow" is probably intended to act as a pat on the back to people on low incomes,

with high mortgages, with bad marriages, with bleak prospects, etc. It is saying "yes, we know your life is dull/bleak/wearying/unrewarding, but … anyhow…"'.

Uses and gratification theory

Uses and gratification theory has a particular relevance to health promotion. It also has the advantage of simplicity. It provides an especially useful explanation of the limitations of the 'hypodermic model' of media operation and also explains why so little of the contents of the 'aerosol' manage to penetrate. In short, it is a mistake of the greatest magnitude to imagine that the audience targeted by media is a passive, homogeneous mass.

Those watching a television programme do not necessarily concentrate on the message alone and in silence. Quite frequently, they will react to programmes by responding to interjections and comments from other viewers; they may switch channels; they may leave the room for refreshments. Even if they do concentrate, there is absolutely no guarantee that they will interpret the messages in the ways intended by the programme's producers (on the basis of research, quite the opposite situation prevails in practice). Moreover, they will not only actively select what they watch, they will interpret it in accordance with the principles of wish fulfilment.

These facts are explained by uses and gratification theory, which follows a kind of 'law of effect'. People *use* the media to *gratify* their desires and satisfy their prejudices. A journalist (Sarler, 1996), commenting on criticisms of a recently deceased 'agony aunt' colleague (Marjorie Proops) for stimulating sexual irresponsibility, made the point rather nicely:

> People knew Miss Proops' views, as surely as they know the views of all journalists who write on a regular basis …When they wrote to her, they knew in advance what she would say … . An estimated 3 per cent of the population did write to her, comfortable in the certainty that she thought what they thought. Not that she could form their thoughts for them … And as one reader said, 'You put that so well; it's just what I have been thinking for ages.'

Berger (1991: 86–91) provides the following comprehensive list of a wide range of typical gratifications offered by the media which clearly illustrates this particular theory of mass media use:

- to be amused
- to see authority figures exalted or deflated
- to experience the beautiful

- to have shared experiences with others/sense of community
- to satisfy curiosity and be informed
- to identify with the deity and the divine plan
- to find distractions and diversion
- to experience empathy
- to experience, in a guilt-free and controlled situation, extreme emotions, such as love and hate, the horrible and the terrible, and similar phenomena
- to find models to imitate
- to gain an identity
- to gain information about the world
- to reinforce our belief in justice
- to believe in romantic love
- to believe in magic, the marvellous and the miraculous
- to see others make mistakes
- to see order imposed on the world
- to participate in history (vicariously)
- to be purged of unpleasant emotions
- to obtain outlets for our sexual drives in a guilt-free context
- to explore taboo subjects with impunity
- to experience the ugly
- to affirm moral, spiritual and cultural values
- to see villains in action.

Implementing policy by means of collaborative consultation

As we observed above, one of health promotion's concerns is with the potentially health-damaging, or, conversely, potentially health-enhancing effects of mass media. In the first instance, of course, the action implication is to control and minimize the effects, while in the second instance, it is to maximize the beneficial effects. The health-damaging consequences of mass media have been well documented and range from the alleged damage inflicted on 'social capital' (as noted above) to specific effects, such as glorifying the use of firearms.

However, there is considerable doubt about the alleged *direct* effects of, say, the portrayal of violence on film or television and, for example, copy cat killings. Indeed, uses and gratification theory would suggest that negative inclinations are already present, that mass media events are merely used as an adjunct to trigger negative behaviour and perhaps shape the form they take. Nonetheless, mass media clearly exert a 'normative effect', as we noted in Chapter 3. Even if they do not exert pressure on individuals to adopt behaviour that they would not otherwise have adopted, they often signal that such behaviour is normal and acceptable. Alcohol consumption is a case in point and one that

has been subjected to substantial research. Before commenting further, it is important to note that we are not necessarily discussing deliberate persuasive advertising. Rather, we are concerned here with 'incidental' effects exerted via a variety of media – of which soap operas are of particular interest.

Soap operas and norm-sending – the case of alcohol

Dorn and South (1983) provided a number of examples of norm-sending, including Breed and Defoe's (1981) extensive examination of media portrayal of alcohol. This latter included not only magazine advertising, but prime-time TV sitcoms, comic books and campus magazines. Finn (1980) reminded us of the range of available media in a study of the way in which greetings cards perpetuate stereotyped images, such as jolly drunks supporting lamp posts. Hansen (1986) provided a thorough and detailed analysis of the portrayal of alcohol on prime-time television in the UK over a fourteen-day period (excluding actual advertising). Unsurprisingly, not only did it figure prominently, but it also had only positive and unrealistic connotations. Later studies have produced similar results and researchers have typically recommended that television companies should adopt a healthier and more responsible approach to alcohol use.

This exhortation has, in fact, been incorporated into approaches concerned with creating 'healthy public policy', using an approach described as 'collaborative consultation'.

Alcohol policy and collaborative consultation

As we observed earlier, there are two possible approaches to health promotion and 'unhealthy' media products. The first is to educate people to critically appraise media and resist its blandishments. The second is the policy implementation route.

As we have seen, policy measures can make the healthy choice the only choice and, in the present instance, would remove the unhealthy, offending representation of alcohol. As we have also seen, there is great reluctance to utilize draconian measures that inpringe on the freedom to choose. However, Defoe and Breed (1989) have argued for the appropriateness of a compromise approach involving 'collaborative consultation', in which health promoters work with media and persuade them to adopt a responsible approach to their programming. According to the authors, this tactic can be effective and they provide an example of a

A SEVEN-POINT CHARTER FOR ALCOHOL PORTRAYAL IN MEDIA

- Try not to glamorize the drinking or serving of alcohol as a sophisticated or an adult pursuit.
- Avoid showing the use of alcohol gratuitously in those cases when another beverage might be easily and fittingly substituted.
- Try not to show drinking alcohol as an activity which is so 'normal' that everyone must indulge. Allow characters a chance to refuse an alcoholic drink by including non-alcoholic alternatives.
- Try not to show excessive drinking without consequences or with only pleasant consequences.
- Demonstrate that there are no miraculous recoveries from alcoholism; normally, it is a most difficult task.
- Don't associate drinking alcohol with macho pursuits in such a way that heavy drinking is a requirement for proving oneself as a man.
- Portray the reaction of others to heavy alcohol drinking, especially when it may be a criticism.

Defoe and Breed, 1989: 257

seven-point code of good practice (see the box) developed with press and television.

To reiterate earlier comments, the success of this policy development resulted from the application of education in a context of negotiation and bargaining. We should also note the limitations of this policy route where compromise is not really possible. While moderate alcohol consumption may actually be beneficial, cigarette consumption is uniquely damaging to health. Given the melancholy history of the mendacity and machinations of the tobacco companies, more draconian actions would be necessary in this case – as we will note in our later discussion of media advocacy.

Soap operas and edutainment

There is considerable evidence of the impacts of soap operas. They illustrate par excellence the uses and gratification theory in practice. Viewers identify with the characters, the characters reappear in other media, such as popular magazines, and so fiction and reality appear to blend seamlessly. Clearly, soap operas are not real – indeed, analysis demonstrates that they caricature reality (for example, in the amount of alcohol apparently consumed and the high incidence of unnatural deaths and criminality!) They do, however, mirror viewers' constructions of reality and focus on common concerns, interests and prejudices.

The potential of soap operas for influencing their audiences has resulted in the invention of the neologism 'edutainment' – defined in the *American Heritage Dictionary of the English Language* (2000) as, 'The act of learning through a medium, particularly media-based, that both educates and entertains' (see also Zeedyk and Wallace, 2003). It is, therefore, of particular interest to place on record Bouman's research into audience responses to a soap in the Netherlands (Bouman et al., 1998, and Bouman, 1999). The programme, *Medisch Centrum West*, a hospital drama, incorporated various health messages about heart disease provided by the Netherlands Heart Foundation.

While it is clearly not possible, nor appropriate, to evaluate such a programme in respect of behaviour change (and certainly not in relation to variations in cardiovascular death rates!), the programme did not trigger any 'reactance' – as might have been expected on the basis of attitude-change theory. Bouman et al.'s (1998: 503) comment on this exercise in 'edutainment' is as follows:

> *Medisch Centrum West* was both entertaining and informative at the same time; although viewers were well aware that the programme included a health message, they did not find it intrusive to their enjoyment of the storyline. It was interesting to learn that fans were more tolerant and positive towards the E & E [entertainment and education] strategy than non-fans. Age, sex and education level explained only 5 per cent of the variance.

MASS MEDIA CAMPAIGNS – PERSUASION AND SOCIAL MARKETING

Discussion of mass media and health promotion probably triggers images of high-profile media work seeking to persuade individuals to abandon unhealthy behaviour and adopt new, healthy behaviour. Apart from any discussion of empowerment and ethics, it is important to ask how effective a media-centred approach of this kind might be. Following our earlier discussion of theories of mass communication, we might expect only very limited effectiveness. The three examples provided below demonstrate different degrees of success. Of course, variations in success will depend on a number of factors, such as the kinds of indicators used, the aspirations embodied in the programme's objectives and the soundness of the theory, practical experience and professionalism, as well as various other factors associated with success, discussed below.

Mass media campaigns – examples of effectiveness

'Be Healthy. Be Active'

The Washington Coalition for Promoting Physical Activity was successful in influencing the target group of adults aged fifty to seventy. There was a 40 per cent increase in awareness of exercise guidelines, a 230 per cent increase in knowledge of yard work, a 116 per cent increase in mentions of vacuuming. There was an increase in beliefs about the benefits of moderate exercise, with a 55 per cent increase in references to 'feeling better', and a 245 per cent increase in those mentioning 'living longer'. Those who were familiar with the campaign were 20 per cent more likely to increase their physical activity in the next six months than those in the control group (see Kotler et al., 2002).

'Five a Day'

This was a Californian programme, funded by the National Cancer Institute, that was designed to promote the recommended dietary measure of eating five portions of fruit and vegetables a day. It demonstrated a number of successful outcomes. From a baseline of 7 per cent, awareness of the programme increased to 15 per cent over a two-year period. Prior to the programme launch, only 8 per cent of a nationally representative sample of American adults reported that, 'five or more was the number of servings of fruit and vegetables to eat each day for good health.' After two years, the proportion had reached 29 per cent.

The proportion of people who believed that eating fruit and vegetables would be 'quite likely' to help prevent cancer had reached 48 per cent after two years. A belief that fruit and vegetable consumption could help with controlling weight increased from 52 per cent to 64 per cent in the same period. However, the percentage of people considering that it would be 'very hard' to eat five

servings a day had actually increased from 8 per cent to 13 per cent (see Lefebvre et al., 1995).

'Safety Leaflet'

A thirty-six-page booklet containing safety advice was produced for carers of young children. It was primarily designed to accompany a series of television programmes.

One and a half million copies of the booklet were distributed (in the UK) over a six-month period. Surveys revealed that some 11 per cent of adults interviewed had seen the publication and 4 per cent claimed to have read it. Of those who had actually viewed the TV programmes, 15 per cent had seen the booklet and 6 per cent reported having read it. Of those who read the publication, 97 per cent were pleased with it and found it useful, while 59 per cent considered that it provided them with new information and understandings (though 76 per cent believed that 'sensible parents would already follow the advice in the booklet'). Around 16 per cent of the 4 per cent who claimed to have read the booklet stated that they, 'now took more safety precautions in the kitchen', 15 per cent were more cautious with medicines and dangerous liquids, 10 per cent took safety action concerning glass, 6 per cent took more fire precautions and checked electrical safety, 4 per cent secured windows, made stairs safer and secured cupboards. By comparison, 9 per cent of a working-class group of child carers who had watched a number of TV programmes adopted one or more of the fifteen possible safety actions that had been advocated. Of a similar group who received a home visit from a public health nurse, 60 per cent had taken some (observed) preventive action (see BBC, 1982, and Jackson, 1983).

Conclusions from these examples

The almost random selection of evaluations of mass media programmes listed above raises a number of questions. The fundamental question might be, 'So, are mass media effective in promoting health?' The answer must, of course, be 'It depends!' A good deal more information would be needed about the programmes, which would come from answers to a further set of questions, thus.

- What were the characteristics of the target group?
- What were the objectives of the programme?
- Which indicators were used to assess effectiveness and efficiency?
- What were the specific components of the programme?

- What could reasonably have been expected and from what theoretical and research base were those expectations derived?

In other words, we would have to assess the extent to which the interventions were based on sound theory and practice before being able to make a valid and reasoned judgement. We can therefore state – not unreasonably – that what you get out depends on what you put in. Probably the most comprehensive and appropriate guidelines for planning mass media programmes have been provided by the art and science of 'social marketing'.

Social marketing and health promotion

According to Solomon (1989), 'The field of social marketing was probably born in 1952, when Wiebe (1952) raised the question, "Why can't you sell brotherhood like you sell soap?" ' He reviewed four examples of what would now be called health promotion campaigns and concluded that their effectiveness was proportional to the extent that they were similar to commercial product marketing. Kotler et al. (2002) identified further seminal events and landmarks in the rise of social marketing. These included an article by himself and Zaltman (1971) and, most recently, the formation of the Social Marketing Institute in 1999.

Kotler et al. (2002: 19–20) define social marketing as follows:

> Social marketing is the use of marketing principles and techniques to influence a target audience to voluntarily accept, reject, modify, or abandon a behaviour for the benefit of individuals, groups, or society as a whole … [it] is largely a mix of economic, communication, and educational strategies … As a last resort, the social marketer may turn to the law or courts to require a certain behaviour.

While it would be generally accepted that mass media campaigns utilize communication and educational strategies, reference to economics and legal measures move beyond the preserve of traditional mass communications. In other words, the important point is made that marketing is more than mass communication and involves interpersonal and policy development. Katz and Lazarsfeld's principle of 'supplementation' mentioned earlier, is relevant here. Mass media are more effective when supplemented by additional interpersonal strategies. Kotler et al. (2002: 20) also identify a number of differences between commercial and social marketing:

> Social marketers focus on selling behaviours, whereas commercial marketers position their products against those of other companies, the social marketer competes with the audience's current behaviour and associated benefits. The primary benefit of a 'sale' in social marketing is the welfare of an individual, a group, or society, whereas in commercial marketing the primary benefit is shareholder wealth.

Kotler et al. (2002: 21–2) also:

> resent the notion that social marketing has the same motivations and therefore the same processes as those found in organizations for profit. Commercial ventures are 'in it' for the shareholders. We're in it for the public good. We don't like the association.

Social marketing and systematic programme planning

One of the undoubted strengths of marketing in general and social marketing in particular is its commitment to systematic programme planning. There is no fundamental difference between the approach described in this book and the various planning strategies that appear in social marketing practice (see, for instance, 'The Montana Model' of systematic coordination', (Linkenbach and D'Atri, 1998)). A more complete review of this and related models is not possible here. However, it is worth recalling our earlier discussion of health needs assessment and the importance of identifying the key characteristics of individuals and communities prior to designing an efficient programme, as well as comparing this with social marketing's key principle of 'audience segmentation'. For instance, Kotler et al. (2002: 125), emphasizing the importance of minimizing the typical 'blunderbuss' approach of much media work, describes the 'American Health Styles Audience Segmentation Project'. This provides a kind of seven-point category caricature scheme of the American population, including an estimate of their percentage prevalence:

- Decent Dolittles 24 per cent
- Active Attractives 13 per cent
- Hard-Living Hedonists 6 per cent
- Tense but Trying 10 per cent
- Non-interested Nihilists 7 per cent
- Physical Fantastics 24 per cent
- Passively Healthy 15 per cent

Ten key marketing concepts

Solomon (1989) listed the following ten key features of social marketing:

- marketing philosophy
- the marketing mix

- a hierarchy of communication effects
- audience segmentation
- understanding relevant markets
- information and rapid feedback systems
- interpersonal and mass media interactions
- utilization of commercial resources
- understanding the competition
- expectations of success.

These points merit some brief discussion.

Marketing philosophy The essential element of marketing philosophy is *exchange*. In other words, the process involves an exchange of something valued by two or more parties. In commercial marketing, it is typically a consumable product that is exchanged for money. In social marketing, it may be an actual product, but, more typically, it will involve ideas or behaviour. Profit is involved and it is defined by Solomon (1989) as, 'what is left over after the expenses are deducted from the revenues for the sale of products or services ... [it] is fairly foreign to social programme planners. But profit need not exist only in monetary terms; it can also be measured in social terms such as increased job satisfaction, happiness, or decrease in mortality.'

The marketing mix The so-called 'marketing mix' refers to four or five 'Ps' – Product, Price, Place, Promotion and, sometimes, Positioning. Kotler et al. (2002) describe three levels of product. These are core products (benefits), actual products (behaviour), augmented products (tangible objects or services).

The main principle for marketing health is that health products should be tangible, attractive and accessible. Unfortunately, health products are frequently intangible, although it is usually possible to translate vague recommendations into precise operations (as noted in our earlier discussion of attitude change in Chapter 6).

Certainly a major problem with many health promotion wish lists is that their accessibility is limited – for instance, a lack of exercise facilities or, more importantly, access to a decent job, money and respect. As for attractiveness, a majority of traditional health promotion goals look distinctly unappetizing or downright painful to the potential customer!

Price is clearly important for all marketing. It may involve actual financial expense, but, typically, the implication for social marketing is, in Kotler et al.'s words, 'managing the costs of behaviour change'. As has been mentioned on more than one

occasion, a major component of the health belief model is a kind of cost–benefit equation. Preventive behaviour will not occur if the anticipated (and real) costs of acting outweigh its perceived benefits. Kotler et al. provide examples of the costs of tangible objects (bike helmets, condoms, sunscreen, earthquake preparedness kits) and services (swimming classes and family planning services). Non-monetary costs include time, effort and energy – for instance, parking one's car before using a mobile phone or using public transport. A third category of non-monetary cost is labelled 'psychological risks and losses', such as embarrassment, fear of rejection. Kotler et al. specifically refer to:

- finding out whether or not a lump is cancerous
- saying no to a second glass of wine
- having a cup of morning tea without a cigarette
- using sunscreen and returning from Hawaii looking pale.

The cost associated with physical discomfort includes activities such as having a mammogram, suffering nicotine withdrawal, taking exercise.

'Place', in commercial marketing would mean retail outlets, distribution systems and motivated, well-trained staff, for example. In social marketing, the importance of having a convenient service is well recognized. It includes not only physical access and convenient appointment systems, but also psychological access, such as a friendly receptionist and a doctor who has such skills as active listening.

The concept of 'promotion' is a rather wideranging one. It includes campaign publicity and, more importantly the complexities of message design and dissemination, together with monitoring and modification. As Solomon (1989: 94) notes:

Promotion is far more than simply and superficially placing advertisements. It is actively reaching out to the right people with the right message at the right time in order to obtain the right effects. And this is not easy to achieve, especially with the large number of competing messages and media.

'Positioning' (the fifth 'P') is substantially concerned with the psychological location of products. It involves framing products or social issues so that target groups will perceive certain characteristics and believe and remember them rather than alternative, less desirable frames.

Other features of marketing With regard to the remainder of Solomon's ten points of social marketing, reference has already been made to audience segmentation and its similarity to what is for health promotion the more conventional notion of needs assessment.

The hierarchy of communication effects is particularly important for health promotion as it is typically expected to deliver totally unrealistic outcomes for the nature of the task and the available resources. Marketing traditionally seeks to assess the impact of its campaigns only in terms of the early stages of the hierarchy – for example, awareness of a campaign, recall of key points and finding the pictures attractive, rather than the tougher 'distal' measures, such as behaviour change. For instance, an award-winning series of TV advertisements for a brand of wholemeal bread achieved a high recognition value but had no impact on sales. Apparently the bakers were quite satisfied that, although sales had not increased, they had maintained their market share in a competitive situation. In a social marketing context, a substantial investment in anti-smoking media advertising that did not achieve any decrease in smoking rates might well be considered an abject failure!

One of Solomon's recommendations is to understand the market. In more conventional health promotion programmes, the parallel would be to assemble appropriate information about the target group (see Chapter 6). Marketing does, however, remind us to think of the existence of multiple markets. For instance, although a primary market might be the general public, a significant secondary market might include politicians or other gatekeepers having the power to veto or sabotage programmes.

The development of a campaign by the English Health Education Council provides a salutary warning. The primary target group was pregnant women who were smokers and the goal of the programme was to persuade them to quit smoking while they were pregnant. A striking image was developed showing a nude, heavily pregnant woman who was smoking. This image had been pretested with the primary group, which was not offended and accepted that it might well be influential. However, it appeared that the community nurses, who were the gatekeepers responsible for displaying posters and leaflets in clinics, were outraged and refused to display the offending nudes!

Information and rapid feedback systems simply urge programme designers to set in place monitoring systems to check the progress of campaigns. For instance, if a monitoring system demonstrates that a programme is having little impact, remedial steps can be taken to increase audience exposure and supplement, say, TV commercials with posters and/or create news stories. In our later discussions of evaluation, we use the more conventional terms of 'process' and 'formative evaluation'.

The requirement to maximize interaction between media and interpersonal interventions merely reiterates Lazarsfeld and Merton's key principle of 'supplementation'. Media campaigns are more successful to the extent that they are supplemented by point-of-sale interpersonal persuasion (or the equivalent in health promotion programmes). As we noted earlier, it is also true that mass media support is likely to accentuate interpersonal education.

The use of commercial resources simply advocates that social marketers utilize existing commercial resources where possible. For instance, Solomon suggests that advertising agents might be persuaded to lend their support (to enhance their own agency's brand image of social responsibility). Such a tactic should be considered with great caution as association with certain commercial ventures might well vitiate the integrity and credibility of health promotion. For instance, to accept the support of antenatal education by manufacturers of powdered milk for babies would be naïve in the extreme. Again, although it can be argued that moderate alcohol consumption is healthy and it may be true that the alcohol industry really does not want to promote binge drinking, considerable care should be exercised before striking up an alliance with that particular agency.

Another of Solomon's ten points will be fully appreciated by health promoters. The recommendation to understand the competition has particular potency. Anti-health competition is not difficult to find – as the running battle between public health and the tobacco industry over many years has demonstrated. At the time of writing, Britain is moving towards a complete ban on advertising of cigarettes. The policy implementation process has been characterized by the need to consistently keep one step ahead of the opposition, to challenge and forestall its manoeuvrings.

The final point concerns expectations of success. This relates to our comments above about the hierarchy of communication effects. Perhaps one of the most useful lessons to be learned from commercial marketing is its recognition that change is difficult to achieve, even with the expenditure of large sums of money. Expectations must be realistic if they are to be achievable. Realistic expectations derive from research and a sound theoretical understanding of what is involved in achieving given results of a particular kind with the specified target groups.

What can we learn from marketing?

As will be apparent from the above observations, those who design health promotion programmes and engage in social marketing can learn a good deal from their commercial counterparts. In general, the lessons are technical, such as the importance of using appropriate techniques in pretesting. In fact, failure to pretest mass media communications is not merely inefficient, it is unethical as the very nature of mass media precludes gaining immediate knowledge of results and, therefore, immediate knowledge of the reactions of clients. In an interpersonal context, the health promoter can virtually instantly determine whether or not clients have misperceived or misunderstood information or if the educator has generated inappropriate levels of counterproductive anxiety. Where this has happened, they can take immediate steps to rectify misperception or inappropriate belief and assuage anxiety. However, in respect of the broader picture, we might usefully consider the somewhat plaintive and rhetorical question embodied in the title of an influential article by Rothschild (1979). He reiterated Wiebe's question, asking why it was so hard to sell brotherhood like soap. The answer, of course, is that brotherhood is not like soap – marketing commercial products is fundamentally and qualitatively different from marketing health.

As we are told by uses and gratification theory, people selectively respond to mass media messages. As exchange theory reminds us, people will exchange money – or, in social marketing terms, effort and behaviour – for something they want. Unfortunately, whereas the audience for chocolate actually likes chocolate, is keen to eat it and will buy the brand image of a particular kind of chocolate that gratifies its needs, but would be quite happy to eat another brand, by and large, health is not a very appealing product except in the abstract. Clearly, few people would claim that they did not want to be healthy, but, equally, they would prefer to avoid what is frequently involved in becoming healthy as they will perceive that this typically involves one or more of the following outcomes: inconvenience, loss of gratification, embarrassment, discomfort or even pain! If a product does not sell and if rebranding is ineffective because people do not actually want the product, manufacturers will cut their losses and sell something else. Health promoters cannot abandon their product: they are committed to fostering individual and public health.

Advocacy for healthy public policy – the role of mass media

One of the most dramatic contrasts between normative theories in health promotion can be seen in the confrontation between the traditional, coercive model of mass media communication and the approach that is now generally called 'media advocacy' (which received some consideration earlier in Chapter 6). It does, however, seem to be the case that *some* interpretations of the concept of social marketing might be located somewhere between these two positions. Nonetheless, in its traditional form, the focus on persuasion and its individualistic orientation is more akin to the coercive model.

One of the more vitriolic condemnations of the persuasive use of mass communication has been provided by Rakow (1989: 169–70) in her discussion of critical theory and information campaigns. She reiterates a point that we made earlier in our discussions of ideology when she comments that:

> Bureaucratic organizations are ... selective about the information they provide, which exposes the myth that simply providing information is a commendable activity. Organizations control which information will be made available to whom because their goal is not really to inform but rather to control... . That one can presume to have even the *right* to persuade someone else, let alone the *responsibility* to do so is never questioned ... . [this] cultural preoccupation with persuasion reflects a conquest mentality that justifies the 'violence' [invasiveness] of strategies to change others, reflecting a larger cultural – masculine – propensity to dominate and conquer.

Rakow (1989: 169–70) also forcefully challenges the downstream tendency to utilize media in the service of individual behaviour change rather than addressing the root causes and determinants of unhealthy outcomes:

> What information is a potential client of a social service agency going to be given? How to beat the system that put her in the situation in the first place? Why behaviour such as drug use or teenage pregnancy are portrayed as the country's most important problems and not militarism, violence against women, or homelessness? Why is the medical profession targeting individuals with health messages such as restriction of cholesterol intake rather than targeting government and industry who are responsible for the actions and policies that put carcinogens in our food, pollute our planet, determine whose health problems get research attention, and the like?

The alternative strategies advocated by Rakow involve community development and participation. As we will see, Wallack and colleagues also emphasize community involvement, but consider that mass media may make a substantial contribution in tandem with community work in advocating healthy public policy. However, before examining this orientation more closely, it is illuminating to consider alternative views of the ways in which mass media might address the fundamental health issue of inequalities.

The health divide – contributions of mass media

In 1997, a working group was established by the English Health Education Authority to consider the most efficient use of mass media in tackling problems of inequality in health (Hastings et al., 1998).

Two conflicting approaches to addressing this fundamental issue for health promotion were identified. The first of these centres on the use of audience segmentation as part of 'database marketing'. The techniques involved are exemplified by the tobacco industry's practice of directly marketing brands to specific target communities and individuals on the basis of such characteristics as their socio-economic status and personal traits, particularly by direct mail. The technique is associated with 'relationship marketing' – that is, the attempt to build a relationship with customers. As Hastings et al. (1998: 49) explain:

> Loyal customers … buy more … products, are easier to satisfy, are less price-sensitive and make positive recommendations to their friends and family. … acquiring new customers through research, promotion and other marketing is up to five or six times more expensive than retaining existing ones. Similarly, research indicates that the average company loses 10 per cent of its customers each year … by contrast unhappy customers are a considerable liability – they stop buying the company's products – usually without warning – often support the competition and complain to their friends and family.

'Emotional branding' is considered to play a major part in selling commercial or social products. As Hastings et al. (1998) note, 'customers buy products to satisfy not only objective, functional needs, but also symbolic needs, e.g. self-enhancement or group identification (Hirshman and Holbrook, 1982) … [for example] the prospective smoker does not have an objective need for nicotine, but rather a symbolic need to display independence or rebellion (Barton, et al. 1982).'

Social marketers should, therefore, ensure that product 'tonality' matches the needs of their target audience. Lower social status and disadvantaged groups require special treatment (Hastings et al., 1998: 52):

> There is also evidence that branding may be a particularly effective way to reach people in deprived communities. Research into how working-class populations use cultural symbols in advertising found that these groups are often poorly informed about the objective merits of different products and therefore tend to rely more heavily than other groups on 'implicit meanings' – context, price, image – to judge products (Durgee, 1986). … de Chernatony (1993) and Cacioppo and Petty (1989) found that people in deprived communities are less likely to evaluate products on a rational objective basis, but look for clues as to the product's value in terms of its price or its image. They argued that the symbolic appeal of brands is particularly effective in targeting those individuals who do not have the time, skills or motivation to evaluate the objective attributes and benefits of a particular campaign.

Method one, then, for reaching disadvantaged groups is careful targeting of health messages, followed by building relationships and then delivering an appropriate brand mix of positive effects. The alternative strategy to address the 'health divide' is to use media advocacy to challenge the social and political system that results in the disadvantage in the first place! Media advocacy is the recommended empowering approach to achieve these ends.

Defining media advocacy – social justice and market justice

Wallack et al. (1993), in their classic text, challenge the individualistic, victim-blaming tendency, asserting that advocacy:

> is necessary to steer public attention away from disease as a personal problem to health as a social issue… [It] is a strategy for blending science and politics with a social justice value orientation to make the system work better, particularly for those with the least resources.

Wallack et al. (1993: 7) make a succinct and coherent distinction between market justice and social justice in a number of observations that chime with our discussion of voluntarism in Chapter 2.

> Market justice suggests that benefits such as healthcare, adequate housing, nutrition, and sustainable employment are rewards for individual effort (on a level playing field), rather than goods and services that society has an obligation to provide. Market justice depends on enlightened self-interest as a guarantor of the distribution of necessary goods and services to those in need.

Wallack illustrates this philosophy, which is so deeply embedded in the USA (and, indeed, many European societies), by citing Galbraith's (1973: 5–6) classic and maverick approach to economics and his critique of American large corporations:

> The corporate economic is not responsible – or is only minimally responsible – for what it does… If the goods that it produces or the services it renders are frivolous

[ADVOCACY – THE STRUGGLE]

If there is no struggle, there is no progress. Those who profess to favour freedom, and yet deprecate agitation, are men who want crops without ploughing up the ground. They want rain without thunder and lightning. They want the ocean without the awful roar of its many waters. This struggle may be a moral one; or it may be a physical one; or it may be both moral and physical; but it must be a struggle. Power concedes nothing without a demand.

Frederick Douglass, 1857, cited by Wallack et al., 1993: 39

or lethal or do damage to air, water, landscape or the tranquility of life, the firm is not to blame. This reflects public choice. If people are abused, it is because they choose self-abuse.

Social justice, on the other hand, 'is concerned with whether conditions in society are fair and whether resources are distributed equitably. Too often they are not.' (Galbraith, 1973.)

A healthy society is a democratic society founded on social justice (Krieger, 1990: 414, cited by Wallack et al., 1993: 15):

Democracy is about having a stake because you are a real participant. It is about knowing whom to hold accountable, and it is about having the power to hold them accountable. Democracy is not about letting priorities be set by a bureaucratic or technocratic élite, or by the 'blind forces' of the market (which always turn a blind eye toward human suffering); it is about constructing a social agenda, based on human need, through informed and active popular participation at every level.

Subscribing to the 'religious mystique' of individualism and market forces is uncontroversial, so social marketing is entirely acceptable within the dominant ideology. The use of media advocacy is not!

Distinctions between traditional media use and media for advocacy

The main differences between traditional media practices in health promotion and the practice of media advocacy are summarized as follows (following Wallack et al., 1993: 75–60). Traditional mass media direct messages from a central source to a mass audience. They involve one-way communication and, typically, limit audience involvement to pretesting and segmentation. Media advocacy, on the other hand, has close links with communities

and 'seeks to provide community groups with skills to communicate their own story in their own words.' Accordingly, media advocacy has been considered to involve 'narrow-casting' rather than broadcasting and is targeted at relatively small audiences and individual decisionmakers. Community members are viewed as potential advocates and change agents. The focus of traditional mass communication is on *individual* attitude and behaviour change, whereas media advocacy seeks to develop 'healthy public policy'. Although advocacy addresses short-term, pressing issues, the goal is to set this within the broader context of general policy change designed to address social and environmental determinants of health. A peculiar feature of media advocacy is its concern with agenda setting and critical consciousness raising. Media advocates are health activists who confront social rather than individual 'pathogens'. They therefore seek to make full use of news channels by reacting to news and creating it. They present themselves as, 'partners in the news-making and gathering processes.' The use of news is supplemented by appropriate use of paid media placements. Public service announcements (PSAs) are viewed with suspicion as they rarely have access to prime-time programming and controversial issues are likely to be censored. In short, media advocacy aims to fill the 'power gap' rather than the 'information gap'.

Agenda setting

Our earlier comments about the 'aerosol model' and mass media strengths and limitations have received support over the years from many distinguished theoreticians and practitioners. Cohen (1963: 13), for example, commented on the power of the press as follows:

[the press] may not be successful much of the time in telling people what to think, but it is stunningly successful much of the time in telling people what to think *about.* [An observation also attributed to Ed Murrow, the distinguished American journalist and radio reporter.]

Cohen continues with an apt observation that both supports the uses and gratification theory and indicates the role of media producers in shaping opinion:

the world looks different to different people, depending not only on their personal interests but also on the map that is drawn for them by the writers, editors, and publishers of the papers they read.

A major function of media advocates is thus to 'draw particular maps' that highlight key social issues following the now well-recognized strategy of 'agenda setting'. Wallack et al. (1993: 61) offer a nice image (from Lippmann, 1965) of the process of agenda setting as 'directing the searchlight':

Mass media are like the beam of a searchlight that moves restlessly about, bringing one episode and then another out of darkness into vision.

The empowerment model of health promotion, discussed in Chapter 1, emphasized the importance of agenda setting. We should, however, perhaps comment that, in addition to Wallack's interpretation of agenda setting, the empowerment model also acknowledges situations when creating a degree of publicity about an issue (putting it on the public's agenda) might allow a government to gauge public reaction before proceeding to implement restrictive policies without losing popularity – and votes.

The empowerment model placed particular emphasis on the process of 'critical consciousness raising' (CCR) as a more potent device than agenda setting – one that often seeks to bring about quite radical political change. CCR will be revisited in our discussion of community development below.

However, to move on, we might ask who or what are the customary agenda setters? As we observed in Chapter 3, opinion leaders will not only react to events, but may also take a lead. For example, Wallack et al. commented that President Bush (the first) seemed to have 'set the agenda' following a major speech announcing a war on drugs. Agencies and organizations can play an important part, too. In the USA, for instance, it has been suggested that newspaper empires such as *The New York Times* frequently fulfil an agenda-setting role.

Narrow-casting

Reference was made above to media advocacy's 'narrow-casting' approach. This is an important characteristic of advocacy's employment of media.

It asserts that, although, ultimately, the general population is the target, the primary goal will typically be decision-makers, legislators, community leaders and community groups. As Wallack et al. (1993: 78) observe:

Media advocacy isn't about a mass audience. It's not about reaching everybody. It's about targeting the two or three per hundred who'll get involved and make a difference. It's about starting a chain reaction.

They also illustrate the narrow-casting function of media advocacy in relation to attempts to challenge the impact of the giant McDonald's chain on the nation's diet. They (1993: 118–19) describe a radio spot produced by Schwartz that:

addressed the CEO of McDonald's by name and told him he could be a hero to children all over the world if he just changed the way his company fried its food. ... when people hear their names or the names of their organizations mentioned in a spot, they not only pay attention but imagine everyone else hearing the spot is paying attention as well. Schwartz wanted to change the behaviour of only one man; his radio message had an intended audience of one.

Media advocacy and civil disobedience – the case of BUGA UP

BUGA UP was an Australian movement that followed a particularly vigorous and radical pathway, adopting tactics that were, on occasions, of dubious legality and included civil disobedience.

The acronym stands for Billboard Utilizing Graffitists Against Unhealthy Promotions and activists set out to alter advertising messages on billboards and other displays with spray cans to replace them with more appropriate healthy messages. Examples of the finished products included changing the messages on a very large billboard located on top of a building at one of Sydney's crossroads. The original was an advertisement for Marlborough cigarettes. After the 'spray can surgery', it read 'It's a Bore'. A rather more risqué (although perhaps not for Australia) facelift was given to a poster advertising Winfield cigarettes, which incorporated the emblematic term 'Anyhow' (see the discussion on page 244 of myth creation). After the improvements it read, 'anyhow ... have a Wank IT'S HEALTHIER'.

The activists were accused of defacing private property. They claimed that they were 're-facing' it.

Chesterfield-Evans and O'Connor (1986: 241) indicate the effects of this 'civil disobedience':

The group has attracted hundreds of people of all ages. Among about fifty arrests there have been five doctors and a university professor. The charges have generally been along the lines of 'malicious damage'. But the definition of 'malicious' involves 'indifference to human life and suffering' and this has been used by the graffitists to deny malicious intent and maintain that the advertisement was malicious prior to its message being altered. Hence the graffiti 'improved' the ad.

Examples of the re-facing of posters can be seen in Figure 8.1.

The quotation from Chesterfield-Evans and O'Connor indicates two of the main strengths of BUGA UP's approach. The activists were eminently respectable people and their facing up to the giant tobacco corporations was readily 'framed' in terms of the myth of David and Goliath. Chapman's description of the origins of BUGA UP reveals that the reasons for its members' dissatisfaction was that existing health education approaches to smoking were having little effect and thay felt that they should 'refocus upstream'.

Chapman and Lupton (1994) described the major achievement of this group as barring the actor Paul Hogan from advertising Winfield cigarettes because of his enormous popularity with children. The success generated headlines that encapsulated the David and Goliath myth – 'MOP UP's slingshot cuts down the advertising ogre'.

It is important to note at this point that media advocacy is one particular strategy within the general armamentarium of public health advocacy (see Chapter 7). However, as with all effective mass media use, it is important to combine media with interpersonal methods – as with the principle of supplementation mentioned earlier. Chapman and Lupton (1994), in their 'A–Z of public health advocacy', describe a full range of detailed tactics that can be employed.

One of the important tactics included in the complete list of sixty-five tactics, but not listed in the box, is 'creative epidemiology', which was reviewed earlier in Chapter 6, together with another item that figured in the full list – 'demonstrations'.

We will now provide a specific illustration of a consciousness raising demonstration that, unusually, is not from Australia or America but the UK. We should perhaps note in passing that, although demonstrations are not media events as such, their impact frequently depends on their attracting (unpaid) media attention.

The demonstration was associated with a display of art. The tobacco manufacturer John Player sponsored an art exhibition at the National Portrait Gallery in London. A UK advocacy organization, AGHAST, decided to enter a specially commissioned portrait entitled 'The Early Death of Jack Filbert'. It showed an emaciated man in his early thirties propped up in a hospital bed, complete with oxygen cylinder. He held a cigarette in his hand.

A slide of the painting was shortlisted for the second round of judging. Tobacco executives were involved in the final shortlisting procedure. Unsurprisingly, they decided that the portrait of a smoker dying from lung cancer was not appropriate for their exhibition!

Accordingly, AGHAST held its own alternative exhibition entitled 'The Lung Slayer Portrait Award' outside the National Portrait Gallery. Good press coverage was achieved and *The Guardian* newspaper provided a photograph of the Jack Filbert portrait, but not the tobacco award winner.

TEN TACTICS FROM AN A–Z OF PUBLIC HEALTH ADVOCACY

Be there! The first rule of advocacy
Crank letters (or how to put your opposition's worst foot forward)
Gatecrashing
Jargon and ghetto language
Media cannibalism (how media feed off themselves)
Networks and coalitions
'Piggy backing'
Shareholders
Talkback (access) radio
Wrestling with pigs

Chapman and Lupton, 1994

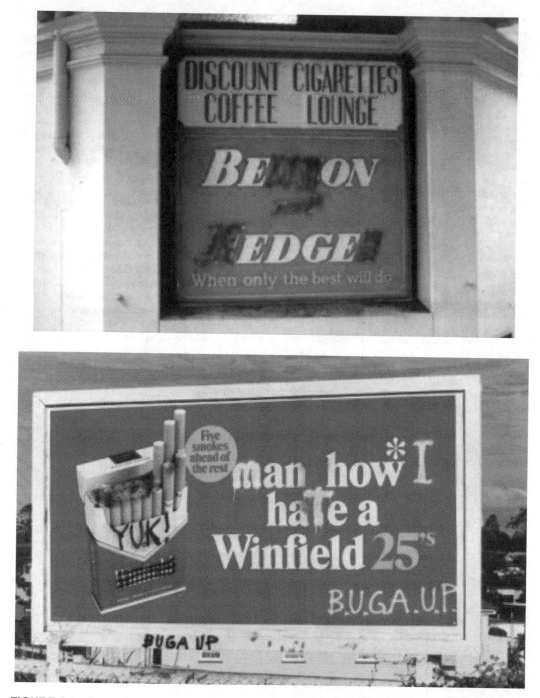

FIGURE 8.1 Examples of the work of BUGA UP's media advocacy work
http://www.bugaup.org/gallery.htm 25/3/02

Key principles and generalizations about mass media

We have hopefully made it clear in this discussion about media advocacy that its philosophy and approach involves close collaboration with communities and community development for social change. Working with communities will constitute our next major health promotion strategy for review. Before we do this, we believe it might be useful to summarize the main principles and generalizations about using mass media for the promotion of health, as follows (Tones and Tilford, 2001: 386–7).

- Mass media should not be used on their own. They should, however, be used to support programmes that centre on interpersonal interactions, such as in schools, workplaces and other settings. They should be considered an integral part of community-wide programmes, working in tandem with supportive policy measures.
- Potentially the most effective use of mass media is in the form of media advocacy – that is, creating public awareness of issues. The following variants are in ascending order of potential effectiveness and radicalism:
  - gaining unpaid advertising by providing newsworthy information
  - agenda setting about health issues as a precursor to later action
  - consciousness raising using creative epidemiology to stimulate actions having a focus on disease and inequalities in health
  - critical consciousness raising about social, economic and environmental issues in the pursuit of equity, supported by various additional advocacy strategies, such as demonstrations and civil disobedience.
- Major policy change may be problematic and 'consultative collaboration' with media funders and producers may be the only possible strategy for health promotion.
- The use of soap operas and other entertainment programmes has a number of particular advantages. They should be used where possible, provided that it is remembered that their main purpose is to entertain (and make money)! Edutainment may be more amenable to fostering health promotion goals as part of its brief as it is, by definition, education.
- Bearing in mind the fundamental differences between marketing commercial products and health products, all mass media work should follow tried and tested marketing principles, in particular the following.

- Audience segmentation, which should be considered an essential element in the process of identifying target groups and needs assessment. The following are especially important:
  (a) database marketing, which increasingly offers scope for moving beyond the description of general demographic variables and assessing psychographic characteristics – beliefs, values and so on
  (b) recognition that it is often necessary to address both primary and secondary audiences, including gatekeepers.
- It is essential to assess the socio-economic and other structural aspects of the target groups that may act as barriers to their responding to the media messages.
- Set realistic objectives, bearing in mind that, although mass media can successfully raise awareness, transmit relatively simple information and produce a positive attitude to message presentation, they cannot create complicated understandings, nor teach the skills needed to support health-related behaviour, nor can they affect beliefs and influence attitudes where these are inconsistent with existing value systems and motivation.
- Plan the delivery of the media programme such that the target receives sufficient exposure. Individuals may need to receive the same messages several times before they manage to absorb and remember it. Also, of course, it should be delivered via media that are used by, and accessible to, the target group.
- Repetition of messages may need to continue for a long period of time if the main purpose is not just to ensure that the message is remembered, but, rather, to act in a norm-sending way – that is, to breed familiarity but not contempt!
- Analyse the nature of the messages to be transmitted, focusing on the audience's likely perceptions of the benefits and costs implicit in the message. Remember that costs are not merely financial, but also have to do with experiencing inconvenience, discomfort, pain or loss of gratification. Even minimal costs are likely to result in a failure to influence behaviour (though the message may set the agenda for subsequent successful interpersonal influence).
- Adopt an appropriate style for message delivery ('branding') – positive affect is

more likely to be successful than negative affect. Take account of the fact that long-term, distal benefits may have zero attraction, especially for young people – short-term gains are more attractive. Beware of using fear appeal – it is hardly ever the most effective strategy in the long run and may create defensive avoidance. If fear is to be aroused, there must be some means of reducing any anxiety generated – for example, by setting up accessible sources, personal support and advice, available either directly or via telephone hotlines.

- The message can often be crafted to provide inoculation against anticipated negative messages and products. When handled with care, this can be a useful function for media work.
- Use an appropriate source, even if this is just a voiceover. The source must be credible and, preferably, provide an attractive model for the adoption of recommended attitudes or behaviour. Credible sources can lose their credibility in a remarkably short period of time. For instance, youth audiences are notoriously fickle in their allegiances.
- Do not patronize, demean or otherwise antagonize the audience!
- More effective campaigns use multiple media.
- All mass media should be pretested following recommended guidelines for formative research.

• The mass media are still frequently seen as a panacea. They are also especially attractive to politicians as the appearance on television of dramatic and attractive 'commercials' (such as on the evils of drug abuse) may at least convince voters that their government is taking positive action (however ineffectively). It is, therefore, essential to submit campaigns that have unrealistic goals to critical appraisal and evaluation.

WORKING WITH COMMUNITIES – ORGANIZATION, DEVELOPMENT AND SOCIAL ACTION

[Community development is] a strategy for the attainment of social policy goals. It is concerned with the worth and dignity of people and the promotion of equal opportunity... [it] is most needed in communities where social skills and resources are at their weakest. [It] involves working with those most affected by poverty, unemployment, disability, inadequate housing and education, and with those who for reasons of class, income,

race or sex are less likely than others to be, or to feel, involved and significant in local community life.

Calouste Gulbenkian Foundation, 1984

We have emphasized in earlier chapters the centrality of community participation in health promotion. Our focus here is on the strategy of community development (CD) and, at first glance, it would appear that there is no strategy more congruent with the ideology of health promotion. Readers doubtless do not need to be reminded of WHO's 'purple passages' referring to the primacy of equity and the importance of active participating communities – and, of course, empowerment. Community development espouses these goals wholeheartedly.

CD, however, is by no means unproblematic. There is, for example, some confusion over terminology and, more importantly, a view that it has serious limitations in achieving equity and empowerment – it may even be counterproductive. Moreover, our description of CD as a 'strategy' might be criticized as many would see it as a 'process' that somehow emerges from within a community and so to talk about strategies implies a deliberate external intervention that may be (wrongly) viewed as a cosmetically concealed top-down, authoritarian attempt at coercion.

We have already recognized, in our comments on communication of innovations theory in Chapter 3, that change may indeed occur within a community without any outside intervention, provided that the community recognizes it has a problem and then generates its own solutions. We are, however, interested here in those situations where communities are relatively powerless – they may not even enjoy the status of communities – and some kind of outside intervention is essential to jump start the empowerment process. This we define as a strategy – to be compared and contrasted with other strategies, particularly with the use of mass communication as described earlier in this chapter.

After defining the concept of community and the nature and history of community development, some consideration is given to ideological issues. A typology of different types of community strategies will be offered prior to critically appraising the strengths and limitations of CD. Finally, we comment on some technical and methodological aspects and present a model that is designed to address some of the concerns about CD while retaining its traditional strengths. We also emphasize the importance as a central component of critical education.

CD – definitions and history

Bivins (1979) described CD as an old and reliable grass-roots approach to health education and gave examples of its use in the 1940s, although its principles and applications were in use at a much earlier date (see also Cox et al., 1979). For instance, Hilton (1988: 3–4), using the synonym 'community organization', sees its origins in the Antigonish movement in the 1920s. The principles of this religious organization are entirely consistent with CD, namely:

- each person is endowed by God with intellectual, volitional (act of will) and physical faculties that must be developed to obtain full and abundant life for all
- major social institutions of society must be transformed to guarantee equal opportunity and full development of all people
- adult education and group action are the most effective means whereby the common people themselves will be able to transform social institutions and this will be done by defining and controlling the nature and direction for social change
- the process begins when common people use adult education and group action to solve their immediate social and economic problems.

Kindervatter (1979: 71) also referred to the origin of CD in the 1920s:

Community organization first appeared in US social work textbooks in the 1920s and 1930s; however, not until the War on Poverty in the sixties did the concept and its application receive much attention. [Its] purpose is to enable communities to improve and change their socio-economic milieu and/or their position in that milieu. [It] developed largely as a response to the conditions of poor people in Western urban settings, but is now practised in a variety of forms in urban and rural locales, in Third World as well as technologically advanced contexts.

The concept of community

The English health policy document 'Our Healthier Nation' (Department of Health, 2002: 1) defines a healthy community as one that, 'contains or enables access to all things which allow people to live a full life.' A community is a 'setting':

- where diversity and local character are celebrated
- where everyone is valued equally, regardless of race, age and gender
- where people are responsible citizens and support each other
- with ready access to the necessities of everyday life, including good work prospects, adequate

shops and high-quality public services, such as schools, and medical and social care

- where people like to be and where they can and do join in
- which is safe and environmentally sound
- which provides healthy housing
- with good transport links
- which has good opportunities for play and recreation.

While the sentiments are undoubtedly appropriate and the implications for creating social capital are of interest, it is misleading to conflate 'community' with 'neighbourhood', as has happened here. A neighbourhood is best defined as a 'setting' whereas a community is characterized by the existence of a network of relationships and a shared sense of identity, predicament and perhaps purpose. Whereas, traditionally, most CD work has operated within a relatively small and self-contained geographical location of similar size to a neighbourhood, the notion of 'virtual community' exists outside of geographical boundaries – note, for instance, the gay community or a professional community of, say, physiotherapists.

Ideological dimensions of community development

We observed earlier that the ideological purpose of CD was akin to the goals of an empowerment model of health promotion and the statements of purpose promulgated by WHO over several years.

The very existence of a genuine community is frequently seen as a desirable goal in its own right – that is, a social system that actually shares a sense of purpose and has a coherent network of social relationships. The idea of a 'sense of purpose', however, would normally be an extension to that of a 'sense of community'. According to the oft-quoted definition of McMillan and Chavis (1986) this latter has four main components:

- **membership** a feeling of belonging
- **influence** a sense of mattering
- **integration and fulfilment of needs**
- **shared emotional connection**.

Where a community also possesses an additional fund of competences such that it can offer social support to its members, it can also be said to be healthy. The currently popular description of this 'fund of competences' is, of course, social capital. One of the more adequately substantiated truths in health promotion is that social support is good for you! For instance, Gottlieb and McLeroy (1992) considered that social support was one of three features of social health. They demonstrated its effectiveness not only for social health, but also for disease prevention. They also remarked that a number of studies from the hundred or so articles published on the subject each year from 1989 to 1991 had demonstrated the beneficial effects of social participation. They summarize these effects as follows:

- the impact of social relationships on physical health is non-specific and is related to all-cause mortality
- risk of dying is increased with very low levels of social interaction
- the impact of social interaction on health varies with community size and gender – it is stronger in urban than in rural areas.

It could reasonably be argued, therefore, that, if this is true, then the mere fact of creating or building communities having social capital where none existed before is quintessentially health-promoting. However, the ultimate ideological goal of health promotion and CD is the achievement of equity and the reduction of inequalities – a point robustly articulated by the report produced by the Calouste Gulbenkian Foundation (1984) on CD cited above.

Typologies of community work

A number of terms have been used, sometimes interchangeably, for a variety of related interventions in the community context. One of the most influential typologies was produced by Rothman (1979).

He separately identified 'locality development', 'social planning' and 'social action'. The main differences between them are as follows:

- **locality development** self-help; community capacity and integration (process goals)
- **social planning** problem solving with regard to community problems (task goals)
- **social action** shifting of power relationships, achievement of social change (task/process goals).

There seems to be general agreement about the meaning of social action as a movement embodying protest and associated with Alinsky's (1969; 1972) radical activities. Kirklin and Franzen (1974: 5) describe this succinctly:

Large numbers of people are organized to bring into being a new power aggregate (or community organization) to force the existing political/economic power structure to change public and private policies. The battle is classically seen to be between the 'power haves' and the 'power have nots'.

Social planning is also generally understood to refer to top-down programmes that involve systematic planning – although Nix (1970) prefers to use the term 'technical planning'. We have described this type of intervention as a Type 5 programme in Figure 8.2.

Twelvetrees (1982) provides another related classification system when he identifies three overlapping approaches to community work:

- **community development** – proper
- **political action** – similar to Alinsky's social action approach
- **social planning** – collaboration between voluntary bodies and the state to change and improve services.

Great confusion exists over the terminology for community development 'proper'. Some would view it as identical to 'locality development', but others see it as equivalent to 'community organization' and yet others may use the term to describe what are essentially social or technical planning programmes. Ross et al. (1967: 40), for instance, prefer the following definition:

Community organization ... is to mean a process by which a community identifies its needs or objectives, orders (or ranks) these needs or objectives, develops the confidence and will to work at these needs or objectives, finds the resources (internal and/or external) to deal with these needs and objectives, takes action in respect to them, and in so doing, extends and develops cooperation and collaborative attitudes and practices in the community.

This particular definition of community organization most nearly approximates to our interpretation of community development – and to European practice.

In the 1960s and early 1970s in the UK, a number of CD 'demonstration projects' were launched and an assessment of the results was published by the national Community Development Project Intelligence and Information Unit (1974). The report is particularly valuable in that it makes it very clear that 'pure' community development rarely happens (always assuming that there is agreement about just what 'pure' CD actually is!). The authors seek to categorize the varieties of approach that might be observed in actual practice. In fact, nine such varieties were identified and categorized in relation to different 'levels' and 'assumptions' (see Table 8.1 on page 262).

In respect of our discussions so far, Type 1 – social planning – approximates to our earlier reference to social or technical planning. On the other hand, Types 3, 6 and 9, which are considered to be

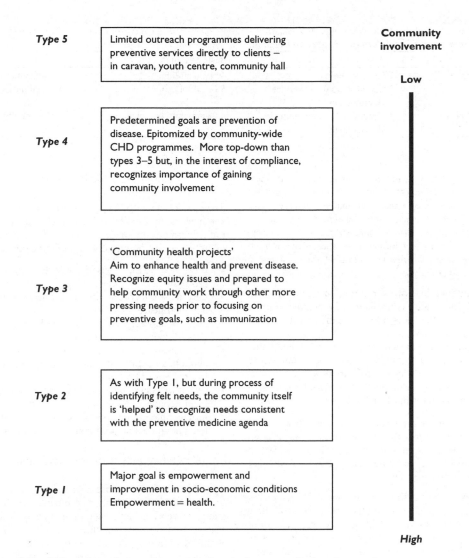

Type 5 — Limited outreach programmes delivering preventive services directly to clients – in caravan, youth centre, community hall

Type 4 — Predetermined goals are prevention of disease. Epitomized by community-wide CHD programmes. More top-down than types 3–5 but, in the interest of compliance, recognizes importance of gaining community involvement

Type 3 — 'Community health projects' Aim to enhance health and prevent disease. Recognize equity issues and prepared to help community work through other more pressing needs prior to focusing on preventive goals, such as immunization

Type 2 — As with Type 1, but during process of identifying felt needs, the community itself is 'helped' to recognize needs consistent with the preventive medicine agenda

Type 1 — Major goal is empowerment and improvement in socio-economic conditions Empowerment = health.

Community involvement

Low

High

Figure 8.2   Categories of programmes by level of community involvement

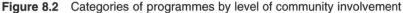

grass roots operations, describe what would normally be considered to be community development 'proper'. The purpose of Type 2 actions is to, 'bring about changes in organizational practices, by managerial and administrative rearrangements.' Types 4 and 5 involve the well-recognized processes of negotiation and bargaining and are central to the factors associated with successful intersectoral collaboration. Types 7, 8 and 9 derive from recognition of the structural conflict between ideologies and different power bases inherent in society.

Political pressure at national and local levels, together with community action, are necessary if substantial political change is to occur.

The national Community Development Project Information and Intelligence Unit (1974: 25) definition of 'traditional' CD is interesting. The authors see it as aiming to:

bring about changes in the functioning of individuals, groups, and 'communities' by facilitating their integration into more coherent wholes. The 'community' is

Table 8.1   *Models of social change and possible strategies on three Levels of operation (Community Development Project Information and Intelligence Unit, February 1974: 24)*

Level		Basic assumptions		
National	1 Social planning	4 National lobby		7 National pressure
Local	2 Organizational and service development	5 Local lobby		8 Local pressure
Grass roots	3 'Traditional' community development	6 Community organization		9 Community action

assumed to be homogeneous in its needs and where conflicts of interest are found, these are reconcilable through better communication and intergroup relations. The process of community development is often seen as more important than any product, that is development of community relationships is seen as an end in itself, rather than primarily as a means of solving common external problems.

The authors do, however, note that structures such as neighbourhood councils may be created in order to represent the community more effectively in relation to external decisionmakers.

'Community organization', on the other hand, was considered to be the closest approximation to the majority of local projects described in the report. The predicaments of the communities in question derive from a lack of power:

> The powerlessness of residents to control their own life situations, or to influence the decisions which affect their areas, is seen to be related partly to their lack of information, access to relevant expertise and advocacy and poor organization.

However, the author (Community Development Project, 1974: 26) questions the success of these endeavours as much of the activity 'has been limited to here-and-now issues, and has been in reaction to agency programmes, rather than any real claiming of initiative for change.'

There seems to have been little evidence of 'community action' (Type 9) – the kind of social action advocated by Alinsky and Freire.

Community development and participation

As we noted earlier, 'pure' CD is relatively rare. In fact, analysis of various community-orientated programmes reveals an often wide divergence in the extent to which the community rather than the external agent or agency is in control. Of course, this is an important issue, bearing in mind our earlier comments about the relationship between community control and adoption of innovations – of all kinds, including taking political action.

Community health projects

The characteristics of Type 3 projects are succinctly summarized by Rosenthal (1983), who reveals their radical dimension in the context of what is frequently a preventive model of public health action:

- they are firmly based outside the health professions
- they are concerned with inequalities in health and healthcare provision
- they are concerned to promote collective awareness of social causes of ill health
- they assert that the monopoly of information about health and ill health by professionals must be challenged both individually and collectively
- activities centre on work with small groups of local people
- projects have a catalyst function in stimulating local health, social and education services.

Community-wide interventions

Type 4 programmes – those often called 'community-wide' – merit some further comment. The best of such interventions have been meticulously designed and evaluated. They include such classics as the Stanford Five City Project, North Karelia Project, Pawtucket Heart Health Programme and Minnesota Heart Health Programme.

It is no coincidence that the major focus of these various interventions is on the prevention of heart disease. This reflects the medical importance of the disease and its general cost to (Western) societies. The agenda is thus predetermined. It would, however, be churlish not to acknowledge that programme designers have recognized the importance of community involvement – both for reasons of ethics and, perhaps more importantly, to maximize the programmes' effectiveness. In fact, Minkler (1990), in a very useful review of community organization and radical community movements, acknowledges the way in which the Minnesota Heart Health Programme (targeting a population of some 250,000 residents) was committed to developing 'community partnerships'.

Attempts to involve community members typically include community representation in broad-based coalitions of the great and good and their involvement in 'citizen boards' and various task-forces (Bracht, and Gleason, 1990). Bracht and Kingsbury (1990) exemplify the composition of these citizen boards as comprising local government officials, local media personnel, schools, commercial and business organizations, unions, health professionals, minority and voluntary groups, hospitals, churches and community groups. However, the extent to which such initiatives are really representative of the community is somewhat questionable and it is highly unlikely that disadvantaged groups will be substantially empowered. On the other hand, Minkler (1990: 279) regards the Minnesota Heart Health Programme's achievements as praiseworthy:

Community participation and involvement has been critically integrated into each step of the process by means of a series of small group structures (board membership, functional taskforces, and committees) used as vehicles through which residents have played major roles in generating action areas to be addressed, specific activities to be undertaken, and appropriate groups to be targeted. Moreover, participation on taskforces and committees has not only enabled community residents to share their knowledge of community needs and resources in the design of concrete strategies, but also promoted the continued diffusion of awareness of and interest in heart disease prevention in the community.

Interestingly, one of the most significant figures in the Minnesota Heart Health Programme, Mittelmark, produced (1999b: 11) a rather bleak assessment of the effectiveness of the 'flagship' heart disease prevention programmes: 'in the final analysis, the main objectives of these studies were not achieved. Risk factors did not on the whole differ between intervention and control communities, and all communities tended to show improvement.'

A discussion of the effectiveness of the programme is not appropriate here, but it is not unreasonable to speculate that the limited success of these well-designed interventions has something to do with failure to address fundamental structural issues and the root social and political determinants of the problem.

Gilding the ghetto? Some limitations of community development

Although criticisms have been directed at 'pseudo' community organizations that operate in a top-down fashion with predetermined agendas, it would certainly be wrong to assume that CD itself should be regarded as a strategy of choice to address social-structural health problems. Indeed, although an advocate of CD, Constantino-David (1982) provides a very thoughtful critique listing the following limitations and potential threats.

• Community members are at risk of becoming dependent on the community workers and when the workers withdraw and/or funding is withdrawn, the project collapses.
• A new élite might be created from indigenous workers/opinion leaders recruited by change agents.
• Community workers may face a dilemma: the community's felt needs may be relatively insignificant in the long term and more fundamental goals, such as empowerment or political change, may be deferred or ignored.
• Following on from this last point, community workers must be on their guard to avoid imposing their own political agenda on the community. They therefore face a 'facilitation v. manipulation' dilemma. Their role is to *facilitate* community decision making in the interest of empowerment. They may, however, yield to the temptation to manipulate or subtly steer the community in the direction of their own choosing. Constantino-David refers to this process as 'facipulation'.

A more important question mark hanging over CD is whether or not it can really have any significant influence on major structural problems such as inequality. The activities of communities and their successes have been described by such metaphors as 'tidying the deckchairs on the Titanic'. Loney (1981), for example, makes this point when referring to the report of the Community Development Project, *Gilding the Ghetto* (1977).

Rahman (1995: 32) discusses the problems associated with the failure of successive approaches to Third World development initiatives and comments specifically on what he describes as a, 'new worldwide culture of development action termed "popular participation in development" or simply "participatory development" (PD)'. He has severe reservations about small-scale PD efforts that, 'seem to be serving the purpose mainly of providing a "safety net" and do not promise fundamental movement toward people's liberation' and do not reflect, 'the values of social activism, building towards a more genuinely participatory approach to transformation.'

Serrano-Garcia discusses the effect of a community development programme in Esfuerzo, a poor rural community in Puerto Rico, and asks the question, 'Did our intervention facilitate the empowerment of the residents of Esfuerzo? What are the limits of empowerment efforts within our colonial context?' She (1984: 197) concludes that:

> the community members had gained new skills, feelings of competency, and insights that should enable them to achieve greater control over some aspects of their community life. [they would probably have] ... a different, more affirmative, perspective on their role in their community.

Her writing, however, reflects concern that they might have 'fostered the illusion' that their society allows for empowerment. She then questions the possibility of creating real social change using CD techniques. Her (1984: 197–8) review of the nature of the society, its power structure and barriers to change is illuminating and iterates the recurring observations we have made throughout this book:

> I am convinced that our society does not allow [empowerment]. Ours is a society which, along with the economic and political facts previously presented, is characterized by an ideology of conservatism and pro-American values. These emphasize (a) an electoral definition of democracy, (b) the prevalence of a conservative vision of law and order, (c) uncritical acceptance of United States dominance over Puerto Rico, (d) rigid value stances that acknowledge only clear-cut definitions of right and wrong, (e) individualism, (f) veneration of the right to private property, (g) the belief in the governmental duty to protect this right, (h) protection of the free market, and (i) intolerance toward dissidence ... demonstrated through the constant and active persecution of pro-independence group members.

The general tenor of all of these various observations is that, unless if can be redefined to become more politically aware and radical, CD is unlikely to bring about necessary fundamental change in society to address 'class, race or gender struggles to transform the existing economic and power structures' (Dixon, 1989: 84).

It is our intention below to address this task of redefinition in the context of briefly considering what is involved in translating CD (and social action) principles into practice.

Devising community programmes for development and social action

A number of texts have provided guidelines for community work. A detailed discussion of these is not possible here, but Henderson and Thomas (1980) offer a thorough exposition of requirements

that relate to the following key steps and stages (derived from the chapter titles in their book):

- **planning and negotiating entry** including orientation/clarification of own goals and purposes and thinking through the problem(s) to be addressed, making contact with groups and agencies
- **getting to know the community** data collection/ needs assessment/acquiring information
- **working out what to do next** prioritization – setting aims and objectives, decisions about role
- **making contacts and bringing people together**
- **forming and building organizations**
- **helping community clarify goals and priorities** for example, following Freirean techniques of consciousness raising
- **keeping the organization going** providing support, resources, training and so on
- **dealing with friends and enemies** making contact with other groups, liaisons, coalitions
- **leavings and endings** evaluation, closure.

Batten (1967) focuses in on a process of awareness raising and changing group members' perceptions of their situation that parallels aspects of Freierean critical consciousness raising (see Figure 8.3).

CD – a Freirean perspective

As we noted in our general discussion of critical education in Chapter 8, Freire and his followers provided quite detailed suggestions for practice. These are consistent with what might be termed a standard approach to CD and the analyses by Batten and Henderson and Thomas that were described above. However, as we emphasized earlier in the discussion centring on the phenomenon of 'ghetto gilding', there are substantial limitations to the potential of CD to effect radical change.

Kindervatter (1979) reinforces these doubts and uncertainties in her discussion of the effectiveness of two projects in Indonesia and Thailand. She asks is it really possible to empower, 'in political settings not committed or even antagonistic to a more equitable sharing of power and resources?' She also raises the important question of the 'balance of power between conflicting parties' and the need for confrontation by less powerful parties. She (1979: 240) makes an important cultural point, too – namely that cultural norms in the two projects she studied were inimical to confrontation:

> Confrontation has been employed by some groups in Asian contexts, such as squatters in the Philippines, but only in reaction to grossly oppressive conditions. In most cases, people would probably seek other means to

Actions of community worker	Reactions of group members
I Stimulates people to think why they are dissatisfied and with what	Vaguely dissatisfied but passive
II Stimulates people to think about what specific changes would result in these needs being met	Now aware of certain needs
III Stimulates people to consider what they might do to bring such changes about by taking action themselves	Now aware of wanting changes of some specific kinds
IV If necessary, stimulates people to consider how best they can organize themselves	Decide for, or against, trying to meet to do what they now want to do for themselves
V Stimulates people to consider and decide in detail just what to do, who will do it, and when and how they will do it	Plan what to do and how they will do it
VI Stimulates people to think through any unforeseen difficulties or problems that they may encounter in the course of what they do	Act according to their planning
VII Satisfied with the results of what they have achieved?	

Figure 8.3 Stages in the thinking process leading to action by a group
(After Batten 1967)

solve a problem, and if that failed, possibly leave the problem unsolved.

She observes that although some gains were achieved in the Thai and Indonesian projects, 'these gains were not those which significantly altered existing power structures or relationships.' In those countries, 'people know that posing real challenges to the political or economic system can have serious consequences [and] people themselves must balance the possible risks and sacrifices with achieving a particular gain, and decide what course of action to follow.'

Taking account of these several difficulties, the redefinition of CD that we called for earlier will need to include an expanded model. It will additionally need to emphasize the importance of identifying ways in which to actively support community members' commitment to action. Figure 8.4 seeks to provide some indication of what might be involved in this task of redefinition.

In short, community workers act as catalysts and occupy a kind of combined counselling and catalyst role. They employ such typical counselling skills as active listening and providing reflective feedback and act in accordance with the 'holy trinity' of counselling – demonstrating respect, empathy and genuineness. Their credibility and perceived status

is clearly important. As we noted in our earlier discussion of communication of innovations theory, the quality of homophily is important in establishing a trusting relationship.

The major difference between this redefined model of CD and standard versions centres on the kinds of support provided to the dialogic process of consciousness raising and praxis. Before the action plans resulting from praxis can be translated into successful actions, community members will need a range of appropriate life skills and action competences if they are to work effectively in groups, act as lobbyists and deploy a range of other confrontational techniques.

Media advocacy – following the precepts described above and associated with Wallack's formulation – enables community members to raise consciousness in the community as a whole. They might, for instance, use media messages based on creative epidemiology or, as described by Wang and Burris (1994), create their own images of community life and predicaments using photography. As Wallack and others have demonstrated, media advocacy is typically associated with the development of coalitions of like-minded people, both within and outside the community. Although the main focus of action might be on a relatively small scale, such as the development of food cooperatives

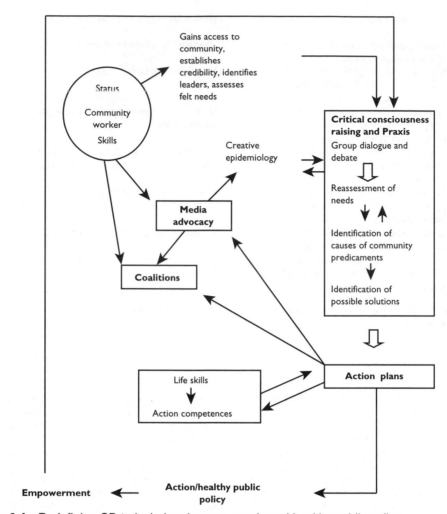

Figure 8.4   Redefining CD to include advocacy, praxis and healthy public policy

or credit unions, by collaborating with broader-based coalitions, such as those operating in the UK's Health Action Zones, local communities may contribute to a more substantial movement for addressing issues such as health inequalities. As Taylor (1995: 109–10) remarks:

it is likely that in a more fragmented 'postmodern' environment, networks and alliances will be the foundation on which empowerment is built. Community work needs to develop a practice which can work with allies across the institutional map to find the possibilities for change in an increasingly turbulent environment.

THE EXPERT'S TASK

Experts should be on tap not on top!

Kindervatter, 1979

The educational dimension

One of the main themes of this book is our assertion that education (broadly defined) is at the very epi-centre of health promotion. Its contribution to CD and its variants is probably self-evident. However, Kindervatter's philosophy and practice is of particular interest as she more or less equates CD/organization with what she calls 'non-formal education'. She (1979: 87–8) defines CD/development as:

- attempting to build local capability by nurturing grass-roots organizations and creating coalitions of organizations
- utilizing natural groups or structures
- starting from people's interests and moving at their pace
- emphasizing the identification and development of 'native' leaders – that is, opinion leaders
- promoting peer support and mutual help
- having an open-ended agenda and aiming to activate people to work together
- building cooperative community problem-solving capacity and a power base from which existing power relationships can be confronted
- emphasizing discussion methods, democratic procedures and action
- having an organizer who serves as a 'process guide' and resource person
- enabling the transfer of initiative and responsibility from community worker to the people to achieve local autonomy.

Non-formal education (NFE) is a process the *raison d'être* of which is identical to WHO's definition of empowerment as people gaining control over their lives (and their health) or, in Kindervatter's words, gaining, 'understanding of and control over social, economic, and/or political forces.' Its methodology includes small group 'teaching' with a community worker as a facilitator rather than instructor, the transfer of responsibility from teacher to participants and an emphasis on participant leadership, as well as the integration of reflection and action (praxis).

In addition to community organization, Kindervatter compares NFE with three related empowering processes – self-management and collaboration, particpatory approaches and education for justice. We will merely remark that self-management and collaboration relate to education in the workplace that has as its goal 'equalizing power in work relationships' and effectively views the workplace setting as a community ripe for democratic development. Its relevance for the 'settings approach', described in the next chapter, will be clear.

Education for justice and related developments

Minkler (1990) reminds us that participatory education featured prominently in the work of Dewey (1946) and Lindeman (1926). Minkler (1990: 271–2) also comments that adult education (or andragogy) can be defined as a process that is centrally concerned with:

> enlarging people's understandings, activating them, and helping them make and implement decisions for themselves. [It is also] ... congruent with the community organization principle of facilitating true involvement and participation by community members at all stages of the organizing process.

This section on achieving socio-political change and empowerment within communities ends now with some final thoughts on Kindervatter's NFE. We have already discussed the radical philosophy of Freire's empowering educational approach and its imperative for socio-political change in pursuit of equity. Kindervatter (1979: 149) incorporates Freire's principles and practice, together with those of Charnofsky (1971), Curle (1972) and Wren (1977), and summarizes them under the rubric 'education for justice':

- development of critical consciousness
- small group discussion (culture circles)
- utilization of a problem stimulus for circle members to decode
- utilization of tools, such as games, to help people reflect on their realities
- a focus on 'system blame' rather than 'person blame' as a cause of problems
- aim to achieve conflict resolution with a win – win outcome
- emphasis on non-hierarchical methods and relationships, dialogue and shared leadership
- utilization of facilitators who are committed to liberation, have faith in people, are humble and who act primarily as problem and question posers.

EDUCATION FOR JUSTICE

Justice calls for the establishment of a society in both a global and national scale where each person has an equal right to the most extensive basic liberties compatible with a like liberty for all, where social and economic inequalities are so arranged that they are to the greatest benefit of the least advantaged, and where they are linked with position and appointments which are open to all through fair equality of opportunity.

Wren, 1977: 55

We commented earlier on the difference between communities and neighbourhoods, arguing that neighbourhoods should be regarded as settings. We have described in some detail different approaches to health promotion within communities – particularly CD in its original and redefined versions. We turn next to a more detailed consideration of settings and discuss the peculiar requirements for effective health promotions in that context – requirements are encapsulated in the notion of a 'settings approach'.

9

Settings and Methods

To me education is a leading out of what is already there in the pupil's soul. To Miss Mackay it is a putting in of something that is not there, and that is not what I call education, I call it intrusion.

Muriel Spark, *The Prime of Miss Jean Brodie*, 1961

INTRODUCTION

We have already considered macro-level strategies for influencing health, notably policy and mass media. At the meso level we have also considered community-based approaches. We now turn our attention to the settings approach.

Throughout this book, emphasis has been placed on the centrality of education and learning to achieving change, regardless of whether the change involves individual behaviour, environment, policy or organizational change. We therefore include in this chapter an analysis of key issues relating to educational methods.

THE SETTINGS APPROACH

The nature of the approach

It is self-evident that a fundamental requirement for health education is access to individuals or groups. The opportunity afforded by different settings for gaining entry has therefore been of considerable interest. The notion of a health career, to which we referred in Chapter 2, is one means of identifying points of contact. The box contains a list of key questions for assessing their potential.

KEY QUESTIONS FOR WORKING IN SETTINGS

- **Regarding access**
  What kind of target group is accessible via this setting?
  How many people will be reached?
  How easy will it be to reach them?

(Continued)

(Continued)

- **Regarding the philosophy and purpose**
  Has the institution with which the strategy is associated a particular philosophy or goal?

- **Regarding commitment**
  How committed are the institution and its members to the preventive philosophy underpinning the aims (of health education)?

- **Regarding credibility**
  How credible are the institution and the people in it who will act as health educators? How will the public respond to them?

- **Regarding competence**
  Irrespective of commitment, do the potential health educators have the necessary knowledge and communication/education/training skills to promote efficient learning?

After Whitehead and Tones, 1990: 19–20

However, there is an important distinction to be made between seeing a setting merely as a location that offers opportunities for delivering health education – that is, 'health education *in* a setting'– and the 'settings for health approach', which involves a more comprehensive and coordinated response.

A key feature of the settings approach is that it involves ensuring that the ethos of the setting and all the activities are mutually supportive and combine synergistically to improve the health and wellbeing of those who live or work or receive care there. It involves integrating health promotion into all aspects of the setting and including within its remit all those who come into contact with that setting.

To illustrate the difference, Table 9.1 provides a comparison of health education provided in a school and the health promoting school.

The emergence of the settings approach has generally been attributed to the Ottawa Charter's (WHO,1986) assertion that, 'health is created and lived by people within the settings of their everyday life; where they learn, work, play and love.'

Commitment to the settings approach was strongly endorsed by the Jakarta Declaration (WHO,1997):

comprehensive approaches to health development are the most effective ... particular settings offer practical opportunities for the implementation of comprehensive strategies. These include megacities, islands, cities, municipalities, local communities, markets, schools, the workplace, and health care facilities.

Kickbush (1998) has emphasized the importance of harnessing the health promoting potential of organizations as a means of achieving health for all in the twenty-first century and also of involving those organizations not traditionally involved in health. The earliest WHO healthy settings initiative was the 'Healthy Cities' project, set up in 1987 and involving some eleven European cities. The settings approach has subsequently expanded rapidly. There are now over 1000 healthy cities and towns in the European region and the principles of the approach have been applied to other settings – some of them linked internationally via WHO networks (see the box). Denman et al. (2002) draw attention to subtle semantic differences in terminology – health promoting schools and hospitals in contrast to healthy cities and prisons. Latterly, there has been some alignment of terminology, with a trend towards using the term 'healthy' schools and hospitals.

EXAMPLES OF SETTINGS FOR HEALTH

Healthy cities
Healthy villages
Healthy islands
Health promoting hospitals
Health promoting schools
Health in prisons
Healthy marketplaces
Workplace health promotion

Table 9.1 *Moving from traditional school health education towards the health promoting school (Young and Williams, 1989: 32)*

Traditional health education	The health promoting school
Considers health education only in limited classroom terms	Takes a wider view, including all aspects of the life of the school and its relationships with the community – for example, developing the school as a caring community
Emphasizes personal hygiene and physical health to the exclusion of wider aspects of health	Based on a model of health that includes the interaction of physical, mental, social and environmental aspects
Concentrates on health instruction and acquisition of facts	Focuses on active pupil participation with a wide range of methods, developing pupils' skills
Lacks a coherent, coordinated approach that takes account of other influences on pupils	Recognizes the wide range of influences on pupils' health and attempts to take account of pupils' preexisting beliefs, values and attitudes
Tends to respond to a series of perceived problems or crises on a one-off basis	Recognizes that many underlying skills and processes are common to all health issues and that these should be preplanned as part of the curriculum
Takes limited account of psycho-social factors in relation to health behaviour	Views the development of positive self-image and individuals taking increasing control of their lives as central to the promotion of good health
Recognizes the importance of the school and its environment only to a limited extent	Recognizes the importance of the physical environment of the school in terms of aesthetics and also direct physiological effects on pupils and staff
Does not consider actively the health and wellbeing of staff in the school	Views health promotion in the school as relevant to staff wellbeing and recognizes the exemplar role of staff
Does not involve parents actively in the development of a health education programme	Considers parental support and cooperation as central to the health promoting school
Views the role of school health services purely in terms of health screening and disease prevention	Takes a wider view of the school health services, which includes screening and disease prevention, but also attempts actively to integrate services within the health education curriculum and helps pupils to become more aware as consumers of health services

Within the UK, the strategic importance of healthy schools, healthy workplaces and healthy neighbourhoods/communities has been recognized as a means of improving health and tackling inequalities (Department of Health, 1999). These settings were identified as providing access to substantial proportions of the population – schools focusing on children, workplaces on adults and neighbourhoods on older people (Department of Health, 1998) – with subsequent recognition that a focus on the community could be relevant to young families, older people, people on low incomes, with disabilities and ethnic minority communities (Department of Health, 2002).

A key consideration, however, is who is left out. Clearly, these settings have limited potential for reaching the unemployed, those who do not or cannot attend school (and, even within schools, those who feel alienated are less likely to be influenced), the homeless – that is, the most disadvantaged groups in society and those who have the greatest health needs. Green et al. (2000: 25) contend that 'health promotion has chosen to privilege some settings (e.g. workplaces, schools, communities) as being more "legitimate" sites of practice than others (e.g. bingo halls, nightclubs, street corners, public washrooms and other "sites of resistance")'.

If the settings approach is to avoid the risk of increasing the health gap in society, it will need to address the needs of marginalized groups and include (as yet) unconventional and challenging settings.

A setting has been defined (WHO, 1998a) as:

where people actively use and shape the environment and thus create or solve problems relating to health. Settings can normally be identified as having physical boundaries, a range of people with defined roles, and an organizational structure.

Green et al. (2000: 23) draw on critical theory to provide a broader conceptualization. They caution against taking a simple, instrumental view of settings as neutral, self-contained environments containing 'target audiences' and argue that settings are more than, 'physically bounded space–times in which people come together to perform specific tasks (usually oriented to goals other than health).'

Instead, consideration needs to be given to the variability between settings, pre-existing social relationships in the setting and the permeability of its boundaries. Furthermore, settings themselves are culturally constructed and mediated via individual interaction and activity – 'Settings are both the medium and the product of human social interaction' (2000: 23).

The view of settings can therefore be expanded (Green et al., 2000: 23) to also include the following:

> arenas of sustained interaction, with pre-existing structures, policies, characteristics, institutional values, and both formal and informal social sanctions on behaviours.

This view resonates with a postmodern conceptualization of organizations that acknowledges the complex interplay of factors that shape them (see the box for Charles Handy's description of the culture of organizations.) In contrast, a modernist view would see organizations as structured and predictable. This clearly has implications for attempts to introduce change. Postmodern interpretations of organizations cast doubt on the capacity of top-down directives to achieve the commitment required to make them become more health promoting and demand a more complex multilevel response.

Ziglio et al. (1995: 2) identify the main features of settings as follows:

- known boundaries of action
- defined populations

- common 'culture' affecting all who learn, work or receive care
- defined set of stressors and resources to reduce or overcome them
- opportunity to observe and measure the impact of health promotion actions.

Baric (1993) suggests that, to achieve the status of a health promoting setting, the following conditions should be met:

- creation of a healthy working and living environment
- integration of health promotion into the daily activities of the setting
- creation of conditions for reaching out into the community.

The settings approach is consistent with an ecological view of health. Green et al. (2000: 16) contend that it sees health as dependent on the interaction between 'individuals and subsystems of the ecosystem'. The settings approach therefore offers the potential for shaping these elements to maximize health gain. It shifts the goals away from specific behaviour change and towards creating the conditions that are supportive of health and wellbeing more generally, with a corresponding shift in focus of activity from risk factors and population groups towards organizational change. Furthermore, it is anticipated that the organizational change will be sustainable so that 'the wheel does not have to be reinvented with each new generation of workers, teachers, nurses' (WHO, 1998a). The box, for example, provides a brief descriptor of a healthy city.

Baric (1993) contends that the settings approach requires an extension of the conceptual framework of health promotion to include:

THE CULTURE OF ORGANIZATIONS

In organizations there are deep-set beliefs about the way work should be organized, the way authority should be exercised, people rewarded, people controlled. What are the degrees of formalization required? How much planning and how far ahead? What combination of obedience and initiative is looked for in subordinates? Do work hours matter, or dress, or personal eccentricities?... Do committees control, or individuals? Are there rules and procedures or only results? These are all part of the culture of an organization.

Handy, 1993: 181

WHAT IS A HEALTHY CITY?

A healthy city is defined by a *process* not an *outcome*.

A healthy city is not one which has achieved a particular health status. A healthy city is conscious of health and striving to improve it. Thus any city can be a 'healthy' city, regardless of its current health status. What is required is a commitment to health and a process and structure to achieve it.

A healthy city is one that is continually creating and improving those physical and social environments and expanding those community resources which enable people to mutually support each other in performing all the functions of life and in developing to their maximum potential.

WHO Regional Office for Europe, 2002b

What is the 'healthy cities' approach?

Successful implementation of this approach requires explicit political commitment, leadership and institutional change, intersectoral partnerships, innovative actions addressing all aspects of health and living conditions, and extensive networking between cities across Europe and beyond. These are characterized as the four elements for action.

A. Explicit political commitment at the highest level to the principles and strategies of the 'Healthy Cities' project.
B. Establishment of new organizational structures to manage change.
C. Commitment to developing a shared vision for the city, with a health plan and work on specific themes.
D. Investment in formal and informal networking and cooperation.

WHO Regional Office for Europe, 2002c

- organizations as systems
- the interactions, behaviour and roles of people in organizations
- accountability – including social responsibility.

Denman et al. (2002) locate the settings approach within Beattie's (1991) model (referred to in Chapter 5) by characterizing it as having a collective focus and negotiated style of working. Similarly, drawing on Caplan and Holland (1990), they see it as concerned with radical change rather than social regulation and based on the view that knowledge is subjective rather than objective – that is, it is consistent with a radical humanist position.

Kickbush (1995: 6) notes that views about healthy organizations equate with modern management theory and that the characteristics of such organizations include:

- goal focus
- communication adequacy
- optimal power equalization

- resource utilization/distribution
- cohesiveness
- morale
- innovativeness
- autonomy
- adaptation.

Consideration of the respective contributions to health of behaviour and environment – that is, agency and structure – has been a major concern of health promotion. Green et al. (2000) draw attention to the reciprocal determinism between environment and behaviour that is integral to ecological perspectives of health promotion and the settings approach. In short, behaviour is influenced by environment and the behaviour of individuals and groups shapes the environment. The settings approach does not, therefore, subscribe to a simple input–output view of intervention and effect, but, rather, presupposes a complex web of interaction between multiple layers of inputs. Poland et al. (2000: 346) identify the key characteristics of settings for health projects as 'integrated, comprehensive, multifaceted, participatory, empowering, partnership, responsive, and tailored'. Whitelaw et al. (2001: 341) suggest that activity in the settings approach is concerned with:

- development of personal competences
- policies
- reshaping environments
- building partnerships
- bringing about sustainable change by means of participation
- developing empowerment
- ownership of change throughout the setting.

Wenzel (1997), however, contends that, despite the rhetoric, the settings approach has amounted to little more than rebadging of traditional health education and that settings are simply a vehicle for individualistic health promotion. This view is challenged by Mittelmark (1997) who notes that the post Ottawa era has been characterized by awareness among practitioners of the complex interaction between settings and behaviour. Furthermore, Green et al. (2000) suggest that any failure to achieve full health promoting setting 'status' may derive not so much from the inherent sophistication of the concept and the lack of comprehension on the part of practitioners, but from practical limitations within the setting. These include the 'competing interests, agendas and interpretations of key "gatekeepers"' (2000: 24). Whitelaw et al. (2001) attribute the relatively modest achievements to health promotion being only one element within the context of wider organizational development and identify a number of practical difficulties:

- competing forces
- translating the philosophy of the approach into practical activity within the setting
- the credibility and status of health promoters as agents of change
- lack of sufficient support.

Whitelaw et al. (2001) note the variation in what is being attempted under the settings banner and the difficulty faced by practitioners in moving beyond a focus on projects and towards achieving broader change across the setting and sustaining activity over a significant period. They raise the issue of whether or not there should be a consensus on what constitutes a settings approach – a one size fits all – given the differences in:

- the scale of what is attempted
- the nature of the setting – from nation states to prisons
- the range of outcomes and emphases.

While a consensus contributes to achieving a common vision, Whitelaw at al. (2001: 341) note that

allowance should be made for practical reality failing to live up to the theoretical ideal. Poland et al. (2000: 346) also suggest that 'a one size fits all approach (the use of identical protocols in similar settings)' may be inappropriate and that local autonomy may be required in relation to adaptation to suit specific needs and circumstances.

Whitelaw et al. (2001: 342–4) identify five broad types of settings activity by considering the ways in which problems are framed and solutions identified – in particular, the respective weight attached to the contributions of agency and structure.

- **The passive model** The problem and solution are dependent on the behaviour and actions of individuals. Traditional health education activity takes place within the setting – the setting itself merely has a subservient role.
- **The active model** The primary problem and part of the solution lie with the behaviour of individuals and part of the solution with the setting. The contribution of the setting is therefore needed to facilitate change in behaviour and the achievement of goals.
- **The vehicle model** The problem lies with the setting and the solution with learning from individually based projects. The primary goal shifts from the individual to changing features of the setting. Working on specific topic-focused projects is the 'vehicle' for achieving this – for example, beginning with an issue such as sun protection as a basis for considering the wider health promoting potential of the organization.
- **The organic model** The problem is seen to lie with the system and the solution with the processes and practices that make up the whole. It focuses on the development of individuals and groups throughout the organization, premised on the assumption that overarching systems are the product of individual actions. The overall aim is to improve the ethos or culture of the setting and strengthen collective participation.
- **The comprehensive model** This aims to change the structure and culture of the setting with the assumption that individuals are relatively powerless to do anything about it. It takes more of a deterministic view that systems change is dependent on 'powerful levers', so the emphasis is on policies and strategies for achieving change.

The latter two are clearly more consistent with the 'ideal' interpretation of the settings approach. However, Whitelaw et al. suggest that the distinctions between these five types of activity should be viewed loosely and that they may overlap in a complementary way or operate sequentially to facilitate progression within an organization.

Variations in practice may, therefore, arise from the extent to which organizations aspire, and are able, to achieve the 'ideal'. The particular characteristics of organizations will also undoubtedly influence the way in which the settings approach is operationalized. Denman et al. (2002) observe that differences in the size and complexity of settings will influence the mode of operation of the settings approach. For example, they refer to healthy cities as macro settings that rely heavily on intersectoral collaboration to achieve their goals. Schools, in contrast, are held to be more self-contained and self-sufficient. While collaboration has undoubted benefits (and is a core principle of the approach) schools will be less dependent on this aspect.

There is also variation within settings. Rivers et al.'s (1999) audit of local healthy schools schemes identified two broad types of schemes – prescriptive and needs-led. The former involve working towards predefined criteria, whereas needs-led approaches are more flexible and responsive to local priorities. The WHO position has been to acknowledge – indeed welcome – diversity in implementation of the settings approach, both between and within settings, provided it is consistent with core principles. In line with notions of subsidiarity, this affords considerable local autonomy and the opportunity to respond to local needs while maintaining the integrity of the approach and commitment to its underpinning values.

Carrots and sticks

A range of factors will impinge on an organization's decision to become a health promoting setting – at the most basic level, these could be the latitude for making change and the resources available. A critical issue is the momentum created by external pressure (or incentives!) and internal motivation. In some instances, formally structured international, national or local programmes may be in place. For example, the introduction of the 'National Healthy School Standard' in the UK outlined minimum criteria that 'healthy' schools would be expected to achieve and aimed to ensure that, by March 2002, all local education authorities would have an accredited scheme in place.

While schools are not *obliged* (as yet) to become health promoting schools, there is an expectation that they will do so and that the ways in which they attempt to promote health will be addressed during quality inspections of schools. In short, national standards have been set, opportunities for accreditation are being established at the local level and strong normative pressure created, including emphasis on the benefits for the whole school community. Furthermore, advocacy for the healthy school concept, via international networks such as the European Network of Health Promoting Schools (ENHPS) and the Global Network, has encouraged a number of other countries to adopt the initiative. Stewart Burgher et al. (1999) document the growth of the ENHPS from four countries in 1991 to thirty-eight by 1999.

The position with regard to workplace health promotion is that, while it is possible to regulate health and safety issues (for example, within the EU, the Framework Directive on safety and health – Council Directive 89/391/EC), the move towards consideration of positive health and full commitment to addressing the factors that would improve health identified by the Luxembourg Declaration (see the box) will necessarily demand a high level of motivation.

'LUXEMBOURG DECLARATION ON WORKPLACE HEALTH PROMOTION IN THE EUROPEAN UNION'

Factors that improve employees' health:

- management principles and methods that recognize employees as a necessary success factor for the organization instead of a mere cost factor
- a culture and corresponding leadership principles that include participation of the employees and encourage motivation and responsibility of all employees
- work organization principles that provide the employees with an appropriate balance between job demands, control over their own work, level of skills and support
- a personnel policy that actively incorporates health promotion issues
- an integrated occupational health and safety service.

(Continued)

(Continued)

Guidelines for workplace health promotion (WHP)

- all staff have to be involved (participation)
- WHP has to be integrated in all important decisions and in all areas of organizations (integration)
- all measures and programmes have to be orientated towards a problem solving cycle: needs analysis, setting priorities, planning, implementation, continuous control and evaluation (project management)
- WHP includes individually directed and environment-directed measures from various fields and combines the strategy of risk reduction with the strategy of the development of protection factors and health potential (comprehensiveness).

European Network Workplace Health Promotion, 1997

Clearly different settings will vary in both their commitment and capacity to prioritize health goals. This might be expected to be a more realistic proposition within the public than the private sector, notwithstanding Kickbush's (1998: 2) assertion that, 'almost all organizations have not only a vested interest, but also a social responsibility, in maintaining and improving their members' health.'

Some of the structural barriers to health promotion in the workplace have been identified by the Faculty of Public Health Medicine (1995: 4) as the:

- problem of access to the very large number of small workplaces
- decentralization and fragmentation of larger organizations
- absence of statutory provision for occupational health in the United Kingdom (unlike other countries such as France, Germany and Holland) – such provision ensures that basic requirements of occupational health and safety are met
- organizational cultures that can discourage the implementation and support of health promotion policies
- financial difficulties – in times of recession, health promotion programmes may be among the first company activities to be cash limited
- continuous organizational change, as lack of formal plans and short-term focus prevent the development of longer-term health promotion initiatives
- failure to assign managerial responsibility and accountability for workplace health promotion to a named individual or department – lack of continuity is common

- lack of facilities, including appropriate accommodation, which may impede the implementation of programmes – this is related to the wider issue of funding
- inadequate basic safety and absent or poor occupational health, which may induce cynicism.

The 'Healthy Workplace Initiative' in the UK makes a point of outlining the benefits to employers (see the box). While purists might be critical of the narrow focus on servicing the needs of productivity, from the perspective of persuasive communication, framing the argument in this way means that it is likely to appeal to the primary motivation of those working in industry. (Note also the use of a respected insider voice – the CBI is quoted!)

An alternative conceptualization of benefits might include improved working relationships, the opportunity to improve the health and wellbeing of the workforce and enhance the corporate image – echoing the tradition of nineteenth-century industrial philanthropists such as Salt, Cadbury and Rowntree! Within the educational context, there is clear recognition of the reciprocal relationship between health and education. Children who are healthy are more able to take advantage of education and education contributes to health. As the Department of Health (1999: 4.16) points out:

Education is vital to health. People with low levels of educational achievement are more likely to have poor health as adults. So by improving education for all we will tackle one of the main causes of inequality in health. Education can build self-esteem and can equip children and young people with the skills to adopt a healthier lifestyle. Education can also contribute to general improvement in health by enhancing people's ability to secure opportunities for work.

BENEFITS OF THE HEALTHY WORKPLACE

Improving health is everybody's business

We recognize that improved health for people at work offers real gains to employers and employees through:

- improved productivity
- lower rates of sickness
- less time to recover and a quicker return to work
- fewer accidents and less illness.

Department of Health, 2000

The case for employer action

The Confederation of British Industry (CBI) estimates of the annual cost to industry of the three major causes of sickness absence:

mental ill health	cost: £3.7 billion/91 million days lost
coronary heart disease and stroke	cost: £2.1 billion/62 million days lost
alcohol and drink-related diseases	cost: £1.7 billion/8 million days lost

Department of Health, 1995

It might be anticipated that an organization's motivation to become a health promoting setting would be influenced by the level of compatibility with:

- its primary goals
- its core values
- its *modus operandi*.

Hospitals, for example, might appear to be obvious contenders in that the core business of hospitals could loosely be defined as being concerned with health. However, the move to becoming a health promoting hospital (see the box) would require traditional organizations to undergo a major reorientation – from curing disease to promoting health, from patient compliance to empowerment, from a narrow concern with patients to including relatives, staff and the wider community and from being inward-looking to outward-looking.

In contrast, while at first sight schools are primarily concerned with educational rather than health goals, commitment to education as a means of developing the whole person has much in common with a positive holistic view of health. Furthermore, the emergence of the 'whole school approach' to education in the 1980s was entirely consistent with the settings approach. This recognized that a child's learning at school is the product not just of what is taught through the planned formal curriculum, but also their total experience at school, which would include the environment, relationships and practices in the school (the hidden curriculum), the activities organized by the school (the informal curriculum) and contact with the school health service (the parallel curriculum).

We have made some general observations about the key features of the settings approach. While it is not possible to discuss the various settings in detail, by way of example, we will provide a brief overview of the health promoting school and the factors that contribute to its development. Although, as we have noted, there are substantial contextual differences between settings, there are still some parallels to be drawn.

THE HEALTH PROMOTING SCHOOL

Bearing in mind our earlier point about the problems of reaching out of school youth and disaffected young people, schools are widely accepted as having considerable potential for influencing the health of young people and future adults. This is not altogether surprising given that the length of time spent in school in industrialized countries has been estimated to be around 15,000 hours (Rutter et al.,

THE VIENNA RECOMMENDATIONS ON HEALTH PROMOTING HOSPITALS (HPHs)

Fundamental principles

Within the framework of the health for all strategy, the Ottawa Charter for Health Promotion, the Ljubljana Charter for Reforming Health Care and the Budapest Declaration on Health Promoting Hospitals, a health promoting hospital should:

1 promote human dignity, equity and solidarity, and professional ethics, acknowledging differences in the needs, values and cultures of different population groups
2 be orientated towards quality improvement, the wellbeing of patients, relatives and staff, protection of the environment and a realization of the potential to become learning organizations
3 focus on health with a holistic approach and not only on curative services
4 be centred on people providing health services in the best way possible to patients and their relatives, to facilitate the healing process and contribute to the empowerment of patients
5 use resources efficiently and cost-effectively, and allocate resources on the basis of contribution to health improvement
6 form as close links as possible with other levels of the healthcare system and the community.

WHO Health Promoting Hospitals Network, 1997

1979). Schools are increasingly recognized as a major setting for health promotion. Not only do they reach a substantial proportion of young people at a formative stage in their development, they also provide opportunities for influencing the health of staff and the wider community. The health promoting school aims to achieve (WHO Euro-EC-CE, 1993):

> healthy lifestyles for the total school population by developing supportive environments conducive to the promotion of health. It offers opportunities for, and requires commitments to, the provision of a safe and health-enhancing social and physical environment.

Futhermore, it is seen to contribute to school improvement by improving 'the whole quality of the school setting. Success here will better equip schools to enhance learning outcomes' (Stewart Burgher et al., 1999: 5).

The 'English National Healthy School Standard' (Department for Education and Employment, 1999) emphasizes the dual benefits of the health promoting school – contributing to health gain and raising levels of pupil achievement. This is consistent with the twin national drivers of 'Saving Lives: Our Healthier Nation' (Department of Health, 1999) and 'Excellence in Schools' (Department for Education and Employment, 1997).

Although the roots of the health promoting school can be traced back much further (for a detailed account, see St Leger, 1999, Tones and Tilford, 2001, and Denman et al., 2002), the origin of the concept is generally attributed to a consensus conference sponsored by WHO in 1989, which led to the publication of *The Healthy School* (Young and Williams, 1989). This identified three main elements of the health promoting school:

- health education taught through the formal curriculum
- the school ethos and environment
- the relationships between the home, school, the surrounding community and services.

It also established as a key principle that the focus should be on addressing the needs of pupils and they should be actively involved. Health education should, therefore, meet the needs of pupils as they mature – revisiting issues at an appropriate level by means of a so-called 'spiral curricular approach' – and use active learning methods. Tones (1996) suggests that a health promoting curriculum should include the following three broad areas:

- **health knowledge** to develop awareness and understanding of key issues
- **life skills** to develop skills and competences
- **social education** to raise consciousness about the social determinants of health.

The ethos and environment should complement what is taught and be health-enhancing in their own right. Furthermore, efforts within the school should be strengthened and supported by strong links with parents and the wider community.

THE TWELVE ENHPS CRITERIA FOR A HEALTH PROMOTING SCHOOL (ENGLISH VERSION)

Ethos and environment

- Provide a safe, secure and stimulating school environment which encourages pupils to be health and safety conscious both in and out of school.
- Actively promote opportunities which develop pupils' self-esteem and self-confidence, enabling them to take initiatives, make choices and exercise responsibility for their own and others' health.
- Foster a whole-school understanding and sharing of the school's aims for health education and the contribution that individuals can make through their respective skills and personal qualities.
- Create a school climate in which good relationships, respect and consideration for others flourish.
- Promote the health and wellbeing of all staff and pupils and consider the role of staff as an exemplar of a healthy lifestyle.

Curriculum

- Formulate a range of health-related policies which are in accord with the school's aims – for example, those concerned with nutrition, physical activity, substance misuse and bullying.
- Implement the health-related policies and monitor any changes in pupils' knowledge, skills, attitudes and behaviour.
- Plan and implement a coherent health education curriculum which complies with statutory requirements and is accessible to all pupils.
- Ensure that teaching is informed, of a consistently high quality and based on a positive approach which recognizes the importance of starting with pupils' existing levels of understanding and experience of health matters.
- Provide stimulating challenges for all pupils through a wide range of physical, academic, social and community activities.

Family and community

- Develop good liaison with other schools, pupils' parents/guardians and the community on a range of health promoting initiatives.
- Make effective use of outside agencies and specialist services to advise, support and contribute to the promotion of health, either directly or through the curriculum.

HEA, 1996

A more detailed specification of criteria for the health promoting school was subsequently developed by the European Network of Health Promoting Schools (see the box). The 'Global School Health Initiative' (GSHI) was launched in 1995 and has also developed related criteria (WHO, 2002). St Leger (1999) notes the similarity of structural frameworks adopted by the different regions. Parsons et al. added management and planning to the basic tripartite model, along with desired impact. Furthermore, they placed the whole within the local, national and international context – referring to it as an ecoholistic model (see Figure 9.1). Management aspects are also included in the operational definition offered by Stewart Burgher et al. (1999: 4–5):

> A health promoting school uses its management structures, its internal and external relationships, its teaching and learning styles and its methods of establishing synergy with its social environment to create the means for pupils, teachers and all those involved in everyday school life to take control over and improve their physical and emotional health.

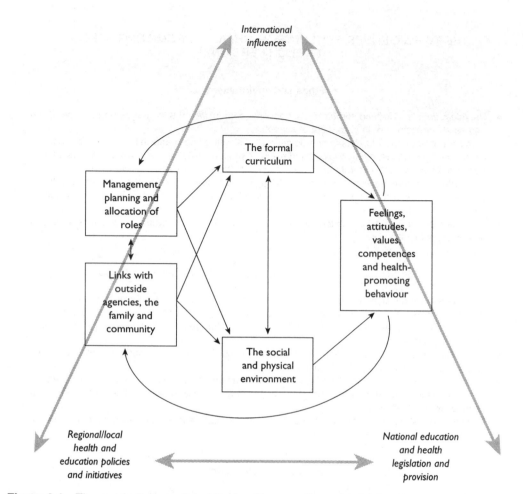

Figure 9.1   The eco-holistic model of the health-promoting school (after Parsons and Stears et al., 1997)

The activities carried out in schools under the health promoting school banner vary enormously. Stewart Burgher et al. (1999) identify five broad categories of activity in ENHPS schools:

- improvements to the physical environment
- education on health topics
- building democracy in schools
- development of policies

- teacher training both topic-based and skills-based – for example, in communication, the use of active learning methods, management, cooperation with parents and so on.

Activities in health promoting schools usually span most, if not all, the categories. The box provides examples of the activities undertaken to promote mental health in Hull and the East Riding in the UK.

EXAMPLES OF ACTIVITIES TO PROMOTE MENTAL HEALTH

- Developing and introducing anti-bullying strategies.
- Setting up a school council to give pupils a voice.

(Continued)

(Continued)

- Introducing 'circle time' – encouraging pupils to speak, listen and empathize with each other.
- Setting up a breakfast club to help pupils concentrate in lessons, socialize and so on.
- Improving the staffroom facilities.
- Creating a playground area for quiet activities.
- Organizing a stress management course for staff.
- Introducing a new school uniform to reduce peer pressure to wear designer labels.
- Introducing new playtime games and equipment to reduce opportunities for bullying at lunchtime.
- Developing and setting up a 'buddy system' to integrate pupils at breaks and lunchtimes, assist new children to feel part of the school.
- Promoting the 'Baby Think It Over' project to highlight the challenges of parenthood to teenagers.
- Introducing a 'skills swap' between pupils and older members of the community to enhance relationships and develop trust.

Cockerill, undated

Developing partnerships is fundamental to this way of working – within schools, involving pupils and all staff, and outside schools, working with parents, the community and other agencies. Commitment to democracy, equity and empowerment are among the core principles established by the First Conference of the European Network of Health Promoting Schools (see the box for the full list).

The emphasis on democratic approaches to education has been spearheaded in Denmark, where the aim of health education is to develop the capacity of pupils to act independently and collectively to promote their own and other's health (Jensen, 1991). This ability to influence one's own life and society is referred to as 'action competence' and its key components have been listed (Jensen, 2000) as:

- insight and knowledge
- commitment

- vision
- experience
- social skills.

Reference to our earlier discussion of empowerment in Chapter 3 will indicate that the notion of action competence links in to the various constructs of empowerment. Within the UK, this constellation of competences has been conceived as 'health skills' by Anderson et al. (1994) or, more broadly, as 'life skills' (see Figure 9.2).

Implementation of the concept

The degree to which the state controls education and the level of national and local support for the concept of the health promoting school will clearly be

PRINCIPLES OF THE HEALTH PROMOTING SCHOOL DEVELOPED BY THE FIRST CONFERENCE OF THE ENHPS

- Democracy.
- Equity.
- Empowerment and action competence.
- School environment – physical and social.
- Curriculum.
- Teacher training.
- Measuring success.
- Collaboration.
- Communities.
- Sustainability.

European Network of Health Promoting Schools, 1997

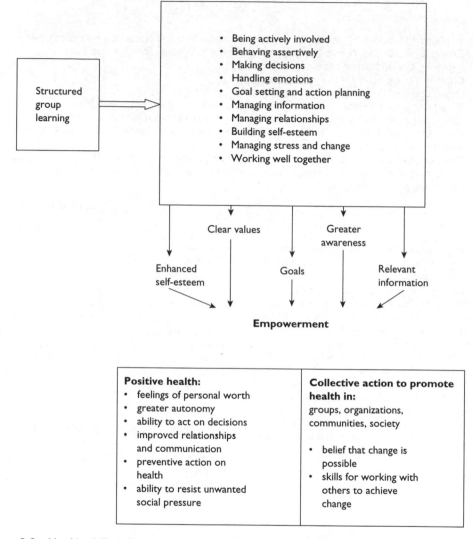

Figure 9.2   Health skills (after Anderson et al., 1994)

influential in relation to implementation. Similarly, cultural and professional norms about the purpose of education, the role of schools and the way in which they function will shape views about the acceptability of the approach. Lawton (1986), for example, identified key factors that influence views about what should be included in the school curriculum. These derive from a number of perspectives – ideological and philosophical perspectives on the aim of education, sociological perspectives on the nature of society and childhood and psychological perspectives on development and learning. Although practical and organizational constraints will also have a

bearing, the various influences will combine to shape views about what ought to be taught and the methods that should be used. An adaptation of Lawton's model is provided in Figure 9.3 and could equally apply more broadly to views about the health promoting school and receptivity to the concept.

The shift in organizational culture integral to the settings approach requires commitment across the board. To avoid the tokenism associated with top-down approaches, it follows that staff and pupils should be involved in decisions and that some staff development may need to take place. Indeed, the basic premise of the health skills project in the UK

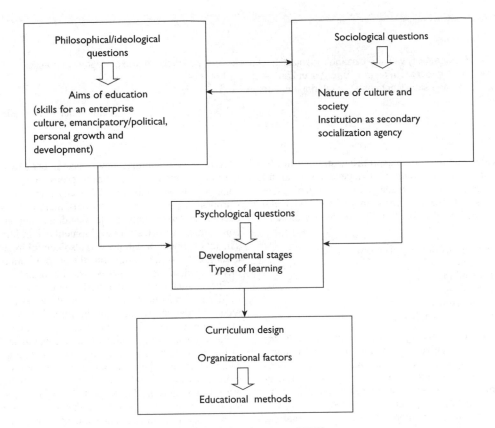

Figure 9.3 Influences on the curriculum (after Lawton, 1986)

(Anderson, undated) was that staff training was a prerequisite for the introduction of a whole school approach to developing health skills.

There is an extensive body of literature on the curriculum and the factors that shape it (for a brief review of the application to health education, see Ryder and Campbell, 1988, Harrison and Edwards, 1994, Tones et al., 1995, Tones and Green, 2000). However, our purpose here is to focus more specifically on the factors associated with organizational change. Tones et al. (1995) draw on Rogers and Shoemaker (1979) to suggest that the adoption of an innovation by schools will depend on:

- the nature of the school as a social system
- the characteristics of individual teachers within the school
- the extent to which the school feels it *owns* the innovation
- the attributes of the innovation
- the characteristics of the change agents.

The features of an innovation that make it more likely to be adopted are summarized in the box (for a more comprehensive review of communication of innovations theory, see Chapter 3).

FEATURES OF AN INNOVATION THAT INFLUENCE THE LIKELIHOOD OF ADOPTION

- Simple, flexible and adaptable, rather than complicated, rigid and teacher-proofed.
- The opportunity to try it out in a limited way and observe results before making a full-scale commitment.

(Continued)

(Continued)

- Compatibility with the existing organization of the school, its timetable and pedagogical practices.
- An improvement on the current situation.
- Lacking significant costs – material and human.

After Tones et al., 1995

The development of an appropriate strategy for the management of change will depend on a careful reading of the key features of the organization. Anderson (undated) draws on the six-box model developed by Weisbord (1978) to identify these as the:

- purpose of the organization
- structure
- leadership
- rewards
- relationships
- helpful mechanisms.

The role of change agents – either internal or external to the organization – will be important in gaining the support of a critical mass of staff. Tones et al. (1995) note that the change agent or 'product champion' is more likely to be effective if they are perceived to have expertise and be similar in most respects to other members of staff – that is, homophilous.

They also need to identify those whose support it would be most expedient to obtain. Anderson (undated) refers to the matrix developed by Elliott-Kemp (see Figure 9.4) for mapping the people in an organization to identify the key people to persuade or work with. The vertical axis represents power or influence, which can be associated with position, expertise, charisma or the power to punish or reward. The horizontal axis represents the degree of concern or interest. A strategy for building support and influence can be developed from an analysis of the positions of staff on the matrix, bearing in mind the need to obtain senior level support. Where those with considerable position and power have little or no interest, generating a groundswell of commitment among the less powerful may provide sufficient leverage.

Anderson also notes Elliot-Kemp's (1982) warning that people cannot support what they don't understand. It is essential, therefore, that people are drawn into what he terms the 'circle of understanding'. Clarity of purpose and the ability to communicate this to others will therefore be instrumental to success.

A number of studies have been undertaken of the implementation of the health promoting school concept. Parsons et al.'s (1997) study involving six European countries found schools that were successful in disseminating ideas and gaining staff commitment valued staff development and training. The involvement of parents was also helpful in generating enthusiasm throughout the school community and celebration of success was important.

The evaluation of the ENHPS pilot project in England (Jamison et al., 1998) made a series of recommendations concerning the initiation, implementation and establishment of change. An essential prerequisite for initiation of change was an audit of the current situation, focusing on both strengths and weaknesses. The contribution of key committed individuals was central to success, particularly having a designated coordinator with the capability and standing among other staff to be able to take the initiative forward. Strong management support provided authority and impetus. Setting clear aims and objectives and adopting a systematic approach to planning also contributed to success. However, the need to be realistic was recognized in relation to what is feasible, timescales and the local and national educational contexts and directives. The flexibility of the settings approach and the ability to adapt it to maximize compatibility with the school's existing priorities was beneficial. The need to consult and keep all stakeholders informed was recognized, along with the importance of good communication mechanisms. The provision of additional funding helped to get activities up and running, but the authors also drew attention to the hidden costs associated with staff putting in a considerable amount of their own time.

In relation to implementation of change, Jamison et al. found that key factors were good communication and management. Allowing time for communication, both within schools and with external agencies, was crucial. Other factors included involving all stakeholders in implementation – pupils, non-teaching staff, parents and outside agencies, as well as teaching staff. Tangible achievements and special events helped to maintain a high profile and

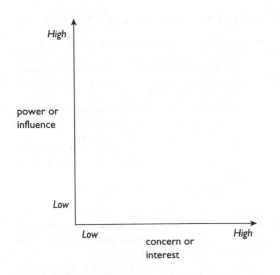

High

power or
influence

Low

Low   High
concern or
interest

Figure 9.4 The Elliott-Kemp matrix
(after Anderson, undated)

provide motivation. This, coupled with time, helped to convince the small core of sceptics within schools who had concerns about the innovation. Flexibility was also important, to respond to new opportunities or competing pressures. Establishing change over the longer term was more likely if linked to the school's development plan. Sustaining ongoing activity was also dependent on having a designated coordinator and ongoing training and support for staff, particularly when there were staff changes. Finally, monitoring and evaluation systems were seen to be important, to check on progress and celebrate achievement.

The audit of healthy schools schemes conducted by Rivers et al. (1999) identified broadly similar factors that facilitated the implementation of healthy schools activities and barriers to success. These are listed in the box. The authors also observed that, frequently, young people are not involved in a systematic way.

Denman et al. (2002) identified the important contributory role of school policies, although St Leger's (1999) study of primary schools found that this aspect of the health-promoting school received comparatively little attention. Referring to the evaluation of the 'Nottinghamshire Towards Health Project', they noted that key factors influencing success included the school's organizational structure, the level of commitment of staff and awareness of the benefits of being involved. They also identified the characteristics of schools which experienced particular difficulty such as:

- starting from a low level of development
- changing their original objectives
- giving the responsibility for coordination to relatively junior members of staff
- few reserves to deal with unanticipated pressures

FACTORS AFFECTING THE IMPLEMENTATION OF HEALTHY SCHOOLS INITIATIVES

Facilitating factors were:

- staff commitment
- support from senior school management
- a concern for pupils' health
- pupils' awareness of the scheme and its work
- outside financial support.

Barriers to success were:

- lack of time and resources
- poor school facilities
- curriculum pressures
- other pressures of work – preparation for OFSTED (Office for Standards in Education) inspection
- ineffective system for internal communication.

Rivers et al., 1999

- a tradition of responding reactively to pressure and crisis management
- unrealistic initial objectives.

Although evidence of the health impacts of the health-promoting schools approach is not yet strong, Lister-Sharp et al.'s (1999) systematic review found the approach to be promising. This view is endorsed by Jamison et al. (1998), Denman et al. (2002) and Parsons et al. (1997). McBride and Midford (1996) demonstrated that relatively modest interventions can achieve change in the management practices of schools to create a structure that enables schools to promote health in a comprehensive manner. Implementation of the concept of the health promoting school, while challenging, clearly has potential for contributing to the health of the whole school community. The growth of the health promoting school movement has been supported by local, national and international networks, which provide opportunities for technical support and information exchange and a forum for collaboration (Rowling, 1996).

Concluding remarks

Organizations and social systems have an enormous impact on health. The settings approach aims to harness that potential to promote health and wellbeing. The advantages offered by the settings approach are that it:

- offers opportunities for working upstream to develop conditions supportive of health
- embeds consideration for health within organizational structures
- has an holistic orientation rather than a focus on problems, risks or specific groups.

However there are also numerous challenges:

- less obvious settings should be considered as well as large-scale mainstream ones to avoid further marginalization of some disadvantaged groups
- the settings approach demands organizational change and commitment – it is not merely a vehicle for more traditional approaches
- it requires a delicate balance between top-down managerial support and the creation of an overall sense of direction on the one hand and, on the other, participation and a sense of ownership at grass roots level
- it demands new ways of working.

The shift in emphasis from behaviour or policy change to organizational change will necessarily draw on a different combination of professional skills and insights (see the box).

Poland et al. (2000: 347) provide a useful summary of key factors contributing to the success of the settings approach that depend on a 'reflexive reading of the particular setting and one's role in it'. These include:

- the institutional organizational culture
- the expectations, attitudes and beliefs of key players – workers, management, patients and physicians, students and teachers, parents and children, community groups and state officials
- the nature of the practice environment – such as incentives and disincentives for undertaking health promotion, such as reward structures, pace of work, competing demands, scepticism, regarding the value or relevance or effectiveness of health promotion, training of key staff
- historical developments in the setting – trends in the organization of work, composition of the family or organization of healthcare

---

REQUIREMENTS FOR ACHIEVING ORGANIZATIONAL CHANGE

- Understanding the influence of organizations on the health and illness of their clients and members.
- Understanding the special logic and dynamics of organizations in different sectors.
- Skills in analysing social structures and processes in organizations.
- Ability to shape their own role within the organizations.
- Social skills for teamwork and team leadership.
- Skills for intervening in organizations.

After Scala, 1996

- internal politics, leadership (formal and informal), past successes and failures
- who controls access to the setting, who has influence within the setting
- broader social, economic and political context – non-setting factors.

The ultimate indicator of the success of the settings approach will be when giving consideration to health is so firmly embedded into the structure and ways of working of organizations that the qualifying term 'healthy' is no longer needed.

METHODS FOR FACILITATING LEARNING

A theme running through this book is that, regardless of whether the focus is on policy, behaviour or empowerment, achieving change is ultimately dependent on learning. Clearly the actors will differ and the type of learning required will vary. It is worth reiterating here our earlier definition of learning as a 'relatively permanent change in capability or disposition'. This might involve:

- change in knowledge, understanding
- change in ways of thinking
- change in beliefs
- clarification of values
- change in attitudes
- acquisition or development of skills.

The adoption of a systematic approach to planning and the application of theory will arrive at a clear specification of what type of learning is required and by whom. For example, this could involve attempts to shift the attitudes of those holding the balance of power in policy development or consciousness raising and the development of community activist skills with a community group or assertiveness skills with young women.

The framework developed by McLeroy (1992) (see Table 9.2) provides a useful overview. Green (2000) contends that, without a full theoretical analysis, interventions risk addressing inappropriate variables or failing to tackle the whole combination of variables required to bring about the desired effect. There is also a developing evidence base on the effectiveness of different methods (see, for example the Contributers to the Cochrane Collaboration and Campbell Collaboration, 2000).

The key questions underpinning the selection of methods are the following:

- What learning is required?
- Who is the target (group)?

- How large is the group
- What are the contextual factors?

The role of health education is to create the conditions necessary to achieving the required learning.

We have already looked at the contribution of mass media and now turn our attention to interpersonal methods. There is a considerable repertoire of methods on which to draw, backed up by numerous manuals on their detailed application. Our purpose here is not to review the utility of specific methods, but, rather, draw out key principles that will inform the selection of methods to promote learning. Reference should also be made to Chapter 7 for the learning theory that provides insight into their *modus operandi*.

As we noted in Chapter 1, the methods used to promote health can be arranged along a spectrum of coercion from brainwashing and coercion at one end to education and voluntarism at the other. Furthermore, educational methods themselves range from formal, top-down, didactic ones to participatory methods. A one-to-one encounter can, similarly, involve authoritarian instruction, as in the archetypal medical advice, or, alternatively, a more empowering interchange, as set out in the box on page 289. Figure 9.5 (see page 290) attempts to order selected educational methods with respect to the size of the target group and the level of participation.

Clearly, ideology will play an important part in the selection of methods (we have already discussed ideology at some length in Chapter 1). Tones (1993) attributes the shift from formal to more participatory methods of health education over the last fifty years to ideological considerations – notably a commitment to participation and empowerment. A further influence has been the development of theory that has supported their use and evidence of greater effectiveness of these approaches. This shift has also been accompanied by an increasing awareness of the importance of process as well as content. Furthermore, there has been a gradual move away from seeing learners as empty vessels to be filled with knowledge and towards acknowledging and building on their prior learning and experience. The role of the health educator has correspondingly changed from expert to facilitator and the role of the learner from passive acceptance to active involvement. Over and above ideological concerns, the selection of an appropriate mix of activities will therefore be governed by:

- the type of learning required
- the characteristics of the learner
- the characteristics of the teacher
- other factors – context, availability of resources, time, feasibility.

Table 9.2   *Targets of change and strategies for different ecological levels (derived from McLeroy, 1992)*

Ecological level	Targets of change	Strategies and skills
Intra-personal	Developmental processes Knowledge Attitudes Values Skills Behaviour Self concept, self-efficacy, self-esteem	Tests and measurements Educational approaches Mass media Social marketing Skills development Resistance to peer pressure
Interpersonal	Social networks Social support Families Workgroups Peers Neighbours	Enhancing social networks Changing group norms Enhancing families Social support groups Increasing access to normative groups Peer influence
Organizational	Norms Incentives Organizational culture Management styles Organizational structure Communication networks	Organizational development Incentive programmes Process consultation Coalition development Linking agents
Community	Area economics Community resources Neighbourhood organizations Community competences Social and health services Organizational relationships Folk practices Governmental structures Formal leadership Informal leadership	Change agents Community development Community coalitions Empowerment Conflict strategies Mass media
Public policy	Legislation Policy Taxes Regulatory agencies	Mass media Policy analysis Political change Lobbying Political organizing Conflict strategies

Type of learning

A fundamental principle of Carl Rogers' approach to education is that we cannot teach, but can only facilitate learning (Barrett-Lennard, 1998). Work undertaken some time ago at the Industrial Training Research Unit at the University of Wales Institute of Science and Technology (Belbin et al., 1981) found that poor learners were characterized by a passive attitude towards learning, used a narrow range of learning methods and frequently inappropriate methods. The active involvement of the learner is therefore essential. Not only does this maximize learning, but it also contributes to empowerment. As we noted in Chapter 7, it is central to Freirean approaches and underpins life and health skills teaching and the development of action competences. A digest on National Standards for School Health Education in the USA (Summerfield, 1995: 3) affirmed that:

the most effective methods of instruction in health are student-centred approaches: hands-on activities, cooperative learning techniques, and activities that include problem solving and peer instruction to help students develop skills in decision making, communication,

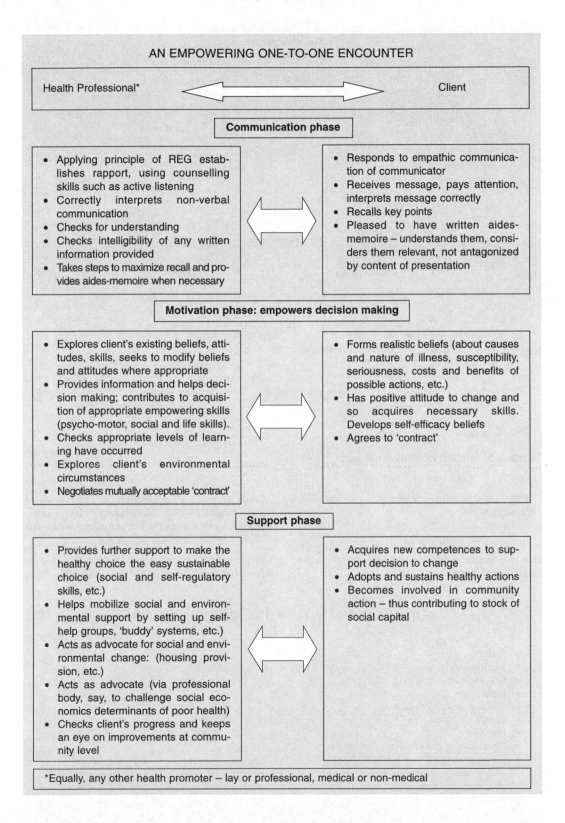

AN EMPOWERING ONE-TO-ONE ENCOUNTER

Health Professional* ⟺ Client

Communication phase

- Applying principle of REG establishes rapport, using counselling skills such as active listening
- Correctly interprets non-verbal communication
- Checks for understanding
- Checks intelligibility of any written information provided
- Takes steps to maximize recall and provides aides-memoire when necessary

- Responds to empathic communication of communicator
- Receives message, pays attention, interprets message correctly
- Recalls key points
- Pleased to have written aides-memoire – understands them, considers them relevant, not antagonized by content of presentation

Motivation phase: empowers decision making

- Explores client's existing beliefs, attitudes, skills, seeks to modify beliefs and attitudes where appropriate
- Provides information and helps decision making; contributes to acquisition of appropriate empowering skills (psycho-motor, social and life skills).
- Checks appropriate levels of learning have occurred
- Explores client's environmental circumstances
- Negotiates mutually acceptable 'contract'

- Forms realistic beliefs (about causes and nature of illness, susceptibility, seriousness, costs and benefits of possible actions, etc.)
- Has positive attitude to change and so acquires necessary skills. Develops self-efficacy beliefs
- Agrees to 'contract'

Support phase

- Provides further support to make the healthy choice the easy sustainable choice (social and self-regulatory skills, etc.)
- Helps mobilize social and environmental support by setting up self-help groups, 'buddy' systems, etc.)
- Acts as advocate for social and environmental change: (housing provision, etc.)
- Acts as advocate (via professional body, say, to challenge social economics determinants of poor health)
- Checks client's progress and keeps an eye on improvements at community level

- Acquires new competences to support decision to change
- Adopts and sustains healthy actions
- Becomes involved in community action – thus contributing to stock of social capital

*Equally, any other health promoter – lay or professional, medical or non-medical

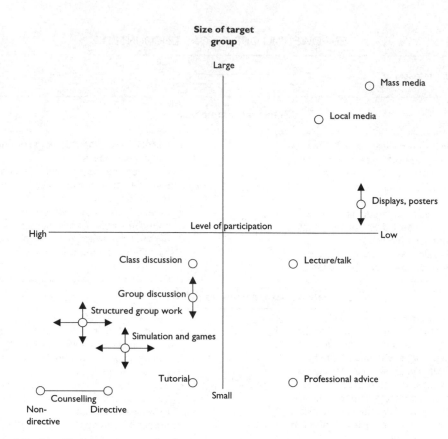

Figure 9.5   Health education methods

setting goals, resistance to peer pressure, and stress management.

Similarly, in England and Wales, curriculum guidance on health education (National Curriculum Council, 1990: 7) states:

While there is a place for direct teaching, the use of audio-visual aids, visits and contributions from visitors, much of the teaching of health education will be based on the active involvement of pupils.

The guidance goes on to list methods suited to this active learning approach (see the box).

TEACHING METHODS SUITED TO ACTIVE LEARNING

- Games
- Simulations
- Case studies
- Role plays
- Problem-solving exercises
- Questionnaires
- Surveys
- Open-ended questions and sentences
- Groupwork of various kinds.

National Curriculum Council, 1990

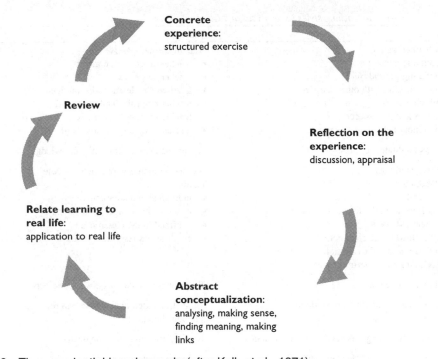

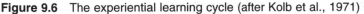

Figure 9.6 The experiential learning cycle (after Kolb et al., 1971)

There are various different terms applied to methods for achieving active learning – 'experiential learning', 'participatory learning', 'active methods', 'student-centred learning', 'confluent education'.

The notion of the 'experiential learning cycle' derives from the work of Kolb et al. (1971), shown in Figure 9.6.

The cycle begins with a new experience or some device for drawing on the learner's past experience, followed by reflection and sharing of learning. This is followed by processing, which involves an analysis of the learning in cognitive, affective and conative domains and its relevance. The learner may appreciate the need for additional skills or knowledge. Anderson (undated) suggests that the role of the teacher or the trainer at this point, can be to provide input that is outside the experience of the group. Provided the input is linked to the learner's needs and experiences, this is not seen as compromising commitment to active learning. Furthermore, if it is to be meaningful, learning should be applied to the real world, with opportunities for subsequent reflection and review.

Ryder and Campbell (1988) draw on the work of Settle and Wise (1986) and Brandes and Ginnis (1986) to contrast experiential methods with more traditional approaches, as shown in Table 9.3.

The mainstay of experiential learning is structured groupwork. The effective functioning of groups as a means of promoting learning is dependent on good facilitation and attention to two broad areas of functioning, although there may be some overlap – namely:

- task-orientated functions – designed to achieve specific leaning
- group-orientated functions – designed to build and maintain the cohesiveness of the group.

The selection of appropriate methods is made easier if learning objectives are formulated precisely – and optimally if framed as behavioural objectives (that is, they specify what the learner will be expected to be able to *do*, under what conditions and over what timescale – see (Hubley, 1993). For example:

Following the groupwork session, participants will:

Table 9.3 *Contrasting teaching styles (after Ryder and Campbell, 1988)*

Experiential	Traditional
Role of learner–active: • negotiating content • negotiating ground rules • communication with other learners • displaying work • management of resources • maintaining behaviour as agreed	Role of learner–passive • teacher determines content • teacher sets rules • talk between learners discouraged • teacher controls display of work • teacher manages resources • teacher maintains standards of discipline
Teacher as facilitator or guide	Teacher as expert – transmits knowledge
Uses active methods: • collaboration • groupwork • starts from what the learner knows or is concerned about • not confined to the classroom • regular review and evaluation (of self and group performance)	Focuses on memory, practice and rote learning: • individual and competitive • concerned with academic standards • confined to the classroom • emphasis on tests and grades
Subject matter integrated	Traditional boundaries between subjects
Uses the intrinsic motivation of students	Motivation external and based on rewards and punishments
Focuses equally on cognitive and affective domains	The affective domain is neglected
Students encouraged to reflect on, and talk about, their learning	Little attention to learning behaviour
Process is valued as well as content	Little attention is paid to process

- when asked, list the main routes of transmission of HIV (knowledge)
- demonstrate to the group, using a condom and banana as visual aids, the correct way to put on a condom (skills)
- in a role-play situation, use three different strategies to refuse pressure to have unprotected sex (skills).

Clearly, the development of knowledge will require different methods from those used in the development of skills. Belbin et al. (1981) produced a simple taxonomy using the acronym MUD to distinguish between appropriate methods for memorizing, understanding and doing (see Figure 9.7). However, Ryder and Campbell observe that, in experiential learning, the affective and cognitive domains tend to flow together to achieve confluent learning. They cite Rogers' (1983) view that the personal involvement in learning central to experiential approaches necessarily touches feelings, even when it has a cognitive orientation or the impetus comes from outside.

In some instances, it will be possible to identify detailed and specific learning objectives, leading to

sharply focused interventions. Furthermore, as we will note below, messages can be tailored with increasing sophistication to match the characteristics and precise learning needs of individuals. This effectively demands greater precision – and potentially control – on the part of those responsible for designing interventions. This approach may be more relevant in the context of vertical rather than horizontal programmes and is certainly less applicable when the objectives are couched in broader terms, such as the development of empowerment or social capital. While it would, in principle, be possible to conduct a detailed analysis of the constructs of empowerment and put together an appropriate collection of methods to address each of these, an alternative approach would be to use methods that are more wideranging and have a multidimensional impact. These allow the learner to take from the learning experience whatever meets his or her own learning needs and achieves confluence between the different learning domains rather than compartmentalization of knowledge. The potential of the creative arts for contributing to community health has begun to receive attention and we will conclude this section with a brief consideration of their role in health promotion.

M **Memorizing**	U **Understanding**	D **Doing**
Facts	Concepts	Skills
Methods of learning		
Association: • visual • verbal Repetition: • written • verbal • aural • visual Self-testing	Listening Questioning: • ourselves • others Discussing Comparing Solving problems Acting out Experiencing Imagining	Practice Demonstration Teaching others Trial and error Doing and reviewing

Figure 9.7 Appropriate learning strategies (after Belbin et al., 1981, in Anderson undated)

The creative arts and health promotion

The capacity of the arts in general to enhance well-being is well recognized, as is their capacity to improve communication by increasing aesthetic appeal and arousing emotions and, indeed to raise awareness of oppression and social inequality. However, in contrast to the visual and performing arts, the explicit use of the arts to promote health is characterized by participation and active involvement in the creative process – hence, the term creative arts projects (see the box for a couple of examples).

EXAMPLES OF WALSALL'S COMMUNITY ARTS TEAM PROJECTS

Truck Stop Rock

A singer/songwriter interviewed forty-two truck drivers and turned the findings into a song entitled '10, 20, 30, 40, 50 a day', about a chain-smoking truck driver. It was felt that the music provided a way into talking to the truck drivers and that they were much more open than they would have been talking to health professionals.

Issues raised included the problems of healthy eating and exercising when on the road and the problem of loneliness. As well as the song raising the awareness of drivers, haulage companies are beginning to talk about work-based clinics.

Comedy

Theatreworkers went into 'spit and sawdust' working men's clubs where they helped members and healthworkers to devise a comedy routine on men's health – including men's reluctance to admit that they are ill and see a doctor.

When the routine was performed, nurses were available to carry out health checks and 200 of the 300 men who saw the routine had a check-up.

The follow-on project is developing a cabaret along similar lines.

Carlisle, 2002

The materials produced may take a number of forms – from posters and leaflets to banners, artworks, music and drama performances – and may or may not have an additional educational purpose. For example, a giant mobile developed by pupils on the importance of clean air and the polluting effects of smoking displayed in the school entrance hall communicated the message to the whole school community without a word being said. However, it is important to distinguish the effects it had on two major constituencies. Those who developed the mobile benefited from having participated in the creative process. On the other hand, for those who had not taken part, it was simply a means of communicating a message – comparable to professionally developed materials, albeit benefiting from local relevance and a certain homophily between the designers and the audience.

Participating in creative arts projects will contribute to the learning of those taking part in a number of ways. Learning may be concerned with substantive content and developing knowledge, raising awareness and changing attitudes. Additionally, the process itself may be empowering as a result of its developing skills, which, together with the concrete evidence provided by the successful production of materials, will contribute to self-efficacy beliefs, confidence and a sense of control. Clearly, if others recognize the value of the 'products' or artefacts, then there will be further enhancement of self-esteem.

These terms above should be familiar to the reader as basic constructs of empowerment. The development of these attributes will apply outside the boundaries of the arts projects to more general areas of people's lives. If those involved feel that they are achieving worthwhile goals, then the meaningfulness of their involvement will lead to an enhanced sense of coherence (Antonovsky, 1984) and the achievement of salutogenic goals. Furthermore, contact with other individuals may generate a sense of social connectedness, contributing to a sense of community and the development of social capital. An illustration of these effects deriving from a community arts project is provided in the box.

The review of good practice in community-based 'arts for health' projects commissioned by the Health Education Authority (now Health Development Agency, HEA, 1999a) noted that the quality of the artefacts was of central importance in generating a sense of pride and influencing the extent to which the participants took the activity seriously. It also saw no conflict between an emphasis on the rigorous teaching of basic skills (and, if necessary, correcting them) and commitment to participation, but, rather, found that this contributed to the quality of the artefacts. The participatory models that were found to work best were, 'well-structured, well-organized and specifically related to the acquisition of skills or of resources for self-expression' (HEA, 1999b: 5).

LANTERN FESTIVAL

A lantern festival was one of a number of creative arts activities set up to tackle social isolation in a new and rapidly growing housing development. The area was characterized by an influx of newcomers, the absence of an infrastructure to support social cohesion and a consequent lack of a sense of community, little social connection and the absence of lay support networks.

Lantern-making workshops to prepare for the 'festival' were led by a professional artist in the local doctor's surgery and schools.

The event itself was highly symbolic and involved a procession around the houses, lighting the streets and drawing people out of the isolation of their own homes, and culminated in a party. From small beginnings with only 15 families taking part in 1990, it went on to become an annual event and, by 1996, 400 families were involved.

Preparation for the festival brought people together in a mutually dependent way. Over and above the social contact, people developed skills – not just in making lanterns, but also all the other activities needed to make the event a success – and frequently passed these skills on to others. Involvement contributed to self-efficacy beliefs, self-confidence, self-esteem and a sense of community. There are clear links between this and the main elements of a sense of community identified by McMillan and Chavis (1986: 6):

- membership – a feeling of belonging
- influence – making a difference
- integration and fulfilment of needs
- shared emotional connection – 'the commitment and belief that members have shared and will share history, common places, time together, and similar experiences'.

Rigler, 1996, and Tones and Green, 1999

Creative arts projects have also been used to explore health needs. Their capacity to put people in touch with their feelings and engage their imagination to envisage how things *might* be is particularly valuable in this regard. The materials produced can themselves have a powerful advocacy function. For example, one community arts project involved different generations in depicting their views about the health of their community through the medium of art. A display of their work was described by one observer as 'chilling' (Tones and Green, 1999). It communicated to policymakers the fear of crime and going out at night, the problem of traffic and the issue of loneliness more graphically than perhaps any other medium could.

The creative arts can also have a role in developing awareness of issues and the motivation to take action about them. This critical consciousness raising is a central concern of Freirian approaches and liberatory education discussed in Chapter 7. In particular, creative arts can contribute to critical reflection on reality and the belief that change is possible. The use of theatre has been popular in this regard and notably forum theatre, which is attributed to Freire's fellow Brazilian, Augusto Boal.

In forum theatre, members of the audience with ideas for change go on stage and act out their ideas, becoming transformed from spectators in to 'spect-actors'. This enables the audience to envisage change, act it out and reflect collectively on outcomes and potentially empowers the audience to take social action. The use of theatre to achieve social change has been referred to as 'theatre of the oppressed' (Paterson, 1999).

Theatre is becoming more widely used in health education – for example in HIV, AIDS and drugs education. However, theatre can only be included under the umbrella of 'creative arts' if the audience actually participates. There is a well recognized repertoire of theatre in education (TIE) activities to encourage such participation – role play, simulation and problem solving. The use of theatre can be particularly relevant to developing empathy, clarifying values and exploring moral dilemmas.

Day (2002) provides an example of the use of forum theatre in schools to enable young people to put themselves in other people's shoes and try out

moral behaviour with regard to the homeless and refugees. Ball (1994) identifies a number of commonalities between health education and theatre to provide a philosophical basis for theatre in health education. These are:

- the need for affective as well as cognitive involvement
- utilization of active learning
- concern to explore attitudes and values
- role-taking
- self-empowerment
- concern with what it is to be human
- a community dimension.

In summary, creative arts offer the potential for enhancing learning in relation to both cognitive and affective issues and have a particular capacity for developing individual empowerment, a sense of community and social capital.

The HEA (now HDA, HEA, 1999b: 2) review of arts for health projects proposes a broad range of possible outcomes, which would include:

- enhanced motivation – within the project and in the participants' lives generally
- greater social connectedness
- people perceiving that they have a more positive outlook on life
- reduced sense of fear, isolation and anxiety
- increased confidence, sociability and self-esteem.

Participation was identified as a key element linking the arts activity with health outcomes and the principal contributions of projects (HEA, 1999b) were seen as:

- development of interpersonal skills
- opportunities to make new friends
- increased involvement.

The study by Comedia (Matarasso, 2001) identified some fifty social impacts deriving from participation in arts projects. While they might all have affected empowerment and health in a general way – for example, in terms of enhanced educational opportunity and increased employability – a selection of immediate relevance to health is provided in the box.

SELECTED SOCIAL IMPACTS OF ARTS PROJECTS

- Increase people's confidence and sense of self-worth.
- Provide a forum to explore personal rights and responsibilities.
- Reduce isolation by helping people to make friends.

(Continued)

(Continued)

- Develop community networks and sociability.
- Build community organizational capacity.
- Encourage local self-reliance and project management.
- Help people extend control over their own lives.
- Be a means of gaining insight into political and social ideas.
- Facilitate effective public consultation and participation.
- Strengthen community cooperation and networking.
- Help feel a sense of belonging and involvement.
- Create community tradition in new towns or neighbourhoods.
- Help community groups to raise their vision beyond the immediate.

After Matarasso, 2001: 159–60

Characteristics of the learner

Using educational approaches and content suited to the age and stage of development of young people is fundamental to good educational practice. The notion of 'cognitive matching' (Bruner, 1971) underpins the concept of the spiral curriculum, which introduces ideas in a simple form and revisits them with increasing sophistication and levels of abstraction as children mature. As noted earlier in our discussion of communication in Chapter 7, Bruner's (1966) categorization of ways of knowing is as follows, corresponding to increasing levels of maturity:

- **enactive** based principally on actual experience and doing
- **iconic** mental pictures can be used to enable thinking about objects
- **symbolic** based on categorization and the ability to develop hierarchies of categories.

The work of Piaget has been influential in relation to understanding the cognitive development of young people. While a full discussion of developmental psychology is beyond the scope of this chapter, there is a summary of Piaget's developmental stages in the box. Ryder and Campbell (1988: 101) characterize the development in reasoning through these stages as:

- taking things at face value
- exploring relationships between tangible entities
- recognizing relationships involving unseen events
- abstract conceptualization.

Approximately 20 per cent of adults do not reach the stage of having developed full formal operational thought and the capacity for hypothetico-deductive reasoning. Kohlberg's analysis of the stages of moral development parallels Piaget's stages of cognitive development and this is included in the second box.

PIAGET'S DEVELOPMENTAL STAGES

Sensory-motor – 0 – 1½/2 years
Pre-operational – 1½/2 – 7/8 years
Concrete operations – 7/8 – 11/12 years
Formal operations – 11/12 – 15 years/adolescence

Piaget, 1969

KOHLBERG'S STAGES OF MORAL DEVELOPMENT

Level 1 Preconventional

Stage 1: *Heteronomous morality*
Motivation: reward and punishment, obedience for its own sake.

(Continued)

(Continued)

Stage 2:   *Individualism, instrumental purpose and exchange*
Motivation: following rules if in one's own interest, fairness and equal exchange.

Level II Conventional

Stage 3:   *Mutual interpersonal expectations, relationships and interpersonal conformity*
Motivation: avoiding disapproval, living up to expectations, trust, loyalty, respect.

Stage 4:   *Social system and conscience*
Motivation: fulfilling agreed duties, contributing to society, group, institution.

Level III Post conventional (principled)

Stage 5:   *Social contract or utility and individual rights*
Motivation: aware of moral relativism.

Stage 6:   *Universal ethical principles*
Motivation: self-chosen ethical principles of universal justice, equality of human rights and respect
               for the dignity of human beings as individuals.

Kohlberg, 1984, in Ryder and Campbell, 1988

As well as consideration of the stage of development, the need to 'start where children are' has informed the development of school-based health education projects. For example, 'Health for Life' (HEA (now HDA) 1989), was based on extensive research into children's conceptualization of health and health-related issues. It used the 'draw and write' technique, which, despite some recent criticism (Backett-Milburn and McKie, 1999), has proved valuable in enabling children to express their views (Williams et al., 1989a, Williams et al., 1989b, and Pridmore, 1996).

While the relevance of didactic methods for teaching young people is questionable, the use of these methods is particularly inappropriate to the needs of adult learners. The idea that adult learners have different learning needs to those of children and the use of the term 'andragogy' to refer to adult learning has been associated particularly with the work of Knowles, who built on the earlier work of Lindeman dating back to the 1920s. Knowles' seminal text, *The Adult Learner: A Neglected Species*, was published in 1973 and is now in its fifth edition (Knowles et al., 1998).

The core principles of adult learning that can usefully inform the development of health education interventions for adults are:

- adulthood is associated with a self concept of being self-directed and in control – adults therefore need to feel responsible for their own learning

- adults have large reserves of experience on which to draw, so learning should utilize this experience
- the willingness to learn is associated with its contribution to carrying out roles and coping with life situations
- the relevance of the learning needs to be clear and immediate rather than deferred
- the motivation to learn is internal and linked to coping with real-life situations.

Over and above the stage of development, within any group there will be differences in preferred learning style, linked to personality.

There are several different instruments for assessing learning styles. Perhaps the best-known of these is the Myers-Briggs Type Indicator (MBTI), developed from Jungian theory and first published in 1962 (see the box). The 'Health Skills Project' used a simpler version, based on two dimensions – 'doer-intuiter' and 'feeler-thinker' – to identify four basic personality types, which were enthusiastic, imaginative, practical and logical (Anderson, undated).

Teaching methods will vary in their appeal according to an individual's learning style. For example, extraverts (spelt as in Myers-Biggs) often learn by explaining to others, whereas this may not appeal to introverts who prefer to have a logical framework to order their learning. The tendency is also to teach in one's own preferred learning style, but, given that in any group there is likely to be a mix of styles, variety is essential to ensure that the needs of all learners are met at some point.

THE MYERS-BRIGGS TYPE INDICATOR

On the basis of the four dimensions below, there are sixteen possible combinations.

- extraversion (E) v introversion (I)
- seeing (S) v intuition (N)
- thinking (T) v feeling (F)
- judging (J) v perceptive (P).

In addition to developmental and personality factors, the effective facilitation of learning also requires sensitivity to issues such as gender, ethnicity and culture. Such sensitivity is central to the core values of health promotion, as well as being instrumental to success. Clearly, educational interventions are more likely to be effective if they are perceived to be personally relevant. A key consideration is the extent to which interventions are designed to suit the specific requirements of individuals – that is, the extent to which they are targeted or individually tailored.

Targeting and tailoring

Reference to social marketing theory would indicate that health education is more likely to be effective if there is a good fit between the message and the characteristics of the target group.

The notion of 'targeting' applies the principle of market segmentation to the design of materials for specific subgroups in relation to particular characteristics, such as age, gender, ethnicity, social class, occupation. In contrast, 'tailoring' refers to adapting the educational approach to meet the needs of the individual (Kreuter and Skinner, 2000):

> Any combination of information or change strategies intended to reach one specific person, based on characteristics that are unique to that person, related to the outcome of interest, and have been derived from an individual assessment.

Kreuter and Skinner provide a useful analogy, comparing off-the-peg clothing (targeted) and bespoke tailored clothing (tailored).

Holt et al. (2000) identify a number of empirical studies that have demonstrated the superior effectiveness of tailored materials, but also note that factors such as personality and locus of control play a part. They suggest that developments in information technology offer considerable potential for tailoring health education materials to suit individual psycho-social and behavioural profiles. However,

their effectiveness will ultimately be dependent upon being able to identify, with some precision, all relevant variables.

Kreuter et al. (2000) contend that tailoring is currently relatively crude and its comparative advantage over targeted or mass-produced material has not been fully revealed. The most commonly used approach is 'behavioural construct' tailoring, which draws on theories of behaviour. Constructs such as stages of readiness to change, identification of barriers to change and self-efficacy for changing behaviour are frequently used. As yet, however, there is little advantage over well-designed non-tailor-made materials that address these constructs. This could, perhaps, be expected, given that little attention is paid to cultural and personality factors. Kreuter et al. suggest that the inclusion of a wider range of variables, including non-behavioural factors such as preferred learning styles, would increase the relative advantage over non-tailored material.

The stages of change model (Prochaska and DiClemente, 1983) offers the possibility of designing interventions that are appropriate to the various stages, so it can be applied to both targeting and tailoring. Miilunpalo et al. (2000) describe the basic elements of the model as being:

- **motivational** concerned with attitudinal readiness, intention building and decision making
- **behavioural** tentative performance up to regular practice.

Progression through the stages of change from precontemplation to contemplation, preparation, action and maintenance is marked by a shift in emphasis from motivation to behaviour. Figure 9.8, developed from Cabanero-Verzosa (1996), indicates how learning needs will vary depending on the stage an individual or group is at.

A key concern is whether or not the individuals at a particular stage are, in fact, a homogeneous group. Miilunpalo et al. (2000), for example, suggest that, in relation to physical activity, the precontemplation

Stages of change

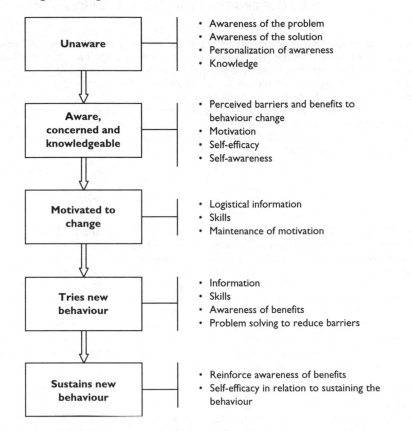

Figure 9.8   Learning needs and stages of change

stage may be subdivided into two groups – 'negative precontemplation' in which individuals may be consciously resistant to change, and 'neutral precontemplation', in which little consideration, if any, has been given to the possibility of change. The findings of Dijkstra and de Vries (2000) also confirm that the precise tailoring of smoking interventions would need to recognize that there are subgroups within the precontemplation stage.

The principles of targeting and tailoring support the development of interventions to suit particular needs. Clearly tailoring is more challenging in that messages are designed for individuals and depend on an analysis of pertinent individual-level factors. However, we should also note that the process of checking out individual characteristics is integral to the interchange that takes place in one-to-one counselling. For example, 'motivational interviewing' (Rollnick et al., 1992) was developed as a means of

helping people to work through ambivalence about behaviour change and is structured to respond to different needs at the various stages of change. Furthermore, well-designed experiential groupwork has the capacity to achieve highly individualized learning outcomes. However, one-to-one counselling or small groupwork may only be feasible in relatively small-scale projects. Targeting and tailoring offer the potential for improving the effectiveness of larger-scale programmes by means of individualization of messages.

Characteristics of the teacher

Social learning theory – which has been a major influence on the development of health education interventions – recognizes the contribution of the characteristics of the teacher to the learning process

---

TO THE COORDINATOR OF A CULTURAL CIRCLE

In order to be able to be a good coordinator for a 'cultural circle', you need, above all, to have faith in man [sic], to believe in his possibility to create, to change things. You need to love. You must be convinced that the fundamental effort of education is the liberation of man, and never his 'domestication'. You must be convinced that this liberation takes place to the extent that man reflects upon himself in relationship to the world in which, and with which, he lives... A cultural circle is a live and creative dialogue, in which everyone knows some things and does not know others, in which all seek, together, to know more. This is why you, as the coordinator of a cultural circle, must be humble, so that you can grow with the group, instead of losing your humility and claiming to direct the group, once it is animated.

Freire, 1972: 61

---

through 'modelling'. Ryder and Campbell (1988) cite McPhail et al.'s (1972) research for the 'Lifeline Project' on moral education, which found that young people were critical of being told how to behave when this was not reflected in the behaviour of their teachers. This applies to a whole range of 'teacher' behaviour, but is particularly pertinent to fundamental principles such as integrity and respect.

These principles are also integral to Rogerian and Freirian approaches. Rogers refers to 'realness' or 'genuineness' as a key attribute of a facilitator, along with acceptance, trust and valuing of the learner. He also notes the importance of being able to empathize with the learner (Rogers, 1967). The 'Health Skills Project' (Anderson, undated) used the acronym REG to summarize these requirements – respect, empathy and genuineness. To avoid any gender bias, it also offered RUBY – respect, understanding and be yourself. Reference to Freire's message to the coordinator of a 'cultural circle' in the box reveals similar views about what makes a good coordinator.

Our discussion of communication of innovations theory in Chapter 3 also highlighted the importance of the change agent's characteristics, particularly the principle of homophily (Rogers and Shoemaker, 1971). The growth in popularity of peer education in recent years is premised on the notion that peer educators will automatically have more credibility than other teachers and that people learn best from those who share similar characteristics. Given the growth in popularity of peer education in recent years and the development of what Frankham (1998) refers to as the 'dogma' of peer education, we will briefly consider its relevance for enhancing learning.

Peer education

Peer education has been defined (Sciacca, 1987, in Milburn, 1995: 407) as, 'the teaching or sharing of health information, values and behaviours by members of similar age or status groups.'

There is some variation in the terminology associated with peer education (see the box), which Milburn (1995) suggests signals subtle difference in roles and styles of working – particularly regarding the level of control and authority.

PEER EDUCATION – THE TERMINOLOGY

- Peer education
- Peer training
- Peer tutoring
- Peer counselling
- Peer facilitation
- Peer leader
- Peer helper

THE 'CHILD-TO-CHILD' PROGRAMME

Basic assumptions:

- Primary education becomes more effective if it is linked closely to things that matter most to children and their families and communities.
- That education in and out of school should be linked as closely as possible so that learning becomes part of life.
- That children have the will, skill and motivation to help educate each other – and can be trusted to do so.

Hawes, in Hubley, 1993: 181

A number of claims have been put forward to support the use of peer education. Turner and Shepherd (1999) identify the following. Peers are:

- a credible source of information
- acceptable sources
- more successful than professionals
- able to reinforce learning through ongoing contact
- positive role models.

Peer education:

- is empowering for those involved
- is beneficial to those involved
- utilizes established channels of communication
- provides access to those who are hard to reach through conventional methods
- is more cost-effective.

Furthermore, the use of peers as educators may enable groups to be reached who would ordinarily be difficult to access. The 'Child-to-Child' movement (Aarons and Hawes, 1979, and Hawes and Scotchmer, 1993), for example, which was set up in 1979 to mark the International Year of the Child and has subsequently expanded to involve more than seventy countries, recognized the potential of children to reach younger brothers and sisters, families, out of school youth and the wider community. A key principle of the programme is that action should be based on children's own observations and conclusions and that there is the opportunity for reflection on action. The assumptions underpinning the programme are summarized in the box and they are particularly concerned with the benefits for those taking part.

Clearly, peer education is more than a device for educating 'others'. Those who take on the role of peer educator stand to benefit from improved knowledge, skills, self-confidence, self-esteem and standing within their social group. This may derive

from the training they receive, but may also stem from their role as 'educators', as summed up in the aphorism *qui docet discit* – he who teaches learns!

Fundamental questions in the development of peer education projects concern who is a peer and who defines this, together with the related issue of how peer leaders/educators are selected. Age has often been seen as a key determining factor – many projects have focused on young people and there has been interest in peer education programmes for senior citizens. However, other commonalities may also be relevant, such as common status (being a pupil in a school, for example, or a member of the workforce of a company) or experience that is relevant to the programme (such as breastfeeding or quitting smoking).

Turner and Shepherd (1999) note that the principles of social learning theory (Bandura, 1986) would suggest that the effectiveness of peers as educators will be influenced by their standing within the group. Michell's (1997) study, for example, revealed that thirteen-year-olds have a very clear grasp of their social map and the pecking order within it. In many instances, peer education projects have paid little regard to this and peer leaders have been volunteers or, alternatively, selected as 'suitable' by project coordinators. In contrast, others have included provision for groups to select their own peer leaders – such as the 'Smoking and Me' project (HEA (now HDA), 1991) or have even used systematic network measurement techniques for identifying those individuals who are most centrally and socially connected (Larkey et al., 1999).

Peer education projects fall into two broad groups – those that tap into existing social and friendship groups and those in which groups are more artificially constructed for the purpose of 'receiving' peer education (Milburn, 1995). Furthermore, the method of delivery can be through 'formal', planned sessions or informal

THEORIES RELEVANT TO PEER EDUCATION

- Social learning theory (Bandura, 1986)
- Social inoculation theory (Duryea, 1991)
- Role theory (Sarbin and Allen, 1968)
- Communication of innovations theory (Rogers and Shoemaker, 1971)
- Differential association theory (Sutherland and Cressy, 1960)
- Subculture theories (for example, Cohen, 1955)

social contacts. There is no rigid boundary between the two approaches and, whichever is used, the involvement of peer leaders in the selection and development of methods helps to ensure relevance. Backett-Milburn and Wilson (2000) noted that young peer leaders were aware of the advantages of informal approaches in that they could choose the right moment and adapt what they said to suit the needs and experience of the person they were speaking to.

Turner and Shepherd (1999) assert that many peer education projects lack a sound theoretical base and that, given its diversity, peer education will need to draw on a number of theories. The box provides a list of the theories that they identify as being relevant to peer education.

A review of the effectiveness of peer education interventions with young people (EPPI-Centre, 1999) found some evidence of their producing positive changes in behaviour. However, it noted that the lack of methodologically sound evaluations meant that the intuitive appeal of the approach was not backed up by much hard evidence. Similarly, Frankham (1998) expresses concern about the way that claims made for the relevance of peer education for young people are repeated as dogma without being substantiated by research evidence. She takes the 'key tenets of the faith' and subjects them to critical scrutiny in relation to peer sex education.

- The claim that young people talk openly to each other about sensitive issues, such as sex and drugs:

  - little factual learning takes place between friends and the content of conversations in groups is limited by the need for girls to protect their reputation and boys to be seen as 'one of the lads'
  - young people are more likely to turn to friends for advice than parents, but friends are not necessarily seen as credible sources
  - giving advice to friends can be seen as 'breaking the unwritten rules of friendship'.

- The claim that peer pressure is a powerful influence on young people's behaviour:

  - young people appear to choose peer groups that suit their preferences, rather than their preferences being dictated by the group (a view endorsed by Michell, 1997) and allegiance to such groups is concerned more with identity formation than being pressured to fit in
  - the portrayal of young people as a homogeneous group or, alternatively, as members of stable subgroups, both appear to be erroneous – there are several subgroups and the boundaries between them are relatively fluid.

- The claim that peer education is participatory and empowering:

  - peer educators facilitating sessions with groups may feel the need to set themselves up as experts and model the behaviour of those who trained them
  - peer educators often see maintaining control of the group as part of their purpose
  - it may, therefore, be difficult for young people to use participatory forms of education
  - peer leaders may not be representative of young people generally and the agenda that they set may reflect their own needs rather than responding to others' needs.

Frankham (1998: 190) concludes that peer education 'seems to sit (often uneasily) at the intersection of two cultural domains – the professional cultures of health education and the peer cultures of young people who are the intended recipients'. Young peer educators are confronted with the challenge of bridging both worlds. She also sees an inherent contradiction in submitting to peer influence in the context of peer education, but resisting it in other areas of life. Milburn (1995) also notes the ethical dilemma of placing peer educators in a position in which they feel responsible for influencing behaviour when the principal determinants of that behaviour are social and environmental factors beyond their control.

The EPPI Centre review (1999) called for a clearer understanding of the processes involved in peer education and the ways in which they impact on outcomes. Backett-Milburn and Wilson (2000) concur with this view. Their process evaluation of a young people's peer education project noted the reluctance of adults to relinquish control to young people and that this was attributed to concerns about passing on inaccurate information. They emphasize the importance of distinguishing between concerns that can be addressed by means of the quality of the training given to peer educators and the more general concerns about handing over power to young people, such as fear that they might talk about sensitive subjects, such as sex, in ways that adults might not approve of.

The insight into the peer education process provided by Backett-Milburn and Wilson (2000) allows us to identify a number of key factors that impinge on it:

- **the recruitment process** the extent to which peer educators are recognized as natural leaders within the group
- **setting** the formality of the setting and consistency with the informality of peer education, the opportunity to maintain protected time for peer education, enthusiasm and commitment of staff, good liaison and evidence of success as a motivational factor
- **organizational context** role of various stakeholders in decision making and the extent to which power rests with the peer educators themselves
- **personal development of participants** the development of the skills and acquisition of information needed to be peer educators

- **ongoing support for peer educators** whether or not this is in place as they carry out their role.

Peer education offers the opportunity to capitalize on the shared characteristics of 'the teacher' and the 'learner' to enhance learning. However, it needs to be based on a full understanding of the social context in which it takes place (Milburn, 1995, and Frankham, 1998). Furthermore, to maximize its potential, the peer educators need to be fully involved in developing the agenda and making decisions about process and content rather than merely acting as agents delivering a professionally defined programme.

Other factors

Educational interventions will necessarily be influenced by contextual factors. These can be thought of as falling into two broad groups. First, there is a set of factors that will determine the practical feasibility and acceptability of different methods and this is largely outside the control of those responsible for implementing interventions. This would include the availability of resources (financial and other), size of the target group, experience of the staff and so on. Cultural and professional norms will also influence the acceptability of programmes – to both recipients and key gatekeepers.

Second, there are several contextual factors that health educators might consciously seek to control to enhance the quality of the learning environment. Ryder and Campbell (1988) see part of the educator's role as that of providing an appropriate learning climate. This can include phycho-social as well as physical factors. Some of the key factors identified by the 'Health Skills Projects' are listed in the box.

SELECTED KEY FACTORS THAT INFLUENCE THE LEARNING CLIMATE

Physical factors

- Space – appropriate for comfort and closeness.
- Seating – to allow eye contact with all participants.
- Bright, stimulating environment.
- Protected from outside distractions.
- Convenient timing for participants – and sufficient for the task.

Psycho-social factors

- Appropriate style of leadership.
- Negotiated ground rules.
- Appropriate size of group.
- Unfinished business' or members' mental baggage cleared away.

(Continued)

(Continued)

- Any conflict is brought into the open and dealt with.
- Clear expectations and purpose.
- Reactions of the group are checked out regularly.
- High levels of trust and cooperation.
- Constructive feedback.
- Appropriate use of humour.
- Interactions between all members of the group – and leader's attention shared evenly.
- Good group management skills.

Adapted from Anderson, undated

Summary

We have noted that the selection of educational methods will be influenced by a combination of different considerations. Ideology and professional values – particularly the level of commitment to participation – will underpin the process. A systematic approach to the selection of methods is based on the clear formulation of learning objectives and specification of the characteristics of the learner. Reference to theory and evidence of effectiveness will identify those methods that offer greatest potential within a specific context. Finally, the effectiveness of the methods will be dependent on the skills and training of those delivering interventions and their capacity to motivate learners.

OVERVIEW AND CONCLUDING COMMENTS

Clearly, there are numerous methods and strategies that might be used in health promotion interventions. Our purpose here has not been to attempt to review the whole range – a task of encyclopaedic proportions – but, rather, to draw out key principles.

Consideration of the relative roles of agency and structure will be important in reaching decisions about the focus of health promotion efforts and the balance of activity – in particular, whether the emphasis should be on environmental and policy change, behaviour change or enabling people to address issues that affect their health, individually or collectively. Given the complexity of the web of factors that impact on health and health behaviour, these options are neither discrete nor mutually exclusive. Ultimately, the choice should be determined by which efforts – or, rather, combination of efforts – are likely to achieve maximum gain and are consistent with the core values of health promotion.

The emergence of the settings approach acknowledged the interplay of factors that influence health. It moved forward from seeing settings merely as a means of providing access to a target population towards harnessing the potential offered at all levels within a setting – policy, environment (in its widest sense, including social relationships and interaction), along with opportunities for education. Furthermore, the settings approach sees the boundaries of settings as permeable, with opportunities to interact in a mutually beneficial way with the wider community and other settings.

A theme that runs through this book is that change – whether it be a policy change or behavioural change or empowerment – is dependent on learning. We therefore concluded this chapter with a consideration of methods for facilitating learning. The methods selected should be appropriate for achieving objectives and suited to the needs of the learner. While we would support the view that the methods used in the learning encounter should, in general, be consistent with principles of empowerment, we would not exclude the use of 'persuasive communication' to attempt to convince policymakers of the need for change. Moreover, the pursuit of overriding empowerment goals, equity and achievement of social justice would provide justification for the use of such methods.

10

Evaluation

When God made Heaven and God made Earth
He [sic] formed the seas and gave them birth;
His heart was full of jubilation;
But he made one error – no EVALUATION!

'Oh!' He said, 'That's good!' and He meant it too,
But now we know that that won't do.
Even something that we know is best,
We've got to PROVE by a PRE-POST test.

Apocryphal wisdom from a NASA Newsletter

Evaluation is a vast, lumbering, overgrown adolescent. It has the typical problems associated with this age group too. It does not know quite where it is going and it is prone to bouts of despair. But it is the future after all …

Pawson and Tilley, 1997: 1

CONTENT OF CHAPTER 10

INTRODUCTION

This chapter addresses one of the key features of programme design – evaluation. Given the insistence of current demands that both medicine and health promotion demonstrate their effectiveness and value for money, we might be forgiven for thinking that it is *the* most important feature.

The European Commission Department of Health and Consumer Protection's (European Commission, undated: 107, drawing on Donabedian, 1980. See Rootman et al., 2001) glossary of public health technical terms defines evaluation as:

The critical and objective assessment of the degree to which services or interventions fulfil stated goals. The achievement must be compared with predetermined standards of expectations. Three components … are usually considered:

- **structure** the framework of the service, the equipment used, etc.
- **process** how the service is organized, and what is done
- **outcome** the result.

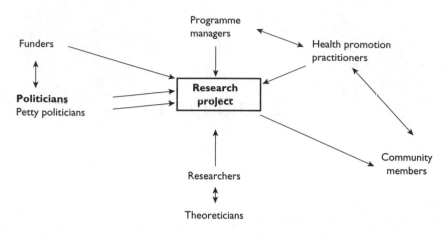

Figure 10.1 The stakeholder community

The evaluation enterprise is, however, not as straight-forward as the above definition might imply – we have merely to note Rootman's (2001) observation that the American Evaluation Association recognizes more than a hundred types of evaluation! Moreover, evaluation is by no means a neutral, technical activity – it is saturated with values, ideological debate and, sometimes, vitriolic argument! Quite obviously then, this chapter must be limited in scope. We therefore include analysis and discussion of those aspects of evaluation that we consider particularly relevant to programme planning.

Fundamental to all evaluation research is the question of validity – the urgent need to 'prove' that any claims made about the effectiveness and effi-ciency of interventions are robust and justifiable. Therefore, a major source of discussion will involve questioning traditional notions of a 'gold standard' for evaluation methodology. This will also involve some consideration of the clash between different research ideologies – the use of the term 'paradigm war' illustrates the intensity of this debate.

A *new* gold standard for evaluating health pro-motion will be proposed. This is based on the adoption of a 'judicial principle' that is applicable to all inter-ventions, but is particularly relevant to complicated community interventions and the radical, empower-ing purpose of health promotion. Consideration will also be given to the ways in which the results of evalu-ation and evidence of effectiveness may be used – or misused – as a basis for influencing policy and practice.

WHY EVALUATE?

At first glance, the above question seems redundant. Clearly, we evaluate to check whether or not an intervention or programme has worked. However, definitions of effectiveness can differ – or, at any rate, the emphasis placed on different definitions can vary. As WHO (1995) has noted, health promo-tion is an investment and evaluation is concerned to address the costs and benefits of this investment. More specifically, evaluators might be concerned to measure programme outcomes and processes in order to assess one or more of the following results of this investment:

- contribution to knowledge base/theory of health promotion
- insights that will result in more effective health promotion practice
- relative costs and benefits in financial terms
- levels of stakeholder satisfaction
- evidence to influence policymakers in respect of:

  - development of health policy
  - continued employment of researchers and health promotion departments

- impact on individual and public health.

WHOSE VALUES?

Essentially, evaluation is concerned with assessing the extent to which certain valued goals have been achieved. However, as the above-mentioned list of reasons for evaluating programmes may suggest, there is often substantial variation between the goals espoused by different stakeholders in the evaluation enterprise. Figure 10.1 provides an overview of the dynamics of the stakeholder community.

IS THE CUSTOMER ALWAYS RIGHT? THE ROTHSCHILD PRINCIPLE

The main principle governing any Government funding of R&D is the Rothschild principle, laid down in Cmd 4814 and reiterated in the White Paper 'Realising Our Potential: A Strategy for Science, Engineering and Technology': '... the customer says what he wants, the contractor does it, if he can, and the customer pays'.

Code of practice, Department of Health, 1993, cited in Pawson and Tilley, 1997: 14

In theory at least, the various stakeholders may all influence evaluation. However, research is typically carried out *on* rather than *with* individuals and the community. Although this is antithetical to the participation imperative inherent in the empowerment model of health promotion, it is currently the most prevalent form of evaluation.

Funders are clearly key stakeholders. As the adage reminds us, 'he who pays the piper calls the tune.' Funder power can operate at both ends of the evaluation enterprise. Allocation of funding can be used to control the research agenda. Funders can also act as gatekeepers in relation to the dissemination of research findings – to the extent of withholding unpalatable findings. A well-known attempt to limit publicity in the UK was when Sir Douglas Black's report on health inequalities was published on an August bank holiday – a release date that would minimize its coverage in the news.

It is, perhaps, not unreasonable that funders should wish to exercise some degree of control. Pawson and Tilley (1997) quote a Department of Health's Code of Practice (see the box) to illustrate this phenomenon.

The authors also refer to Stufflebeam's (1980: 90, cited in Pawson and Tilley, 1997: 13) concern at the 'standards' produced by the US Joint Committee on Standards for Educational Evaluation:

[these have] four features... *utility, feasibility, propriety* and *accuracy* [in that order] .... and evaluation should not be done at all if there is no prospect for its being useful to some audience. Second, it should not be done if it is not feasible to conduct it in political terms, or practicality terms, or cost-effectiveness terms. Third, they do not think it should be done if we cannot demonstrate that it will be conducted fairly and ethically. [If it has utility, feasibility and propriety] ... they said we could turn to the difficult matters of the technical accuracy of the evaluation.

The authors object to this kow-towing to customer demands, which, in their view, is characteristic of what they call 'pragmatic evaluation'. This mode of

evaluation is seen as 'methodologically rootless' and, epistemologically speaking, knowledge is considered to be valid to the extent that it is pragmatically acceptable, so, ontologically, the social world centres on 'power-play'. Political astuteness and technical proficiency rule (Pawson and Tilley, 1997: 14).

The political dimension

The question of power is central to the dynamics of the stakeholder community. Evaluation is inherently political – it is rooted in some stakeholders' concerns to achieve change (and, of course, to provide justificatory feedback for preferred policies and actions!). In many instances the political agenda is written large. For example, a critical theory stance in health promotion is manifestly concerned to bring about social change involving, ultimately, a challenge to many aspects of capitalist economies. However, most programmes – even those having a radical agenda – tend to operate *within* systems rather than directly challenge them. For instance, community development might typically concentrate on creating food cooperatives rather than developing a popular movement designed to confront the power of the web of agencies and government departments involved in food production and, indeed, the retail profit motive. Pawson and Tilley have coined the term 'petty political' to refer to the operations involved in the former, limited pressure for change. We have retained the term in Figure 10.1 and expanded its meaning somewhat to refer to the various minor processes and all actors involved in jostling for power at different levels of influence.

Health promotion values – the seal of approval

While there may be conflicting values, both explicit and implicit, in the stakeholder community, it is worth emphasizing the research-related values that

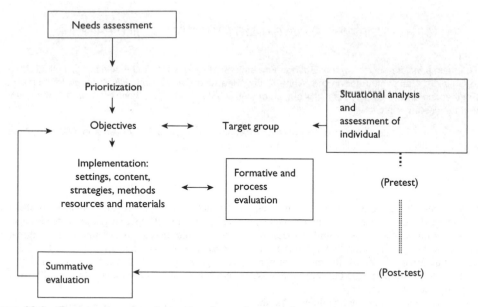

Figure 10.2   Programme planning – the place of research

must be upheld if an evaluation is to follow ideological commitments to an empowerment model of health promotion. The following guiding principles encapsulate this ideological commitment and have additional significance as they incorporate the endorsement of WHO European Working Group on Health Promotion Evaluation (Rootman et al., 2001) Health promotion programmes, policies and other organized activities should be:

- **empowering** enabling individuals and communities to assume more power over the personal, socio-economic and environmental factors that affect their health
- **participatory** involving all concerned at all stages of the process
- **holistic** fostering physical, mental, social and spiritual health
- **intersectoral** involving the collaboration of agencies from relevant sectors
- **equitable** guided by a concern for equity and social justice
- **sustainable** bringing about changes that individuals and communities can maintain once initial funding has ended
- **multi-strategy** using a variety of approaches, including policy development, organizational change, community development, legislation, advocacy, education and communication, in combination.

EVALUATION AND PROGRAMME DESIGN

Evaluation is an integral element of systematic programme planning. The model adopted here centres on the key elements described in Figure 10.2.

Three varieties of evaluation are included in Figure 10.2 – summative, formative and process. 'Summative' refers to an end-on assessment of the extent to which the programme has achieved its purpose. 'Process' evaluation consists of recording information collected throughout the programme and will be used for 'illumination'. 'Formative' evaluation also involves using information acquired throughout the programme. However, this information is used *during* the programme to make changes designed to maximize outcomes.

The construction of objectives is used to formulate specific goals based on information about the 'client group' and also the nature of the desired outcomes. The actual selection of research methodology and methods will depend on the nature of the evaluation task and, of course, the ethical/ideological appropriateness of that methodology. At this juncture, we will consider the ideological issues associated with the choice of research methodology. In essence, this will involve discussing approaches that have competing value positions rather than technical matters – and these trigger quite heated debate!

PARADIGM – A DEFINITION

A paradigm is a worldview built on implicit assumptions, accepted definitions, comfortable habits, values defended as truths, and beliefs projected as reality. As such, paradigms are deeply embedded in the socialization of adherents and practitioners: paradigms tell them what is important, legitimate, and reasonable. Paradigms are also normative, telling the practitioner what to do without the necessity of long existential or epistemological consideration. But it is this aspect of paradigms that constitutes both their strength and their weakness – their strength in that it makes action possible, their weakness in that the very reason for action is hidden in the unquestioned assumptions of the paradigm.

Patton, 1997: 267

PARADIGM WARS – POSITIVISM AND ITS ALTERNATIVES

Paradigm conflicts not only apply to the nature and philosophy of health promotion, but are reflected in different stances about what should or should not constitute appropriate and ethical evaluation. The major debate centres on the battle between positivism and a collection of approaches associated with qualitative methodology. More particularly, it is revealed in challenges to the 'medical model'.

'Epistemology' is at the very centre of disagreements about which research approach and its concomitant methods are acceptable. Epistemology is concerned with beliefs about knowledge – about how we know our world. It is associated with the concept of 'ontology'.

Denzin and Lincoln (1994: 99) succinctly describe the relationship between paradigms and the above-mentioned concepts, along with their specific application in methodologies.

> A paradigm encompasses three elements: epistemology, ontology and methodology. Epistemology asks, how do we know the world? What is the relationship between the enquirer and the known? Ontology raises basic questions about the nature of reality. Methodology focuses on how we gain knowledge about the world.

Accordingly, some approaches to evaluation would be considered inherently flawed and incapable of revealing the 'truth'. Furthermore, advocates of some approaches might argue that there are different forms of truth, while others might deny that truth exists.

The positivist paradigm

By way of simplifying an exceedingly complicated field of philosophical analysis and criticism related to conceptualizations of research and practice, three different paradigms will be discussed below. These are positivism, interpretivism and a 'third way' – arguably a compromise position that espouses critical realism and a utilization-focused perspective. While various factions take different stances within the field of interpretivism, the most heated debates occur between advocates of interpretivism (and other allies that tend to espouse qualitative methodology) and what has been until recently the dominant paradigm of positivism. The third way paradigm might be subject to challenge, largely because of its alleged compromise position and, because, arguably, it is not a paradigm at all. For health promotion, however, the positivism v. interpretivism debate is of special importance as a positivist approach has characterized the medical model and underwritten the alleged 'gold standard' for evaluating programmes – the randomized controlled trial (RCT).

Positivism defined

Positivist philosophy can be traced to Auguste Comte (1798–1857), who compared and contrasted three constructions of reality – theological, metaphysical and positive. Positivism was equated with science, which was seen as the sole way forward to gaining a true understanding of the world. Comte's ideas were adopted by the logical positivists, whose philosophy rested on the assumption that we could gain an accurate representation of the world through our senses (and various devices that would increase the power of our senses); this 'scientific knowledge' would form the basis for progressive and cumulative advances in knowledge that would be free from partial interpretations and superstitious interpretations of reality.

Positivist science was viewed as having a values-free, 'neutral' status. It was objective rather than subjective. Moreover, the positivist approach was more than mere empiricism – a procedure, 'involving the production of accurate data – meticulous, precise, generalizable – in which the data themselves constitute the end for the research. It is summed up by the catchphrase "the facts speak for themselves"' (Dulmer, 1982). While accurate data collection and generalizability is also characteristic of positivist research, unlike empiricism, it is theory-driven. The ultimate goal is the construction of general laws.

Experiment is central to positivist methodology, although Popper has challenged its capacity to achieve verification. His centrally important concept of falsifiability is now inevitably considered to be at the heart of 'scientific method'. In other words, a theory holds until disproved, so the logical method of science is falsification and continual checking of claims to knowledge. In short, the key features of Popper's perspective are as follows:

- critical of 'induction'
- it is impossible to verify a universal theory with any degree of certainty but it *is* possible to disprove a theory and therefore only one convincing 'disproof' will result in the rejection of theory regardless of how much supporting evidence already exists
- therefore, theory (a set of hypotheses) only survives until disproved – Popper was critical of those who cling to their preferred theories and ignore contrary evidence
- accordingly, the method employed by 'science' must be falsification
- therefore, the 'gold standard' results of a properly constructed randomized controlled trial would also only hold until disproved.

Knowledge is therefore always provisional. As the procedure involves deduction rather than induction and is based on the confirmation or falsification of hypotheses, the scientific model adopted has been described as 'hypothetico-deductive' (Popper, 1945, 1959).

Perhaps unsurprisingly, social and behavioural scientists seeking to enhance the credibility of their activities and professions looked to the natural sciences and positivism as the way forward. The application within medicine and public health has been subject to quite intense criticism in association with the increasing challenge to medical hegemony. Health promotion has been at the forefront of this challenge.

Interpretivism – an alternative to positivism

While positivism is relatively easy to define, it is much more difficult to pick one's way through the plethora of paradigms, methodologies and methods that constitute the opposition! Perhaps the most frequently used overarching terms are 'interpretivism' and 'constructivism'.

'Interpretivism' – a concept virtually identical to 'constructivism' (Guba and Lincoln, 1989) – centres on people's ways of interpreting/making sense of reality. It is essentially inductive – theory tends to be generated from data rather than data being used to test theory. Interpretivism derives from 'phenomenology' and is thus concerned with the 'lived experience' of people (Spiegelberg, 1960). It also has roots in 'ethnomethodology'. As Holloway (1997: 93) notes, interpretivism:

> can be linked to Weber's *Verstehen* (German for 'empathetic' understanding) approach ... 'understanding' in the social sciences is inherently different from 'explanation' in the natural sciences. [Weber] differentiates between *nomothetic,* rule-governed methods of the latter and *idiographic* methods focusing on individual cases and not linked to the general laws of nature but to the actions of human beings ... Most qualitative research has its origin in the interpretive perspective.

A further variation on the interpretivist approach has been termed 'hermeneutics' (from the Greek god Hermes, the messenger, who interpreted messages from Zeus to human beings). Holloway (1997: 87) again:

> Researchers ... gather data from language, texts and actions. They have to return to the data frequently, and ask the participants what the data mean to them.

Guba and Lincoln (1989) add the term 'dialectic' to their version of the approach. As Schwandt (1994: 128) explains:

> They believe that the best means of achieving researcher and client constructions of reality is the 'hermeneutic-dialectic' process, so called because it is interpretive and fosters comparing and contrasting divergent constructions in an effort to achieve a synthesis of same. They strongly emphasize that the goal of constructivist enquiry is to achieve a consensus (or, failing that, an agenda for negotiation) on issues and concerns that define the nature of the enquiry.

Apart from the constructions of the research reality embodied in this latter constructivist approach, it will be apparent that 'subjects' of the research are not 'objects' but, rather, participants. This commitment is also apparent in what Guba and Lincoln (1989) called 'fourth generation research', which entails stakeholder involvement, exploration of different perspectives and issues, negotiation to achieve consensus, development of reports communicating the nature of consensus and proposed actions to participants and an iterative process of reviewing and revisiting the evaluation to address perceptions, concerns and issues that have not been resolved.

New paradigm research

It will probably be apparent to those readers who have not already been immersed in the wealth of conceptualizations associated with the paradigm wars that the battlefield is immense! By way of a resumé of the key features of the paradigms opposed to positivism, we might usefully summarize the 'manifesto' of new paradigm research, according to Reason and Rowan (1981) as shown in the box.

Pawson and Tilley (1997: 19) provide a useful graphic summary of constructivist research and its rationale (see Figure 10.3).

Participatory research

As we noted earlier, the participative convictions of interpretivism chime with health promotion's ideological commitment to involving client and community. Whyte (1997) provides an interesting

historical slant on the development of 'participatory research' and 'action research'. He notes the possible confusion between the terms 'action research', 'participatory research' and 'participatory action research' and proceeds to remind us that it is possible to have action research without participation and participatory research without action. Moreover, participation and action can 'emerge' from social research and Whyte recalls how, in his classic research on *Street Corner Society* (Whyte, 1943), two participants, Doc and Sam Franco, 'became in a very real sense participant observers'. Moreover, 'We all hoped that publication of the book would eventually be helpful to the district and to others like it ... (although there were no specific action or policy recommendations.) Certain individuals begin as informants, then become key informants and ended up as co-participant observers, helping the professional field worker to interpret what they are learning from interviewing and observation.' Whyte (1991) defined 'participatory action research' (PAR) as follows:

> In participatory action research (PAR), some of the people in the organization or community under study participate actively with the professional researcher throughout the research process from the initial design to the final presentation of results and discussion of action implications.

He subsequently felt that it was necessary to expand this definition to take account of emancipatory values (which he considered had always been implicit in the first definition). The addendum (Whyte, 1997: 111–12) states:

A MANIFESTO OF NEW PARADIGM RESEARCH

- Research is never neutral – either it accepts or rejects the status quo.
- Research may be beneficial, but it may also be harmful.
- A close relationship between researcher and researched is essential. Both are equal in the research process. They are partners in defining the scope and nature of the research.
- Researcher and researched should have equal ownership of the products of the research.
- Research should be particularly concerned with knowledge having a practical, action-orientated outcome.
- Research should encourage people to take action – new paradigm research supports the politics of self-determination.
- New paradigm research rejects a traditional 'objective' approach and associated quantitative methods. It seeks a new kind of synthesis of subjectivity and objectivity.
- New paradigm researchers are committed to a holistic view of people and the environments and contexts in which they live their lives.

After Reason and Rowan, 1981

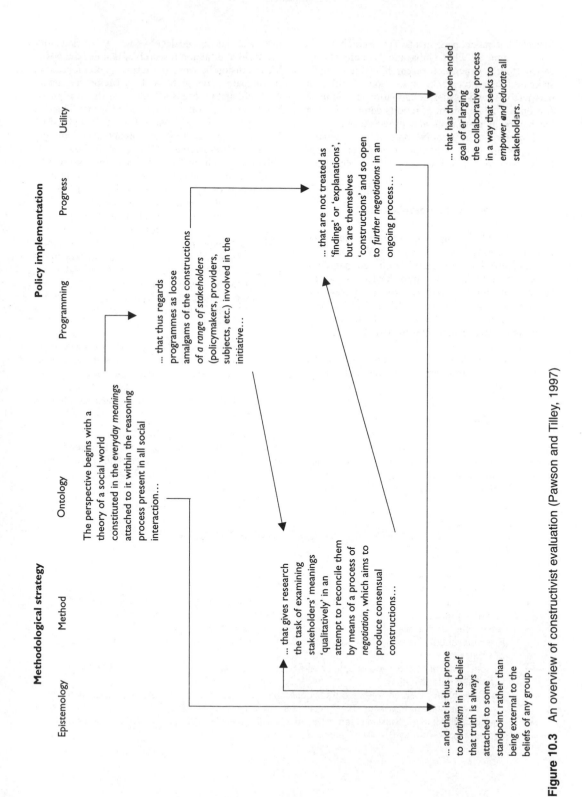

Figure 10.3 An overview of constructivist evaluation (Pawson and Tilley, 1997)

The social purpose underlying PAR is to empower low-status people in the organization or community to make decisions and take actions which were previously foreclosed to them.

Macauley et al., (1999: 774), discussing research imperatives in the health context, reiterate the nature and importance of participation:

Participatory research attempts to negotiate a balance between developing valid generalizable knowledge and benefiting the community that is being researched and to improve research protocols by incorporating the knowledge and expertise of community members ... these goals can best be met by the community and researcher collaborating in the research as equals ... Participatory research began as a movement for social justice in international development settings. It was developed to help improve social and economic conditions, to effect change, and to reduce the distrust of the people being studied. [Participatory research] ... provides a framework to respond to health issues within a social and historical context.

Realistic v. utilization-focused evaluation

Pawson and Tilley (1997) have launched a vigorous, and influential, challenge to both traditional, positivist research paradigms and, at the same time, to the constructivists' equally constraining insistence that, in the words of (Guba and Lincoln 1989: 17), 'no accommodation is possible between positivist and constructivist belief systems as they are now formulated.' To do this was to throw out the evaluation baby with the positivist bathwater! On the other hand, they questioned what they describe as a purely 'pragmatic approach', which they felt was exemplified in Patton's (1982: 49) alleged lack of interest in the epistemological basis of research and his overemphasis on an all-purpose methodological 'toolbox'. They disapprovingly cite the following statement:

If a funding mandate calls for a summative outcomes evaluation, then the evaluator had better be prepared to produce such an animal, complete with a final report that includes that terminology right there on the front page, in big letters in the title.

This is perhaps rather unfair. Patton (1997) in a recent text on 'utilization-focused evaluation', acknowledges the value of both positivist and interpretivist paradigms. He considers that discussions about paradigm wars, 'are now primarily about philosophy rather than methods.' He (1997: 296) adds,

I disagree, then, that philosophical assumptions necessarily require allegiance by evaluators to one paradigm or the other. Pragmatism can overcome seemingly logical contradictions ... the flexible and open evaluator can view the same data from the perspective of each paradigm and can help adherents of either paradigm interpret data in more than one way.

From our particular perspective on the inherently political nature of health promotion, we should also record Patton's belief that evaluation is not values-free and, 'politics is omnipresent in evaluation.' (see the box).

Patton also adds that, as utilization-focused evaluation is pragmatic (and 'useful'), it can be applied to a variety of situations having different ideological commitments. Accordingly, he (1997: 103) states that, 'Using evaluation to mobilize for social action, empower participants, and support social justice are options on the menu of evaluation process uses.'

An interesting indicator of Patton's 'pragmatic paradigm' is provided by his apparent affection for Rudyard Kipling's (*Just So Stories*, 1902) well-known aphorism:

I keep six honest serving men,
(They taught me all I knew);

WHEN IS EVALUATION NOT POLITICAL?

Evaluation is *not* political under the following conditions:

- no one cares about the programme
- no one knows about the programme
- no money is at stake
- no power or authority is at stake
- and no one in the programme, making decisions about the programme, or otherwise involved in, knowledgeable about, or attached to the programme, is sexually active.

Patton, 1997: 352

Their names are What and Why and When
and How and Where and Who.

He translates this as:

Who is the evaluation for?
What do we need to find out?
Why do we want to find that out?
When will the findings be needed?
Where should we gather information?
How will the results be used?

Further consideration of the philosophy and ideology
of pragmatism requires much more space than is at
our disposal here. However, we would certainly wish
to insist that, within the medical/health promotion
field, we have not seen the end of the debate, we may
not even have seen the beginning of the end, but we
may have seen the end of the beginning!

Realistic evaluation

Pawson and Tilley's approach to 'realistic evaluation'
has been particularly influential in evaluating 'social
programmes' and, thus, is especially relevant to the
complicated interventions and collaborations characteristic of health promotion. The approach can be
termed 'post positive' and recognizes the existence of
realities that can be investigated in robust fashion and
used to implement social policy. At the same time, the
narrow positivist approach epitomized by randomized
controlled trials are determinedly discarded. On this
occasion, the authors approvingly quote Guba and
Lincoln's (1989: 60, cited by Pawson and Tilley,
1997: 22) observation that true experimental design
'effectively strips away the context and yields results
that are valid only in other contextless situations'.
Realistic evaluation rejects this 'succesionist' logic
and argues for a 'generative logic'. The essence of
realistic evaluation is to be found in a simple formula:

$$Outcome = mechanisms + context$$

Part of the rationale for Pawson and Tilley's rejection of the simplistic causal underpinning of the
RCT is the fact that physical science and its many
advances depend on recognition of a 'stratified reality' and inherently complicated 'mechanisms'.
Observations of 'regularities' in both physical and
social science can be understood and influenced
only by understanding these mechanisms. We will
later, in discussing health promotion programmes,
make reference to the 'black box' that must be illu-
minated if understanding is to be gained and efficient programmes achieved. Moreover, the
individual choices resulting from the interplay of
'mechanisms' take place within 'contexts' – in

other words, within various settings and their
associated sets of norms and social rules. Accordingly (Pawson and Tilley, 1997: 216–8):

> Evaluators need to acknowledge that programmes are
> implemented in a changing and permeable social world,
> and that programme effectiveness may thus be sub-
> verted or enhanced through the unanticipated intrusion
> of new contexts and new causal powers. Evaluators
> (also) need to focus on how the causal mechanisms
> which generate social and behavioural problems are
> removed or countered through the alternative causal
> mechanisms introduced in a social programme...

Before leaving our brief description of realistic
evaluation, it is worth noting that qualitative/inter-
pretivist methodology is central to its philosophy
and practice. One particularly interesting aspect is
the authors' argument that a central part of the collaboration of researcher and participants involves a
'teaching-learning' process: stakeholders are
'taught' by the researchers so that they gain understandings of programmes and their attributes in
order to participate fully in (empowered) decision
making. Also, of course, the researchers need to be
taught by the stakeholders to gain maximum insight
into the social and psychological realities and constructions of reality.

Before proceeding to consider the factors associated with selecting indicators of programme success
within the kinds of complicated contexts discussed
above, we should perhaps end this section on paradigm wars by asking where we stand. Which paradigms and ideologies and methodologies would
seem to be most appropriate to health promotion?
We would wish to avoid postmodern pessimism and
consider that it is, in fact, possible to develop understandings of the world. On the other hand, we recognize that multiple interpretations occur as a result
of psychological and social constructions of reality.
Our stance is thus post positive. Life and health are
complicated and we must gain in-depth understandings if we are to exert influence over the development of health promotion. We are firmly committed
to participative, emancipatory research designed to
empower and address social injustice and health
inequalities. We are thus perhaps concerned not so
much with an ideology of research, but, rather with
research for an ideology of health promotion.

EFFECTIVENESS, EFFICIENCY
AND EFFICACY

In the last analysis, evaluation is concerned with
whether or not an intervention has been successful.
Two standards are typically used in assessing the

extent of success – or failure. These are 'effectiveness' and 'efficiency'. The former term simply refers to the extent to which a programme has achieved its goals, while 'efficiency' is a measure of *relative* effectiveness – that is, how successful a programme has been in comparison to competing strategies or methods. For instance, if a course of drugs could lower population cholesterol levels more quickly, completely and safely than dietary change, it would be more efficient (although possibly less cost-effective) to prescribe that drug.

The efficacy paradox

The concept of efficacy has also been used, albeit less commonly, as a measure of effectiveness. It describes effectiveness and efficiency when interventions operate under ideal conditions: 'Effectiveness has all the attributes of efficacy except one: it reflects performance under ordinary conditions...' (Brook and Lohr, 1985: 711).

The concept of efficacy relates to the notion of programme fidelity, which means the extent to which an intervention is delivered in accordance with recommended best practice. It has particular significance for evaluating health promotion programmes in relation to what we describe here as the 'efficacy paradox'. For instance, if an intervention has been shown to be effective when it has been constructed according to an *ideal* specification and implemented with complete fidelity, the chances are that *ordinary* practitioners working under *average* conditions will not be able to achieve the same degree of success. Indeed the programme might fail. Conversely, when a programme has not met its objectives and, consequently, has been considered ineffective, that evaluation judgement is flawed as the programme was doomed to fail due to inadequate implementation. We will consider the implications of such flawed judgement when discussing the question of validity later in the chapter. For now, we should merely note that programme design must clearly identify what might be achieved within existing limitations and set the objectives accordingly. If these limited results are judged to be not worthwhile, the proposed programme should be scrapped. In the last analysis, the decision is

grounded in health economics – do the programme gains justify the expenses incurred?

On cost-effectiveness

One of the most important criteria for appraising the efficiency of health promotion programmes involves calculating the relative financial costs of competing interventions. Godfrey (2001) notes the tendency for using 'partial' economic assessments – for example, merely describing the cost of an intervention. Clearly this situation would be seen as far from satisfactory by health economists and Godfrey lists four different types of 'full' economic evaluation.

- **Cost-minimization** The costs of two or more interventions assumed to achieve identical outcomes are calculated. The intervention that minimizes costs is judged to be the intervention of choice.
- **Cost-effectiveness analysis** In addition to measuring the cost of programmes, benefits are assessed in quantifiable terms, such as the numbers of individuals exercising regularly or uptake of immunization against childhood diseases. It would, of course, be meaningless to make judgements about relative value for money unless indicators of health common to all programmes are employed (for instance, life years gained).
- **Cost utility analysis** This mode of analysis seeks to measure the utility or values attached to particular health gains. QALYs (quality adjusted life years) are typically used to assess utility.
- **Cost–benefit analysis** CBA not only states the costs in monetary terms, but also seeks to place a price tag on the benefits accruing from the programme. A calculation of the cost per given benefit is then possible, typically expressed as a cost–benefit ratio.

Following these observations, it is both clear and logical that if two or more programmes prove to be equally effective, then the intervention that costs least should be selected. The box provides examples of the calculated benefits against costs of selected health promotion measures.

HEALTH PROMOTION – INSTANCES OF ECONOMIC EFFECTIVENESS

- A hypertension and screening programme resulted in a saving of 7.81 dollars per dollar invested. A group discussion used to educate patients on controlling their asthma achieved a cost–benefit ratio of 1:5 (Green, 1974).

(Continued)

(Continued)

- The economic benefits of a family planning service were substantial:
  - prevention of 'typical unplanned pregnancies' – cost–benefit ratio 1.3:1
  - preventing pregnancies among mothers of three or more children – cost–benefit ratio 4.5:1
  - preventing unplanned premarital conceptions – cost–benefit ratio 5.3:1.

  '... for every £100 spent on [the above] family planning services, the public sector can expect a benefit of £130, £450 and £530 respectively' (Laing, 1982).

- The benefits from legislation requiring cycling-helmet use in Israel (over a five-year period) are considerable and exceed costs by a ratio of 3:1 (total benefits were estimated at $40,544,770) (Ginsberg and Silverberg, 1994).

Godfrey et al. (1989) calculated that, for a budget of £1 million, a relatively straightforward and simple intervention involving GPs providing advice to their patients not to smoke might 'notch up' some 59,888 QALYs compared with a mere 302 QALYs for breast screening. Again, a comparison of the highly beneficial surgical procedure of hip replacement cost some £750 per QALY compared with a mere £167 for GP-provided smoking-related advice.

Other evidence can be found to support these claims for the cost-effectiveness of health promotion. For instance, following a different kind of calculation, Warner (1981: 730) described the benefits of anti-smoking campaigns in the USA in terms of the anticipated level of smoking that would have prevailed without health education as follows:

In the absence of the anti-smoking campaign, adult per capita cigarette consumption in 1987 would have been an estimated 78–89 per cent higher than the level actually experienced... [As a result,] ...an estimated 789,200 Americans avoided or postponed smoking-related deaths and gained an average of 21 additional years of life expectancy each.

Although this type of analysis may, at first sight, be very seductive for those keen to demonstrate effectiveness and cost-effectiveness, there are several problems. While costing 'input' is relatively unproblematic, the appropriateness and ethicality of costing 'output' – that is, assessing and assigning a value to quality of life – poses major ethical problems, as noted in Chapter 2. Furthermore, these examples fall within the domain of prevention and treatment and involve comparatively simple interventions targeted at individuals. Raphael (2001a) noted in reference to Lindström's (1994) quality of life model, that it questioned the relevance of cost–benefit analysis to more holistic interpretations of health and interventions operating at interpersonal, community, social and environmental levels that are more typical of health promotion.

A fundamental problem involved in applying cost–benefit analysis to health promotion is that, *if* it is effective in deferring death (often accompanied by a deteriorating quality of life and an increase in the cost of care), then health promotion will actually generate an increasing financial burden on society. Therefore, from a purely cynical point of view – which ignores totally the precept of 'adding life to years as well as years to life' – the most economic scenario would involve individuals staying fit and healthy until they retired (at a later age than that currently prevailing). They should then die peacefully and expeditiously! Alternatively, perhaps we should reconsider Cohen's (1981) reflections on Musgrave's (1959) notion of 'merit want' and 'merit good' (see the box).

THE ADMIRABLE NOTION OF MERIT GOOD

Merit wants are, 'so meritorious that their satisfaction is provided for through the public budget over and above what is provided for through the market and paid for by private buyers'. A merit good satisfies a merit want. A common interpretation of merit wants is that individuals (and politicians?) frequently make 'wrong' choices – that is, choices that do not reflect their 'true' preferences. Some 'élite' is capable of seeing the meritorious nature of the underconsumed good that is not seen by the individual (or, perhaps, is seen by politicians but ignored because of its potential expense?). The élite is therefore justified in interfering with the economist's sacred concept of consumer sovereignty.

After Cohen, 1981: 19

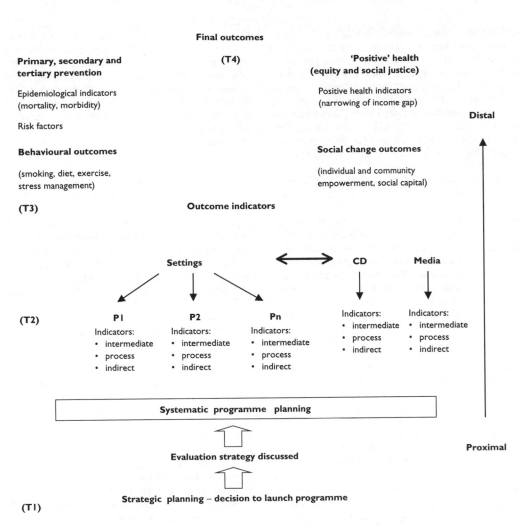

Figure 10.4   An overview of a health promotion programme

DISENTANGLING COMPLEXITY – SELECTING INDICATORS OF SUCCESS

We noted in Chapter 4 the centrality of objectives to programme planning. The attempt to identify coherent and appropriate objectives is an important feature of disentangling the complexity inherent in many, if not most, health promotion interventions. Rigorously formulated objectives will also provide a secure basis for identifying indicators of success – particularly if they define standards and conditions. Although, at first sight, a straightforward task, like much in evaluation, it can be quite challenging. Figure 10.4 provides an overview of a hypothetical, large-scale health promotion programme.

First, it is assumed that the programme has been designed according to the principles of systematic planning discussed earlier in this book. It is launched at a particular time (T1) and will achieve its final goals (if ever) at another point in time (T4). Temporal progress is also indicated by a proximal–distal spectrum – that is, activities occurring at T1 are proximal to the start of the programme, whereas final outcomes at T4 and all other events in between will be more or less distal.

Two kinds of final outcomes – the ultimate strategic goals – are shown in Figure 10.4. They include, on the one hand, the traditional goals of a preventive model of health promotion – namely, primary, secondary and tertiary prevention – and, on the other, the ultimate outcomes of a strategy seeking to address 'positive health'. For reasons discussed in Chapter 1, it is more difficult to explicate these 'positive health' goals than the much more common and precise goals of preventive medicine. The label 'positive health' is therefore used to refer to any outcomes related to 'quality of life' or, even more broadly, 'the good life'. By contrast, the achievement of 'equity' and 'social justice' are more readily conceptualized and operationalized. Indeed, they figure prominently in many community-based initiatives.

The two outcomes levels at T4 are not, of course, completely discrete as the quality of life is typically damaged by disease and enhanced by its prevention. Moreover, as has also been clearly demonstrated, the achievement of wellbeing and, more demonstrably, the reduction of inequalities, may have a major impact on preventive outcomes.

Indicators of successful preventive outcomes are readily available – for example, in the form of mortality and morbidity data. However, we would argue that such epidemiological indicators should not be used to evaluate the effectiveness of health promotion, but, rather, justify its use (Green and Tones, 1999: 136). It is less clear whether or not a similar assertion should be made about the final outcomes of positive health promotion – largely due to the vagueness of many formulations of positive health. However, similar arguments do apply to the achievement of equity – for example, narrowing the income gap between rich and poor.

The reasons for not using final outcome indicators are doubtless evident. There is frequently a substantial time gap between particular health promotion inputs and the final outcomes. For example, it may take many years for the benefits of a school-based healthy eating and exercise programme to become apparent in reduced mortality from coronary heart disease – the gap between T1 and T4 in such a case being thirty or forty years. To use an epidemiological indicator to assess the effectiveness of the teaching programme would thus be entirely unrealistic!

A related objection is based on the fact that many successful health education/promotion interventions may be necessary but not sufficient to influence final outcomes. Typically, a complicated web of inputs over time would be needed. For instance, effective life skills training, together with an efficient sex education programme in schools might only have an impact on sexual risk-taking if policy measures have been implemented to ensure ready access to condoms and, say, a user-friendly drop-in centre for young people.

However, in the last analysis, epidemiological indicators should, quite simply, not be necessary. If there is a robust link between the behavioural outcomes targeted by health promotion (such as smoking, diet, exercise and stress level), then it is only necessary to measure those behavioural outcomes – or some combination in the form of risk factors. If there is *not* a robust relationship with mortality and morbidity, then there is no justification for putting people to the inconvenience of changing their lifestyle!

Intermediate, indirect and process indicators

Figure 10.4 shows a number of hypothetical subordinate programmes that contribute to outcomes at T3 – adoption of exercise, dietary change and so on. These programmes might be located in a number of settings, such as schools, the workplace, hospitals and general medical practice, and be accompanied by non-formal work in the community, together with strategically employed mass media. The settings-based programmes would involve both education and supportive policy. Indicators of success might be identified for each programme. Outcomes might, for example, include smoking cessation in general practice and the implementation of a non-smoking policy in workplaces.

Intermediate indicators could consist of any of the measures derived from relevant sections of the HAM, such as beliefs about the relationship between exercise and heart disease, how the disadvantages of changing diet could be countered by improved body image and attractiveness to the opposite sex and how healthy food can be quite delicious! They could also, of course, be self-efficacy beliefs that individuals could actually avoid temptation and lose weight (with consequent benefits from reduced risk of heart disease and feeling fit).

Process indicators would be used to record the fidelity of the programme and identify needs for improvement and refinement. Consider, for instance, the hypothetical empowering face-to-face counselling interaction between doctor and patient mentioned earlier in Chapter 9 (see Figure 10.5).

The indicators included under the client task in Figure 10.5 would be called 'intermediate indicators' as they contribute, in various degrees, to the behavioural outcomes of stopping smoking and maintaining that behaviour for a year (the indicator normally used to establish ex-smoker status). In the event of failure, these intermediate indicators would provide some insight into possible reasons for the client not achieving non-smoking status. The details of the educational task provide indicators of the

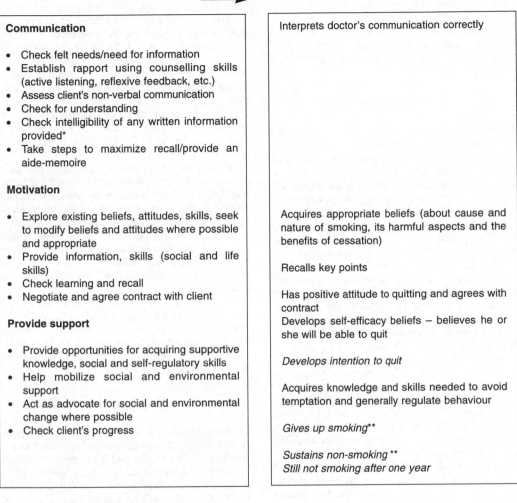

Doctor's task (process indicators) ← Client's task (intermediate and outcome indicators)

Communication

- Check felt needs/need for information
- Establish rapport using counselling skills (active listening, reflexive feedback, etc.)
- Assess client's non-verbal communication
- Check for understanding
- Check intelligibility of any written information provided*
- Take steps to maximize recall/provide an aide-memoire

Motivation

- Explore existing beliefs, attitudes, skills, seek to modify beliefs and attitudes where possible and appropriate
- Provide information, skills (social and life skills)
- Check learning and recall
- Negotiate and agree contract with client

Provide support

- Provide opportunities for acquiring supportive knowledge, social and self-regulatory skills
- Help mobilize social and environmental support
- Act as advocate for social and environmental change where possible
- Check client's progress

Interprets doctor's communication correctly

Acquires appropriate beliefs (about cause and nature of smoking, its harmful aspects and the benefits of cessation)

Recalls key points

Has positive attitude to quitting and agrees with contract
Develops self-efficacy beliefs – believes he or she will be able to quit

Develops intention to quit

Acquires knowledge and skills needed to avoid temptation and generally regulate behaviour

Gives up smoking**

Sustains non-smoking **
Still not smoking after one year

*An indirect indicator
**Outcome indicators

Figure 10.5 An interaction between GP and patient – intermediate, process and indirect indicators of success (after Tones and Tilford, 2001)

counselling process and serve as a kind of quality control. Indications of the failure of this process can both provide evidence for the client's lack of success in giving up smoking and, also, may suggest a training deficit.

Figure 10.5 provides one example of an *indirect indicator*. In so far as written materials, such as a booklet of hints and tips on how to stop smoking, are important to the encounter, it is essential that they have been pretested or otherwise tested for

intelligibility and acceptability before use. Evidence of suitability then provides an indirect indicator of success.

We should perhaps note at this juncture – to add to the complexity – that many indicators may be defined as either intermediate indicators or outcome indicators, depending on the programme in question and its goals. For example, self-empowerment and social capital may be deemed to be outcomes worth pursuing in their own right, so evidence of their effectiveness, provided by measures of confidence and control, could rightly be called *outcome* indicators. On the other hand, it seems increasingly clear that empowerment is a major determinant of adopting behaviour consistent with preventive outcomes. In this latter case, evidence of empowerment would provide *intermediate* indicators of success.

Choosing indicators

Indirect, intermediate and outcome indicators should be viewed as providing evidence at various stages along a complicated and often convoluted pathway leading from proximal interventions to ultimate outcomes (if everything proceeds according to plan!). In such a situation, on what basis can indicators be selected?

In short, the selection of particular indicators should be guided by research and associated theory. Hopefully, this book has provided some insight into the planning process, its underlying ideologies and the theoretical bases for developing appropriate interventions. To reiterate an earlier aphorism, there is nothing so practical as a good theory! The same maxim applies to evaluation. Having identified useful indicators of effectiveness, we should, however, exercise great care to ensure that the evidence revealed by these indicators is valid. In other words, if the combined results of our indirect, intermediate and outcome indicators indicate a certain level of effectiveness, we must be satisfied that the evidence is robust and our claims of success can be justified. Given the political realities of evaluation that we discussed above, how could this be otherwise? We will, therefore, now turn to the matter of validity. In doing so, we will follow up earlier critiques of the application of positivism in health promotion by questioning the positivist gold standard of evaluation of research design – the randomized controlled trial (RCT).

RELIABILITY, VALIDITY AND THE RCT

The two standard criteria for assessing the quality of research measures are reliability and validity. Reliability is concerned with consistency and replicability – that is, the extent to which research techniques will produce consistent results, regardless of how, when and where the research is carried out. For example, a completely reliable questionnaire should yield identical scores, whoever administers the questionnaire. Moreover, if individuals are retested, they should receive the same scores

(provided, of course, that they have not actually changed during the time that elapses between test and retest). Similarly, if individuals or groups are interviewed or observed, then different interviewers or observers should draw the same conclusions.

Validity is, quite simply, the extent to which investigators and their instruments actually measure what they intend to measure – and nothing else. It describes the truth and authenticity of research findings. An unreliable evaluation cannot be valid. Equally an evaluation might demonstrate highly reliable results, but lack validity – it might merely have measured the wrong things, but done so very consistently.

In the context of evaluation of research, two varieties of validity are distinguished – internal and external. 'Internal validity' refers to the degree of certainty that the results of an evaluation are due to the intervention under investigation and not to other factors.

'External validity' describes the generalizability of the results – that is, the extent to which a given intervention can be expected to produce similar results in other populations and, therefore, be of use to other practitioners and planners.

As we will see, the classic RCT is strong on internal validity, but weak on external validity. On the other hand, interpretivist approaches are, perhaps arguably, more likely to generate results that can be used by other practitioners. However, special efforts must be made to ensure rigour.

The RCT – strengths and limitations

The RCT conforms to the principles of true experimental design. Within the domain of medicine, the popularity of the RCT – and the current movement for evidence-based medicine – have been ascribed to the influential work of Cochrane (1972, cited by McPherson 1994: 6), who argued that evaluation of effectiveness should be the first priority of the NHS in the UK and decided, 'to concentrate on one simple idea – the value of randomized controlled trials in improving the NHS – and to keep the book short and simple'.

Cochrane's rationale was certainly convincing, as was his demonstration that many routinely performed medical interventions were not based on evidence of effectiveness. The argument for evidence-based practice – and the use of experimental method – was by no means confined to medicine. Indeed, as Shacklock Evans (1962) points out, the use of experimental designs of the kind Cochrane espoused can be attributed primarily to Fisher (1949) and the field of agricultural biology and subsequently applied to education by Lindquist (1940).

The emphasis of the experimental approach on avoiding threats to internal validity can be seen in Fisher's (1949: 19) observation:

> Whatever degree of care and experimental skill is expended in equalizing the conditions, other than the one under test, which are liable to affect the result, this equalization must always be to a greater or less extent incomplete and in many important practical cases will be grossly defective.

Let us note the obvious limitations of some approaches to making claims that programmes have been effective where the validity of the results can be severely challenged!

Inadequacies in judging programme effectiveness

Situation 1 below is so limited in its utility that it cannot really be called a research design, as there is no indication of the status of the group before the intervention – 'X'.

Situation 1

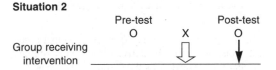

The result of the assessment (observation 'O') might therefore be due to a positive effect of the intervention. Alternatively, the intervention might have had no effect at all. Indeed, it might have made things worse! Situation 2 – a simple pre–post test design – provides more information.

Situation 2

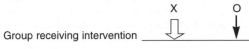

However, although it would be possible to record any changes occurring between the pretest and post-test, it would not be possible to demonstrate with any degree of certainty that the changes were due to the intervention.

Situation 3, on the other hand, uses a control group that does not receive the intervention and, so, assuming that there is a statistically significant difference between pre- and post-test and no such difference in the control group, it is reasonable to conclude that the intervention had had an impact. Unfortunately, there can be no certainty that the

experimental and control groups were identical in all key respects before the intervention. Accordingly, the apparently superior performance of the experimental group might, by chance, have been due to the superiority of the group rather than the effectiveness of the intervention. This design is, therefore, typically described as a quasi-experimental design.

Situation 3

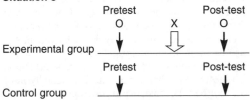

Situation 4, however, is a TRUE experimental design. This is symbolized here by the use of the traditional 'OXO' terminology initiated and elaborated by Campbell and Stanley (1963) and Cook and Campbell (1979). The essential difference is that 'subjects' are randomly assigned to experimental and control situations, thus partialling out differences of any kind. Randomization is the key to the superior status of the RCT and the justification for its gold standard accolade.

Situation 4

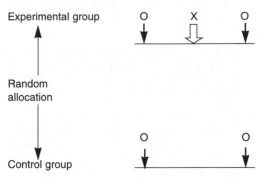

Furthermore, the rigour of RCT versions of true experimental design have been enhanced by the use of additional measures, such as the 'double blind trial', in which neither researchers nor subjects know who is receiving the active, experimental ingredient. (One wag, incidentally, has suggested that 'triple blind trials' occasionally occurred in which no one at all had any idea who had received what!) At all events, the additional extensions to the RCT may well make little if any contribution to dealing with another error to which evaluation is exposed.

Type 1 and 2 errors and true experimental design

The major strength of true experimental designs is their capacity to avoid 'Type 1 error'. In other words, to avoid claiming that a given intervention has been effective when apparent differences between experimental and control groups might have resulted from extraneous factors. The success of the research design is thus due to its capacity to exclude all possible rival causes of an observed effect so that only one robust causal agent remains.

This particular virtue may be achieved at the expense of incurring a 'Type 2 error' – that is drawing an erroneous conclusion that an intervention was ineffective when it may, in fact, actually have had an effect. For instance, a programme may actually have had an impact on the target group, but the instruments might have been insufficiently sensitive to discriminate between the effect on experimental and control groups. Similarly, failure to detect change may also occur when there are mixed populations and the positive effect of an intervention in one section of the population is diluted by a zero effect in the rest of the population or even a negative 'reactance' effect. (See the box on page 323 for additional comments on types of errors.)

Green and Lewis (1986: 264–7), while cautioning evaluators against the, 'fallacy of assuming inexorable forward movement', list the following situations that may also distort understanding of the effectiveness of interventions and contribute to Type 1 and 2 errors.

- **Delay of impact (or sleeper effect)** an intervention actually has an impact, but this does not emerge until later – perhaps quite a long time after the evaluation when circumstances are favourable.
- **Decay of impact (or backsliding effect)** the intervention produces an effect, but this decays more or less rapidly. Without continuing measurement, the programme might have been judged a success when it had, for all practical purposes, been a failure.
- **Borrowing from the future** the intervention triggers changes in behaviour that would have happened anyway, the programme merely hastening the inevitable.
- **Secular trends** a positive secular trend may result in overestimating programme effects, while a negative secular trend may result in discounting an influence that had delayed the decline.
- **Contrast effects** premature termination of a programme may create a backlash resulting in a

slowing or reversal of behavioural outcomes that would have occurred had the programme continued.

The limitations of the RCT have been recognized even within a biomedical context. Charlton (1991: 355) argued that the RCT was:

> vital but of restricted applicability to medicine. [He reminded readers that] … it should only be employed in conditions of clinical unpredictability. When an obviously effective treatment emerges there is no need for a controlled trial to establish its usefulness.

On the other hand, he noted that (1991: 356), 'Gain in objectivity is achieved by simplification and at the cost of completeness … the patient is depersonalized, the doctor is deskilled.'

McPherson (1994: 12), while generally lauding the approach, notes that human volition and decision making can challenge the apparent objectivity of some trials. He concludes that, 'choice itself can dramatically affect important measures of outcome.'

The former UK government chief scientist Sir Douglas Black (1998: 23) is equally, if not more, sceptical. Although he considered the RCT, 'a brilliant response to the increasing problems set by the proliferation of agents that are highly effective but also potentially hazardous from their side-effects…' he considered it appropriate only in the following situations (p. 25):

> when a clinical situation is common, so that the trial can be carried out in one centre; easily defined so that inclusion and exclusion are simple; and has little variation between patients. [Therefore] …the quality of evidence should be assessed not by the method by which it is obtained but by its strength or weakness. I suggest that we are more commonly persuaded by a balance of likelihoods than we are driven forward by the iron laws of evidence.

It is interesting to note that Black argued that clinical decisions should be derived from many sources in many complicated medical situations. Given the much greater complexity prevailing in most educational and health promotion programmes, the use of true experimental designs would seem to be even less relevant. Black adopts a position that is not dissimilar to the stance we take about the use of the judicial principle.

Are RCTs ever relevant for evaluating health promotion?

We are inclined to respond to this question by saying, 'Well, not never, but hardly ever!' More particularly, we might say that the RCT or, more properly, the true experimental design is likely to be useful to the extent that the health promotion intervention approximates to the clinical trial. In other words, that, first, the intervention is simple and, second, we do not know the answer already nor have better ways of finding it. This is rare within the overall complexity of the health promotion enterprise. Furthermore, following our earlier discussion of realistic and utilization-focused evaluation, if the trial strips away consideration of contextual factors, the findings will have little relevance to other situations.

Although not unique to RCTs, the emphasis in evaluation design is on assessing outcomes rather than the quality of the intervention itself. A 'Type 3 error' occurs when an intervention could not possibly succeed – or reach minimal standards of acceptability – because of its inherent inadequacy. The Type 3 error relates to the concept of efficacy that was defined earlier in this chapter. Tones (1997: 190–1) offers a summary of the key features of sound programme design that, assuming fidelity in programme implementation, should reduce the risk of Type 3 errors. Programmes should:

- be based on relevant theory and, where possible, prior research
- be based on a sophisticated diagnosis of the social, psychological and environmental determinants of the health- or illness-related behaviour in question

- the focus should not only be on knowledge, but also beliefs and relate to the individual's developmental stage
- full account should be taken of the various 'pushes and pulls' of competing motivations on intention to act
- the importance of social pressures should be acknowledged
- barriers to adoption and maintenance should be identified – especially environmental barriers
- empowerment factors should be emphasized
- education must be complemented by achieving a supportive environment
- interventions should be maximized by creating coalitions between different settings and stakeholders – maximum participation should be a major goal
- coalitions should be supported by appropriate use of mass media
- a sophisticated behavioural diagnosis should be matched by the use of appropriate methods and learning resources
- health staff must be trained to use the appropriate educational methods.

The 'Type 5 error' is a well-known phenomenon, but not normally labelled in this way. However, it is not unknown for research to yield very respectable p-values by simply using very large numbers of subjects! Practical significance is undoubtedly of more relevance to those working in the field than such artificially constructed statistical significance.

FIVE TYPES OF ERRORS

Type 1 error

An erroneous conclusion that an intervention has achieved significant change when, in fact, it has failed to do so.

Type 2 error

An erroneous conclusion that an intervention has failed to have a significant impact when, in fact, it has actually done so.

Type 3 error

Asserting that an intervention has failed to achieve successful results when it was so poorly designed that it could not possibly have had a desired effect.

(Continued)

(Continued)

Type 4 error

Conducting an evaluation of a programme that no one cares about and is irrelevant to decisionmakers. Evaluation for the sake of evaluation is central to this error.

Type 5 error

An intervention is shown to produce a genuine statistically significant effect, but the change is so slight as to have no practical significance.

After Basch and Gold, 1986: 300–1

Ideological and illuminative difficulties with experimental design

Although researchers wedded to positivist experimental design have made sterling efforts to take account of complexity, it is our view that the complexities of most health promotion ventures will defeat even sophisticated positivist approaches. We concur with the conclusions of the WHO European Working Group on Health Promotion Evaluation (WHO, 1998a: 3):

> *Conclusion 4* The use of randomized control [sic] trials to evaluate health promotion initiatives is, in most cases, inappropriate, misleading and unnecessarily expensive.
>
> For a better understanding of the impact of health promotion initiatives, evaluators need to use a wide range of qualitative and quantitative methods that extend beyond the narrow parameters of randomized controlled trials.

In a follow-up to these recommendations, Rootman et al. (2001) assembled a substantial body of theory, argument and opinion in support of alternative paradigms and practices.

Opening the black box

One of health promotion's major requirements is illumination. In other words, we need to know not just whether or not a programme has been effective, but also why it has been effective or why it has failed. We are committed to the idea of formative evaluation and, thus, need information to help us with the task of modifying and improving programmes, both during and after their delivery. The more complicated the programme, the greater our need for illuminative insights. Lang's (in Cohen and Cohen, 1960) acerbic comment would seem to be appropriate here: 'He uses statistics as a drunken man uses lampposts – for support rather than illumination.'

Again, the significance of illumination in evaluation is not a discovery of health promotion, as workers in the field of educational research who questioned the value of experimental design also argued the case for gaining insights through illumination. Parlett and Hamilton (1972), for example, proposed an 'illuminative, social-anthropological paradigm' that took account of the wider contexts in which educational programmes function. They cited Trow (1970: 302):

> Research on innovation can be enlightening to the innovator and to the whole academic community by clarifying the processes of education and by helping the innovator and other interested parties to identify those procedures, those elements in the educational effort, which seem to have had desirable results.

Parlett and Hamilton (1972) use an analogy with the theatre to point out that, without such insights, evaluators risk being 'rather like a critic who reviews a production on the basis of the script and applause-meter readings, having missed the performance'!

In short, illuminative evaluation uses 'thick (rich) description' – a term coined by Ryle (1949). As will be apparent later, thick description is central to disentangling the complicated realities and perceptions of reality that characterize major community interventions concerned with addressing complicated goals, such as the achievement of equity. Figure 10.6 illustrates what might be called the 'black box problem'.

Figure 10.6 simulates an experimental evaluation of a school-based programme designed to reduce the incidence of unwanted pregnancies by comparing its long-term results with one of a number of control schools lacking such an intervention. Apart from demonstrating that there were no important curricular elements in the control schools that might contribute to the reduction of future pregnancies, an evaluator would need detailed information about

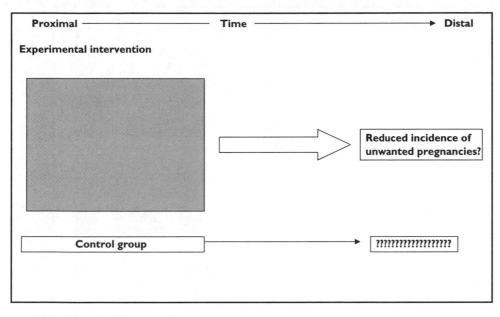

Figure 10.6   The black box problem

the intervention and its dynamics. Figure 10.7 reveals the kinds of complexity that might be revealed if the black box were opened!

In short, we would expect to observe a complicated reality of synergistic clements – all of which would require separate evaluation. It also demonstrates that a number of additional, cumulative inputs would be needed over quite a lengthy period of time if success were to be achieved. Moreover, as a school setting would be only one component of a community-wide programme, Figure 10.7, in fact, substantially underestimates the level of complexity there would actually be. Illumination is therefore essential. The RCT is irrelevant.

Evaluating complicated community initiatives

Most interventions, then, are more or less complicated and, perhaps, the most complicated of all are those that operate within a relatively large geographical area and seek to enhance the health of all its inhabitants. The classic heart disease prevention projects are good examples of such a situation (see, for example, Tones and Tilford, 2001: 447 ff).

Evaluation of such programmes has been attempted by assigning whole communities to experimental and control groups (or, to be more accurate, comparison or reference groups). Various studies have demonstrated that such studies are, in many ways, problematic. Contamination of the comparison group is a major challenge. Nutbeam et al. (1993), for instance, reported that reference areas used by the 'Heartbeat Wales' heart disease prevention programme rapidly became independently involved in establishing their own heart health initiatives, thus compromising their value as controls. Furthermore, Mackenbach (1997) has argued that it is almost impossible to provide an adequate control in situations where the impetus for the intervention originates in the community itself. Problems are not, however, limited to technical design factors – they also involve ideological issues and fundamental flaws in the conceptual basis of the programme (Mittelmark, 1999b).

Increasingly, 'horizontal programmes' (see Chapter 4) are being developed that seek to address social, economic, environmental and general structural determinants of health and illness. These 'complicated community initiatives' (CCIs) are indeed decidedly complicated (Connell et al., 1995, and Aspen Institute, 1997). They tackle some of the most difficult challenges in bringing about social change, operate across a variety of agencies, institutions and non-formal settings, while also recognizing that a longitudinal approach must be adopted as major outcomes will not be achieved in the short term.

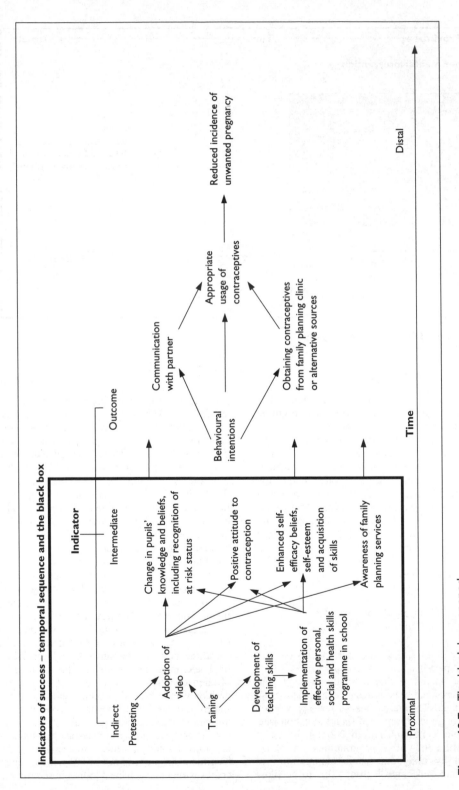

Figure 10.7 The black box, opened

A good example of the CCI is provided by the development of 'Health Action Zones' in England (Secretary of State for Social Security, 1999). These new initiatives aim, 'to bring together organizations within and beyond the NHS to develop and implement a locally agreed strategy for improving the health of local people'. Their goal is to tackle inequalities in health and develop services that are more responsive to patients and users (Department of Health, 1997).

The three defining characteristics of CCIs (Judge, 2000: 2) are:

- they aim to promote positive change in individual, family and community circumstances
- they develop a variety of mechanisms to improve social, economic and physical circumstances, services and conditions in disadvantaged communities
- they place a strong emphasis on community building and neighbourhood empowerment.

Unsurprisingly, given the complexities of the programmes and the paramount need for insights into process, qualitative methods and illuminative evaluation associated with the interpretivist paradigm are typically employed. More particularly, Pawson and Tilley's 'realistic evaluation' (discussed earlier in this chapter) is taken as a model for programme evaluation, together with the insights offered by Weiss' (1995) 'theories of change' approach – one that is consistent with the model of systematic planning promoted in this book.

Health promotion, ideological imperatives and the RCT – an overview

Before summarizing our concerns about the relevance of the RCT to health promotion evaluation, we will raise one final objection. Because this objection is ideological, it cannot be challenged, as to do so would be to challenge the avowed overriding philosophy and goal of health promotion – namely, participation of patients, learners, clients and communities – and participation is not possible within the narrow framework of the RCT.

By way of summary, the limitations of RCTs are, therefore, that they:

- are difficult to establish, artificial and randomization is difficult outside the laboratory, so, although they are efficient at addressing problems of Type 1 errors, they are prone to Type 2 errors and, particularly, Type 3 errors
- are unable to cope with the complexity of health promotion programmes

- are of limited use in community programmes as 'control' communities are frequently contaminated
- may yield *statistical* significance but have little *practical* significance, thus contributing little to effectiveness reviews and policy implementation
- do not offer illumination
- cannot use formative evaluation, which is essential to achieving effective action outcomes in an efficient manner
- are ideologically unsound and incompatible with such imperatives as:
  - 'active' individual and community participation in the research process
  - health promotion's political and 'emancipatory' role and its use of research as a tool for achieving political and social change.

A NEW GOLD STANDARD – THE JUDICIAL PRINCIPLE

We have asserted the need for adopting a particular kind of post positivist paradigm for health promotion research. The rejection of a positivist approach, together with its gold standard RCT design, does not mean that we should abandon the pursuit of reliability and validity. Quite the reverse. A critical realist model, as we have seen, has no difficulty in addressing Type 2 and 3 errors, but it is imperative that it replace the techniques intrinsic to true experimental design with robust alternatives that will maximize internal validity – that is, provide strong evidence that will substantiate claims that programmes or parts of programmes have produced change.

Reliability, replicability, dependability and validity

As qualitative methodology is central to the interpretivist aspects of critical, realistic evaluation, it makes sense to give some thought to the methods recommended by qualitative researchers to achieve reliability and validity. It is, of course, possible to adopt the kinds of measure to achieve reliability that were mentioned earlier in this chapter. Although a 'test–retest' approach may be difficult given the 'formative' concerns of much health promotion to react to change with more change in pursuit of action goals, it is not difficult to check for consistency. For instance, as semi-structured interviews and observation are commonplace in qualitative research, it is not difficult to arrange for more than one interviewer or observer to observe the same events and compare notes. The question of validity is somewhat more complicated. Lincoln and Denzin (1994: 579), for example, comment that:

> a text is valid if it is sufficiently grounded, triangulated, based on naturalistic indicators, carefully fitted to a theory [and its concepts], comprehensive in scope, credible in terms of member checks, logical, and truthful in terms of its reflection of the phenomenon in question. The text's author then announces the validity claims to the reader. Such claims now become the text's warrant to its own authoritative representation of the experience and social world under inspection.

Reliability and validity are often assessed simultaneously and qualitative researchers tend to use such terms as 'replicability', 'dependability', 'confirmability', 'trustworthiness', 'transferability' and 'authenticity' to assess the consistency of interventions and the extent to which their results actually measure the constructs that they are claiming to measure.

According to Denzin (1994: 508):

> The foundation for interpretation rests on triangulated empirical materials that are trustworthy. *Trustworthiness* consists of four components: credibility, transferability, dependability, and confirmability (these are the constructionist equivalents of internal and external validity, reliability and objectivity).

Various specific techniques have also been devised to provide a basis for demonstrating credibility and providing transparent results that allow judgements to be made about the reliability and validity of research data. Three such techniques are member checks, the use of thick description and the provision of audit trails.

Member checks

In general, the rationale for this technique is testing results of research against the perceptions of audience members. Guba and Lincoln (1981: 316) suggest that the evaluator should, for example:

- draw a sample from informants
- check data derived (from interviews, for example) with the interviewees
- ask them to point out any errors of fact.

Apart from checking reliability and validity, the researcher's categorization of interviewees' responses can be reassessed and incomplete categories can be fleshed out.

Member checks provide what elsewhere might be described as 'respondent validation'.

Thick description

Denzin (1994: 505) compares 'thin description' to 'thick description'. The former:

> simply reports facts, independent of intentions or circumstances. A thick description, in contrast, gives the context of an experience, states the intentions and meanings that organized the experience, and reveals the experiences as a process. Out of this process arise ... claims for truth, [and its] verisimilitude.

In short, thick, rich detail makes it possible to gain illuminative insights and allow others to check a researcher's claims.

Audit trails

This interpretivist research technique is designed to provide a detailed account of how researchers/evaluators have reached their decisions about the categories that they have constructed from raw data and the conclusions they have reached and, perhaps, about the theories they have derived from these. As Morse puts it, 'interested parties can reconstruct the process by which the investigators reached their conclusion.'

She (1994: 230) cites the following list of six types of documentation for an audit trail (developed by Halpern, 1983):

> raw data, data reduction and analysis products, data reconstruction and synthesis products, process notes, materials relating to intentions and dispositions, and instrument development information.

Transferability

This is the alternative version of external validity. Again, providing thick descriptions can provide sufficiently detailed information for people to make judgements about the relevance of findings to different but related situations and to know how to proceed.

'Purposive/purposeful sampling' is considered to yield the most useful data. Situations and/or individuals are deliberately selected in the expectation that they will prove to be a rich source of relevant data. Deliberate selection implies choosing from alternatives. Choices should be made on the basis of both previous research and, of course, sound theoretical understandings.

Authenticity

Lincoln and Guba (1985) offer authenticity as an alternative concept to validity. Research is not only authentic when the strategies it uses will ensure true reporting of participants' feelings and ideas, it should also demonstrate that it is consistent with these ethical and ideological principles. The components of authenticity would typically include:

- notions such as fairness and equity
- ontological authenticity – that is, participants gain some insight into their human condition
- understandings that help with insight and relating to other people
- catalytic authenticity/validity – the research method itself should achieve its substantive ideological goals so that, for example, in participative health promotion research, it should contribute to empowerment.

The judicial principle – assessing the validity of evidence

The business of evaluating health promotion, with all its contradictions and complexities, requires a new approach – a new gold standard. Decisions must of course still be made on the basis of evidence, but the criteria for making the vigilant decisions that would be used by real people in real life when addressing problems and making policy must be reassessed. Accordingly, we propose here the use of a 'judicial principle'. As the words suggest, we draw a parallel with the judicial system and argue that decisions should be made on the basis of a pot pourri of evidence derived from different sources. Two degrees of judicial certainty should be employed. Where the level of certainty for action must be of a higher order, the criterion used in criminal law should be used – that is, it must be beyond reasonable doubt. Where the consequences of decision making are less serious and the demand for evidence is, therefore, less stringent, the criterion employed in civil law might be used – that is, take into account the balance of probabilities.

These two levels of probability could loosely be compared with their quantitative equivalents – p-values of $p < 0.01$ (or less if the evidence is especially compelling) and $p < 0.05$ for balance of probability estimates.

Evidence and causality

Although Pawson and Tilley questioned the utility of assumptions of causality based on linearity – that is, the notion that whatever precedes an event is presumed to have caused it (*post hoc ergo propter hoc*) – cause–effect evidence is important in applying the judicial principle. As we noted in Chapter 2, several criteria are generally accepted as providing

evidence of causality in the medical arena. In addition to identifying strong, specific, consistent associations that are temporally correct, health promotion research would, ideally, seek evidence that better results were achieved when interventions were relevant, comprehensive and of sufficient intensity – and theoretically plausible.

The question of triangulation

In the last analysis, the question of causality and internal validity rests on the nature and quality of the evidence that has been assembled by the evaluation research. It is our view that the judicial principle should make substantial use of triangulation of evidence to maximize researchers' and decision-makers' conviction that cause has been demonstrated to at least the level of a balance of probabilities.

Triangulation is of central significance for qualitative research methodology. Essentially, triangulation is a metaphor derived from surveying or navigation. It is a technique involving two or more sightings of a particular target to then accurately establish its geographical position. In the same way, using different 'research sightings' should contribute to valid interpretations of reality or realities. The idea is very attractive and has the virtue of common sense. However, some researchers and theoreticians have struck a cautionary note. For instance, Blaikie (1991: 131) makes the following point:

> The failure to recognize the implications of using incompatible ontologies and epistemologies has led either to muddy confusions about bias and validity … or false pretensions about what combining quantitative and qualitative methods means … It should also be clear that triangulation means many things to many people and none of the uses in sociology bears any resemblance to its use in surveying.

To provide an extreme illustration, consider a situation in which one group of researchers believes that it is not possible to know the world, but only a variety of different interpretations of it, whereas another group believes that the world is real and knowable. If these contradictory beliefs are well founded, then it has to be admitted that using evidence based on one perspective could not be used to support evidence based on the other! However, as Blaikie implies, researchers adopting a post positive realist position *can* legitimately accumulate evidence from many different sources and, in principle, these sources of data can all offer valid insights into whatever issue or problem is under investigation. As is hopefully clear by now, we concur with the realist position. Accordingly, we believe that a considered use of triangulation is justified. A number of varieties have traditionally been identified (Denzin, 1970):

- data triangulation
- investigator triangulation
- theory triangulation
- methodological triangulation.

In short, our confidence in the validity of observations and findings is proportional to the extent that information from different sources is congruent and compatible. For instance, from different data sources (such as, GP records of drug use over a period of time and interview data from patients and data from observations of patients in social settings), reports of different investigators (such as interview reports from other investigators), consistency between analyses of findings derived from different (and appropriately selected) theories (such as consistency between communication of innovations theory and the health belief model) and achieving similar results from different methods (such as questionnaire data, semi-structured interviews and, sources of 'unobtrusive measures').

As Stake (1995) points out, the acceptance of triangulation has not been limited to qualitative researchers or realist evaluators. He cites Campbell and Fiske (1959: 81, in Stake 1995: 114): 'The achievements of useful hypothetically realistic constructs in a science requires multiple methods focused on the diagnosis of the same construct from independent points of observation through a kind of triangulation.'

Finally, in this chapter, we need to consider how evidence might be translated into policy and practice.

EVIDENCE-BASED HEALTH PROMOTION

The movement towards evidence-based practice has been heavily influenced by evidence-based medicine, the origins of which Sackett et al. (1996) trace back to mid nineteenth-century Paris. Its basic tenets are summarized in the box.

As we noted in Chapter 5, there is increasing recognition of the importance of evidence-based practice within the wider public health arena and considerable current interest in evidence-based health promotion. Nutbeam (1999) points to the significant inclusion of the words 'evidence-based' in the call for member states to 'adopt an evidence-based approach to health promotion policy and practice' in the Resolution on Health Promotion passed at the Fifty-first World Health Assembly (WHO, 1998c). He takes this to imply the need to justify health promotion activity with greater reference to research evidence on effectiveness in achieving 'predetermined outcomes'.

Raphael (2000) suggests that the increasing emphasis on evidence-based practice derives, in part, from 'economic rationalism' and the need to justify expenditure and ensure that funds are deployed to maximum effect. However there is also a strong ethical imperative to adopt the principles of evidence-based practice to ensure that health promotion does no harm – either directly or indirectly by wasting limited funds on ineffective or inappropriate interventions or by raising unrealistic expectations about what might be achieved. We might also add that incorporating evidence into decisions about practice is a key aspect of 'reflective practice' and fundamental to the provision of *quality* health promotion. The basic premise of this text is that the systematic planning of health promotion requires a series of decisions to be made at each stage and that these should be informed by a thorough appraisal of available evidence.

THE BASIC TENETS OF EVIDENCE-BASED MEDICINE

- Clinical decisions should be based on the best available scientific evidence.
- The clinical problem determines the evidence to be sought.
- Identifying the best evidence involves epidemiological and biostatistical ways of thinking.
- Conclusions based on the available evidence are useful only if put into action for individual patients or for population healthcare decisions.
- Performance should be constantly evaluated.

Davidoff et al., 1995, in Jacobson et al., 1997: 449

Perkins et al. (1999) note that, 'like motherhood and apple pie', evidence-based health promotion has come to be seen as a good thing. However, they identify a number of tensions in implementing it. First, the tension between reflection and action and the issue of how much evidence is required before action can be taken and what level of uncertainty can be tolerated.

Second, the tension between evidence and practice and the theory–practice gap that arises from failure to translate research findings into practice. This, they suggest, can have a number of origins, which include shortcomings on the part of practitioners in accessing, interpreting and acting on relevant evidence or on the part of researchers in addressing relevant issues and disseminating their findings in ways that meet practitioners' needs. An alternative explanation is the lack of acknowledgement of the 'uniqueness of practice contexts and the processes of social, organizational and educational change' (1999: 7).

Third, the tension between different types of knowledge – not only between different research paradigms, which we have discussed above, but also between empirical evidence and professional judgement.

Fourth, the tension between values and evidence and the complex interplay between the two, particularly in relation to the selection and interpretation of evidence.

Finally, the tension between inspiration and evidence and the relative emphasis on tried and tested methods in contrast to innovative and creative solutions to problems.

A particular area of contention concerns attempts to apply the principles of evidence-based medicine to health promotion. This derives from a conceptualization of evidence-based medicine as being associated with the use of the RCT as the gold standard of evaluation and taking a narrow biomedical view of outcomes – an interpretation that has been challenged even by the proponents of evidence-based medicine. The key issues that we will consider at this point are what evidence of effectiveness is relevant to health promotion practice and how that evidence can be accessed – in particular via systematic reviews.

What is evidence?

Evidence-based health promotion has been defined (Wiggers and Sanson-Fisher, 1998: 141) as: 'the systematic integration of research evidence into the planning and implementation of health promotion activities.'

We have questioned the utility of experimental methods for assessing the effectiveness of health promotion. MacIntyre and Pettigrew (2000) suggest that resistance to applying the principles of evidence-based medicine – and by this they are essentially referring to systematic reviews and experimental designs – to social or public health settings derives from a number of misconceptions:

- systematic reviews and experimental designs have a biomedical provenance
- the real world is too complex for evidence-based medicine principles
- social and public health interventions do not have the capacity to do harm
- it is sufficient to know that an intervention does good in a general sense without the necessity of analysing how much, for which subgroups and at what cost
- plausibility is an adequate basis for policy making
- experimental methods define outcomes narrowly and use too short a time frame.

A particular concern is the capacity to do harm. The authors cite a study by Carlin and Nolan (1998) that demonstrated that a bicycle safety education programme doubled the risk of injury in boys. Furthermore, they note that plausibility is not necessarily sufficient justification. For example, putting babies to sleep in the prone position would seem to make sense in that it resembles the recovery position, but has been shown to be associated with increased risk of sudden infant death syndrome. They argue that systematic evaluation offers the opportunity to identify the wider effects of interventions, both positive and negative. While agreeing with these concerns and upholding the need for rigour in evaluation research, our contention is that this is best achieved by means of triangulation and the judicial principle.

Sackett et al. (1996: 72) support the use of randomized trials and systematic reviews to assess the effectiveness of therapy: 'It is when asking questions about therapy that we should try to avoid the non-experimental approaches, since these routinely lead to false-positive conclusions about efficacy.' However they contend that evidence-based medicine is not restricted to randomized trials and meta analyses, but 'involves tracking down the best external evidence with which to answer our clinical questions'.

There is a growing consensus that the best evidence in relation to health promotion interventions includes both quantitative and qualitative research and addresses process and context as well as outcomes. This adoption of a more catholic and methodologically plural approach to evidence runs

counter to attempts to create hierarchies of evidence
topped by the RCT (see the box on page 171 for an
example). It also acknowledges that the answer to
the simple question 'Does it work?' is not enough
and that evidence is needed in relation to process as
well as outcomes. A whole series of supplementary
questions require answers, such as the following.

- How does it work?
- Were there any unanticipated outcomes?
- What components are essential for success?
- What components are redundant?
- Why does it work in this context (or, equally
  importantly, *not* work)?
- Can it be replicated?
- Is this an appropriate and acceptable way of
  tackling the problem?

A Health Development Agency's (HDA, undated)
consultation exercise on the development of an evidence base found support for the inclusion of a
broader range of research than that provided by
RCTs, notwithstanding some concern among a
minority about any overemphasis on 'grey' evidence. The decision to adopt an inclusive approach
to sources of information acknowledged the complex interplay of factors that influence health, the
need to understand what works in particular contexts and why and the inability of narrowly focused
experimental methods to capture the breadth of
information required. Sources of evidence were
identified (HDA, undated) as:

- evidence maps
- expert working groups reports
- literature reviews
- meta analyses
- research summaries
- reviews
- syntheses
- systematic reviews of effectiveness.

Raphael (2000) suggests that decision making
should still draw on local evidence, even when there
is a strong accumulated evidence base. On the one
hand – and particularly at the needs assessment
stage – this helps to secure local ownership. On
the other hand, it ensures and checks out local
relevance.

Wiggers and Sanson-Fisher's definition referred
to above presupposes that evidence derives from
research. However Sackett et al.'s (1996: 71) discussion of evidence-based medicine, while calling
for the 'conscientious, explicit and judicious use of
current best evidence in making decisions about the
care of individual patients', also recognizes the
importance of integrating evidence with clinical
expertise (1996: 72):

Without clinical expertise, practice risks becoming
tyrannized by evidence for even excellent external evidence may be inapplicable or inappropriate for an individual patient. Without current best evidence, practice
risks becoming rapidly out of date to the detriment of
patients.

They see the application of professional expertise as
a means of avoiding evidence-based medicine
becoming merely 'cookbook' medicine. Equally,
professional judgement that incorporates familiarity
with the context and constraints is important in relation to assessing what health promotion interventions are likely to be successful in particular
situations and with specific groups.

Sackett et al. also note the importance of integrating guidelines on practice with individual
patient preferences and choice. The issue of choice
is perhaps particularly relevant to health promotion,
given its emphasis on participation and empowerment rather than control and compliance. Making
informed choices will necessarily require access to
non-prejudicial information and the accurate interpretation of risk. Jacobson et al. (1997) draw attention to the problem of incomplete and partial
reporting, citing as an example the media coverage
of early research findings on the association
between third-generation oral contraceptive pills
and venous thrombosis. The selective reporting of
risk by the press ignored any protective effects in
relation to cardiovascular risk and the increased
risks associated with pregnancies arising as a result
of discontinuing oral contraception, which tends to
occur following such scare stories.

Green (2000: 125) has argued that empirical evidence alone is 'insufficient to direct practice and
that recourse to the explanatory and predictive
capability of theory is essential to the design of both
programmes and evaluations'. When there is no
empirical evidence available, then recourse to
theory will be the only option. However, even when
there is ample empirical evidence, the application
of theoretical principles remains important for a
number of reasons. Identification of appropriate
indicators of outcome and process is reliant on
theory. Reference to theory, as we have noted, can
also ensure that all the necessary elements of a programme are in place and, therefore, reduce the risk
of intervention failure and Type 3 errors in evaluation. Consideration of the extent to which they are
based on theory therefore becomes an essential criterion in assessing the quality of interventions and
evaluation designs. Not only should evaluation be
informed by theory, but the findings of evaluations
should contribute to the further development and
refinement of theory in a constantly evolving cycle.
Without the extraction of general theoretical principles,

empirical evidence of effectiveness risks offering little more than a menu of, often context-specific, proven interventions. General principles may be of more relevance to practitioners in that they allow adaptation to suit specific situations.

Clearly the interpretation of evidence will be value-laden – note, for example, the different interpretations of ways for achieving better health in the box. Raphael (2000: 335) argues that, given the commitment of health promotion to enabling and empowerment, evidence relevant to health promotion should encompass consideration of whether or not these goals have been achieved, contending that 'ethical health promotion practice requires explicit recognition of the interactions among ideologies, values, principles and rules of evidence'.

A further example of the way in which values may lead to different opinions about evidence is provided by Jacobson et al. (1997) in the context of evidence-based medicine. They refer to the widely quoted study by Russell et al. (1979), which demonstrated that brief advice to stop smoking from a GP during routine consultations with a warning of follow-up, achieved a 5 per cent rate of quitting. This could be interpreted by some as highly effective and worth the small amount of additional time, whereas for others 5 per cent may be seen as too small an effect to justify action. Furthermore, we could speculate that some would see offering such unsolicited advice as intrusive and interfering with individual freedom or, alternatively, as motivating people to give up a demonstrably health-threatening habit. It is interesting to note the Cochrane Collaboration's (2002) disclaimer about Cochrane reviews that acknowledges interpretations of the evidence may vary:

ALTERNATIVE INTERPRETATIONS OF THE ROUTE TO BETTER HEALTH

Ten tips for better health (Donaldson, 1999)

1　Don't smoke. If you can, stop. If you can't, cut down.
2　Follow a balanced diet with plenty of fruit and vegetables.
3　Keep physically active.
4　Manage stress by, for example, talking things through and making time to relax.
5　If you drink alcohol, do so in moderation.
6　Cover up in the sun and protect children from sunburn.
7　Practise safer sex.
8　Take up cancer-screening opportunities.
9　Be safe on the roads: follow the highway code.
10　Learn the First Aid ABC – airways, breathing, circulation.

An alternative ten tips for better health (Gordon, 1999)

1　Don't be poor. If you can, stop. If you can't, try not to be poor for long.
2　Don't have poor parents.
3　Own a car.
4　Don't work in a stressful, low-paid manual job.
5　Don't live in damp, low-quality housing.
6　Be able to afford to go on a foreign holiday and sunbathe.
7　Practise not losing your job and don't become unemployed.
8　Take up all the benefits you are entitled to, if you are unemployed, retired or sick or disabled.
9　Don't live next to a busy major road or near a polluting factory.
10　Learn how to fill in the complicated housing benefit/asylum application forms before you become homeless and destitute.

Raphael, 2000

The results of a Cochrane Review can be interpreted differently, depending on people's perspectives and circumstances. Please consider the conclusions presented carefully. They are the opinions of review authors, and are not necessarily shared by the Cochrane Collaboration.

The Research and Evaluation Division of HEBS (1996: 359) suggests that there are different demands when assessing the outcomes of health promotion interventions in comparison to medical interventions as 'outcomes might be difficult to specify tightly or measure consistently, and indeed differ according to the agendas of particular stakeholders'.

By way of example, let us consider Wight et al.'s (2002) rigorous cluster randomized trial of a theoretically based sex education programme for adolescents (SHARE). The findings were reported by the press as evidence of the ineffectiveness of sex education – for example, in *The Independent,* was the headline 'Classes in safe sex are ineffective, says study' (Duckworth, 2002). The objective of the study was to compare the effectiveness of the SHARE programme with current practice in reducing unsafe sexual intercourse. The main outcome measures used were self-reported exposure to sexually transmitted disease, use of condoms and contraceptives in most recent sexual intercourse and unwanted pregnancies. The conclusions drawn by the authors were that '*compared with conventional sex education* [our emphasis] this specially designed intervention did not reduce sexual risk taking in adolescents' (2002: 1430). It is worth noting in passing that a process evaluation of the delivery of sex education and the broader features of each school enabled the authors to discount differences in quality of delivery as a factor in the lack of effectiveness. However, they also found that pupils in the intervention arm of the trial were more knowledgeable than those in the control arm of the trial. Furthermore, the SHARE programme was rated more positively by pupils than comparison programmes, did not encourage earlier sexual activity and had some beneficial effects on the quality of young people's sexual relationships – outcomes that may variously be judged as more relevant by teachers and young people than behavioural outcomes.

Nutbeam (2000) notes that different stakeholders have different perspectives on what constitutes success and may have different views about the evidence needed:

- policymakers and budget managers may be concerned about the likely short-term achievement of returns on the level of investment in relation to health gain

- health promotion practitioners need to assess the feasibility of achieving defined objectives within particular contexts
- the population that is to benefit from health promotion intervention may be concerned about whether or not the programmes address recognized priorities and felt needs and are participatory
- academic researchers may be concerned with epistemological considerations and methodological rigour in making judgements about success.

Access to evidence of effectiveness

A key requirement for getting evidence into practice involves access to evidence. It is worth noting at this point that there may be a mismatch between the needs and interests of those generating research evidence and the end-users of that evidence. Furthermore, comparatively little attention has been given to the dissemination of research findings.

The development of electronic databases and search tools has done much to improve access to published research papers. However, Jacobson et al. (1997) draw attention to a number of limitations. They note, for example, that databases such as Medline have only 50–80 per cent recall of relevant literature. Furthermore, accessing grey literature, such as unpublished reports, theses and conference proceedings, can be difficult. Given the wideranging and multidisciplinary nature of health promotion, the numerous journals that publish papers on relevant issues and the variety of different databases that cover these, locating *all* published papers on a particular topic can be particularly problematic.

Clearly, journal editors and peer reviewers of articles occupy key gatekeeper positions. Not only do they control quality standards for published material and establish what would be regarded as minimal reporting criteria, but they also arbitrate on matters of current interest. Lister-Sharp et al.'s (1999: v) review of health promoting schools made the following recommendations for these groups:

Ensure, in publications of studies of school health promotion interventions, that the following are reported: the theoretical basis or assumptions underpinning the interventions; the content of the interventions; and the process of delivery.

Oakley et al. (1995) call for journals to refuse to accept methodologically flawed papers. Jacobson et al. (1997) suggest that negative findings are less likely to be published. Studies that yield negative findings are also less likely to be submitted for publication: 'current emphasis on success stories may deter the dissemination of cautionary tales regarding tales of things that have gone wrong' (Research and Evaluation Division HEBS, 1996: 360).

Conversely, multiple reporting of some studies can distort the picture. The pressure on academics to publish papers has fuelled the practice of publishing a number of separate papers on different stages of a single project. This so-called 'salami slicing' inflates the visibility of individual projects, but, at the same time, can fail to provide a complete view of the whole.

Even presupposing that information is readily available, coping with the plethora of published material can be problematic for practitioners. Some years ago, Davidoff et al. (1995) estimated that doctors would need to read seventeen articles a day, every day of the year to keep up to date. It is clear that the demands of practice make it impossible for practitioners to keep on top of the ever-growing literature on effectiveness. It is not surprising, therefore, that increasing emphasis is being placed on reviews of evidence that attempt to synthesize the literature.

Tones and Tilford (2001) distinguish between commentary reviews and systematic reviews. The former bring together the findings of available studies and, hence, are subject to the vagaries of access to and selection of information and, in some instances, interpretation. There is clearly a risk that, consciously or unconsciously, such commentaries will be based on studies selected to suit a particular agenda or argument. Clearly, objectivity would demand that an attempt is made to seek out and, if appropriate, discount contradictory findings. Overreliance by commentators on a few key studies can inflate their importance in influencing decisions about practice.

Cummins and McIntyre (2002) use the term 'factoids' to refer to assumptions or speculations that are reported and repeated until they are considered to be true. They examine the current policy emphasis in the UK on tackling food deserts – areas of deprivation where it is difficult for families on low income to gain access to affordable healthy food – to illustrate that, when the social climate is right, facts can become assumed and decisions made on comparatively little evidence. Without questioning the quality of the studies themselves – or, indeed, the existence of food deserts – the authors are concerned that the evidence is heavily influenced by three key studies. They (2002: 438) conclude that:

> The overinterpretation of a few small-scale studies undertaken up to ten years ago could end up being used to make policy decisions supported by major central government groups and agencies, because the findings

are understood to fit in with the current way of thinking...

This paper illustrates how factoids can easily and uncritically become part of the apparatus of government health policy when they fit in with broader policy objectives. The key problem is that the burden of proof, or demand for evidence, may vary according to a policy's perceived fit with the prevailing collective worldview about issues of popular topical interest. One of the main messages of the evidence-based movement needs to be emphasized: when making any health policy (or other) decisions, we need to move away from an unquestioning acceptance of conventional wisdom and 'expert' advice and cast a more critical and objective eye over the facts.

Jacobson et al. (1997) suggest that the same papers may be used to support *different* conclusions or not used at all. To illustrate the point they note that the same three papers on screening and intensive management in patients over seventy-five have been used as evidence to demonstrate both benefit and no benefit and that they did not feature at all in other reviews. They (1997: 449) also contend that, 'the quality of review articles is inversely related to the expertise of the reviewer in the clinical topic, and practitioners are justified in maintaining some scepticism about their conclusions.' This inverse relationship might at first sight appear surprising. However, a high level of clinical expertise may militate against pure objectivity in reviewing the evidence.

Systematic reviews attempt to address the shortcomings of commentary reviews by bringing together all the published and unpublished material on a particular issue and drawing objective conclusions. Both the selection of studies and extraction of data should conform to explicit criteria so that the process is essentially replicable.

The development of the methodology for conducting systematic reviews has been pioneered by the Cochrane Collaboration, which focuses particularly on healthcare interventions. There is also a Cochrane health promotion and public health field. In an attempt to apply similar evidence-based principles to the development of social policy, the Campbell Collaboration has been established more recently. Within the UK, the NHS Centre for Reviews and Dissemination and the Evidence for Policy and Practice Information and Coordinating Centre (EPPI Centre) have been involved in the development of systematic reviews.

The process of conducting a systematic review involves a number of stages. An overview of the stages identified by the NHS Centre for Reviews and Dissemination is provided in the box.

STAGES IN THE SYSTEMATIC REVIEW PROCESS

Stage 1: Planning the review

Phase 0 Establishing the need for a review

Phase 1 Preparation of a proposal for a review

Phase 2 Development of a review protocol

Stage 2: Conducting a review

Phase 3 Identification of research

Phase 4 Selection of studies

Phase 5 Study quality assessment

Phase 6 Data extraction and monitoring progress

Phase 7 Data synthesis

Stage 3: Reporting and dissemination

Phase 8 The report and recommendations

Phase 9 Getting evidence into practice

NHS Centre for Reviews and Dissemination, 2001

Ensuring that the selection of articles is free from bias and replicable is fundamental to the systematic reviewing process. It is therefore important that written criteria for inclusion and exclusion are established at the outset. Guidance on undertaking systematic reviews developed by the NHS Centre for Reviews and Dissemination (2001) suggests that criteria should be defined in terms of the:

• population
• interventions
• outcomes
• study designs of interest.

The Campbell Collaboration Guidance lists questions that reviewers should consider in establishing criteria about which studies are relevant to the review (see the box).

The studies ultimately selected should meet all the inclusion and none of the exclusion criteria. Although decisions should be based on explicit criteria, there will inevitably be a certain amount of subjectivity. Reliability is enhanced if papers are independently assessed by more than one reviewer. A further stage in the selection may involve identifying those papers that would be included in a narrative review only and those that might be included in a meta analysis.

Oakley et al.'s (1995) review of sexual health interventions for young people initially identified 270 papers reporting sexual health interventions. Of these, 73 reported evaluations of sexual health interventions examining their effectiveness in changing knowledge, attitudes or behaviour, of which 65 were identified as separate outcome evaluations – 45 (69 per cent) lacked random control groups, 44 (68 per cent) failed to present pre-intervention data and 38 (59 per cent) post-intervention data and

CONSIDERATIONS WHEN ESTABLISHING INCLUSION AND EXCLUSION CRITERIA

• What characteristics of studies will be used to determine whether or not a particular effort was relevant to the topic of interest?
• What characteristics of studies will lead to exclusion?
• Will relevance decisions be based on a reading of report titles, abstracts, full reports?
• Who will make the relevance decisions?
• How will the reliability of relevance decisions be assessed?

Campbell Collaboration, 2001

26 (40 per cent) omitted to discuss the relevance of loss of data caused by drop-outs. Only 12 (18 per cent) of the 65 outcome evaluations were judged to be methodologically sound.

Similarly, Lister-Sharp et al.'s (1999) review of primary studies of the health promoting schools approach found 1067 titles and abstracts that were initially selected as evaluations of interventions or providing useful background material. However, only 12 finally met the inclusion criteria. Furthermore, of the 200 reviews of the effectiveness of school health promotion, only 32 met the inclusion criteria.

Thus, commenting on the lack of methodologically sound evaluations for inclusion is a common feature of systematic reviews. Notwithstanding the explicit rational basis for rejecting papers, there are questions about the feasibility of drawing generalizable conclusions from the final batch of papers, which frequently, as we have seen, constitute only a minute proportion of the literature available.

Clearly, it is important that the reviews bring together robust evidence, which will inevitably be related to the quality of the study design. There has been concern that, despite increasing recognition of the value of qualitative studies, the criteria for inclusion of studies within systematic reviews of health promotion have tended to replicate those adopted by evidence-based medicine, with over-emphasis on RCTs and experimental studies (see the box on page 171).

Tilford (2000) suggests that the selection of studies has, in fact, been broader than is often supposed, while still acknowledging the dominance of positivist studies and criteria relevant to these.

Speller et al. (1997) contend that inclusion tends to be based on the quality of the research only and overlooks the quality of the health promotion intervention. They note that Oakley's systematic review of the effectiveness of sexual health interventions for young people did not use criteria on the appropriateness of the interventions included in the review. Speller at al. also refer to problems arising from 'pooling' dissimilar interventions and cite a comparison of 'brief interventions' on alcohol misuse with more extensive approaches (NHS Centre for Reviews and Dissemination, 1993). The interpretation of what constituted a 'brief' intervention was very broad, ranging from five minutes' advice to structured sessions provided by a general practitioner over six months.

Tilford (2000) also notes the lack of attention to the process of implementation and the tendency for reviews to be conducted on narrowly focused health education interventions rather than more complex initiatives that have come to be more typical of health promotion. This disparity between the types of reviews produced and the types of activity in which practitioners are involved clearly limits their utility.

There are signs that some of these concerns are beginning to be addressed. The *Campbell Collaboration Guidelines* (2001), for example, state:

A Campbell Review can include evidence from studies of the implementation of an intervention. These studies can identify factors that enable/impede the implementation process and they can describe the subjective experience of the people providing and/or receiving the intervention or the process of implementing a particular intervention. This evidence can derive from studies using a range of methods and include both qualitative and quantitative data.

The *Guidelines* (2001) also suggest that qualitative research can:

• contribute to the development of a more robust intervention by helping to define an intervention more precisely
• assist in the choice of outcome measures and assist in the development of valid research questions
• help to understand heterogeneous results from studies of effects.

Furthermore, the guidance on undertaking systematic reviews developed by the NHS Centre for Reviews and Dissemination (2001) proposes criteria for assessing the quality of qualitative research as well as experimental and observational studies and economic evaluations (see Khan et al., 2001).

We have focused here particularly on the selection of papers for inclusion in systematic reviews. However, it is worth noting that subjectivity and human error can influence the data extraction process. This can be minimized by using clear data extraction forms and more than one assessor (Khan and Kleijnen, 2001). Synthesizing findings can also be problematic, particularly when there is lack of consistency and wide divergence in the findings. Information about process and context, if available, can offer some insight into the origins of the variation. The issue of contradictory findings arose in a review of the effectiveness of peer-delivered programmes for young people (EPPI Centre, 1999), which found five studies comparing the effects of peer-delivered and teacher-delivered interventions. Two of these found peers to be more effective than teachers, two found them to be neither more nor less effective and one concluded that neither peers nor teachers were effective.

Pawson and Tilley (1997) refer to the much-quoted review by Martinson (1974) which provides a summary of all published reports on attempts at rehabilitation of offenders between 1945 and 1967 and the conclusions of which are equivocal. While acknowledging the importance of accumulating sound evidence, Pawson and Tilley contend that answers are both complicated and may lack uniformity.

Although systematic reviews aspire to seek out and provide an objective and transparent synthesis of *all* evidence, we have noted a number of limitations. We might add that the search for evidence is frequently restricted to one language – usually English – which clearly inhibits the international exchange of information and cross-fertilization of ideas. The utility of reviews to professional, organizational and policy decisions will necessarily be dependent on the reliability of the review process. Sheldon et al. (1998) propose a number of criteria that increase the reliability of systematic reviews (see the box).

Evidence into practice

We have already commented in Chapter 5 on the way practitioners use evidence. Clearly, it is essential that evidence meets the needs of practitioners and due attention is given to the dissemination of evidence of effectiveness. Oldenburg et al.'s (1999) analysis of the extent to which health promotion research provides an empirical basis for the diffusion and institutionalization of effective interventions involved an audit of articles in twelve selected journals. They found that:

- less than 11 per cent of studies could be classified as diffusion or institutionalization research

- most research was on behaviour associated with cardiovascular disease and cancer
- most published research was on interventions directed at behaviour change in individuals or small groups rather than social, environmental, ecological or policy approaches.

They conclude that these findings support the view that health promotion research is not relevant to the issues that practitioners are dealing with and the methods they use and is difficult to apply to real-life practice situations.

It would seem that, to improve the translation of public health intervention and health promotion research into practice and relevant policy, it will be important to encourage:

> intervention research directed at those targeted behaviours that have not been studied adequately to date; appropriately staged research to ensure that efficacy and effectiveness are proven prior to policy and community-wide implementation; and, most importantly, research which directly addresses methods of diffusing effective programmes and implementing social and environmental strategies to promote better health. (1999: 128)

In the UK, a number of attempts have been made to facilitate access to evidence of effectiveness. *Effectiveness Matters,* for example, is produced by the NHS Centre for Reviews and Dissemination and provides short, journalistic-style summaries of high-quality systematic reviews to update practitioners and decision makers in the NHS on the effectiveness of important health interventions.

The Contributors to the Cochrane and Campbell Collaborations (2000) have produced summaries of

---

CRITERIA THAT INCREASE THE RELIABILITY OF A SYSTEMATIC REVIEW

- Explicit inclusion and exclusion criteria that specify the population, intervention, outcome and methodological criteria for studies used in the review.
- Comprehensive and systematic search methods to locate all relevant studies, including searching a wide range of computerized databases using a mixture of appropriate key words and free text.
- Assessment of the validity of primary studies, which should be reproducible and attempt to avoid bias.
- Exploration of variation between the findings of the different studies.
- Appropriate synthesis of primary studies.

After Sheldon et al., 1998

evidence related to implementing the wider public health agenda and, in particular, achieving the targets of the national health strategy 'Saving Lives: Our Healthier Nation'. Furthermore, the HDA (undated) is developing an evidence base. The quality standards adopted for judging the quality of evidence are:

- transparency in relation to:
  - collation
  - sources consulted
  - full disclosure of analysis and findings
  - who was involved in collating evidence
  - sources of funding
- systematicity
  - clear display of the process of gathering and assessing evidence
- relevance
  - relevance to public health and particularly 'Saving Lives: Our Healthier Nation'.

However Wilson et al. (2001) suggest that it is naïve to suppose that if information is made available to practitioners it will automatically be accessed, appraised and integrated into practice. Indeed, it is hardly surprising that the forces of inertia affecting changes in professional practice are not dissimilar to those influencing changes in individual behaviour. This resistance to change has been graphically encapsulated by Tyrrell (1951):

The human mind is in the grip of an unconscious urge which makes it cling desperately to the world of familiar things and resists all that threatens to tear it away from its moorings.

Some time ago, Gibson (undated) developed a checklist, based on his personal experience, of some fifty ploys used to avoid change in the school curriculum (see the box).

In our earlier consideration of the factors influencing behaviour change in Chapters 3 and 7, we made the important distinction between increasing awareness and actually changing behaviour. Dissemination of information, however effective, cannot be expected, in itself, to achieve changes in practice. A review of strategies for getting knowledge into practice and improving the quality of healthcare (NHS Centre for Reviews and Dissemination, 1999) concluded that:

- routine mechanisms are essential for achieving individual and organizational change
- individual beliefs, attitudes and knowledge influence professional behaviour, together with other important factors, such as the organizational, economic and community environments in which practitioners are working
- attempts to achieve change should be based on a 'diagnostic analysis' to identify factors that will affect the proposed change

HOW TO AVOID CURRICULUM CHANGE!

It's been done before.
It has never been done before.
The parents wouldn't like it.
It doesn't fit into any syllabus.
It's too vague and I haven't got time anyway.
We don't have suitable staff.
The Head wouldn't go along with it.
I am personally in favour, but the Unions you know …
It's not a multidisciplinary thing is it?
Not if it means another committee.
Only if we can have another committee.
I don't have the power to implement it.
You don't have the right to suggest it.
Who are you anyway?
Have you had any experience of this sort of thing?
etc.
etc.

Gibson, undated

Plus ça change!!

- multifaceted interventions that tackle different barriers to change are more likely to be successful than single interventions
- adequate resources are needed along with people with appropriate knowledge and skills
- systematic strategies for achieving change should include monitoring and evaluation, along with plans to consolidate change.

Evidence-based health promotion holds out the promise of ensuring that energy and resources are directed to maximum effect by enabling effective interventions to be identified. It can also support practitioners' attempts to resist pressure to adopt ill-conceived, although politically appealing, stratagems or programmes. Middleton et al. (2001), for example, have made their concerns known to the Home Office about the introduction into the UK of the 'Scared Straight' programme from the USA. They base their objection on the fact that systematic

reviews of the programme have shown adverse outcomes. Furthermore, rather than being the cost-cutting exercise that some feared, evidence-based practice enables a realistic assessment to be made of the scope of the intervention necessary to achieve desired effects. It can therefore be used to generate arguments to secure sufficient funding. However, whether or not these potential benefits are realized will ultimately be dependent on the quality of the evidence base and in particular:

- relevance to practitioners
- identification of appropriate outcomes
- attention to process and context as well as outcomes
- recognition of the need for methodological pluralism
- consistency with the core values of health promotion
- effective dissemination.

Epilogue

Promoting health is a complex and multifaceted enterprise characterized by diverse opinions about goals and the means of achieving them. It necessarily involves a range of different sectors, all of which can legitimately lay claim to being part of the wider public health workforce. The emergence of health promotion as a specialist discipline in the 1980s was accompanied by debate about its core values and purpose as it strove to position itself in relation to other key players – not least biomedicine. One of our major aims in this book has been to capture the 'distinctive voice' of health promotion in order to provide a meaningful framework for action based on analysis of values, theory and empirical evidence.

Hopefully we have indicated our unequivocal commitment to systematic planning as a *sine qua non* for achieving programme aims in an effective and efficient manner. We have also emphasized that the term 'programme' can be applied to a wide variety of initiatives from national and international policy change to community development, settings based approaches and, indeed, one-to-one encounters. The principles are the same and involve developing action-orientated programmes based on assessments of need and rigorous analysis of the social, environmental and psychological factors influencing health and health choices. In addition to having clear objectives, successful interventions require critical appraisal of contextual factors. Intervention strategies should be appropriate and incorporate judiciously selected methods. Evaluation should be an integral part of the programme and should be used not only to assess ultimate success but also to provide insight into process and serve as a basis for ongoing modification of the various programme components to maximize the likelihood of achieving that success.

We have indicated that one of the weaknesses of many health promotion programmes is the lack of an appropriate theoretical base and believe that successful programmes tend to be rooted in robust and relevant theory. Given its breadth, diversity and ambitions, assembling a 'theory of health promotion'

is no easy task. The theory of health promotion inevitably incorporates principles based on knowledge acquired from research into the determinants of health, the factors influencing social change and the manifold social, environmental and psychological factors determining individual health choices. We will hopefully have convinced readers that, given our present knowledge, we already have a plethora of theories to guide planning and practice.

One of the most significant aspects of health promotion is its action orientation and the values on which this is grounded. In a recent research report on the value base of health promotion and public health (Tilford et al., 2003), we referred to MacDonald and Mussi's (1998) observations about the 'distinctive voice of the health promotion *profession*' (our emphasis). Their tripartite analysis referred to:

- the theory of the problem – a social and economic analysis of health and its determinants
- principles of the solution – commitment to a clear set of principles
- integration of response – bridging the boundary between strategy development and hands-on implementation of strategy.

Using this framework we can conceptualize health promotion in the following way:

- the theory of the problem – involves a holistic view of health, including wellbeing, a socio-ecological analysis of the determinants of health and an 'upstream approach' to prevention
- principles of the solution – including empowerment; participation; a collaborative approach to working with individuals, communities and organizations; a comprehensive approach
- integration of response – requires working at all levels and across all sectors.

Above all there is commitment to health – as a fundamental human right – and to equity. We have attempted to demonstrate how programme planning should not only be systematic, but must be based on an acceptable ideology (symbolized by the twin notions of equity and empowerment) and should incorporate the principles outlined above. We have supported participation as being healthy in its own right but also as contributing to the achievement of other health goals. Furthermore, we paid special attention to the values-base of different strategies, for instance, by comparing different mass media approaches and their ideological rationales, and by focusing on the values – implicit and explicit – in different community-orientated approaches. We also noted how specific methods that might operate within settings or in the context of broader strategic interventions could either militate against the key values of health promotion or enhance and reinforce them.

A final observation about the incorporation of key health promotion values into programme planning: the ideological dimension of evaluation. In our final chapter we attempted to demonstrate how evaluation was one of the most contested features of programme design. Indeed, we made reference to the notion of 'paradigm wars' to describe the ideological and ethical clash between an 'interpretivist' approach and a 'positivist' approach, indicating that the latter was typically inconsistent with the major ideological features of health promotion – not only in its lack of concern for community participation, but in the intrinsic commitment to social change that characterizes action research – arguably the most significant imperative for evaluating health promotion.

Apart from the contribution of values, we have argued that a new role for health education is a central feature of health promotion's 'distinctive voice'. We repeated the observation that, in operational terms, it is useful to consider health promotion as a multiplicative relationship between healthy public policy and health education. Moreover, we have argued that a 'new' version of health education should take pride of place in this synergistic relationship.

We have acknowledged that certain 'traditional' approaches to health education were guilty of 'victim blaming'. Health promotion was a kind of 're-badging' exercise which sought to remedy this victim-blaming tendency by shifting the focus of attention 'upstream' and emphasizing the primacy of creating 'healthy public policy'. Arguably, this laudable development resulted in discarding the health education baby with the victim-blaming bathwater! We have readily acknowledged that health education needs a supportive environment to achieve its goals. However, the converse has frequently been ignored. In other words, the creation

of healthy public policy – especially where this is politically unacceptable – needs education to overcome political barriers and generate popular pressure for change.

This is not to say that the traditional role of health education should be totally rejected. There are many varieties of learning and individual clients, students or patients will always need efficient education to provide them with the knowledge and skills they need to make and sustain decisions. We have endeavoured in this book to provide a thorough theoretical analysis of education as a process that supplies the conditions for learning. Indeed, we struggled to find any type of health promoting change that was not dependent on learning of some kind. We argue here that the kind of learning provided by the New Health Education involves a number of major shifts of focus.

Rather than focusing on individual behaviour change the New Health Education is concerned to influence policymakers and politicians (both large and small) and professionals – and may need to take advantage of the extensive armamentarium of attitude change devices currently available! Similarly, traditional health education has sought to disseminate the results of effective (usually behaviour change) interventions; the New Health Education is also concerned with dissemination but the interventions will often be different.

Most important of all, the major concern of New Health Education and its specialist corpus of knowledge and competences is with achieving social and political change by education of the public. Drawing on 'critical theory', its purpose is radical – that is, addressing the root causes of health and illness, their social and environmental determinants. Key features of the approach include critical consciousness raising achieved by diverse means such as community activism and media advocacy.

The New Health Education is, of course, overtly political and therefore potentially problematic to those who do not acknowledge health as a basic human right. We commented above that health promotion is a complex, multisectoral enterprise and there is evidence of an emerging coalition among the wider public health workforce – and in some countries evidence of general political support for addressing the broader determinants of health. Quite clearly intersectoral working, one of the cardinal principles of health promotion, will be essential for success – especially when working way 'upstream'.

In short, this 'new', 'critical' health education is empowering: it is radical and political in intent. It should be the *distinctive* voice of health promotion.

References

Aarons, A. and Hawes, H. (1979) *Child-to-child*. London: Macmillan.

Abbasi, K. (1999) 'The World Bank and world health under fire', *British Medical Journal*, 318: 1003–6.

Abel-Smith, B. (1994) *An Introduction to Health Policy: Planning and Financing*. London: Longman.

Abramson, L.Y., Seligman, M.E.P. and Teasdale, J.D. (1978) 'Learned helplessness in humans: critique and reformulation', *Journal Abnormal Psychology*, 87: 49–74.

Acheson, D. (1998) *Independent Inquiry into Inequalities in Health: Recommendations*. London: Department of Health.

Adams, L. and Armstrong, E. (1995) *From Analysis to Synthesis II: The Revenge*, report of the Penrith Symposium. Sheffield: Sheffield Health.

Advocacy Institute (1992) *Telling Your Story*. Washington, DC: Advocacy Institute. (*Website:* www.advocacy.org/publications.htm)

Advocacy Institute (2001) 'What is "Advocacy"?' *(*definition on website). Washington, DC: Advocacy Institute. (*Website:* www.advocacy.org/definition.htm)

Ahmad, O.B., Boschi-Pinto, C., Lopez, A.D., Murray, C.J.L., Kozano, R. and Inoue, M. (2001) *Age Standardization of Rates: A New WHO Standard*. Geneva: WHO, GPE Discussion Paper Series: No. 31.

Ajzen, I. (1991) 'The theory of planned behavior', *Organizational Behavior and Human Decision Processes*, 50: 179–211.

Alberoni, F. (1962) 'L'élite irresponsable; theorie et recherche sociologique sur "le divismo"', *Ikon*, 12–40/1: 45–62, (Translated by McQuail.)

Alinsky, S. (1969) *Reveille for Radicals*. New York: Vintage Books.

Alinsky, S.D. (1972) *Rules for Radicals*. New York: Random House.

Allport, G.W. (1961) *Pattern and Growth in Personality*. NewYork: Holt, Rinehart & Winston.

American Heritage Dictionary of the English Language (2000, 4th edn) New York: Houghton Mifflin.

Amidei, N. (1991) *So You Want to Make a Difference: Advocacy is the Key*. Washington, DC: OMB Watch.

Anderson, J. (1975) 'Public policy making', in F. Delaney *Policy and Health Promotion, Journal of the Institute of Health Education*, 32 (1): 5–9.

Anderson, J. (undated) *The HEA Health Skills Dissemination Project: A Whole School Approach to Life Skills and Health Education*. Leeds: Counselling and Career Development Unit.

Anderson, J., Beels, C. and Powell, D. (1994) *Health Skills for Life*. Walton-on-Thames: Nelson.

Annett, H. and Rifkin, S. (1990) *Improving Urban Health*. Geneva: WHO.

Anonymous. (1994) 'Population health looking upstream', *Lancet*, 343: 429–30.

Ansari, W.E. (1998) 'Partnerships in health: how's it going to work?' *Target*, 29 July: 18.

Antonovsky, A. (1979) *Health, Stress and Coping*. San Francisco, CA: Jossey-Bass.

Antonovsky, A. (1984) 'The sense of coherence as a determinant of health', in J.D. Matarazzo, S.M. Weiss, J.A. Herd, N.E. Miller and S.M. Weiss (eds) *Behavioural Health: A Handbook of Health Enhancement and Disease Prevention*. New York: John Wiley: 114–129.

Antonovsky, A. (1987) *Unraveling the Mystery of Health*. San Francisco: Jossey-Bass.

Antonovsky, A. (1996) 'The salutogenic model as a theory to guide health promotion', *Health Promotion International*, 11 (1): 11–18.

Appleton, J. (1992) 'Notes from a food and nutrition PRA in a Guinean fishing village', *RRA Notes (No. 16): Special Issue on Applications for Health*: 77–85.

Argyle, M. (1978) *The Psychology of Interpersonal Behaviour* (3rd edn). Harmondsworth: Penguin.

Argyle, M. and Kendon, A. (1967) 'The experimental analysis of social performance', *Advances in Experimental Social Psychology*, 3: 35–98.

Arnstein, S.R. (1971) 'Eight rungs on the ladder of citizen participation', in S.E. Cahn, and B.A. Passett, *Citizen Participation: Effecting Community Change*. New York: Praeger Publications.

Aronson, E. (1976) *The Social Animal*. San Francisco: W.H. Freeman.

Aronson, E. and Mettee, D. (1968) 'Dishonest behavior as a function of low levels of self-esteem', *Journal of Personality and Social Psychology*, 9: 121–7.

ASH (1999) *Bad for Business? Smoking and the Hospitality Trade*. London: ASH.

ASH (2001) *Factsheet No. 2: Smoking Statistics: Illness and Death*. London: ASH.

ASH (2002) *Basic Facts No. 1: Smoking Statistics*. London: ASH.

ASH (2002a) *British American Tobacco – The other report to society*. London: ASH.

ASH (2002b) *Fact Sheet No. 19: Tobacco Advertising and Promotion.* London: ASH.

ASH (undated) *Action on Smoking and Health,* – Home page (on website). *Website:* www.ash.org.uk

Ashton, J. and Seymour, H. (1988) *The New Public Health.* Buckingham: Open University Press.

Aspen Institute (1997) *Voices from the Field: Learning from the Early Work of Comprehensive Community Initiatives.* Washington, DC: The Aspen Institute.

Association of Public Health Observatories (2002) *Focusing on the Health of England: Background.* (*Website:* www.pho.org.uk, Stockton on Tees: APHO.

Baan, C., Barendregt, J., Bonneux, L., Brønnum-Hansen, H., Gunning-Schepers, L., Kamper-Jørgnsen, F., van der Maas, P., Marang van de Mheen, P., Mooy, J., McPherson, K., Naidoo, B., Rosen, M., Stenbeck, M., Thorogood, M. and Welvaart (1999) *Public Health Models: Tools for Health Policy Making at National and European Level.* Amsterdam: Instituut voor Sociale Geneeskunde, Universteit van Amsterdam.

Bachrach, P. and Baratz, M.S. (1970) *Power and Poverty: Theory and Practice.* New York: Oxford University Press.

Backett-Milburn, K. and McKie, L. (1999) 'A critical appraisal of the draw and write technique', *Health Education Research,* 14 (3): 387–98.

Backett-Milburn, K. and Wilson, S. (2000) 'Understanding peer education: insights from a process evaluation', *Health Education Research,* 15 (1): (85–96).

Baelz, P.R. (1979) 'Philosophy of health education', in I. Sutherland (ed.), *Health Education: Perspectives and Choices.* Allen & Unwin, London.

Bales, R.F. (1951) *Interaction Process Analysis.* New York: Addison Wesley.

Ball, S. (1994) 'Theatre and health education: meeting of minds or marriage of convenience?', *Health Education Journal,* 53: 222–5.

Bandura, A. (1977) 'Self-efficacy toward a unifying theory of behavioural change', *Psychological Review,* 64 (2): 191–225.

Bandura, A. (1982) 'Self-efficacy mechanism in human agency', *American Psychologist,* 37 (2): 122–47.

Bandura, A. (1986) *Social Foundations of Thought and Action: A Social Cognitive Theory.* Englewood Cliffs, NJ: Prentice-Hall.

Bandura, A. (1989) 'Human agency in social cognitive theory', *American Psychologist,* 44 (9): 1175–84.

Bandura, A. (1992) 'Exercise of personal agency through the self-efficacy mechanism', in R. Schwarzer (ed.), *Self-Efficacy: Thought Control of Action.* Washington, DC: Hemisphere Publishing.

Banfield, E.C. (1958) *The Moral Basis of a Backward Society.* New York: Free Press.

Banken, R. (2001) *Strategies for Institutionalizing HIA.* ECHP Health Impact Assessment Discussion Papers, No. 1. Brussels: European Centre for Health Policy.

Baric, L. (1969) 'Recognition of the "at-risk" role', *International Journal of Health Education,* XII (1): 2–12.

Baric, L. (1974) 'Acquisition of the smoking habit and the model of "smokers" careers', *Journal of the Institute of Health Education,* 12 (1): 9–18.

Baric, L. (1975) 'Conformity and deviance in health and illness', *International Journal of Health Education* (supplement to Vol. XVIII): 1–12.

Baric, L. (1993) 'Health promotion – the settings approach', *Journal of the Institute of Health Education,* 31 (1): 17–24.

Baric, L., McArthur, C. and Sherwood, M. (1976) 'A study of health education aspects of smoking in pregnancy', *International Journal of Health Education,* XIX (2): 1–17.

Barker, D.J.P. and Rose, G. (1984) *Epidemiology in Medical Practice* (3rd edn) Edinburgh: Churchill Livingstone.

Barker, P. (1990) 'Breaking the shell', *Nursing Times,* 86 (46): 36–8.

Barnard, H.C. (1961) *A History of English Education.* London: University of London Press.

Barnes, R. and Scott-Samuel, A. (2000) *Health Impact Assessment – A Ten Minute Guide.* Liverpool: Liverpool Public Health Observatory.

Barrett-Lennard, G.T. (1998) *Carl Rogers' Helping System: Journey and Substance.* London: Sage.

Bartholomew, L.K., Parcel, G.S., Kok, G. and Gottlieb, N.H. (2001) *Intervention Mapping: Designing Theory- and Evidence-Based Health Promotion Programs.* Mountain View, CA: Mayfield.

Bartlett, R.V. (1989) 'Policy through impact assessment: institutionalised analysis as a policy strategy', in R. Banken *Strategies for Institutionalizing HIA.* Brussels: European Centre for Health Policy.

Barton, J., Chassin, L. and Presson, C.C. (1982) 'Social image factors as motivators of smoking initiation in early and middle adolescence', *Child Development,* 53: 1499–1511.

Basch, P.F. (1990) *Textbook of International Health.* Oxford: Oxford University Press.

Basch, C.E. and Gold, R.S. (1986) 'Type V errors in hypothesis testing', *Health Education Research,* 1 (4): 299–305.

Batten, T.R. (1967) *The Non-Directive Approach in Group and Community Work.* Oxford: Oxford University Press.

Bauld, L. and Judge, K. (2000) 'Strong theory flexible methods: emergent approaches to health promotion evaluation', British Heart Foundation Health Promotion Research Group Workshop, 'Evaluating Health Promotion Interventions: Beyond the Dialogue', Ilkley 8th and 9th May.

Baum, F. (2001) 'Healthy Public Policy', in T. Heller, R. Muston, M. Sidell and C. Lloyd (eds), *Working for Health.* London: Sage.

BBC (1982) '*Play it Safe*': *Child Accident Prevention Campaign.* BBC Broadcasting Research Special Report. London: BBC.

Beaglehole, R., Bonita, R. and Kjellström, T. (1993) *Basic Epidemiology*. Geneva: WHO.

Beattie, A. (1991) 'Knowledge and control in health promotion: a test case for social policy and social theory', in J. Gabe, M. Calnan, and M. Bury (eds) *The Sociology of the Health Service*. London: Routledge.

Beattie, A. (1993) 'The changing boundaries of health', in A. Beattie, M. Gott, L. Jones and M. Sidell (eds) *Health and Wellbeing: a Reader*. London Macmillan.

Beauchamp, D.E. (1976) Public health as social justice, *Inquiry*, 13: 3–14.

Beauchamp, T.L. (1978) 'The regulation of hazards and hazardous behaviors', *Health Education Monographs*, 6 (2): 242–56.

Becker, M.H. (ed.) (1984) *The Health Belief Model and Personal Health Behavior*. Thorofare, NJ: Charles B. Slack.

Belbin, E., Downs, S. and Perry, P. (1981) 'How do I learn?' in J. Anderson, *The HEA Health Skills Dissemination Project: A Whole School Approach to Life Skills and Health Education*. Leeds: Counselling and Career Development Unit.

Bell, S. (2001) *LogFrames: Improved NRSP research project planning and monitoring*. Hemel Hempstead: DFID, NRSP.

Benjamin, H. (1971) 'The saber-toothed curriculum', in R. Hooper (ed.) *The Curriculum: Context, Design and Development*. Edinburgh: Oliver & Boyd in association with the Open University. (Originally published in 1939 under the pseudonym J.A. Peddiwell.)

Bennett, P. and Murphy, S. (1997) *Psychology and Health Promotion*. Buckingham: Open University Press.

Berensson, M.K., Carlsson, P., Granath, M. and Urwitz, V. (2001) 'Quality indicators for health promotion programmes', *Health Promotion International*, 16 (2): 187–95.

Berger, A.A. (1991) *Media Analysis Techniques*. Newbury Park, CA: Sage.

Berkman, L.F. and Syme, S.L. (1979) 'Social networks, host resistance, and mortality: a nine-year follow-up study of Alameda County residents', *American Journal of Epidemiology*, 109: 186–203.

Berndt, T.J. and Burgy, L. (1996) 'Social self concept', in B.A. Bracken (ed.) *Handbook of Self Concept: Developmental, Social and Clinical Considerations*. New York: Wiley.

Berne, E. (1964) *Games that People play*. New York: Grove Press.

Bernhard, J. (2001) *Health Education Research: Special Issue on Health Education and the Internet*, 16 (6).

Bivins, E.C. (1979) 'Community organisation – an old but reliable health education technique', in P.M. Lazes, (ed.) *Handbook of Health Education*. New York: Aspen.

Black, D. (1998) 'The limitations of evidence' *Journal of the Royal College of Physicians of London*, 32 (1): 23–6.

Blackwell, S. and Kosky, M. (2000) *The Role of 'Citizens' Juries' in Decisions About Equity in Health Care*. Perth, Australia: Medical Council.

Blaikie, N.W.H. (1991) 'A critique of the use of triangulation in social research', *Quality and Quantity*, 25: 115–36.

Blaxter, M. and Paterson, S. (1982) *Mothers and Daughters: A Three Generational Study of Health Attitudes and Behaviour*. London: Heinemann.

Blazer, D.G. (1982) 'Social support and mortality in elderly community populations', *American Journal of Epidemiology*, 115: 684–94.

Bloxham, S. (1997) 'The contribution of interagency collaboration to the promotion of young people's sexual health', *Health Education Research*, 12 (1): 91–101.

Boster, F.J. and Mongeau, P.A. (1984) 'Fear arousing persuasive messages', in R. Bostrom (ed.) *Communication Yearbook* (Vol. 8): 330–75. Newbury Park, CA: Sage.

Botvin, G.J. (1984) 'The life skills training model: a broad spectrum approach to the prevention of cigarette smoking', in G. Campbell (ed.), *Health Education and Youth: A Review of Research and Developments*. Lewes, East Sussex: Falmer Press.

Bouman, M. (1999) *The Turtle and the Peacock: The Entertainment Education Strategy on Television*. Wageningen, Netherlands: Wageningen Agricultural University.

Bouman, M., Maas, L. and Kok, G. (1998) 'Health education in television entertainment – Medisch Centrum West: A Dutch Drama Serial', *Health Education Research*, 13 (4): 503–18.

Bourdieu, P. (1980) *Questions de Sociologie*. Paris: Les Editions des Minuit.

Bowling, A. (1997a) *Measuring Health: A Review of Quality of Life Measurement Scales* (2nd edn). Buckingham: Open University Press.

Bowling, A. (1997b) *Research Methods in Health*. Buckingham: Open University Press.

Bracht, N. (ed.) (1999) *Health Promotion at the Community Level: New Advances*. Thousand Oaks, CA: Sage.

Bracht, N. and Gleason, J. (1990) 'Strategies and structures for citizen partnerships', in N. Bracht (ed.), *Health Promotion at the Community Level*. Thousand Oaks, CA: Sage.

Bracht, N. and Kingsbury, L. (1990) 'Community organization principles in health promotion: a five stage model' in N. Bracht (ed.), *Health Promotion at the Community Level*. Thousand Oaks, CA: Sage.

Bracht, N., Kingsbury, L. and Rissel, C. (1999) 'A five-stage community organization model for health promotion', in N. Bracht (eds), *Health Promotion at the Community Level: New Advances*. Thousand Oaks, CA: Sage.

Bradshaw, J. (1972) 'The concept of social need', *New Society*, 30 March.

Bradshaw, J. (1994) 'The conceptualization and measurement of need: a social policy perspective', in J. Popay and G. Williams (eds), *Researching the People's Health*. London: Routledge.

Brager, C. and Specht, H. (1973) *Community Organizing*. New York: Columbia University Press.

Brandes, D. and Ginnis, P. (1986) 'A guide to student-centred learning', in J. Ryder and C. Campbell, *Balancing Acts in Personal, Social and Health Education*. London: Routledge.

Braybrooke, D. and Lindblom, C.E. (1963) *A Strategy of Decision*. New York: Free Press.

Breed, W. and Defoe, J.R. (1981) 'The portrayal of the drinking process on prime-time television', *Journal of Communication*, 31: 48–58.

Brehm, J.W. (1966) *A Theory of Psychological Reactance*. New York: Academic Press.

Brehm, S.S. and Brehm, J.W. (1981) *Psychological Reactance: A Theory of Freedom and Control*. New York: Academic Press.

British Standards Institute (1978) 'BS 4778 British Standard quality vocabulary', in Society of Health Education and Health Promotion Specialists, *Developing Quality in Health Education and Health Promotion*. Society of Health Education and Health Promotion Specialists.

Brook, R.H. and Lohr, K.N. (1985) 'Efficacy, effectiveness, variations, and quality: boundary-crossing research', *Medical Care*, 23 (5): 710–22.

Broughton, B. (2001) *How LogFrame Approaches Could Facilitate the Planning and Management of Humanitarian Operations*. http://www.mande.co.uk/docs/bblogframe.pdf [accessed 22/05/02].

Brown, C. (1984) 'The art of coalition building: a guide for community leaders', in F.D. Butterfoss, R.M. Goodman and A. Wandersman, 'Community coalitions for prevention and health promotion', *Health Education Research*, 8 (3): 315–30.

Brown, E.R. and Margo, G.E. (1978) 'Health education: can the reformers be reformed?', *International Journal of Health Services*, 8 (1): 3–23.

Bruner, J. (1966) *Towards a Theory of Instruction*. Cambridge, MA: Harvard University Press.

Bruner, J. (1971) *The Relevance of Education*. New York: Norton & Co.

Brunner, E. (1996) 'The social and biological basis of cardiovascular disease in office workers', in D. Blane, E. Brunner and R. Wilkinson (eds) *Health and Social Organization: Towards a Health Policy for the 21st Century*. London: Routledge.

Buchan, H., Gray, M., Hill, A. and Coulter, A. (1990) 'Needs assessment made simple', *Health Service Journal*, (100): 240–1.

Buchanan, D.R. (1994) 'Reflections on the relationship between theory and practice', *Health Education Research*, 9 (3): 273–83.

Buchanan, D.R. (2000) *An Ethic for Health Promotion: Rethinking the Sources of Human Well-Being*. New York: Oxford University Press.

Bulmer, M. (1982) *The Use of Social Research: Social Investigations in Public Policy Making*. London: Allen & Unwin.

Bunton, R. (1992) 'Health promotion as social policy', in R. Bunton and G. Macdonald (eds), *Health Promotion: Disciplines and Diversity*. London: Routledge.

Bunton, R. and Burrows, R. (1995) 'Consumption and health in the "epidemiological" clinic of late modern medicine', in R. Bunton, S. Nettleton and R. Burrows (eds) *The Sociology of Health*. London: Routledge.

Bunton, R. and Macdonald, G. (eds) (1992) *Health Promotion: Disciplines and Diversity*. London: Routledge.

Butcher, K. and Kievelitz, U. (1997) 'Planning with PRA: HIV and STD in a Nepalese mountain community', *Health Policy and Planning*, 12 (3): 253–61.

Butterfoss, F.D., Goodman, R.M. and Wandersman, A. (1993) 'Community coalitions for prevention and health promotion', *Health Education Research*, 8 (3): 315–30.

Cabanero-Verzosa, C. (1996) *Communication for Behavior Change*. Washington, DC: The World Bank.

Cacioppo, J.T. and Petty, R.E. (1989) 'The elaboration likelihood model: the role of effect and affect laden information processing in persuasion', in P. Cafferata and A. Tybout (eds), *Cognitive and Affective Responses to Advertising*. Lexington, MA: Lexington Books.

Calman, K.C. (1997) 'Equity, poverty and health for all', *British Medical Journal*, 314 (7088): 1187–91.

Calouste Gulbenkian Foundation (1984) *A National Centre for Community Development* (report of a working party). London: Gulbenkian Foundation.

Campbell Collaboration (2001) *Campbell Collaboration Guidelines*. University of Pennsylvania, Philadelphia, PA: Campbell Collaboration. *Campbell Systematic Reviews: Guidelines for the Preparation of Review Protocols. (Website:* www.campbellcollaboration.org/Fraguidelines.html)

Campbell, C., Wood, R. and Kelly, M. (1999) *Social Capital and Health*. London: Health Development Agency.

Campbell, D. and Fiske, D. (1959) 'Convergent and discriminant validation by the multitrait-multimethod matrix', *Psychological Bulletin*, 56: 81–105.

Campbell, D. and Stanley, J. (1963) *Experimental and Quasi Experimental Evaluations in Social Research*. Chicago: Rand McNally.

Campbell, O., Cleland, J., Collumbien, M. and Southwick, K. (1999) *Social Science Methods for Research on Reproductive Health*. Geneva: WHO.

Canadian Council on Social Development (2001) 'Defining and Redefining Poverty: a CCSD Perspective', Position Paper, Ottawa, Ontario: CCSD. (*Website:* www.ccsd.ca/pubs/2001/povertypp.htm)

Cantril, H. (1958) 'The invasion from Mars', in E.E. Maccoby, T.M. Newcomb and E.L. Hartley, (eds) *Readings in Social Psychology*. New York: Henry Holt.

Caplan, R. and Holland, J. (1990) 'Rethinking health education theory', *Health Education Journal*, 49: 10–12.

Care Sector Consortium (1997) *National Occupational Standards*. London: Local Government Management Board.

Carlin, J.P.T. and Nolan, T. (1998) 'School-based bicycle safety education and bicycle injuries in children', in S. MacIntyre and M. Petticrew, 'Good intentions and received wisdom are not enough', *Journal of Epidemiology and Community Health*, 54: 802–3.

Carlisle (2002) '*Artful Approach to Joint Working*', *Health Development Today*. (*Website:* www.hda-online.org.uk)

Carr-Hill, R. and Dixon-Chalmers, P. (2002) *A Review of Methods for Monitoring and Measuring Social Inequality, Deprivation and Health Inequalities*. Oxford: South East Public Health Observatory. (*Website:* www.sepho.org.uk)

Catford, J. (1983) 'Positive health indicators – towards a new information base for health promotion', *Community Medicine*, 5: 125–32.

Catford, J. (1993) 'Auditing health promotion: what are the vital signs of quality', *Health Promotion International*, 8 (2): 67–8.

Cattell, R.B. (1966) *The Scientific Analysis of Personality*. Chicago: Aldine.

Chapman, S. (1994) 'The A–Z of public health advocacy', in S. Chapman and D. Lupton, (eds), *The Fight for Public Health: Principles and Practice of Media Advocacy*. London: BMJ Publishing Group.

Chapman, S. and Egger, G. (1983) 'Myth in cigarette advertising and health promotion', in S. Chapman and D. Lupton, (1994), *The Fight for the Public Health: Principles and Practice of Media Advocacy*. London: BMJ Publishing Group.

Chapman, S. and Lupton, D. (1994) *The Fight for Public Health: Principles and Practice of Media Advocacy*. London: BMJ Publishing Group.

Charlton, B.G. (1991) 'Medical practice and the double-blind, randomized controlled trial', (editorial) *British Journal of General Practice*, 42 (350): 355–6.

Charnofsky, S. (1971) *Educating the Powerless*. Belmont, CA: Wordsworth Publishers.

Chave, S.P.W. (1958) 'John Snow, the Broad Street pump and after', in J. Ashton, *The Epidemiological Imagination*. Buckingham: Open University Press.

Chesterfield-Evans, A. and O'Connor, B. (1986) 'Billboard utilizing graffitists against unhealthy promotions (BUGA UP) – its philosophy and rationale and their application in health promotion', in D.S. Leathar, G.B. Hastings and J.K. Davies (eds), *Health Education and the Media*. London: Pergamon Press.

Cochrane, A.C.L. (1972) *Effectiveness and Efficiency: Random Reflections on the Health service*. London: Nuffield Provincial Hospitals Trust.

Cochrane Collaboration (2002) *Cochrane Collaboration Disclaimer about Cochrane Reviews*. Oxford: Cochrane Collaboration. (*Website:* www.cochrane.org/cochrane/revabstr/mainindex.htm)

Cockerill, A. (undated) *Promoting Mental Health in Schools*. Hull: HAZNET, Hull and East Riding Community Health NHS Trust. (*Website:* www.haznet.org.uk/hazs/hazmap/hull_mental-hlth-schools.pdf)

Cohen, A.K. (1955) *Delinquent Boys: The Culture of the Gang*. New York: Free Press.

Cohen, B. (1963) *The Press and Foreign Policy*. Princeton, NJ: Princeton University Press.

Cohen, D. (1981) *Prevention as an Economic Good*. Aberdeen: Health Economics Research Unit.

Cohen, J.M. and Cohen, M.J. (1960) *The Penguin Dictionary of Quotations*. Harmondsworth: Penguin.

Colebatch, H.K. (1998) *Policy*. Buckingham: Open University Press.

Coleman, J. (1988) 'Social capital in the creation of human capital', *American Journal of Sociology*, 94 (supplement): S25–S120.

Coleman, J. (1990) *Foundations of Social Theory*. New York: Free Press.

Community Cohesion Review Team (2001) *Community Cohesion*. London: Home Office.

Community Development Project Information and Intelligence Unit, (1974) *Models of Social Change and Possible Strategies on Three Levels of Operation*. London: Community Development Project.

Community Development Project (1977) *Gilding the Ghetto*. London: Community Development Project.

Connell, J.P., Kubisch A.C., Schorr, L.B., Weiss, C.H. (eds) (1995) *New Approaches to Evaluating Community Initiatives: Concepts, Methods and Contexts*. Washington, DC: The Aspen Institute.

Connelly, J. (2001) 'Critical realism and health promotion: effective practice needs an effective theory' (editorial), *Health Education Research*, 16 (2): 115–9.

Conner, M. and Norman, P. (1996) (eds) *Predicting Behaviour*. Buckingham: Open University Press.

Conner, M. and Sparks, P. (1996) 'The theory of planned behaviour and health behaviours', in M. Conner and P. Norman (eds), *Predicting Behaviour*. Buckingham: Open University Press.

Constantino-David, K. (1982) 'Issues in community orgnization', *Community Development Journal*, 17: 190–201.

Constantino-David, K. (1992) 'The Philippine experience in scaling-up', in G. Walt, *Health Policy: An Introduction to Process and Power*. London: Zed.

Contributors to the Cochrane Collaboration and the Campbell Collaboration (2000) *Evidence from Systematic Reviews of Research Relevant to Implementing the 'Wider*

Public Health' Agenda. University of York: NHS Centre for Reviews and Dissemination. (*Website:* www.york.ac.uk/inst/crd/wph.htm)

Cook, T.D. and Campbell, D.T. (1979) *Quasi-Experimentation*. Chicago: Rand McNally.

Cooper, H., Arber, S., Fee, L. and Ginn, J. (1999) *The Influence of Social Support and Social Capital on Health*. London: Health Development Agency.

Cornwall, A., Musyoki, S. and Pratt, G. (2001) *IDS Working Paper 131: In search of a new impetus: pra titioners' reflections on PRA and participation in Kenya*. University of Sussex, Brighton: Institute of Development Studies. (*Website:* www.ids.ac.uk/ids/bookshop/details.asp?id=639)

Cornwell, J. (1984) *Hard-earned Lives*. London: Tavistock.

Corwin, R.G. (1978) 'Power', in E. Sagarin (ed.), *Sociology: The Basic Concepts*. New York: Holt, Rinehart & Winston.

Coulthard, M., Walker, A. and Morgan, A. (2001) *Assessing People's Perceptions of Their Neighbourhood and Community Involvement* (Part 1). London: Health Development Agency.

Coulthard, M., Walker, A. and Morgan, A. (2002) *People's Perceptions of Their Neighbourhood and Community Involvement: Results From the Social Capital Module of the General Household Survey 2000*. London: The Stationery Office. (*Website:* www.statistics.gov.uk/products/p9233.asp)

Cox, F.M., Erlich, J.L., Rothman, J. and Tropman, J.E. (eds) (1979) *Strategies of Community Organization: A Book of Readings* (3rd edn). Itasca, IL: F.E. Peacock.

Crawford, R. (1980) 'Healthism and the medicalization of everyday life', *International Journal of Health Services*, 10 (3): 365–88.

Crick, B. and Lister, I. (1978) 'Political literacy', in B. Crick and A. Porter (eds), *Political Education and Political Literacy*. London: Longman.

Croft, S. and Beresford, P. (1992) 'The politics of participation', *Critical Social Policy*, 26: 20–44.

Culyer, A.J. (1977) 'Need, values and health status measurement', in A.J. Culyer and K.G. Wright (eds), *Economic Aspects of Health Services*. London: Martin Robertson.

Cummins, S. and MacIntyre, S. (2002) ' "Food deserts" – evidence and assumption in policy making', *British Medical Journal*, 325: 436–8.

Cunningham, G. (1963) 'Policy and practice', *Public Administration*, 41.

Curle, A. (1972) *Education for Liberation*. New York: John Wiley.

Dahlgren, G. and Whitehead, M. (1991) *Policies and Strategies to Promote Social Equity in Health*. Stockholm: Institute of Futures Studies.

Dahlgren, G., Nordgren, P. and Whitehead, M. (1996) *Health Impact Assessment of the EU Common Agricultural Policy*. Stockholm: The Swedish National Institute of Public Health.

Daniel, P. and Dearden, P.N. (2001) *Integrating a Logical Framework Approach to Planning into the Health Action Zone Initiative*. Hull: HAZNET, Hull and East Riding Community Health NHS Trust.

Daniels, N. (1985) *Just Health Care*. New York: Cambridge University Press.

Davey Smith, G. (1996) 'Income inequality and mortality: why are they related?' *British Medical Journal*, 312: 987–8.

Davidoff, F., Haynes, B., Sackett, D.L. and Smith, R. (1995) 'Evidence-based medicine: a new journal to help doctors identify the information they need', *British Medical Journal*, 310: 1085–6.

Davie, R., Butler, N. and Goldstein, H. (1972) *From Birth to Seven*. London: Longman.

Davies, J.B. (1992) *The Myth of Addiction*. Switzerland: Harwood.

Davis, H. and Walton, P. (eds) (1983) *Language, Image and Media*. Oxford: Blackwell.

Day, I. (2002) ' "Putting yourself in other people's shoes": the use of forum theatre to explore refugee and homeless issues in schools', *Journal of Moral Education*, 31 (1): 21–34.

de Chernatony, L. (1993) 'Categorizing brands: evolutionary process underpinned by two key dimensions', *Journal of Marketing Management*.

De Kadt, E. (1982) 'Ideology, social policy, health and health services: a field of complex interactions', *Social Science and Medicine*, 16: 741–52.

De Leeuw, E. (1993) 'Health policy, epidemiology and power: the interest web', *Health Promotion International*, 8 (1): 49–52.

de Vries, H. (1989) *Smoking Prevention in Dutch Adolescents*. Maastricht: University of Limburg.

Deetz, S.A. (1992) *Democracy in an Age of Corporate Colonization: Developments in Communication and the Politics of Everyday Life*. Albany: State University of New York Press.

Defoe, J.R. and Breed, W.R. (1989) 'Consulting to change media contents: two cases in alcohol education', *International Quarterly of Community Health Education*, 9: 257–72.

Delaney, F. (1994a) 'Making connections: research into intersectoral collaboration', *Health Education Journal*, 53: 474–85.

Delaney, F. (1994b) 'Muddling through the middle ground: theoretical concerns in intersectoral collaboration and health promotion', *Health Promotion International*, 9 (3): 217–25.

Delaney, F. (1994c) 'Policy and health promotion', *Journal of the Institute of Health Education*, 32 (1): 5–9.

Delk, J.L. (1980) 'High-risk sports as indirect self-destructive behavior', in N.L. Farberow (ed.), *The Many Faces of Suicide*. New York: McGraw-Hill.

Denman, S., Moon, A., Parsons, C. and Stears, D. (2002) *The Health Promoting School: Policy Research and Practice*. London: Routledge Falmer.

Denzin, N.K. (1970) *The Research Act in Sociology.* London: Butterworths.

Denzin, N.K. (1994) 'The art and politics of interpretation', in N.K. Denzin and Y.S. Lincoln (1994) (eds) *Handbook of Qualitative Research.* Thousand Oaks, CA: Sage.

Denzin, N.K. and Lincoln, Y.S. (1994) (eds) *Handbook of Qualitative Research.* Thousand Oaks, CA: Sage.

Department for Education and Employment (1997) *Excellence in Schools.* London: The Stationery Office.

Department for Education and Employment (1999) *National Healthy School Standard: Guidance.* Nottingham: DfEE Publications.

Department for Environment Food and Rural Affairs (2001) *Indicators of Sustainable Development – health.* http://www.sustainable-development.gov.uk/indicators/headline/h6.htm [accessed 23/3/02].

Department of Health (1991) *The Health of the Nation: A Consultative Document for Health in England.* London: HMSO.

Department of Health (1992) *The Health of the Nation.* London: HMSO.

Department of Health (1993) *The Code of Practice for the Commissioning and Management of Research and Development.* London: HMSO.

Department of Health (1995) *ABC of Health Promotion in the Workplace.* Wetherby: Department of Health.

Department of Health (1995a) *Variations in Health: What Can the Department of Health and NHS Do? Report of the Variations Sub-group of the Chief Medical Officer's Health of the Nation Working Group.* London: HMSO.

Department of Health (1996) *Policy Appraisal and Health.* London: Department of Health.

Department of Health (1997) *The New NHS: Modern Dependable.* London: The Stationery Office.

Department of Health (1998) *Our Healthier Nation.* London: Department of Health. (*Website:* www.ohn.gov.uk/ohn/ohn.htm)

Department of Health (1998a) *Smoking Kills: A White Paper on Tobacco.* London: The Stationery Office.

Department of Health (1998b) *The Health of the Nation – A Policy Assessed.* London: The Stationery Office.

Department of Health (1999) *Saving Lives: Our Healthier Nation.* London: The Stationery Office.

Department of Health (2000) *Information About the Healthy Workplace Initiative* (from website). London: Department of Health. (*Website:* www. signupweb.net/about.htm)

Department of Health (2001) *Our Healthier Nation: Health Inequalities – Some Key Facts* (from website). London: Department of Health. (*Website:* www.ohn.gov.uk/ohn/inequ.htm health)

Department of Health (2002) *Our Healthier Nation: Healthy Neighbourhoods* (from website). London: Department of Health. (*Website:* www.ohn.gov.uk/ohn/people/neighb.htm)

Department of Health and Social Security (1976) *Prevention and Health: Everybody's Business.* London: HMSO.

Department of Health and Social Security (1980) *Inequalities in Health: Report of a Research Working Group Chaired by Sir Douglas Black.* London: DHSS.

Department of Social Security Analytical Services Division (1999) *Opportunity for All: Tackling Poverty and Social Exclusion: Indicators of Success: Definitions, Data and Baseline Information.* London: DHSS.

DETR (2000) *Index of Multiple Deprivation 2000.* London: DETR.

DETR (2001) *Local Strategic Partnerships: Government Guidance.* London: DETR. (*Website:* www.local-regions.dtlr.gov.uk/lsp/guidance)

Dewey, J. (1910) *How We Think.* Boston, MA: Heath.

Dewey, J. (1946) *The Public and Its Problems: An Essay in Political Inquiry.* Chicago: Gateway Books.

Dickson, D.A., Hargie, O. and Morrow, N.C. (1989) *Communication Skills Training for Health Professionals: An Instructor's Handbook.* London: Chapman & Hall.

Dignan, M.B. and Carr, P.A. (1992) *Program Planning for Health* (2nd edn) Malvern, PA: Lee & Febiger.

Dijkstra, A. and de Vries, H. (2000) 'Subtypes of pre-contemplating smokers defined by different long-term plans to change their smoking behavior', *Health Education Research*, 15 (4): 423–34.

Dixon, J. (1989) 'The limits and potential of community development for personal and social change', *Community Health Studies*, XII (1) 82–92.

Doll, R., Peto, R., Wheatley, K., Gray, R. and Sutherland, I. (1994) 'Mortality in relation to smoking: 40 years' observations on male British doctors', *British Medical Journal*, 309: 901–11.

Donabedian, A. (1980) *Explorations in Quality Assessment and Monitoring,* (Vol. 1). Ann Arbor, MI: Health Administration Press.

Donaldson, L. (1999) *Ten Tips for Better Health.* London: The Stationery Office. (*Website:* www.archive.official-documents.co.uk/document/cm43/4386/4386-tp.htm)

Dorn, N. and South, N. (1983) *Message in a Bottle.* Aldershot: Gower.

Douglas, M.J., Conway, L., Gorman, D., Gavin, S. and Hanlon, P. (2001) 'Developing principles for health impact assessment', *Journal of Public Health Medicine*, 23 (2): 148–54.

Downie, R.S., Tannahill, C. and Tannahill, A. (1996) *Health Promotion Models and Values* (2nd edn) Oxford: Oxford University Press.

Downie, R.S. and Macnaughton, J. (1998) 'Images of health', *Lancet*, 351: 823–5.

Doyal, L. and Gough, I. (1991) *A Theory of Human Need.* London: Macmillan.

Doyal, L. and Pennell, I. (1979) *The Political Economy of Health.* London: Pluto.

Draper, R. (1988) 'Healthy public policy: a new political challenge', *Health Promotion*, 2 (3): 217–18.

Drever, F., Whitehead, M. and Roden, M. (1996) 'Current patterns and trends in male mortality by social class (based on occupation)', *Population Trends*, 86: 15–20.

Dubos, R. (1965) *Man Adapting*. New Haven, CT: Yale University Press.

Dubos, R. (1979) *The Mirage of Health*. New York: Harper Colophon.

Duckworth, L. (2002) 'Classes in safe sex are ineffective, says study', *The Independent*, 14 June.

Duncan, J.S. and Duncan, N.G. (1992) 'Ideology and bliss: Roland Barthes and the secret history of landscape', in T.J. Barnes and J.S. Duncan (eds) *Writing Worlds: Discourse, Text and Metaphor in the Representation of Landscape*. London: Routledge.

Durfee, W. and Chase, T. (1999) *Brief Tutorial on Gantt Charts* (on website). Minneapolis, MN: University of Minnesota. (*Website:* www.me.umn.edu/courses/me4054/assignments/gantt.html)

Durgee, J.F. (1986) 'How consumer sub-cultures code reality: a look at some code types', *Advances in Consumer Research*, 13: 332–7.

Duryea, E.J. (1991) 'Principles of non-verbal communication in efforts to reduce peer and social pressure', *Journal of School Health*, 61: 5–10.

Dworkin, G. (1972) 'Paternalism', *Monist*, 56 (1): 64–84.

Eagleton, T. (1991) *An Introduction to Ideology*. London: Verso.

Edgar, A., Salek, S., Shickle, D. and Cohen, D. (1998) *The Ethical QALY: Ethical Issues in Healthcare Resource Allocations*. Haslemere: Euromed Communications Ltd.

Ehrenreich, B. and English, D. (1979) *For Her Own Good: 150 Years of Experts' Advice to Women*. London: Pluto Press.

Eiser, J.R. and Eiser, C. (1996) *Effectiveness of Video for Health Education: A Review*. London: HEA.

Elliott-Kemp, J. (1982) 'Managing Organizational Change', in Anderson, J., *HEA Health Skills Project*. Leeds: Counselling and Career Development Unit.

EPPI-Centre (1999) *A Review of the Effectiveness and Appropriateness of Peer-delivered Health Promotion Interventions for Young People*. London: Institute of Education, University of London. (*Website:* http://eppi.ioe.ac.uk/EPPIWeb/home.aspx?page=/hp/reports/peer_health/peer-delivered_health_promotion_intro.htm)

Etzioni, A. (1967) 'Mixed scanning: a third approach to decision making', *Public Administration Review*, 27: 385–92.

European Centre for Health Policy (1999) *Gothenburg Consensus Paper: Health Impact Assessment*. Copenhagen: WHO Regional Office for Europe. (*Website:* www.who.dk./eprise/main/WHO/Progs/HPA/HealthImpact/20020319_1)

European Commission (undated) *Glossary of Public Health Technical Terms*. Brussels. European Commission, Directorate-General 'Health and Consumer Protection', Directorate General Public Health. (*Website:* http://europa.eu.int/comm/health/index_en.html)

European Network of Health Promoting Schools (1997) *Conference Resolution. First Conference of the European Network of Health Promoting Schools*, Thessaloniki-Halkidiki, 1–5 May, WHO Regional Office for Europe.

European Network Workplace Health Promotion (1997) 'Luxembourg Declaration on Workplace Health Promotion in the European Union', *WHP-Net-News*, 4.

EuroQol (undated) *EQ-5D*. Rotterdam, The Netherlands: EuroQol Group. (*Website:* www.euroqol.org/content.htm)

Evans, D., Head, M.J. and Speller, V. (1994) *Assuring Quality in Health Promotion: How to Develop Standards of Good Practice*. London: HEA.

Evans, G. and Newnham, J. (1992) 'The dictionary of world politics: a reference guide to concepts, ideas and institutions', in G. Walt, *Health Policy: An Introduction to Process and Power*. London: Zed.

Evans, R.I. (1976) 'Smoking in children: developing a social psychological strategy of deterrence', *Preventive Medicine*, 5: 122–7.

Ewart, C.K. (1992) 'Role of physical self-efficacy in recovery from heart attack', in R. Schwarzer (ed.), *Self-efficacy: Thought Control of Action*. Washington: Hemisphere Publishing.

Eysenck, H.J. (1960) *The Structure of Human Personality*. London: Methuen.

Faculty of Public Health Medicine (1995) 'Health Promotion in the Workplace', *Guidelines for Health Promotion*, 40.

Faden, R.R. and Faden, A.I. (1978) 'The ethics of health education as public health policy', *Health Education Monographs*, 6 (2): 180–97.

Fairclough, N. (1995) *Ideology*. London: Arnold.

Feigherty, E., Rogers, T., Thompson, B. and Bracht, N. (1992) 'Coalition problem solving guide', in N. Bracht, *Health Promotion at the Community Level – New Advances*. Thousand Oaks, CA: Sage.

Feighery, E. and Rogers, T. (1989) 'Building and Maintaining Effective Coalitions', in F.D. Butterfoss, R.M. Goodman and A. Wandersman, 'Community coalitions for prevention and health promotion', *Health Education Research*, 8 (3): 315–30.

Festinger, L. (1957) *A Theory of Cognitive Dissonance*. Stanford, CA: Stanford University Press.

Fien, J. (1994) 'Critical theory, critical pedagogy and critical praxis in environmental education', in B.B. Jensen and K. Schnack (eds), *Action and Action Competence as Key Concepts in Critical Pedagogy*. Copenhagen: Royal Danish School of Educational Studies.

Fien, J. (2000) 'Education for sustainable consumption: towards a framework for curriculum and pedagogy', in B.B. Jensen, K. Schnack and V. Simovska (eds)

Critical Environmental and Health Education. Copenhagen: Research Centre for Environmental and Health Education, Danish University of Education.

Fien, J. and Trainer, T. (1993) 'Education for sustainability', in J. Fien (ed.) *Environmental Education: A Pathway to Sustainability.* Geelong, Australia: Deakin University Press.

Finn, P. (1980) 'Attitudes toward drinking conveyed in studio greeting cards', *American Journal of Public Health*, 70: 826–9.

Finnegan, J.R. and Viswanath, K. (1999) 'Mass Media and Health Promotion: Lessons Learned, with Implications for Public Health Campaigns', in N. Bracht (ed.), *Health Promotion at the Community Level.* Thousand Oaks, CA: Sage.

Fishbein, M. (1976) 'Persuasive Communication', in A.E. Bennett (ed.) *Communication Between Doctors and Patients.* London: Oxford University Press for Nuffield Provincial Hospitals Trust.

Fishbein, M. and Ajzen, I. (1975) *Belief, Attitude, Intention and Behavior: An Introduction to Theory and Research.* Reading, MA: Addison-Wesley.

Fisher, R. (1949) *The Design of Experiments* (5th edn). Edinburgh: Oliver & Boyd.

Flesch, R. (1948) 'A new readability yardstick', *Education Research Bulletin*, 27 (37): 11–20.

Fletcher, C.M. (1973) *Communication in Medicine.* (The Rock Carling Fellowship, 1972.) London: Nuffield Provincial Hospitals Trust.

Foreman, A. (1996) 'Health needs assessment', in J. Percy-Smith (eds), *Needs Assessments in Public Policy.* Buckingham: Open University Press.

FOREST (2002) *FOREST Home page.* (*Website:* www.forestonline.org)

Forrest, R. and Kearns, A. (2000) 'Social Cohesion, Social Capital and the Neighbourhood', in C.C.R. Team, *Community Cohesion.* London: Home Office.

Fowler, H.W. (1929) *The Concise Oxford Dictionary of Current English.* Oxford: Oxford University Press.

Frank, R.H. (2000) 'Why living in a rich society makes us feel poor', *New York Times Magazine*, October 15.

Frankel, S., Davison, C. and Davey Smith, G. (1991) 'Lay epidemiology and the rationality of responses to health education', *British Journal of General Practice*, 41: 428–30.

Frankena, W.K. (1970) 'A model for analyzing a philosophy of education', in J.R. Martin (ed.), *Readings in Philosophy of Education: A Study in Curriculum.* Boston, MA: Allyn & Bacon.

Frankham, J. (1998) 'Peer education: the unauthorised version', *British Educational Research Journal*, 24 (2): 179–93.

Freidson, E. (1961) *Patients' Views of Medical Practice.* New York: Russell Sage.

Freire, P. (1972) *Pedagogy of the Oppressed.* Harmondsworth: Penguin.

French, J. (2000) 'Understanding health promotion through its fault lines', PhD thesis. Leeds: Leeds Metropolitan University.

French, J. and Milner, S. (1993) 'Should we accept the status quo?', *Health Education Journal*, 52 (2): 98–101.

French, J.R.P. and Raven, B.H. (1959) 'The bases of social power', in D. Cartwright (ed.), *Studies in Social Power.* Ann Arbor, MI: University of Michigan Press.

Freudenberg, N. (1978) 'Shaping the future of health education: from behavior change to social change', *Health Education Monographs*, 6 (4): 372–7.

Freudenberg, N. (1981) 'Health education for social change: a strategy for public health in the US', *International Journal of Health Education*, XXIV (3): 1–7.

Freudenberg, N. (1984) 'Training health educators for social change', *International Quarterly of Community Health Education*, 5 (1): 37–52.

Friedman, M. and Rosenman, R.H. (1974) *Type A Behavior and Your Heart.* New York: Knopf.

Fukuyama, F. (1999) *Social Capital and Civil Society.* Fairfax, VA: The Institute of Public Policy, George Mason University, IMF Conference of Second Generation Reforms. (*Website*: www.imf.org/pubs/ft/seminar/1999/reforms/fukuyama.htm)

Funnell, R., Oldfield, K. and Speller, V. (1995) *Towards Healthier Alliances.* London: HEA.

Gagne, R.M. (1985) *The Conditions of Learning and Theory of Instruction* (4th edn). New York: Holt Saunders.

Galbraith, J. (1973) *Economics and the Public Purpose.* New York: Mentor.

Gallie, W.B. (1955) 'Essentially contested concepts', *Proceedings of the Aristotelian Society*, 56: 167–98.

Garcia, I., March, J.C. and Piette, D. (1999) 'Report of the Delphi study', in E. Ziglio, S. Hagard, L. McMahon, S. Harvey and L. Levin, 'Principles methodology and practices of investment for health', *Promotion & Education.* VII (2): 4–15.

Garmezy, N. (1983) 'Stressors of childhood', in N. Garmezy and M. Rutter (eds) *Stress, Coping and Development in Children.* New York: McGraw-Hill.

Gibson, M. (undated) 'How to avoid curriculum change', personal communication.

Gibson, R. (1986) *Critical Theory and Education.* London: Hodder & Stoughton.

Giddens, A. (1989) *Sociology.* Cambridge: Polity Press.

Giddens, A. (1991) *Modernity and Self Identity: Self and Society in the Late Modern Age.* Cambridge: Polity Press.

Gillam, S. and Murray, S. (1996) *Needs Assessment in General Practice.* London: RCGP.

Gillies, P. (1998) 'Effectiveness of alliances and partnerships for health promotion', *Health Promotion International*, 13 (2): 99–120.

Ginn Daugherty, H. and Kammeyer, K.C.W. (1995) *An Introduction to Population* (2nd edn). New York: Guilford.

Ginsberg, G. and Silverberg, D. (1994) 'A cost–benefit analysis of legislation for bicycle safety helmets in Israel', *American Journal of Public Health*, 84 (4): 653–6.

Godfrey, C. (2001) 'Economic evaluation of health promotion', in I. Rootman, M. Goodstadt, B. Hyndman, D.V. McQueen, L. Potvin, J. Springett and E. Ziglio (eds) *Evaluation in Health Promotion: Principles and Perspectives*. Copenhagen: WHO.

Godfrey, C., Harman, G. and Maynard, A. (1989) *Priorities for Health Promotion: An Economic Approach*, Discussion Paper 59. York: Centre for Health Economics, University of York.

Goodman, R.M., Steckler, A. and Kegler, M.C. (1997) 'Mobilizing organizations for health enhancement: theories of organizational change', in K. Glanz, F.M. Lewis and B.K. Rimer (eds) *Health Behavior and Health Education: Theory, Research, and Practice* (2nd edn). San Francisco: Jossey-Bass.

Gordon, D. (1999) 'An alternative ten tips for staying healthy', in D. Raphael, 'The question of evidence in health promotion', *Health Promotion International*, 15 (4): 355–67.

Gordon, D., Adelman, L., Ashworth, K., Bradshaw, J., Levitas, R., Middleton, S., Pantazis, C., Patsios, D., Payne, S., Townsend, P. and Williams, J. (2000) *Poverty and Social Exclusion in Britain*. York: Joseph Rowntree Foundation.

Gordon, I. (1958) 'That damned word health', *Lancet*, 2: 638–9.

Gottlieb, N. and McLeroy, K.R. (1992) 'Social Health', in M.P. O'Donnell (ed.), *Health Promotion in the Workplace* (2nd edn). New York: Delmar Publishing.

Gottlieb, N.H., Brink, S.G. and Levenson Gingis, P.L. (1993) 'Correlates of coalition effectiveness: the "Smoke Free Class of 2000" program', *Health Education Research*, 8 (3): 375–84.

Gough, I. (1992) 'What are human needs?' in J. Percy-Smith and I. Sanderson (eds), *Understanding Local Needs*. London: Institute for Public Policy Research.

Grace, V.M. (1991) 'The marketing of empowerment and the construction of the health consumer: a critique of health promotion', *International Journal of Health Services*, 21 (2): 329–43.

Graham, H. (1987) 'Women's smoking and family health', *Social Science and Medicine*, 25 (1): 47–56.

Green, J. (1995) 'School sex education policies: a qualitative analysis of the process of policy development', *Journal of the Institute of Health Education*, 32 (4): 106–11.

Green, J. (1997) 'A survey of sex education in primary schools in the Northern & Yorkshire Region', *International Journal of Health Education*, 35 (3): 81–6.

Green, J. (1998) 'School sex education and education policy in England & Wales: the relationship examined', *Health Education Research*, 13 (1): 67–72.

Green, J. (2000) 'The role of theory in evidence-based health promotion practice' (editorial), *Health Education Research*, 15 (2): 125–9.

Green, J. and Tones, K. (1999) 'Towards a secure evidence base for health promotion', *Journal of Public Health Medicine*, 21 (2): 133–9.

Green, L.W. (1974) 'Toward cost–benefit evaluations of health education: some concepts, methods and examples', *Health Education Monographs*, 2: 34–64.

Green, L.W. (1996) 'Bringing people back to health', *Promotion & Education*, III (1): 23–6.

Green, L.W. and Kreuter, M.W. (1991) *Health Promotion Planning: An Educational and Environmental Approach*. Mountain View, CA: Mayfield.

Green, L.W. and Kreuter, M.W. (1999) *Health Promotion Planning: An Educational and Ecological Approach*. (3rd edn). Mountain View, CA: Mayfield.

Green, L.W., Glanz, K., Hochbaum, G.M., Kok, G., Kreuter, M.W., Lewis, F.M., Lorig, K., Morisky, D., Rimer, B.K. and Rosenstock, I.M. (1994) 'Can we build models on, or must we replace, the theories and models in health education?', *Health Education Research*, 9 (3): 397–404.

Green, L.W. and Lewis, F.M. (1986) *Measurement and Evaluation in Health Education and Health Promotion*. Palo Alto, CA: Mayfield.

Green, L.W., Poland, B. and Rootman, I. (2000) 'The Settings Approach to Health Promotion', in B. Poland, L.W. Green and I. Rootman (eds), *Settings for Health Promotion: Linking Theory and Practice*. Thousand Oaks, CA: Sage.

Green, L.W., Simons-Morton, D. G. and Potvin, L. (1997) 'Education and life-style determinants of health and disease', in R. Detels, W.W. Holland, J. McEwen and G.S. Omenn (eds), *Oxford Textbook of Public Health*. (Vol. 1, 3rd edn). Oxford: Oxford University Press.

Gruder, C.L., Cook, T.D., Hennigan, K.M., Flay, B.R., Alessis, C. and Halamay, J. (1978) 'Empirical tests of the absolute sleeper effect predicted from the discount-cue hypothesis', *Journal of Personality and Social Psychology*, 36: 1061–74.

Guba, E.G. and Lincoln, Y.S. (1981) *Effective Evaluation*. San Francisco: Jossey-Bass.

Guba, E.G. and Lincoln, Y.S. (1989) *Fourth Generation Evaluation*. Newbury Park, CA: Sage.

Guttman, N. (2000) *Public Health Communication Interventions: Values and Ethical Dilemmas*. Thousand Oaks, CA: Sage.

Habermas, J. (1972) *Knowledge and Human Interests*. London: Heinemann.

Hagard, S. (2000) 'Benchmarking to promote better health', *Promotion & Education*, VII (2): 2–3.

Haglund, B., Weisbrod, R.R. and Bracht, N. (1990) 'Assessing the community: its services, needs, leadership, and readiness', in N. Bracht (eds), *Health Promotion at the Community Level*. London: Sage.

Haglund, B.J.A., Pettersson, B., Finer, B. and Tillgren, P. (1993) *The Sundsvall Handbook, 'We Can Do It!'*,

Third International Conference on Health Promotion, Sundsvall, Sweden, 9–15 June 1991.

Haglund, B.J.A., Jansson, B., Pettersson, B. and Tillgren, P. (1998) 'A quality assurance instrument for practitioners', in J.K. Davies, and G. Macdonald (eds), *Quality, Evidence and Effectiveness in Health Promotion*. London: Routledge.

Hale, J.L. and Dillard, J.P. (1995) 'Fear appeals in health promotion campaigns: too much, too little, or just right?' in E. Maibach and R.L. Parrott, (eds) *Designing Health Messages*. Thousand Oaks, CA: Sage.

Halpern, E.S. (1983) 'Auditing Naturalistic Inquiries: The Development and Application of a Model', unpublished doctoral dissertation, Indiana University.

Hancock, T. (1982) 'Beyond health care', *The Futurist*, August 4–13.

Hancock, T. (1998) 'Caveat partner: reflections on partnership with the private sector', *Health Promotion International*, 13 (3): 193–5.

Handy, C. (1993) *Understanding Organizations* (4th edn). Harmondsworth: Penguin.

Hansen, A. (1986) 'The portrayal of alcohol on television', *Health Education Journal*, 45 (3): 127–31.

Hansen, S. and Jensen, J. (1969) *The Little Red School Book*. London: Stage 1.

Hardin, G. (1968) 'The tragedy of the commons', *Science*, 162: 1243–8.

Harris, A. and Harris, T. (1986) *Staying OK*. London: Pan.

Harrison, C. (1980) *Readability in Classrooms*. Cambridge: Cambridge University Press.

Harrison, J. and Edwards, J. (1994) *Developing Health Education in the Curriculum*. London: David Fulton.

Hart, J.T. (1971) 'The inverse care law', *Lancet*, (i): 405–12.

Harter, S. (1985) 'Manual for the Self-perception Profile of Children', unpublished, University of Denver, cited in T.J. Berndt and L. Burgy (1996), 'Social self concepts', in B.A. Bracken (ed.), *Handbook of Self Concept: Developmental, Social and Clinical Considerations*, New York: Wiley.

Harter, S. (1993) 'Causes and consequences of low self-esteem in children and adolescents', in R.F. Baumeister, (ed.) *Self-esteem: The Puzzle of Low Self Regard*. New York: Plenum.

Harvey, L. (1990) *Critical Social Research*. London: Unwin-Hyman.

Hastings, G.B., Stead, M., Whitehead, M., Lowry, R., MacFadyen, L., McVey, D., Owen, L. and Tones, K. (1998) 'Using the media to tackle the health divide: future directions', *Social Marketing Quarterly*, IV (3), 41–67.

Hattie, J. (1992) *Self Concept*. Hillsdale, NJ: Erlbaum.

Hawes, H. and Scotchmer, C. (1993) *Children for Health*. London: Child-to-Child Trust/UNICEF.

HDA (undated) *Putting public health evidence into practice: working definition of evidence and criteria for inclusion*. London: HDA.

HEA (1989) *Health for Life*. London: HEA.

HEA (1991) *Smoking and Me: A Teacher's Guide* (2nd edn). London: HEA.

HEA (1996) *European Network of Health Promoting Schools*. London: HEA.

HEA (1999a) *Art for Health: A Review of Good Practice in Community-based Arts Projects and Interventions Which Impact on Health and Well-being: Report*. London: HDA.

HEA (1999b) *Art for Health: A Review of Good Practice in Community-based Arts Projects and Interventions which Impact on Health and Well-being. Summary Bulletin*. London: HDA.

Health Promotion Authority Wales (1992) *Health Promotion: Challenge for the 1990s*. Cardiff: Health Promotion Authority Wales.

Heaver, R. (1992) 'Participatory rural appraisal: potential application in family planning, health and nutrition programmes', *RRA Notes Number 16: Special Issue on Applications for Health*: 13–21.

Henderson, P.D. and Thomas, D.N. (1980) *Skills in Neighbourhood Work*. London: Allen & Unwin.

Herman, K.A., Wolfson, M. and Forster, J.L. (1993) 'The evolution, operation and future of Minnesota SAFPLAN: a coalition for family planning', *Health Education Research*, 3 (8): 331–44.

Herzlich, C. (1973) *Health and Illness*. London: Academic Press.

Higbee, K.L. and Jensen, L.C. (1978) *Influence: What It Is and How to Use It*, Provo, UT: Brigham Young University Press.

Hilton, D. (1988) 'Community-based or oriented: the vital difference', *Contact*, 106, December: 1–4.

Hirschmann, E. and Holbrook, D. (1982) 'Hedonic consumption: emerging concepts, methods and propositions', *Journal of Marketing*, summer, 135–45.

Hirst, P. (1969) 'The logic of the curriculum', *Journal of Curriculum Studies*, 1 (2): 142–58.

Hochbaum, G.M. (1958) *Public Participation in Medical Screening Programs: A Socio-psychological Study*. Washington, DC: Public Health Service Publication No. 572, US Government Printing Office.

Hoge, R.D. and McScheffrey, R. (1991) 'An investigation of self concept in gifted children', *Exceptional Children*, 57: 238–45.

Hogwood, B.W. and Gunn, L.A. (1984) *Policy Analysis for the Real World*. Oxford: Oxford University Press.

Hogwood, B.W. and Gunn, L.A. (1997) 'Why "perfect implementation" is unattainable', in M. Hill (ed.), *The Policy Process: A Reader*. London: Prentice Hall/Harvester Wheatsheaf.

Holloway, I. (1997) *Basic Concepts for Qualitativen Research*. Oxford: Blackwell.

Holman, H. and Lorig, K. (1992) 'Perceived self-efficacy in self-management of chronic disease', in R. Schwarzer (ed.), *Self-efficacy: Thought Control of Action*. Washington, DC: Hemisphere Publishing.

Holt, C.L., Clark, E.M., M.W., K. and Scharff, D.P. (2000) 'Does locus of control moderate the effects of tailored health education materials', *Health Education Research*, 15 (4): 393–403.

Hopson, B. and Scally, M. (1981) *Lifeskills Teaching*. Maidenhead: McGraw-Hill.

Hopson, B. and Scally, M. (1980–2) *Lifeskills Teaching Programmes 1–5*. Leeds: Lifeskills Associates.

Horrobin, D.F. (1978) *Medical Hubris: A Reply to Ivan Illich*. Edinburgh: Churchill Livingstone.

Hospers, H.J., Kok, G.J. and Strecher, V.J. (1990) 'Attributions for previous failures and subsequent outcomes in a weight reduction program', *Health Education Quarterly*, 17: 409–15.

House, J.S., Robbins, C. and Metzner, H.L. (1982) 'The association of social relationships and activities with mortality: prospective evidence from the Tecumseh Community Health Study', *American Journal of Epidemiology*, 116: 123–40.

Hovland, C.I. and Weiss, W. (1951) 'The influence of source credibility on communication effectiveness', *Public Opinion Quarterly*, 15: 635–50.

Hovland, C.I., Janis, I.L. and Kelley, H.H. (1953) *Communication and Persuasion*. New Haven, CT: Yale University Press.

Howlett, A. (1985) 'Problem solving and the art of teacher maintenance', Peterborough Group Secondary Science Curriculum Review, October.

Hubley, J. (1993) *Communicating Health: An Action Guide to Health Education and Health Promotion*. London: Macmillan.

Huff, D. (1979) *How to Lie with Statistics*. Harmondsworth: Pelican.

Hughes, J. (1976) *Sociological Analysis: Methods of Discovery*. London: Nelson.

Huxley, A. (1958) *Brave New World Revisited*. London: HarperCollins.

Hyppä, M.T. and Mäki, J. (2001) 'Why do Swedish-speaking Finns have longer active life? An area for social capital research', *Health Promotion International*, 16 (1): 55–63.

Ignatieff, M. (1992) 'The grey emptiness inside John Major', in G. Walt, *Health Policy: An Introduction to Process and Power*. London: Zed.

Illich, I. (1976) *The Limits to Medicine Medical Nemesis: The Expropriation of Health*. Harmondsworth: Penguin.

International Union for Health Education (1992) *Advocacy for Health*. Paris: International Union for Health Education.

Irvine, E.D. (1948) 'Healthy Discontent', *Health Education Journal*, VI: 173.

Jackson, R.H. (1983) ' "Play it Safe": A campaign for the prevention of children's accidents', *Community Development Journal*, 18: 172–6.

Jackson, S., Cleverly, S., Poland, B., Robertson, A., Burnam, D., Goodstadt, M. and Salsberg, L. (1997) 'Half full or half empty?: Concepts and research design for a study of indicators of community capacity', in N. Smith, L.B. Littlejohns and D. Thompson, 'Shaking out the cobwebs: insights into community capacity and its relation to health outcomes', *Community Development Journal*, 36 (1): 30–41.

Jacobson, L.D., Edwards, A.G.K., Granier, S.K. and Butler, C.C. (1997) 'Evidence-based medicine and general practice', *British Journal of General Practice*, 47: 449–52.

Jamison, J., Ashby, P., Hamilton, K., Lewis, G., Macdonald, A. and Saunders, L. (1998) *The Health Promoting School: Final Report of the ENHPS Evaluation Project in England*. London: HEA.

Janis, I.L. (1975) 'Effectiveness of social support for stressful decisions', in M. Deutsch, and H.S. Hornstein (eds), *Applying Social Psychology: Implications for Research, Practice and Training*. NJ: Erlbaum.

Janis, I.L. and Feshback, S. (1953) 'Effects of fear-arousing communications', *Journal of Abnormal and Social Psychology*, 48 (1): 78–92.

Janis, I.L. and Mann, L. (1964) 'Effectiveness of role playing in modifying smoking habits and attitudes', *Journal of Experimental Research in Personality*, 1: 84–90.

Janis, I.L. and Mann, L. (1977) *Decision Making: A Psychological Analysis of Conflict, Choice, and Commitment*. New York: Free Press.

Jenkins, W.I. (1978) *Policy Analysis: A Political and Organisational Perspective*. London: Martin Robertson.

Jensen, B.B. (1991) *The Action Perspective in School Health Education*. Proceedings from Satellite Congress in Copenhagen 13–14 June, Research Centre for Environmental and Health Education.

Jensen, B.B. (2000) 'Health knowledge and health education in the democratic health-promoting school', *Health Education*, 100 (4): 146–53.

Jitsukawa, M. and Djerassi, C. (1994) 'Birth control in Japan: Realities and prognosis', *Science*, 2675: 1048–51.

John, P. (1998) *Analysing Public Policy*. London: Continuum.

Johns Hopkins Center for Communication Programs (undated) *'A' Frame for Advocacy*. Baltimore, MA: Johns Hopkins Bloomberg School of Public Health, Center for Communication Programs. (*Website*: www.jhuccp.org/pr/advocacy)

Jones, E.E. (1964) *Ingratiation*. New York: Appleton-Century-Crofts.

Jones, L. and Sidell, M. (1997) *The Challenge of Promoting Health*. London: Macmillan.

Jordan, J., Dowsell, T., Harrison, S., Lilford, R.J. and Mort, M. (1998) 'Whose priorities? Listening to users and the public', *British Medical Journal*, 316: 1668–770.

Joseph Rowntree Foundation: (2000) *Findings: Poverty and Social Exclusion in Britain*. York: Joseph Rowntree

Foundation. (*Website:* www.jrf.org.uk/knowledge/findings/socialpolicy/930.asp)

Judge, K. (2000) 'Testing evaluation to the limits: the case of English Health Action Zones', *Journal of Health Services Research and Policy*, 5 (1), January. (*Website:* www.haznet.org.uk/hazs/evidence/judge.asp)

Kanfer, F.H. and Karoly, P. (1972) 'Self-control: a behavioristic excursion into the lion's den', *Behavior Therapy*, 3: 398–416.

Kaplan, G.A., Salonen, J.T., Cohen, R.D., Brand, R.J., Syme, L. and Puska, P. (1988) 'Social connections and mortality from all causes and cardiovascular disease: prospective evidence from eastern Finland', *American Journal of Epidemiology*, 128: 370–80.

Kaplan, G.A., Wilson, T.W., Cohen, R.D., Brand, R.J., Syme, L. and Puska, P. (1994) 'Social functioning and overall mortality: prospective evidence from the Kuopio ischemic heart disease risk factor study', *Epidemiology*, 5: 495–500.

Karasek, R.A. and Theorell, T. (1990) *Healthy Work: Stress, Productivity, and the Reconstruction of Working Life*. New York: Basic Books.

Kasperson, R.E., Renn, O., Slovic, P., Brown, H.S. (1988) 'The social amplification of risk: a conceptual framework', *Risk Analysis*, 8: 177–87.

Katz, E. and Lazarsfeld, P. (1955) *Personal Influence: The Part Played by People in the Flow of Mass Communication*. Glencoe, IL: Free Press.

Kawachi, I. (1997) 'Long Live Community', *The American Prospect*, 8 (35).

Kawachi, I., Colditz, G.A. and Ascherio, A. (1996) 'A prospective study of social networks in relation to total mortality and cardiovascular disease in relation to men in the USA', *Journal of Epidemiology and Community Health*, 50: 245–51.

Keijsers, J.F.E.M. and Saan, J.A.M. (1998) 'The development of two instruments to measure the quality of health promotion interventions', in J.K. Davies and G. Macdonald (eds), *Quality, Evidence and Effectiveness in Health Promotion*. London: Routledge.

Keith, L.K. and Bracken, B.A. (1996) 'Self concept instrumentation: a historical and evaluative review', in B.A. Bracken (ed.) *Handbook of Self Concept: Developmental, Social and Clinical Considerations*. New York: Wiley.

Kelleher, D., Gabe, J. and Williams, G. (1994) 'Understanding medical dominance in the modern world', in J. Gabe, D. Kelleher and G. Williams (eds), *Challenging Medicine*. London: Routledge.

Kelly, M.P. and Charlton, B. (1995) 'The modern and the postmodern in health promotion', in R. Bunton, S. Nettleton and R. Burrows (eds), *The Sociology of Health Promotion*. London: Routledge.

Kemm, J.R. (1993) 'Towards an epidemiology of positive health', *Health Promotion International*, 8 (2): 129–34.

Kemm, J. (2001) 'Health impact assessment: a tool for healthy public policy', *Health Promotion International*, 16 (1): 79–85.

Kerrison, S. and Macfarlane, A. (2000) *Official Health Statistics: An Unofficial Guide*. London: Arnold.

Keys, D. (2000) *Catastrophe: An Investigation into the Origins of the Modern World*. London: Arrow.

Khan, K.S. and Kleijnen, J. (2001) 'Phase 6: Data extraction and monitoring progress', in NHS Centre for Reviews and Dissemination, *Undertaking Systematic Reviews of Research Effectiveness*. York: NHS Centre for Reviews and Dissemination.

Khan, K.S., ter Riet, G., Popay, J., Nixon, J. and Kleijnen, J. (2001) 'Phase 5: Study quality assessment', in NHS Centre for Reviews and Dissemination, *Undertaking Systematic Reviews of Research Effectiveness*. York: NHS Centre for Reviews and Dissemination.

Kickbush, I. (1995) *An Overview of the Settings Approach to Health Promotion*. 'The Settings-based Approach to Health Promotion', An International Working Conference in Collaboration with WHO Regional Office for Europe, 17–20 November 1993. London: NHS Executive/HEA.

Kickbush, I. (1997) 'Think health: what makes the difference?' address at the Fourth International Conference on Health Promotion, Jakarta 21–25 July, in E. Ziglio, S. Hagard, L. McMahon, S. Harvey and L. Levin, 'Principles methodology and practices of investment for health', *Promotion & Education*, VII (2): 4–12.

Kickbush, I. (1998) 'Health promotion in the 21st century: an era of partnerships to achieve health for all', *Press Release*. (WHO/47). Geneva: WHO.

Kidd, R. and Kumar, K. (1981) 'A critical analysis of pseudo-Freirean adult education', *Economic and Political Weekly*, January 3–10, 1981: 27–36.

Kieffer, C. (1984) Citizen empowerment: a developmental perspective', in J. Rappaport, C. Swift and R. Hess (eds) *Empowerment: Steps Toward Understanding and Action*. New York: Haworth Press.

Kindervatter, S. (1979) *Non-formal Education as an Empowering Process*. Amherst, MA: University of Massachusetts, Center for International Education.

Kingdon, J. (1984) 'Agendas, alternatives and public policies', in G. Walt, *Health Policy: An Introduction to Process and Power*. London: Zed.

Kirklin, M.J. and Franzen, L.E. (1974) *Community Organization Bibliography*. Chicago, IL: Institute on the Church in Urban Industrial Society.

Kirscht, J.P. (1972) 'Perceptions of control and health beliefs', *Canadian Journal of Behavioral Science*, 4: 225–37.

Klapper, J.T. (1960) *The Effects of Mass Communication*. Glencoe, IL: Free Press.

Klapper, J.T. (1995) 'The effects of mass communication', in O. Boyd-Barrett and Newbold, C. (eds) *Approaches to Media: A Reader*. London: Arnold.

Knowles, M.S., Holton, F. and Swanson, R.A. (1998) *The Adult Learner: The Definitive Classic in Adult Education and Human Resource Development* (5th edn). Houston, TX: Gulf Publishing.

Kobasa, S.C. (1979) 'Stressful life events, personality and health: an inquiry into hardiness', *Journal of Personality and Social Psychology*, 37: 1–11.

Kohlberg, L. (1984) 'The psychology of moral development: the nature and validity of moral stages', in J. Ryder and C. Campbell *Balancing Acts in Personal, Social and Health Education*. London: Routledge.

Kok, G., Den Broer, D-J., De Vries, H., Gerards, F., Hospers, H.J. and Mudde, A.N. (1992) 'Self-efficacy and attribution theory in health education', in R. Schwarzer (ed.), *Self-Efficacy: Thought Control of Action*. Washington, DC: Hemisphere Publishing.

Kolb, D.A., Rubin, I.M. and McIntyre, J.M. (1971) *Organisational Psychology: An Experiential Approach*. London: Prentice-Hall.

Kotler, P. and Zaltman, G. (1971) 'Social marketing and public health intervention', *Journal of Marketing*, 45 (2): 3–12.

Kotler, P., Roberto, N. and Lee, N. (2002) *Social Marketing: Improving the Quality of Life*. Thousand Oaks, CA: Sage.

Kreiger, N. (1990) 'On becoming a public health professional: reflections on democracy, leadership, and accountability', *Journal of Public Health Policy*, 11: 412–19.

Kreuter, M.W. and Skinner, C.S. (2000) 'Tailoring: what's in a name?' (editorial), *Health Education Research*, 15 (1): 1–4.

Kreuter, M.W., Oswald, D.L., Bull, F.C. and Clark, E. (2000) 'Are tailored health education materials always more effective than non-tailored materials?' *Health Education Research*, 15 (3): 305–15.

Krieger, N. (2001) 'A glossary for social epidemiology', *Journal of Epidemiology and Community Health*, 55: 693–700.

Krisher, H.P., Darley, S.A. and Darley, J.M. (1973) 'Fear-provoking recommendations, intentions to take preventive actions, and actual preventive actions', *Journal of Personality and Social Psychology*, 26 (2): 301–18.

Kroeger, A. (1997) *The Use of Epidemiology in Local Health Planning: A Training Manual*. London: Zed.

Kuhn, T.S. (1970) *The Structure of Scientific Revolutions* (2nd edn). Chicago: University of Chicago Press.

Labonte, R. (1993) 'Community development and partnerships', in L. Jones and M. Sidell, *The Challenge of Promoting Health*. London: Macmillan.

Labonte, R. and Laverack, G. (2001a) 'Capacity building for health promotion, Part 1: for whom? And for what purpose?', *Critical Public Health*, 11 (2): 112–27.

Labonte, R. and Laverack, G. (2001b) 'Capacity building in health promotion, Part 2: whose use? and with what measurement?', *Critical Public Health*, 11 (2): 129–38.

Laing, W.A. (1982) *Family Planning: The Benefits and Costs*, 607. London: Policy Studies Institute.

Lalonde, M. (1974) *A New Perspective on the Health of Canadians*. Ottawa: Ministry of National Health and Welfare.

Larkey, L.K., Alatorre, C., Buller, D.B., Morrill, C., Klein Buller, M., Taren, D. and Sennott-Miller, I. (1999) 'Communication strategies for dietary change in a worksite peer educator intervention', *Health Education Research*, 14 (6): 777–90.

Lasswell, H.D. (1948) 'The structure and function of communication in society', in L. Bryson (ed.), *Communication of Ideas*. New York: Harper.

Last, J.M. (1963) 'The iceberg: completing the clinical picture in general practice', *Lancet*: 28–31, reprinted in J. Ashton (1994), *The Epidemiological Imagination*. Buckingham: Open University Press.

Last, J.M. (1988) *A Dictionary of Epidemiology* (2nd edn). Oxford: Oxford University Press.

Laverack, G. and Labonte, R. (2000) 'A planning framework for community empowerment goals within health promotion', *Health Policy and Planning*, 15 (3): 255–62.

Lawton, D. (1986) *School Curriculum Planning*. London: Hodder & Stoughton.

Lazarsfeld, P.F. and Merton, R.K. (1955) 'Mass communication, popular taste and organized social action', in W. Schramm (ed.), *Mass Communications*. Urbana, IL: University of Illinois Press.

Lefebvre, R.C., Doner, L., Johnston, C., Loughrey, K., Balch, G.I. and Sutton, S.M. (1995) 'Use of database marketing and consumer-based health communication in message design', in E. Maibach and R.L. Parrott (eds) *Designing Health Messages*. Thousand Oaks, CA: Sage.

Leichter, H.M. (1979) 'A comparative approach to policy analysis: healthcare policy in four nations', in G. Walt, *Health Policy: An Introduction to Process and Power*. London: Zed.

Lenin, I. (1969) *Collected Works* (volume 42). London: Lawrence & Wishart.

Leon, D.A., Walt, G. and Gilson, L. (2001) 'International perspectives on health inequalities and policy', *British Medical Journal*, 322: 591–4.

Lerer, L.B. (1999) 'How to do (or not to do) ... Health impact assessment', *Health Policy and Planning*, 14 (2): 198–203.

Leventhal, H. (1980) 'The common sense representation of illness danger', in S. Rachman (ed.), *Contribution to Medical Psychology*, (Vol. II). London: Pergamon.

Leventhal, H. and Cleary, P.D. (1980) 'The smoking problem: a review of the research and theory in behavioural risk modification', *Psychological Bulletin*, (88) 2: 370–405.

Levin, L. and Ziglio, E. (1997) 'Health promotion as an investment strategy: a perspective for the 21st century', in M. Sidell, L. Jones, J. Katz and A. Peberdy (eds), *Debates and Dilemmas in Promoting Health*. London: Macmillan.

Lewin, R.W. (1951) *Field Theory in Social Science*. New York: Harper.

Lewis, F.M. (1987) 'The concept of control: a typology and health-related variables', *Advances in Health Education and Promotion*, 2: 277–309.

Lichtenstein, S., Slovic, P., Fischoff, B., Layman, M. and Combs, B. (1978) 'Judged frequency of lethal events', *Journal of Experimental Psychology*: Human Learning and Memory, 4 (6): 551–78.

Lincoln, Y.S. and Guba, E.G. (1985) *Naturalistic Inquiry*. Beverly Hills, CA: Sage.

Lincoln, Y.S. and Denzin, N.K. (1994) 'The fifth moment', in N.K. Denzin and Y.S. Lincoln (eds), *Handbook of Qualitative Research*. Thousand Oaks, CA: Sage.

Lindblom, C.E. (1959) 'The science of muddling through', *Public Administration Review*, 19: 79–99.

Lindblom, C.E. (1979) 'Still muddling, not yet through', *Public Administration Review*, 39: 517–25.

Lindblom, C.E. (1980) *The Policy-making Process* (2nd edn). Englewood Cliffs, NJ: Prentice Hall.

Lindblom, C.E. (1987) 'How to think about the policy-making process', in F. Delaney, 'Muddling through the middle ground: theoretical concerns in intersectoral collaboration and health promotion', *Health Promotion International*: 9 (3): 217–25.

Lindblom, C.E. and Woodhouse, E.J. (1993) *The Policy-making Process* (3rd edn). Englewood Cliffs, NJ: Prentice Hall.

Lindeman, E. (1926) *The Meaning of Adult Education*. New York: New Republic.

Lindquist, E.F. (1940) *Statistical Analysis in Educational Research*. New York: Houghton Mifflin.

Lindström, B. (1994) *The Essence of Existence: On the Quality of Life of Children in the Nordic Countries*. Gothenburg: Nordic School of Public Health.

Linkenbach, J. and D'Atri, G. (1998) *The Montana Model*. Unpublished training manual for the Montana Social Norms Project.

Lippmann, W. (1965) *Public Opinion*. New York: Free Press. (Originally published 1922.)

Lipsky, M. (1997) 'Street-level bureaucracy: an introduction', in M. Hill, (ed.), *The Policy Process: A Reader* (2nd edn). Hemel Hempstead: Prentice-Hall/Harvester Wheatsheaf.

Liss, P.-E. (1990) *Health Care Need. Meaning and Measurement*. Linkoping: Linkoping Studies in Arts and Science 53.

Lister, H., Simpkin, M. and Jones, M. (1994) *Redressing the Balance*. Leeds: Leeds Health for All.

Lister-Sharp, D., Chapman, S., Stewart-Brown, S. and Sowden, A. (1999) 'Health promoting schools and health promotion in schools: two systematic reviews', *Health Technology Assessment*, 3 (22).

London Health Economics Consortium (1996) *Local Health and the Vocal Community*. London: London Primary Health Care Forum.

London, H. (1973) *Psychology of the Persuader*. Morristown, NJ: General Learning Press.

Loney, M. (1981) 'The British community development projects: questioning the state', *Community Development Journal*, 16: 55–67.

Lukes, S. (1974) *Power: A Radical View*. London: Macmillan.

Lupton, D. and Chapman, S. (1994) 'Two studies of public health news', in S. Chapman and D. Lupton (eds), *The Fight for the Public Health: Principles and Practice of Media Advocacy*. London: BMJ Publishing.

Lynch, J., Davey Smith, G., Kaplan, G.A. and House, J.S. (2000) 'Income inequality and mortality: importance to health of individual income, psycho-social environment, or material conditions', *British Medical Journal*, 320: 1200–4.

Lyng, S. (1990) 'Edgework: a social psychological analysis of voluntary risk taking', *American Journal of Sociology*, 95 (4): 851–86.

Lyotard, J. (1984) *The Postmodern Condition: A Report on Knowledge*. Manchester: Manchester University Press.

Macauley, A.C., Commanda, L.E., Freeman, W.L., Gibson, N., McCabe, L., Robbins, C.M. and Twohig, L. (1999) 'Participatory research maximises community and lay involvement', *British Medical Journal*, 319: 774–8.

MacDonald, G. and Mussi, A. (1998) *Health Promotion Specialists: The Key Profession for Unlocking the Health Agenda Beyond 1998*. Managing Health Promotion: 8th National Conference, Penrith, October.

Macdonald, J.U. and Warren, W.G. (1991) 'Primary health care as an educational process: a model and a Freirean perspective', *International Quarterly of Community Health Education*, 12 (1): 35–50.

MacDonald, M.A. and Green, L.W. (2001) 'Reconciling concept and context: the dilemma of implementation in school-based health promotion', *Health Education and Behavior*, 28 (6): 749–68.

Mackenbach, J. (1997) 'Beyond the RCT? CIT!', *Report of the Expert Meeting Beyond the RCT – Towards Evidence-based Public Health*. Rotterdam: GGD.

Machiavelli, N. (1950) *Discourses*. New York: Humanities. (Originally published 1531.)

Machiavelli, N. (1961) *The Prince*. Harmondsworth: Penguin.

MacIntyre, S. and Pettigrew, M. (2000) 'Good intentions and received wisdom are not enough', *Journal of Epidemiology and Community Health*, 54: 802–3.

Mager, R.F. (1975) *Preparing Instructional Objectives*. Belmont, CA: Fearon.

Manderson, L. and Aaby, P. (1992) 'An epidemic in the field? Rapid assessment procedures and health research', *Social Science and Medicine*, 35: 839–50.

Mao Tse-tung (1967) 'Selected works of Mao Tse-tung, (1967)' (Vol. III), *The United Front in Cultured Work*. Peking.

Mappes, T.A. and Zembary, J.S. (1991) *Biomedical Ethics* (3rd edn). New York: McGraw-Hill.

Marrow, A.J. (1969) *The Practical Theorist: The Life and Work of Kurt Lewin*. New York: Basic Books.

Marsh, H.W. and Holmes, I. (1990) 'Multidimensional self-concepts: construct validation of responses by children', *American Educational Research Journal*, 27: 89–118.

Marsh, A. and Matheson, J. (1983) *Smoking Attitudes and Behaviour.* London: HMSO.

Martin, J. (1978) *Infant Feeding 1975: Attitudes and Practices in England and Wales*. London: HMSO.

Martinson, R. (1974) 'What works? Questions and answers about prison reform', in R. Pawson and N. Tilley, *Realistic Evaluation*. London: Sage.

Maslow, A.H. (1954) *Motivation and Personality*. New York: Harper.

Maslow, A.H. (1970) *Motivation and Personality* (2nd edn). New York: Harper & Row.

Masters, R. (1992) 'The damming graph that killed tobacco sponsorship', *Sydney Morning Herald*, 2 April.

Matarasso, F. (2001). 'The health and social impact of participation in the arts', in T. Heller, R. Muston, M. Siddell and C. Lloyd (eds), *Working for Health*. London: Sage.

Maton, K.I. and Rappaport, J. (1984) 'Empowerment in a religious setting: a multivariate investigation', in J. Rappaport, C. Swift and R. Hess (eds), *Studies in Empowerment: Steps Toward Understanding and Action*. New York: Haworth Press.

May, T. (1993) *Social Research: Issues Methods and Processes*. Buckingham: Open University Press.

Maycock, B., Howat, P. and Slevin, T. (2001) 'A decision-making model for health promotion advocacy: the case for advocacy of drunk driving control measures', *Promotion & Education*, VIII (2): 59–64.

Mayo, M. and Craig, G. (1995) 'Community participation and empowerment: the human face of structural adjustment or tools for democratic transformation?', in G. Craig and M. Mayo (eds), *Community Empowerment: A Reader in Participation and Development*. London: Zed Books.

McBride, N.T. and Midford, R. (1996) 'Assessing organisational support for school health promotion', *Health Education Research*, 11 (4): 509–18.

McDougall, W. (1926) *An Introduction to Social Psychology*. Boston, MA: John W. Luce.

McGuire, G. (1970) 'A vaccine for brainwash', *Psychology Today*, 3: 36–9.

McGuire, G. (1989) 'Theoretical foundations of ca paigns', in R.E. Rice and C.K. Atkin (eds), *Public communication Campaigns* (2nd edn). Newbury Park, CA: Sage.

McKeown, T. (1979) *The Role of Medicine: Dream, Mirage or Nemesis?* Oxford: Blackwell.

McKeown, T. and Lowe, C.R. (1974) *An Introduction to Social Medicine*. London: Blackwell.

McKinlay, J.B. (1975) 'A case for refocusing upstream: the political economy of illness', in A.J. Enelow and J.B. Henderson (eds), *Applying Behavioral Science to Cardiovascular Risk*. Washington, DC: American Heart Association.

McLaughlin, G. (1969) 'SMOG grading: a new readability formula', *Journal of Reading*, 12: 639

McLeroy, K. (1992) 'Editorial: Health education research: theory and practice – future directions', *Health Education Research*, 7 (1–8).

McLeroy, K. (1996) 'Community capacity: What is it? How do we measure it? What is the role of the Prevention Centers and CDC?', in L.K. Bartholomew, G.S. Parcel, G. Kok and N.H. Gottlieb, *Intervention Mapping: Designing Theory- and Evidence-based Health Promotion Programs*. Mountain View, CA: Mayfield.

McLeroy, K., Steckler, A.B., Simons-Morton, B., Goodman, R M., Gotlieb, N. and Burdine, J.N. (1993) 'Editorial: Social science theory in health education: time for a new model', *Health Education Research*, 8 (3): 305–11.

McMillan, D.W. and Chavis, D.M. (1986) 'Sense of community: a definition and theory', *Journal of Community Psychology*, 16: 6–23.

McPhail, P., Ungoed-Thomas, J.R. and Chapman, H. (1972) 'Moral education in the secondary school', in J. Ryder and C. Campbell, *Balancing Acts in Personal, Social and Health Education*. London: Routledge.

McPherson, K. (1994) 'The best and the enemy of the good: randomised controlled trials, uncertainty, and assessing the role of patient choice in medical decision making', *Journal of Epidemiology and Community Health*, 48: 6–15.

McQuail, D. (1994) *Mass Communication Theory: An Introduction* (3rd edn). London: Sage.

McQuail, D. (ed.) (1972) *Sociology of Mass Communications*. Harmondsworth: Penguin.

Mencken, H.L. (2001) cited in 'Thought for the Day', *The Independent*, 31 August.

Mendelsohn, H. (1968) 'Which shall it be? Mass education or mass persuasion for health?', *American Journal of Public Health*, 58: 131–7.

Michell, L. (1997) 'Loud, sad or bad: young people's perceptions of peer groups and smoking', *Health Education Research*, 12 (1): 1–14.

Michener, J. (1971) *Kent State: What Happened and Why*. New York: Random House.

Middleton, J., Reeves, E., Lilford, R., Howie, F. and Hyde, C. (2001) 'Collaboration with the Campbell Collaboration', *British Medical Journal*, 323: 1252.

Miilunpalo, S., Nupponen, R., Laitakari, J., Martila, J. and Paronen, O. (2000) 'Stages of change in two modes of health-enhancing physical activity: methodological aspects and promotional implications', *Health Education Research*, 15 (4): 435–48.

Milburn, K. (1995) 'A critical review of peer education with young people with special reference to sexual health', *Health Education Research*, 10 (4): 407–20.

Milgram, S. (1963) 'Behavioral study of obedience', *Journal of Abnormal and Social Psychology*, 67: 371–8.

Milio, N. (1981) *Promoting Health Through Public Policy*. Philadelphia: F.A. Davis.

Milio, N. (1986) 'Promoting health through public policy', in B. Abel-Smith, *Introduction to Health: Policy, Planning and Financing*. Harlow: Longman.

Milio, N. (1988) 'Making healthy public policy: developing the science by learning the art: an ecological framework for policy studies', *Health Promotion*, 2 (3): 263–74.

Mill, J.S. (1961) *On Liberty*, reprinted in *Essential Works of John Stuart Mill*. New York: Bantam Books.

Miller, I. and Norman, W. (1979) 'Learned helplessness in humans: a review and attribution theory model', *Psychological Bulletin*, 86: 93–118.

Mills, C.W. (1959) *The Sociological Imagination*. New York: Oxford University Press.

MIMAS (2001) *Health Survey for England*. Manchester: MIMAS, The University of Manchester. (Available from the UK Data Archive *Website:* www.data-archive.ac.uk)

Mindell, J., Hansell, A., Morrison, D., Douglas, M. and Joffe, M. (2001) 'What do we need for robust, quantitative health impact assessment?', *Journal of Public Health Medicine*, 23 (3): 173–8.

Minkler, M. (1990) 'Improving health through community organization', in K. Glanz, F.M. Lewis and B.K. Rimer (eds), *Health Behavior and Health Education: Theory Research and Practice*. San Francisco: Jossey-Bass.

Minkler, M. and Cox, K. (1980) 'Creating critical consciousness in health: applications of Freire's philosophy and methods to the health care setting', *International Journal of Health Services*, 10 (4): 311–22.

Minkler, M. and Wallerstein, N. (1997) 'Improving health through community organization and community building', in K. Glanz, F.M. Lewis and B.K. Rimer (eds), *Health Behavior and Health Education: Theory, Research, and Practice* (2nd edn). San Francisco: Jossey-Bass.

Mittelmark, M.B. (1997) 'Health promotion settings' (editorial), *Internet Journal of Health Promotion*. (*Website:* http://elecpress.monash.edu.au/IJHP)

Mittelmark, M.B. (1999a) 'Social ties and health promotion: suggestions for population-based research' (editorial), *Health Education Research*, 14 (4): 447–51.

Mittelmark, M.B. (1999b) 'Health promotion at the community-wide level: lessons from diverse perspectives', in N. Bracht (ed.), *Health Promotion at the Community Level: New Advances*. Thousand Oaks, CA: Sage.

Mittelmark, M.B. (2001) 'Promoting social responsibility for health: health impact assessment and healthy public policy at the community level', *Health Promotion International*, 16 (3): 269–74.

Mittelmark, M.B., Aarø, L.E., Annus, R., Brænde, Å., Christie, M. and Vorsi, M. (2000) 'Benchmarking for investment for health', *Promotion & Education*, VII (2): 24–32.

Mogensen, F. (1997) 'Critical thinking: a central element in developing action competence in health and environmental education', *Health Education Research*, 12 (4): 429–36.

Monahan, J.L. (1995) 'Using positive affect when designing health messages', in E. Maibach and R.L. Parrott, *Designing Health Messages*. Thousand Oaks, CA: Sage.

Mongeau, P.A. (in press) 'Fear-arousing persuasive messages = a meta-analysis re-visited', in M. Allen and R. Press (eds), *Persuasion: Advances Through Meta-Analysis*. Thousand Oaks, CA: Sage.

Moon, G. and Gould, M. (2000) *Epidemiology: An Introduction*. Buckingham: Open University Press.

Mooney, G. and Leeder, S.R. (1997) 'Measuring health needs', in R., Detels, W.W. Holland, J. McEwen and G.S. Omenn (eds), *Oxford Textbook of Public Health*. (Vol. 3, 3rd edn). Oxford: Oxford University Press.

Morgan, D. (1998) 'Health and environmental impact assessment', in J. Kemm, 'Health Impact Assessment: a tool for Healthy Public Policy', *Health Promotion International*, 16 (1): 79–85.

Morrow, R.A. and Brown, D.D. (1994) *Critical Theory and Methodology*. Thousand Oaks, CA: Sage.

Morrow, V. (2001) 'Using qualitative methods to elicit young people's perspectives on their environments: some ideas for community health initiatives', *Health Education Research*, 16 (3): 255–68.

Morse, J.M. (1994) 'Designing funded qualitative research', in N.K. Denzin and Y.S. Lincoln (eds), *Handbook of Qualitative Research*. Thousand Oaks, CA: Sage.

Murphy, S.T. and Zajonc, R.B. (1993) 'Affect, cognition, and awareness: affective priming with suboptimal and optimal stimulus', *Journal of Personality and Social Psychology*, 64 (5): 723–39.

Murray, D.M. (1984) 'Towards an effective smoking prevention programme', in G. Campbell (ed.), *Health Education and Youth: A Review of Research and Developments*. Lewes, East Sussex: Falmer Press.

Murray, S.A. (1999) 'Experiences with "rapid appraisal" in primary care: involving the public in assessing health needs, orienting staff, and education medical students', *British Medical Journal*, 318: 440–4.

Murray, S. and Graham, L.J.C. (1995) 'Practice-based health needs assessment: use of four methods in a small neighbourhood', *British Medical Journal*, 310: 1443–8.

Musgrave, R. (1959) *The Theory of Public Finance*. New York: McGraw-Hill.

Naidoo, J. and Wills, J. (1994) *Health Promotion Foundations for Practice*. London: Baillière Tindall.

Nancholas, S. (1998) 'How to do (or not to do) … a logical framework', *Health Policy and Planning*, 13 (2): 189–93.

National Assembly for Wales (1999) *Developing Health Impact Assessment in Wales*. Cardiff: National Assembly for Wales.

National Assembly for Wales (2002) *Health Impact Assessment*. Cardiff: National Assembly for Wales.

National Cancer Institute (1997) *Theory at a Glance: A Guide for Health Promotion Practice*. Bethesda, MD: National Cancer Institute. (*Website:* http://oc.nci.nih.gov/services/Theory_at_glance/HOME. html)

National Cancer Institute (1998) *Making Health Communication Programs Work: A Planners Guide*. Bethesda, MD: Information Project Branch Office.

National Civic League (2002) *A New Approach to Improving Community Life*. Denver, CO: National Civic League. (*Website:* www.ncl.org/cs/articles/okubo1.html)

National Curriculum Council (1990) *Curriculum Guidance 5: Health Education*. York: National Curriculum Council.

National Statistics (2001) *The National Statistics Socio-economic Classification*. London: National Statistics. (*Website:* www.statistics.gov.uk/nsbase/methods_quality/ns_sec/default.asp)

National Statistics (undated a) *Factsheet 4: Counting Everyone In –The Big Challenge*. London: National Statistics (*Website:* www.statistics.gov.uk/census2001/Introfactsheets.asp)

National Statistics (undated b) *Factsheet 9: The Census Questions*. London: National Statistics. (*Website:* www.statistics.gov.uk/census2001/Introfactsheets.asp)

Navarro, V. (1976) 'The underdevelopment of health of working America: causes, consequences and possible solutions', *American Journal of Public Health*, 66: 538–47.

Newcastle Healthy City Project (1997) 'Taking a Whole Systems Approach or Why Elephants Matter', *Whole Systems Newsletter*, 2.

NHS Centre for Reviews and Dissemination (1993) 'Brief interventions and alcohol use', in V. Speller, A. Learmonth and D. Harrison, 'The search for evidence of health promotion', *British Medical Journal*, 315: 361–3.

NHS Centre for Reviews and Dissemination (1996) *Undertaking Systematic Reviews of Research on Effectiveness: CRD Guidelines for Those Carrying Out or Commissioning Reviews*. York: NHS Centre for Reviews and Dissemination.

NHS Centre for Reviews and Dissemination (1999) 'Getting evidence into practice', *Effective Health Care*, 5 (1).

NHS Centre for Reviews and Dissemination (2001) *Undertaking Systematic Reviews of Research Effectiveness*. CRD Report No.4 (2nd edn). York: NHS

Centre for Reviews and Dissemination. (*Website:* www.york.ac.uk/inst/crd/report4.htm)

Nichols, T. (1979) 'Social class: official, sociological and Marxist', in R. Levitas and W. Guy (eds), *Interpreting Official Statistics*. London: Routledge.

Niebuhr, R. (1960) *Moral Man and Immoral Society*. London: Scribner

Nikku, N. (1997) *Informative Paternalism: Studies in the Ethics of Promoting and Predicting Health*. Linkoping, Sweden: University of Linkoping.

Nix, H.L. (1970) *The Community and its Involvement in the Study Planning Action Process*. Atlanta, GA: US Department of Health, Education and Welfare.

Nkosi Johnson AIDS Foundation (undated) 'About Nkosi' and 'Nkosi's speech' on website. Johannesburg, South Africa: Nkosi Johnson AIDS Foundation. (*Website:* http://nkosi.iafrica.com)

Norman, P. and Bennett, P. (1996) 'Health locus of control', in P. Conner and M. Norman (eds), *Predicting Health Behaviour*. Buckingham: Open University Press.

Nuffield Institute for Health (1993) *Directions for Health: New Approaches to Population Health Research and Practice – The Leeds Declaration*. Leeds: Nuffield Institute for Health.

Nutbeam, D. (1996) 'Achieving "best practice" in health promotion: improving the fit between research and practice', *Health Education Research*, 11 (3): 317–26.

Nutbeam, D. (1998a) 'Evaluating health promotion – progress, problems and solutions', *Health Promotion International*, 13 (1): 27–43.

Nutbeam, D. (1998b) *Health Promotion Glossary*. Geneva: WHO.

Nutbeam, D. (1999) 'The challenge to provide "evidence" in health promotion', *Health Promotion International*, 14 (2): 99–101.

Nutbeam, D. (2000) 'Health promotion effectiveness – the questions to be answered', in International Union for Health Promotion and Education, *The Evidence of Health Promotion Effectiveness: Shaping Public Health in a New Europe*. Paris: IUHPE.

Nutbeam, D., Smith, C., Murphy, S., Catford, J. (1993) 'Maintaining evaluation designs in long-term community-based health promotion programmes', *Journal of Epidemiology and Public Health*, 47: 127–33.

Oakley, A., Fullerton, D., Holland, J., Arnold, S., France-Dawson, M., Kelley, P. and McGrellis, S. (1995) 'Sexual health education interventions for young people: a methodological review', *British Medical Journal*, 310 (6973): 158–62.

O'Brien, M.O. (1995) 'Health and lifestyle: a critical mess?', in R. Bunton, S. Nettleton and R. Burrows (eds), *The Sociology of Health Promotion*. London: Routledge.

Oldenburg, B., Hardcastle, D.M. and Kok, G. (1997) 'Diffusion of innovations', in K. Glanz, F.M. Lewis and B.K. Rimer (eds), *Health Behavior and Health*

Education: Theory, Research, and Practice (2nd edn). San Francisco: Jossey-Bass.

Oldenburg, B.F., Sallis, J.F., Ffrench, M.L. and Owen, N. (1999) 'Health promotion research and the diffusion and insitutionalization of interventions', *Health Education Research*, 14 (1): 121–30.

O'Neill, O. (2002) *Reith Lectures 2002: A Question of Trust*. London: BBC. (*Website:* www.bbc.co.uk/radio4/reith2002/5.shtml)

Ong, B.E., Humphris, G., Annett, H. and Rifkin, S. (1991) 'Rapid appraisal in an urban setting, an example from the developed world', *Social Science and Medicine*, 32 (8): 909–15.

Ong, B.N. and Humphris, G. (1994) 'Prioritising needs with communities: rapid appraisal methodologies in health', in J. Popay and G. Williams (eds), *Researching the People's Health*. London: Routledge.

Orth-Gomér, K. and Johnson, J.V. (1987) 'A six-year follow-up study of a random sample of the Swedish population', *Journal of Chronic Disease*, 40: 949–57.

Packard, V. (1981) *The Hidden Persuaders: A New Edition for the 1980s*. Harmondsworth: Penguin.

Pahl, R. (1995) 'Friendly society', in C. Campbell, R. Wood and M. Kelly, *Social Capital and Health*. London: Health Education Authority.

Parcel, G.S. and Meyer, M.P. (1978) 'Development of an instrument to measure children's health locus of control', *Health Education Monographs*, 6 (2): 149–59.

Parcel, G.S., Perry, C.L. and Taylor, W.C. (1990) 'Beyond demonstration: diffusion of health promotion innovations', in N. Bracht (ed.), *Health Promotion at the Community Level*. Newbury Park, CA: Sage.

Parlett, M. and Hamilton, D. (1972) *Evaluation as Illumination: A New Approach to the Study of Innovatory Programmes*', Occasional Paper No. 9. Edinburgh: Centre for Research in the Educational Sciences, University of Edinburgh.

Parsons, C., Stears, D., Thomas, C., Thomas, L. and Holland, J. (1997) *The Implementation of ENHPS in Different National Contexts*. Canterbury: Centre for Health Education and Research, Canterbury Christchurch College.

Parsons, T. (1958) 'Definitions of health and illness in the light of American values and social structure', in E. Jaco (ed.), *Patients, Physicians and Illness*. New York: Free Press.

Parsons, T. (1967) *Sociological Theory and Modern Society*. New York: Free Press.

Paterson, D. (1999) *Augusto Boal: A brief Biography* (on website). Omaha, NE: Pedagogy and Theatre of the Oppressed. (*Website:* www.unomaha.edu/~pto/augusto.htm)

Patton, M.Q. (1982) *Practical Evaluation*. Beverly Hills, CA: Sage.

Patton, M.Q. (1997) *Utilization Focused Evaluation*. Thousand Oaks, CA: Sage.

Pawson, R. and Tilley, N. (1997) *Realistic Evaluation*. London: Sage.

Pellegrino, E.D. (1993) 'The metamorphosis of medical ethics: a 30-year retrospective', *Journal of the American Medical Association*, 269 (9): 1158–62.

Perkins, E.R., Simnett, I. and Wright, L. (1999) *Evidence-based Health Promotion*. Chichester: John Wiley.

Perry, G. and Markwell, S. (2000) 'Promoting health in Wales – strengthening partnerships for investment for health', *Promotion & Education*, VII (2): 33–7.

Petersen, A. and Lupton, D. (1996) *The New Public Health: Health and Self in the Age of Risk*. London: Sage.

Pfau, M. (1995) 'Designing messages for behavioral inoculation', in E. Maibach and R.L. Parrott (eds), *Designing Health Messages*. Thousand Oaks, CA: Sage.

Pfau, M. and Van Bockern, S. (1994) 'The persistence of inoculation in conferring resistance to smoking initiation among adolescents: the second year', *Human Communication Research*, 20: 413–30.

Piaget, J. and Inhelder, B. (1969) *The Psychology of the Child*. London: Routledge & Kegan Paul.

Pickin, C. and St Leger, S. (1993) *Assessing Health Needs: Using the Lifecycle Framework*. Buckingham: Open University Press.

Poland, B., Green, L.W. and Rootman, I. (2000) *Settings for Health Promotion: Linking Theory and Practice*. Thousand Oaks, CA: Sage.

Poland, B., Green, L.W. and Rootman, I. (2000) 'Reflections on settings for health promotion', in B. Poland, L.W. Green and Rootman, I. (eds), *Settings for Health Promotion: Linking Theory and Practice*. Thousand Oaks, CA: Sage.

Pollard, M.R. and Brennan, J.T. (1978) 'Disease prevention and health promotion initiatives: some legal considerations', *Health Education Monographs*, 6 (2): 211–22.

Pool, H. (1992) *Illness Behaviour and Utilisation of the INF TB Clinic in Surkhet, Nepal*. Leeds: unpublished MSc Dissertation, Leeds Metropolitan University.

Popham, W.J. (1978) 'Must all objectives be behavioural?', in D. Hamilton and M. Parlett (eds), *Beyond the Numbers Game*. London: Macmillan.

Popper, K. (1945) *The Open Society and Its Enemies*. London: Routledge.

Popper, K. (1959) *The Logic of Scientific Discovery*. London: Hutchinson.

Postman, N. and Weingartner, C. (1969) *Teaching as a Subversive Activity*. Harmondsworth: Penguin.

Powles, J. (1988) 'Victoria's food and nutrition policy', *Health Promotion*, 2 (3): 240–42.

Prandy, K. (1990) 'The revised Cambridge scale of occupations: Sociology', *Sociology*, 24: 629–55.

Pressman, J. and Wildavsky, A. (1973) *Implementation: How Great Expectations in Washington are Dashed in Oakland*. Berkeley, CA: University of California Press.

Pridmore, P. (1996) 'Visualising health: exploring perceptions of children using the draw and write method promotion and education', *Promotion & Education*, III (4): 11–15.

Prochaska, J.O. and DiClemente, C.C. (1983) 'Stages and processes of self-change of smoking: toward an integrative model of change', *Journal of Consulting and Clinical Psychology*, 51: 390–5.

Prochaska, J.O. and DiClemente, C.C. (1984) *The Transtheoretical Approach: Crossing Traditional Boundaries of Therapy*. Homewood, IL: Dow Jones Irwin.

Prochaska, J.O. Redding, C.A. and Evers, K.E. (1997) 'The transtheoretical model and stages of change', in K. Glanz, F.M. Lewis and B.K. Rimer (eds), *Health Behavior and Health Education: Theory, Research, and Practice* (2nd edn). San Francisco: Jossey-Bass.

Pruger, R. and Specht, H. (1972) 'Assessing theoretical models of community organization practice: Alinsky as a case in point', in G. Zaltman, P. Kotler and I. Kaufman (eds), *Creating Social Change*. New York: Holt, Rinehart & Winston.

Putnam, R.D. (1993) *Making Democracy Work: Civic Traditions in Modern Italy*. Princeton, NJ: Princeton University Press.

Putnam, R.D. (1995) 'Bowling alone: America's declining social capital', *Journal of Democracy*, 6 (1): 65–79.

Putnam, R.D. (1996) 'The strange disappearance of civic America', *The American Prospect*, 7 (24) (*Website:* www.prospect.org/print/V7/24/putnam-r.html)

Quinn, S.C. (1999) 'Teaching community diagnosis: integrating community experience with meeting graduate standards for health educators', *Health Education Research*, 14 (5): 685–96.

Radical Statistics Health Group (1987) *Facing the Figures*. London: Radical Statistics Health Group.

Raeburn, J.M. and Rootman, I. (1989) 'Towards an expanded health field concept: conceptual and research issues in an era of health promotion', *Health Promotion*, 3 (4): 383–92.

Rahman, M., Kenway, P. and Howarth, C. (2000) *Monitoring Poverty and Social Exclusion 2000*. York: Joseph Rowntree Foundation.

Rahman, M.A. (1995) 'Participatory development: toward liberation or co-optation?', in G. Craig and M. Mayo (eds), *Community Empowerment: A Reader in Participation and Development*. London: Zed Books.

Rakow, L.F. (1989) 'Information and power: toward a critical theory of information campaigns', in C.T. Salmon (ed.), *Information Campaigns: Balancing Social Values and Social Change*. Newbury Park, CA: Sage.

Rankin, S.H. and Stallings, K.D. (2001) *Patient Education: Principles and Practice*. Philadelphia: Lippincott.

Raphael, D. (2000) 'The question of evidence in health promotion', *Health Promotion International*, 15 (4): 355–67.

Raphael, D. (2001) *Inequality is Bad for Our Hearts: Why Low Income and Social Exclusion are Major Causes of Heart Disease in Canada*. Toronto: North York Heart Health Network.

Raphael, D. (2001a) 'Evaluation of quality-of-life initiatives in health promotion', in I. Rootman, M. Goodstadt, B. Hyndman, D.V. McQueen, L. Potvin, J. Springett and E. Ziglio (eds), *Evaluation in Health Promotion: Principles and Perspectives*. Copenhagen: WHO

Rappaport, J. (1987) 'Terms of empowerment/exemplars of prevention: toward a policy for community psychology', *American Journal of Community Psychology*, 15 (2): 121–47.

Rawson, D. (1992) 'The growth of health promotion theory and its rational reconstruction', in R. Bunton and G. Macdonald (eds), *Health Promotion: Disciplines and Diversity*. London: Routledge.

Reardon, K.K. (1981) *Persuasion: Theory and Context*. Beverley Hills, CA: Sage.

Reason, P. and Rowan, J. (eds) (1981) *Human Enquiry: A Sourcebook of New Paradigm Research*. Chichester: Wiley.

Reich, M.R. (2002) *The Politics of Reforming Health Policies*. 5th European Conference on Effectiveness and Quality of Health Promotion, London, 11–13 June.

Research and Evaluation Division HEBS (1996) 'How effective are effectiveness reviews?' (editorial), *Health Education Journal*, 55: 359–62.

Rhodes, A. (1976) *Propaganda: The Art of Persuasion, World War II*. London: Angus & Robertson.

Rifkin, S. (1992) 'Rapid appraisals for health: an overview', *RRA Notes Number 16: Special Issue on Applications for Health*: 7–12.

Rigler, M. (1996) *Withymoor Village Surgery – a Health Hive*. Dudley: Dudley Priority Health NHS Trust.

Rissel, C. and Bracht, N. (1999) 'Assessing community needs, resources and readiness', in N. Bracht (eds), *Health Promotion at the Community Level: New Advances* (2nd edn). Thousand Oaks, CA: Sage.

Rivers, K., Aggleton, P., Chaise, E., Downie, A., Milvihill, C., Sinkler, P., Tyrer, P. and Warwick, I. (1999) *Learning Lessons: A Report on Two Research Studies Informing the National Healthy School Standard*. London: Department of Health and Department for Education and Employment.

Roberts, A.H. (1969) 'Self control procedures in modification of smoking behaviors: replication', *Psychological Reports*, 24: 675–6.

Roberts, H. (1990) *Women's Health Counts*. London: Routledge.

Roberts, H. (1998) 'Empowering communities: the case of childhood accidents', in S. Kendall (ed.), *Health and Empowerment*. London: Arnold.

Roberts, I. and Power, C. (1996) 'Does the decline in child injury mortality vary by social class? A comparison of class-specific mortality in 1981 and 1991', *British Medical Journal*, 313: 784–6.

Robinson, J. and Elkan, R. (1996) *Health Needs Assessment: Theory and Practice*. London: Churchill Livingstone.

Rogers, C. (1967) 'The interpersonal relationship in the facilitation of learning', in H. Kirschenbaum and V.L. Henderson (eds) (1990 edn) *The Carl Rogers Reader*. London: Constable.

Rogers, C. (1983) 'Freedom to learn for the eighties', in J. Ryder and L. Campbell, *Balancing Acts in Personal, Social and Health Education: A Practical Guide for Teachers*. London: Routledge.

Rogers, E.M. (1995) *The Diffusion of Innovations* (4th edn). New York: The Free Press.

Rogers, E.M. and Shoemaker, F.F. (1971) *Communication of Innovations*. New York: The Free Press.

Rogers, E.M. and Shoemaker, F.F. (1979) *Communication of Innovations: A Cross-Cultural Approach*. New York: Free Press.

Rogers, R.W. (1975) 'A protection motivation theory of fear appeals and attitude change', *Journal of Psychology*, 91: 93–114.

Rogers, T., Howard-Pitney, B., Feighery, E.C., Altman, D.G., Endres, J.M. and Roeseler, A.G. (1993) 'Characteristics and participants' perceptions of tobacco control coalitions in California', *Health Education Research*, 8 (3): 345–57.

Rokeach, M. (1965) 'The nature of attitudes', in D.L. Sills (ed.), *International Encyclopaedia of the Social Sciences*. New York: Macmillan and The Free Press.

Rokeach, M. (1973) *The Nature of Human Values*. New York: Free Press.

Rollnick, S., Heather, N. and Bell, A. (1992) 'Negotiating behavior change in medical settings: the development of brief motivational interviewing', *Journal of Mental Health*, 1: 25–37.

Rootman, I. (2001) 'Introduction', in I. Rootman, M. Goodstadt, L. Potvin and J. Springett (2001), in 'A framework for health promotion evaluation', in I. Rootman, M. Goodstadt, B. Hyndman, D.V. McQueen, L. Potvin, J. Springett and E. Ziglio (eds), *Evaluation in Health Promotion: Principles and Perspectives*. Copenhagen: WHO.

Rootman, I., Goodstadt, M., Potvin, L. and Springett, J. (2001) 'A framework for health promotion evaluation', in I. Rootman, M. Goodstadt, B. Hyndman, D.V. McQueen, L. Potvin, J. Springett and E. Ziglio (eds), *Evaluation in Health Promotion: Principles and Perspectives*. Copenhagen: WHO.

Rose, G. (1992) *The Strategy of Preventive Medicine*. Oxford: Oxford Medical Publications.

Rosenman, R.H., Brand, R.J., Friedman, M., Straus, R., and Wurm, M. (1975) 'Coronary heart disease in the Western Collaborative Group Study: final follow-up experience of 8 and a half years', *Journal of the American Medical Association*, 233: 872–7.

Rosenstock, I.M. (1966) 'Why people use health services', *Millbank Memorial Fund Quarterly*, 44: 94–124.

Rosenstock, I.M. (1974) 'Historical origins of the health belief model', *Health Education Monographs*, 2: 1–8.

Rosenthal, H. (1983) 'Neighbourhood health projects: some new approaches to health and community work in parts of the UK', *Community Development Journal*, 13: 122–31.

Ross, H.S. and Mico, P.R. (1980) *Theory and Practice in Health Education*. Palo Alto, CA: Mayfield.

Ross, M.G. and Lappin, B.W. (1967) *Community Organization: Theory, Principles and Practice*. New York: Harper & Row.

Rothman, J. (1979) 'Three models of community organization in practice', in F.M. Cox, J.L. Erlich, J. Rothman and J.E. Tropman (eds), *Strategies of Community Organization: A Book of Readings* (3rd edn). Itasca, IL: Peacock.

Rothschild, M.L. (1979) 'Marketing communications in non-business situations, or why it's so hard to sell brotherhood like soap', *Journal of Marketing*, 43: 11–20.

Rotter, J.B. (1966) 'Generalized expectancies for internal versus external control of reinforcement', *Psychological Monographs*, 80 (1): 1–28.

Rowling, L. (1996) 'The adaptability of the health promoting school concept: a case study from Australia', *Health Education Research*, 11 (4): 519–26.

Royle, J. and Speller, V. (1996) 'Assuring quality in health promotion', paper presented at 'Quality Assessment in Health Promotion and Education', the Third European Conference on Effectiveness, Turin, Italy, September 1996, in V. Speller, L. Rogers and A. Rushmere, 'Quality assessment in health promotion settings', in J.K. Davies and G. Macdonald, *Quality Evidence and Effectiveness in Health Promotion*. London: Routledge.

Russell, M.A.H., Wilson, C., Taylor, C. and Baker, C.D. (1979) 'Effect of general practitioners' advice against smoking', *British Medical Journal*, 2, 231–5.

Rutter, M., Maughan, B., Mortimore, P. and Ouston, J. (1979) *Fifteen Thousand Hours*. London: Open Books.

Ryan, W. (1976) *Blaming the Victim*. New York: Vintage Books.

Ryder, J. and Campbell, L. (1988) *Balancing Acts in Personal, Social and Health Education: A Practical Guide for Teachers*. London: Routledge.

Ryle, G. (1949) *The Concept of Mind*. London: Hutchinson.

Sacker, A., Firth, D., Fitzpatrick, R., Lynch, K. and Bartley, M. (2000) 'Comparing health inequality in men and women: prospective study of mortality 1986–96', *British Medical Journal*, 320: 1303–7.

Sackett, D.L., Rosenberg, W.M.C., Gray, J.A.M., Haynes, R.B. and Richardson, W.S. (1996) 'Evidence-based medicine: what it is and what it isn't', *British Medical Journal*, 312: 71–2.

Sarafino, E.P. (1990) *Health Psychology: Biopsychosocial Interactions*. New York: John Wiley.

Sarbin, T.R. and Allen, V.L. (1968) 'Role theory', in G. Lindzey and E. Aronson, *Handbook of Social Psychology* (Vol. 1). Reading: Addison-Wesley.

Sarler, C. (1996) 'Dear Marje!', *The Independent*, 15th November.

Saussure, F. de (1915) *Course in General Linguistics*. London: Peter Owen. (English translation, 1960.)

Scala, K. (1996) *Health Promotion as Intervention in Social Settings*. Late European Summer School: Stratechniques for Health Promotion 6–11 October, Zeist, The Netherlands, NIGZ.

Scheeran, P. and Abraham, C. (1996) 'The health belief model', in M. Conner and P. Norman (eds), *Predicting Health Behaviour*. Buckingham: Open University Press.

Schnack, K. (2000) 'Action competence as a curriculum perspective', in B.B. Jensen, K. Schnack and V. Simovska, *Critical Environmental and Health Education: Research Issues and Challenges*. Copenhagen: Danish University of Education.

Schramm, W. and Roberts, D.F. (1972) *The Process and Effects of Mass Communication*. Urbana, IL: University of Illinois Press.

Schwandt, T.A. (1994) 'Constructivist, interpretivist approaches to human inquiry', in N.K. Denzin and Y.S. Lincoln (eds), *Handbook of Qualitative Research*. Thousand Oaks, CA: Sage.

Schwartzer, R. and Leppin, A. (1992) 'Possible impact of social ties and support on morbidity and mortality', in M.B. Mittelmark, 'Editorial: Social ties and health promotion: suggestions for population-based research', *Health Education Research*, 14 (4): 447–51.

Sciacca, J. (1987) 'Student peer health education: a powerful yet inexpensive helping strategy', *The Peer Facilitator Quarterly*, 5: 4–6, in K. Milburn, 'A critical review of peer education with young people with special reference to sexual health', *Health Education Research*, 10 (4): 407–20.

Secretary of State for Social Security (1999) *Opportunity for All: Tackling Poverty and Social Exclusion*. London: The Stationery Office.

Seligman, M.E.P. (1975) *Helplessness: On Depression, Development and Death*. San Francisco: W.H. Freeman.

Serrano-Garcia, I. (1984) 'The illusion of empowerment: community development within a colonial context', in J. Rappaport (ed.), *Studies in Empowerment: Steps Toward Understanding and Action*. New York: The Howarth Press.

Settle, D. and Wise, C. (1986) 'Choices: materials and methods for personal and social education', in J. Ryder and C. Campbell, *Balancing Acts in Personal, Social and Health Education*. London: Routledge.

Shacklock Evans, E.G. (1962) 'The design of teaching experiments in education', *Educational Research*, V (1): 37–52.

Shavelson, R.J. and Marsh, H.W. (1986) 'On the structure of self concept', in RT. Schwarzer (ed.), *Anxiety and Cognitions*. Hilssdale, NJ: Erlbaum.

Shaw, M., Dorling, D. and Davey Smith, G. (1999) 'Poverty, social exclusion and minorities', in M. Marmot and G. Wilkinson (eds), *Social Determinants of Health*. Oxford: Oxford University Press.

Sheldon, T.A., Guyatt, G.H. and Haines, A. (1998) 'When to act on the evidence', *British Medical Journal*, 317: 139–42.

Signal, L. (1998) 'The politics of health promotion', *Health Promotion International*, 13 (3): 257–63.

Silberstein, E. (1970) 'Ingratiating behavior in persuaders', senior honors paper, Brandeis University.

Sills, D.L. (ed.) (1965) *International Encyclopedia of the Social Sciences*. New York: Macmillan and The Free Press.

Sindall, C. (1997) 'Intersectoral collaboration: the best of times, the worst of times', *Health Promotion International*, 12 (1): 5–6.

Skinner, B.F. (1971) *Beyond Freedom and Dignity*. New York: Knopf.

Slovic, P., Fischoff, B. and Lichtenstein, S. (1982) 'Why study risk perception?', *Risk Analysis*, 2 (2): 89–93.

Smith, A. (1977) 'The unfaced facts', *New Universities Quarterly*, spring, 135–6.

Smith, N.J. (1997) 'Policy Networks', in M. Hill (ed.), *The Policy Process: A Reader*. London: Prentice Hall/Harvester Wheatsheaf.

Smith, N., Littlejohns, L.B. and Thompson, D. (2001) 'Shaking out the cobwebs: insights into community capacity and its relation to health outcomes', *Community Development Journal*, 36 (1): 30–41.

Sobel, M.E. (1981) *Lifestyle and Social Structure: Concepts, Definition, Analyses*. New York: Academic Press.

Social Exclusion Unit (1999) *Teenage Pregnancy*. London: The Stationery Office.

Society of Health Education and Health Promotion Specialists (1997) *Code of Professional Conduct for Health Education and Health Promotion Specialists*. Principles and Practice Standing Committee, Society of Health Education and Health Promotion Specialists.

Solomon, D.S. (1989) 'A social marketing perspective on communication campaigns', in R.E. Rice and C.K. Atkin (eds), *Public Communication Campaigns* (2nd edn). Newbury Park, CA: Sage.

Song, I.S. and Hattie, J.A. (1984) 'Home environment, self concept and academic achievement: a causal modeling approach,' *Journal of Educational Psychology*, 76: 1269–81.

SOPHE (Society for Public Health Education) (1976) *Code of Ethics*. Washington, DC: SOPHE.

SOPHE (2001) *Code of Ethics for the Health Education Profession*. Washington, DC: SOPHE. (*Website:* www. sophe.org/about/ethics.html)

South, J. and Tilford, S. (2000) 'Perceptions of research and evaluation in health promotion', *Health Education Research*, 15 (6): 729–41.

Speller, V. (1998) 'Quality assurance programmes: their development and contribution to improving effectiveness in health promotion', in D. Scott and R. Weston (eds), *Evaluating Health Promotion*. Cheltenham: Stanley Thornes.

Speller, V., Evans, D. and Head, M.J. (1997) 'Developing quality assurance standards for health promotion practice in the UK', *Health Promotion International*, 12 (3): 215–24.

Speller, V., Learmonth, A. and Harrison, D. (1997) 'The search for evidence of effective health promotion', *British Medical Journal*, 315: 361–3.

Speller, V., Rogers, L. and Rushmere, A. (1998) 'Quality assessment in health promotion settings', in J.K. Davies and G. Macdonald (eds), *Quality, Evidence and Effectiveness in Health Promotion*. London: Routledge.

Spiegelberg, H. (1960) *The Phenomenological Movement: A Historical Introduction* (Vols. 1 and 2). The Hague: Nijhoff.

Springett, J. (1998) 'Quality measures and evaluation of Healthy City policy initiatives', in J.K. Davies and G. Macdonald (eds), *Quality, Evidence and Effectiveness in Health Promotion*. London: Routledge.

Sprinthall, N.A. (1980) 'Guidance and new education for schools,' *Personnel and Guidance Journal*, March: 485–9.

St Leger, S. (1999) 'The opportunities and effectiveness of the health promoting primary school in improving child health – a review of the claims and evidence', *Health Education Research*, 14 (1): 51–70.

Stacey, M. (1994) 'The power of lay knowledge', in J. Popay and J. Williams (eds), *Researching the People's Health*. London: Routledge.

Stake, R.E. (1995) *The Art of Case Study Research*. Thousand Oaks, CA: Sage.

Stansfield, S.A. (1999) 'Social support and social cohesion', in M. Marmot and R.G. Wilkinson (eds), *Social Determinants of Health*. Oxford: Oxford University Press.

Stenhouse, L. (1975) 'A critique of the objectives model', in Stenhouse, L. (ed.), *An Introduction to Curriculum Research and Development*. London: Heinemann.

Sternberg, P. (2002) *Nicaraguan Men's Involvement in Sexual and Reproductive Health Promotion*, unpublished PhD thesis. Leeds: Leeds Metropolitan University.

Stewart Burgher, M., Rasmussen, V.B. and Rivett, D. (1999) *The European Network of Health Promoting Schools: The Alliance of Education and Health*. Copenhagen: WHO Regional Office for Europe.

Stufflebeam, D. (1980) 'An interview with Daniel L. Stufflebeam', *Educational Evaluation and Policy Analysis*, 2 (4).

Summerfield, L.M. (1995) 'National Standards for School Health Education', *ERIC Digest* (ED 387483) ERIC Clearinghouse on Teaching and Teacher Education,

Washington, DC. (*Website:* www.ericfacility.net/databases/ ERIC-Digests/index)

Sutcliffe, T. (1994) 'Don't blame him, he's just a poor sex addict', *The Independent*, June 1994.

Sutherland, E.H. and Cressy, D.R. (1960) *Principles of Criminology*. Philadelphia: Lippincott.

Sutherland, I. (1979) *Health Education: Perspectives and Choices*. London: Allen & Unwin.

Sutherland, I. (1987) *Health Education: Half A Policy: The Rise and Fall of the Health Education Council*. Cambridge: National Extension College.

Sutton, S.R. (1982) 'Fear-arousing communication: a critical examination of theory and research', in J.R. Eiser (ed.), *Social Psychology and Behavioural Medicine*. London: Wiley.

Tagdhisi, E.M. (1992) unpublished PhD thesis. Salford: University of Salford.

Talbot, R.J. (1991) 'Underprivileged areas and healthcare planning: implications of use of Jarman indicators of urban deprivation', *British Medical Journal*, 302: 383–6.

Tannahill, A. (1992) 'Epidemiology and health promotion: a common understanding', in R. Bunton and G. Macdonald (eds), *Health Promotion Disciplines and Diversity*. London: Routledge.

Taylor, L. and Blair-Stevens, C. (2002) *Introducing Health Impact Assessment (HIA): Informing the Decision-making Process*. London: Health Development Agency.

Taylor, M. (1995) 'Community work and the state: the changing context of UK practice', in G. Craig and M. Mayo (eds), *Community Empowerment: A Reader in Participation and Development*. London: Zed Books.

Teenage Pregnancy Unit (2000) *A Guide to Local Campaigning: Information on Using the Media*. London: Department of Health.

Terence Higgins Trust (2001) *Social Exclusion and HIV: A Report*. London: Terence Higgins Trust.

Terris, M. (1996) 'Concepts of health promotion: dualities in public health theory', in J. French, *Understanding Health Promotion Through Its Fault Lines*. PhD thesis. Leeds: Leeds Metropolitan University.

Tesh, S., Tuohy, C., Christoffel, T., Hancock, T., Norsigian, J., Nightingale, E. and Robertson, L. (1988) 'The meaning of healthy public policy', *Health Promotion*, 2 (3): 257–62.

Thoresen, C.E. and Mahoney, M.J. (1974) *Behavioral Self-control*. New York: Holt, Rinehart & Winston.

Thuen, F. (1994) 'Injury-related behaviours and sensation seeking: an empirical study of a group of 14-year-old Norwegian schoolchildren', *Health Education Research*, 9 (4): 465–72.

Tilford, S. (2000) 'Evidence-based health promotion', *Health Education Research*, 15 (6): 659–63.

Tilford, S., Green, J. and Tones, K. (2003) *Values, Health Promotion and Public Health*. Leeds: Centre for Health Promotion Research, Leeds Metropolitan University.

Tones, B.K. (1979) 'Past achievement, future success', in I. Sutherland (ed.), *Health Education: Perspectives and Choices*. London: Allen & Unwin.

Tones, B.K. (1981) 'Affective education and health', in J. Cowley, K. David and T. Williams (eds), *Health Education in Schools*. London: Harper & Row.

Tones, B.K. (1987) 'Health promotion, affective education and the personal–social development of young people', in K. David and T. Williams (eds), *Health Education in Schools*, London: Harper & Row.

Tones, K. (1974) 'A systems approach to health education', *Community Health*, 6: 34–9.

Tones, K. (1986) 'Preventing drug misuse: the case for breadth, balance and coherence', *Health Education Journal*, 45 (4): 223–30.

Tones, K. (1993) 'Changing theory and practice: trends in methods, strategies and settings in health education', *Health Education Journal*, 52 (3): 125–39.

Tones, K. (1996) 'The health promoting school: some reflections on evaluation', *Health Education Research*, 11 (4): i–viii.

Tones, K. (1997) 'Health education: evidence of effectiveness', *Archives of Disease in Childhood*, 77: 189–95.

Tones, K. and Delaney, F. (1995) *Commissioning Health Promotion: A Consultancy Document*. Cambridge: Cambridge and Huntingdon Health Commission.

Tones, K. and Green, J. (1999) *A Case Study of Withymoor Village Surgery – a Health Hive: Health Promotion and Creative Arts in General Practice*. Leeds: Health Promotion Design.

Tones, K. and Green, J. (2000) 'Health education and the health-promoting school: addressing the drugs issue', in B. Moon, M. Ben-Peretz and S. Brown (eds), *Companion to Routledge International Education*. London: Routledge.

Tones, K. and Tilford, S. (1994) *Health Education: Effectiveness, Efficiency and Equity*. London: Chapman & Hall.

Tones, K. and Tilford, S. (2001) *Health Promotion: Effectiveness, Efficiency and Equity* (3rd edn). London: Nelson Thornes.

Tones, K., Dixey, R. and Green, J. (1995) 'Developing and evaluating the curriculum of the health-promoting schools', in European Network of Health Promoting Schools (eds), *Towards an Evaluation of The European Network of Health-Promoting Schools: The EVA Project*. Copenhagen: European Network of Health Promoting Schools, WHO Regional Office for Europe, European Commission and Council for Europe.

Totten, C. (1992) *Developing Quality in Health Education and Health Promotion*. Society of Health Education and Health Promotion Specialists.

Trow, M.A. (1970) 'Methodological problems in the evaluation of innovation', in M.C. Wittrock and D.E. Wiley (eds), *The Evaluation of Instruction*. New York: Holt, Rinehart & Winston.

Trower, P., Bryant, B. and Argyle, M. (1978) *Social Skills and Mental Health*. London: Methuen.

Turner, C. (2001) 'The beginning of health education at WHO', in M.A. Modolo and J. Mamon (eds), *A Long Way to Health Promotion Through IUHPE Conferences, 1951–2001*. University of Perugia, CSESI: IUHPE.

Turner, C.M. (1978) *Interpersonal Skills in Further Education*. Blagdon: Further Education Staff College, Coombe Lodge.

Turner, G. and Shepherd, J. (1999) 'A method in search of a theory: peer education and health promotion', *Health Education Research*, 14 (2): 235–47.

Twelvetrees, A. (1982) *Community Work*. London: Macmillan.

Tyrrell, G.N.M. (1951) *Homo Faber*. London: Methuen.

UNESCO-EPD (1997) *Educating for a Sustainable Future: A Transdisciplinary Vision for Concerted Action*. Background document prepared for the UNESCO International Conference on Environment and Society: Education and Public Awareness for Sustainability, Thessaloniki, Greece, 8–12 December.

United Nations Economic Commission for Europe and Statistical Office of the European Communities (undated) *Recommendations for the 2000 Censuses of Population and Housing in the ECE Region*. Statistical Standards and Studies (No. 49) Geneva: United Nations. (*Website:* www/unece.org/stats/documents/census/2000)

United Nations Statistics Division (2002) *World Population Housing and Census Programme*. New York: United Nations Statistics Division. (*Website:* http://unstats.un.org/unsd/demographic/census/index.htm)

Unwin, N., Carr, S., Leeson, J. and Pless-Mulloli, T. (1997) *An Introductory Study Guide to Public Health and Epidemiology*. Buckingham: Open University Press.

Vallely, A., Scott, C. and Hallums, J. (1999) 'The health needs of refugees: using rapid appraisal to assess needs and identify priority areas for public health action', *Public Health Medicine*, 1 (3): 103–7.

Vlassoff, C. and Tanner, M. (1992) 'The relevance of rapid assessment to health research and interventions', *Health Policy and Planning*, 7 (1): 1–9.

VSO Netherlands (undated) 'Position Paper: VSO Netherlands, The Current Status', Utrecht, The Netherlands: VSO Netherlands. (*Website:* www.vso.nl/download/Samenvatting_discussie.doc)

Wallack, L.M. (1980) *Mass Media Campaigns: The Odds Against Finding Behavior Change*. Berkeley, CA: University of California Social Research Group.

Wallack, L. (1998) 'Media advocacy: a strategy for empowering people and communities', in M. Minkler (eds), *Community Organizing and Community Building for Health*. New Brunswick: Rutgers University Press.

Wallack, L., Dorfman, L., Jernigan, D. and Makani, T. (1993) *Media Advocacy and Public Health: Power for Prevention*. Thousand Oaks, CA: Sage.

Wallerstein, N. and Bernstein, E. (1988) 'Empowerment education: Freire's ideas adapted to health education', *Health Education Quarterly*, 15 (4): 379–94.

Wallerstein, N. and Sanchez-Merki, V. (1994) 'Freirian praxis in health education: research results from an adolescent prevention program', *Health Education Research*, 9 (1): 105–18.

Wallston, B.S., Wallston, K.A., Kaplan, G.D. and Maides, S.A. (1976) 'A development and validation of the health locus of control (HLC) scale', *Journal of Consulting and Clinical Psychology*, 44: 580–5.

Wallston, K.A. and Wallston, B.S. (1982) 'Who is responsible for your health?: The construct of health locus of control', in G.S. Sanders and J. Suls (eds), *Social Psychology of Health and Illness*. Hillsdale, NJ: Erlbaum.

Wallston, K.A. (1991) 'The importance of placing measures of health locus of control beliefs in a theoretical context', *Health Education Research*, 6 (2): 251–2.

Wals, A.E.J. and Jickling, B. (2000) 'Process-based environmental education seeking standards without standardizing', in B.B. Jensen, K. Schnack and V. Simovska, *Critical Environmental and Health Education*. Copenhagen: Danish University of Education.

Walt, G. (1994) *Health Policy: An Introduction to Process and Power*. London: Zed.

Wang, C. and Burris, M.A. (1994) 'Empowerment through photo novella: portraits of participation', *Health Education Quarterly*, 21 (2): 171–86.

Wanless, D. (2002) *Securing Our Future Health: Taking a Long-term View*. London: HM Treasury. (*Website:* www.hm-treasury.gov.uk/Consultations_and_Legislation/wanless/consult_wanless_final.cfm)

Warner, K.E. (1981) 'Cigarette smoking in the 1970s: the impact of the anti-smoking campaign on consumption', *Science*, 211: 729–31.

Warwick, D.P. and Kelman, H.C. (1973) 'Ethical issues in social intervention', in G. Zaltman (ed.), *Processes and Phenomena of Social Change*. New York: Wiley.

Watson, J., Speller, V., Markwell, S. and Platt, S. (2000) 'The Verona benchmark: applying evidence to improve the quality of partnership', *Promotion & Education*, VII (2): 16–23.

Watson, M.C. (2002) 'Normative needs assessment: is this an appropriate way in which to meet the new public health agenda?', *International Journal of Health Promotion and Education*, 40 (1): 4–8.

Weber, M. (1968) *Economy and society* (Vol. 1). New York: Bedminster Press.

Weinstein, N.D. (1982) 'Unrealistic optimism about susceptibility to health problems', *Journal of Behavioral Medicine*, 5 (4): 441–60.

Weinstein, N.D. (1984) 'Why it won't happen to me: perceptions of risk factors and susceptibility', *Health Psychology*, 3 (5): 431–57.

Weisbord, M. (1978) 'Organisational diagnosis: a workbook of theory and practice', in J. Anderson, *HEA*

Health Skills Project. Leeds: Counselling and Career Development Unit.

Weiss, C.H. (1995) 'Nothing as practical as good theory: exploring theory-based evaluation for community initiatives for children and families', in J.P. Connell, A.C. Kubisch, L.B. Schorr and C.H. Weiss (eds), *New Approaches to Evaluating Community Initiatives: Concepts, Methods and Contexts*. Washington, DC: The Aspen Institute.

Welin, L., Tibblin, G. and Tibblin, B. (1985) 'Prospective study of social influence on mortality: the study of men born in 1913 and 1923', *Lancet*, 1: 915–18.

Wenzel, E. (1997) 'A comment on settings in health promotion', *Internet Journal of Health Promotion*, http://www.monash.edu.au/health/IJHP/1997/1.

Werner, D. (1980) 'Health care and human dignity', in S.B. Rifkin (ed.), *Health, the Human Factor: Readings in Health, Development and Community Participation*. (CONTACT Special Series No. 3). Geneva: WCC.

Werner, E.E. (1987) 'Resilient children', in E.E. Fitzgerald and M.G. Walraven (eds), *Annual Editions Human Development 87/88*. Guilford, CT: Dushkin.

Whitehead, M. (1987) *The Health Divide*. London: Health Education Council.

Whitehead, M. (1990) *The Concepts and Principles of Equity and Health*. Copenhagen: WHO.

Whitehead, M. (1992) *Policies and Strategies to Promote Equity*. Copenhagen: WHO.

Whitehead, M. and Tones, K. (1990) *Avoiding the Pitfalls: Notes on the Planning and Implementation of Health Education Strategies and the Special Role of the HEA*. London: HEA.

Whitelaw, S., Baxendale, A., Bryce, C., MacHardy, L., Young, I. and Witney, E. (2001) ' "Settings"-based health promotion: a review', *Health Promotion International*, 16 (4): 339-53.

WHO (1946) *Constitution*. Geneva: WHO.

WHO (1978) *Declaration of Alma Ata*. International Conference on Primary Health Care, Alma Ata 6–12 September. Geneva: WHO.

WHO (1984) *Health Promotion: A Discussion Document on the Concepts and Principles*. Copenhagen: WHO.

WHO (1985) *Targets for Health for All*. Copenhagen: WHO Regional Office for Europe.

WHO (1986) *Ottawa Charter for Health Promotion*. First International Conference on Health Promotion, Ottawa 17–21 November, Copenhagen: WHO Regional Office for Europe.

WHO (1988) *The Adelaide Recommendations*. Geneva: WHO. (*Website:* www.who.int/hpr/archive/docs/ adelaide.html)

WHO (1991) *Sundsvall Statement on Supportive Environments for Health*. Geneva: WHO.

WHO (1995) *Securing Investment in Health: Report of a Demonstration Project in the Provinces of Bolzano and Trento*. Copenhagen: WHO.

WHO (1997) *The Jakarta Declaration on Leading Health Promotion into the 21st Century.* Geneva: WHO. (*Website:* www/who.int/hpr/archive/docs/jakarta/english.html)

WHO (1998) *Health for All in the Twenty-first Century* (A51/5). Geneva: WHO.

WHO (1998a) *Health Promotion Evaluation: Recommendations to Policymakers: Report of the WHO European Working Group on Health Promotion Evaluation.* Copenhagen: WHO Regional Office for Europe.

WHO (1998b) *Health Promotion in the 21st Century: An Era of Partnerships to Achieve Health for All (WHO/47).* Geneva: WHO.

WHO (1998c) *Fifty-first World Health Assembly (WHA51.12): Health Promotion.* Copenhagen: WHO.

WHO (1998d) *The WHO Approach to Health Promotion: Settings for Health.* Geneva: WHO.

WHO (1999) *World Health Report 1999.* Geneva: WHO.

WHO (2000a) *Mexico Ministerial Statement for the Promotion of Health: From Ideas to Action.* Fifth Global Conference on Health Promotion: Bridging the Equity Gap, Mexico 5–9 June. Geneva: WHO.

WHO (2000b) *Report of the Technical Programme.* Fifth Global Conference on Health Promotion: Bridging the Equity Gap, Mexico 5–9 June. Geneva: WHO. (*Website:* www.who.int/hpr/conference/products/Conferencereport/conferencereport.html)

WHO (2001) 'Climate and health', Factsheet, 266. Geneva: WHO.

WHO (2002) *What is a Health-promoting School?* Geneva: WHO. (*Website:* www5.who.int/school-youth-health/main.cfm?p=0000000642)

WHO Euro-EC-CE (1993) *The European Network of Health Promoting Schools.* Copenhagen: WHO European Region.

WHO Health Education Unit (1993) 'Lifestyles and health', in A. Beattie, M. Gott, L. Jones and M. Sidell (eds), *Health and Wellbeing: A Reader.* London: Macmillan.

WHO Health Promoting Hospitals Network (1997) *The Vienna Recommendations on Health Promoting Hospitals.* Copenhagen: WHO European Region. (*Website:* www.univie.ac.at/hph/vierec.html)

WHO Regional Committee for Europe (1998) *Regional Health for All Targets.* Copenhagen: WHO European Region. (*Website:* alpha.mpl.uoa.gr/aspasia/Documents/Regional%20Health.htm)

WHO Regional Committee for Europe (2002) *Technical Briefing: Health Impact Assessment.* Copenhagen: WHO. (*Website:* www.euro.who.int/document/rc52/ ebd3.pdf)

WHO Regional Office for Europe (2002a) *What Is A Healthy City?* (on website). Copenhagen: WHO Regional Office for Europe. (*Website:* www.who. dk/healthy-cities/How2MakeCities/20020114_1)

WHO Regional Office for Europe (2002b) *Health Impact Assessment.* Copenhagen: WHO Regional Office for Europe.

WHO Regional Office for Europe (2002c) *What is the Healthy Cities Approach?* (on website). Copenhagen: WHO Regional Office for Europe. (*Website:* www. who.dk/healthy-aties/How2MakeCities/0020114_2)

Whyte, W.F. (1943) *Street Corner Society.* Chicago: Chicago University Press.

Whyte, W.F. (1991) *Social Theory for Action: How Individuals and Organizations Learn to Change.* Thousand Oaks, CA: Sage.

Whyte, W.F. (1997) *Creative Problem Solving in the Field: Reflections on a Career.* Walnut Creek, CA: AltaMira Press.

Wiebe, G. (1952) 'Merchandising commodities and citizenship on television', *Public Opinion Quarterly,* 15: 679–91.

Wiggers, J. and Sanson-Fisher, R. (1998) 'Evidence-based health promotion', in R. Scott and R. Weston (eds), *Evaluating Health Promotion.* Cheltenham: Stanley Thornes.

Wight, D., Raab, G.M., Henderson, M., Abraham, C., Buston, K., Hart, G. and Scott, S. (2002) 'Limits of teacher-delivered sex education: interim behavioural outcomes from randomised trial', *British Medical Journal,* 324 (7351): 1430.

Wikler, D.I. (1978) 'Coercive measures in health promotion: can they be justified?', *Health Education Monographs,* 6 (2): 223–41.

Wilkinson, G. (1994) 'Divided we fall', *British Medical Journal,* 308: 1113–14.

Wilkinson, R.G. (1997) 'Socio-economic determinants of health: health inequalities: relative or absolute material standards', *British Medical Journal,* 314 (7080): 591–5.

Williams, A. and Kind, R. (1992) 'The present state of play about QALYS', in A. Hopkins (ed.), *Measure of the Quality of Life and the Uses to Which Such Measures May be Put.* London: Royal College of Physicians.

Williams, G. and Popay, J. (1994) 'Lay knowledge and the privilege of experience', in J. Gabe, D. Kelleher and G. Williams (eds), *Challenging Medicine.* London: Routledge.

Williams, R. and Wright, J. (1998) 'Epidemiological issues in health needs assessment', *British Medical Journal,* 316 (2 May): 1379–82.

Williams, R.G.A. (1983) 'Concepts of health: an analysis of lay logic', *Sociology,* 17 (2): 185–204.

Williams, T., Wetton, N. and Moon, A. (1989a) *A Picture of Health.* London: HEA.

Williams, T., Wetton, N. and Moon, A. (1989b) *A Way In: Five Key Areas of Health Education.* London: HEA.

Wilson, P., Richardson, R., Sowden, A.J. and Evans, D. (2001) 'PHASE 9: Getting evidence into practice', in NHS Centre for Reviews and Dissemination, *Undertaking Systematic Reviews of Research Effectiveness* (CRD Report, No. 4, 2nd edition). York: NHS Centre for Reviews and Dissemination.

Winett, R.A., King, A.D. and Altman, D.G. (1989) *Health Psychology and Public Health*. New York: Pergamon.

Winton, W.M. (1987) 'Do introductory textbooks present the Yerkes-Dodson law correctly?', *American Psychologist*, (42): 202–3.

Wise, M. (2001) 'The role of advocacy in promoting health', *Promotion & Education*, VIII (2): 69–74.

World Bank (1993) *World Health Report 1993*. New York: Oxford University Press.

Wren, B. (1977) *Education for Justice*. London: SCM Press.

Wright, C. and Whittington, D. (1992) 'Quality assurance: an introduction for health care professionals', in D. Evans, M.J. Head and V. Speller, *Assuring Quality in Health Promotion*. London: HEA.

Yerkes, R.M. and Dodson, J.D. (1908) 'The relation of strength of stimulus to rapidity of habit formation', *Journal of Comparative Neurology and Psychology*, (18): 459–82.

Young, I. and Williams, T. (1989) *The Healthy School*. Edinburgh: Scottish Health Education Group.

Zacharakis-Jutz, J. (1988) 'Post-Freirean adult education: a question of empowerment and power', *Adult Education Quarterly*, 39 (1): 41–7.

Zajonc, R.B. (1980) 'Feeling and thinking: preferences need no inferences', *American Psychologist*, 35: 151–75.

Zeedyk, M.S. and Wallace, L. (2003) 'Tackling children's road safety through edutainment: an evaluation of effectiveness', *Health Education Research* (in press).

Ziglio, E., Rivett, D. and Rasmussen, V.B. (1995) *The European Network of Health Promoting Schools: Managing Innovation and Change*. Copenhagen: WHO Regional Office for Europe.

Ziglio, E., Hagard, S. and Griffiths, J. (2000) 'Health promotion development in Europe: achievements and challenges', *Health Promotion International*, 15 (2): 143–54.

Ziglio, E., Hagard, S., McMahon, L., Harvey, S. and Levin, L. (2000a) 'Principles, methodology and practices of investment for health', *Promotion & Education*, VII (2): 4–15.

Ziglio, E., Hagard, S., McMahon, L., Harvey, S. and Levin, L. (2001) *Investment for Health*. Geneva: WHO. (*Website:* www.who.int/hpr/conference/products/Techreports/Investment.pdf)

Zimbardo, P.G., Ebbesen, E.B. and Maslach, C. (1977) *Influencing Attitudes and Changing Behavior, second edition*. Reading, MA: Addison-Wesley.

Zuckerman, M. (1990) 'The psychophysiology of sensation seeking', *Journal of Personality*, 58 (1): 313–45.

Index